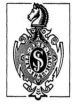

Intracranial Pressure VII

Edited by
J. T. Hoff and A. L. Betz

With 266 Figures and 124 Tables

Springer-Verlag Berlin Heidelberg New York
London Paris Tokyo Hong Kong

Julian T. Hoff, MD
Professor of Surgery
Chief, Section of Neurosurgery
University of Michigan Hospitals
1500 E. Medical Center Dr.
Ann Arbor, MI 48109-0338
USA

A. Lorris Betz, MD, PhD
Professor of Pediatrics,
Neurology, and Surgery
Director, Crosby Laboratories
Section of Neurosurgery
University of Michigan Hospitals
1500 E. Medical Center Dr.
Ann Arbor, MI 48109-0338
USA

ISBN-13: 978-3-642-73989-7   e-ISBN-13: 978-3-642-73987-3
DOI: 10.1007/978-3-642-73987-3

2122/3130-543210 – Printed on acid-free paper

Proceedings of the Seventh International Symposium
on Intracranial Pressure
Held in Ann Arbor, USA, June 19–23, 1988

Honorary Board	Advisory Board
J. Beks	A. Baethmann, Munich
P. Janny	D. P. Becker, Los Angeles
B. Jennett	M. Brock, Berlin
N. Lundberg	S. Ishii, Tokyo
	T. W. Langfitt, Philadelphia
	A. Marmarou, Richmond
	J. D. Miller, Edinburgh
	G. M. Teasdale, Glasgow

List of Contributors

You will find the addresses at the beginning of the respective contribution

Preface

This book is a compilation of scientific papers presented at the Seventh International Symposium on Intracranial Pressure and Brain Injury, held in Ann Arbor, Michigan, USA, June 20–23, 1988. The symposium explored both clinical and basic science aspects of intracranial pressure dynamics and their clinical application. Neuroscientists including neurologists, neurosurgeons, neuroanesthesiologists, neuroradiologists, neurochemists, biophysicists and physiologists contributed to the state-of-the-art presentations and discussions.

Open exchange of ideas characterized this meeting as it did the initial meeting in Hanover, Germany in 1972 and subsequently at tri-annual meetings in Lund, Sweden; Groningen, Holland; Williamsburg, Virginia; Tokyo, Japan; and Glasgow, Scotland. The next Intracranial Pressure Symposium, to be held in Rotterdam, Holland, in 1991, will continue this tradition.

The papers in this book have been grouped for the reader's convenience. Clinical and basic science papers focus on the same subject, consequently they appear together. Subjects include monitoring; biophysics; CSF dynamics and hydrocephalus; control of intracranial pressure; trauma, hemorrhage, and inflammation; free radicals; cerebral perfusion and metabolism; and brain edema.

The science of intracranial pressure and its relevance to human illness continues to provide fascination for investigators throughout the world. This book reflects the research of many of them and, hopefully, will stimulate new and innovative inquiries.

Ann Arbor   J.T. Hoff
                                                                         A.L. Betz

Contents

XVI

Session II: Biophysics Session

Chairmen: H.D. Portnoy and J. Rowan

Session IV: Control of ICP

Chairmen: D.P. Becker and S. Cotev

Session V: Trauma, Hemorrhage and Inflammation

Chairmen: M. Brock, J.T. Hoff, H.M. Eisenberg, P. Reilly, L.F. Marshall,
and H.J. Reulen

XXVIII

Session VI: Free Radicals

Chairmen: A.L. Betz and D.P. Becker

Session VII: Cerebral Perfusion and Metabolism

Chairmen: M. Rosner and A. Tamura

Session I: Monitoring

Chairmen: G. M. Teasdale, C. P. Mc Graw, A. Marmarou, and M. R. Gaab

1

Measuring ICP in Patients – Its Value Now and in the Future?

J.D. Miller

Department of Clinical Neurosciences, Western General Hospital, University of Edinburgh (UK)

Introduction

In reviews of the status of ICP monitoring in patients, presented at past ICP symposia, it has been emphasised that ICP monitoring is the only reliable indicant of intracranial hypertension, provides a means of continuously evaluating an important aspect of brain support in the comatose patient who is paralysed and artificially ventilated, indicates when therapy for raised ICP is needed and whether the treatment has been effective, or if further therapy is necessary. Finally, the peak ICP helps in arriving at a prognosis in the severely head injured patient; it adds confidence in identifying at an early stage patients who will die, and others who will survive with severe disability, and who therefore are in the most need of early rehabilitation measures.

Before congratulating ourselves on having achieved acceptance of these principles of clinical ICP monitoring, we should try to answer two simple questions. How should we measure ICP? What evidence is there that monitoring and control of raised ICP affects the outcome of severe head injury, or any other condition in which ICP monitoring is commonly carried out? At this Seventh International ICP Symposium in 1988, sixteen years after the First Symposium in Hanover, we must admit that we still do not have the final answer to these two simple questions. That should stop us from becoming too self-congratulatory, for another 3 years at least.

A number of issues remain important in the clinical area, particularly as they relate to head injury. These are the choice of methods for measuring ICP, the prevalence of raised ICP requiring action; the common causes of raised ICP and how they may be distinguished at the bedside, and lastly the concept of specific ICP therapy targeted at the cause.

Choice of a Method for Monitoring ICP

Despite the many systems and devices that have been proposed for continuous monitoring of ICP, the intraventricular catheter, fluid filled and connected to an externally mounted transducer, described more than thirty years ago by Guillaume and Janny (1951) and by Nils Lundberg (1960), remains the "gold stan-

Intracranial Pressure VII
Eds.: J.T. Hoff and A.L. Betz
© Springer-Verlag Berlin Heidelberg 1989

5

dard", against which all other systems have to be judged. The system produces accurate measurements of central CSF pressure and its waveform, can be re-zeroed and recalibrated while in situ including zero point positioning of the transducer, permits CSF drainage as a form of therapy for raised ICP and permits volume challenges to the CSF space. The risk of intracranial haemorrhage is very low, and the risk of infection is under 5% in the best hands (Sundbärg et al. 1987). The risk of infection appears to be higher if there is blood in the CSF, and if the system is entered frequently for withdrawal of CSF without taking adequate sterile precautions. The duration of monitoring appears to be less important, provided that the system is carefully handled by doctors and nurses familiar with its use.

In circumstances where repeated measurements of ICP may be necessary over an extended period of time, as in hydrocephalus, we favour the use of a closed CSF reservoir connected to a catheter in the frontal horn of the lateral ventricle. The system can be accessed simply through the overlying scalp by inserting a fine "butterfly" needle bent at a right angle. Such a system is employed in every patient in whom we insert a ventriculo-peritoneal shunt. In this way it is possible to avoid touching the shunt itself, when shunt blockage or infection is suspected and ICP monitoring is needed. In a recent survey of 56 patients with CSF access devices, followed for an average of 4.8 years, we found no evidence that the use of such devices increased the incidence of infection, intracerebral haemorrhage or epilepsy. There was no mortality or morbidity attributable to the insertion of a CSF access device (Leggate et al., in press).

In head injury, because the lateral ventricles are usually small, subdural measurements are often used. The case against the use of subdural screws, bolts and catheters is well known. All three systems tend to underestimate ICP when this exceeds 20 to 30 mm Hg (Barlow et al. 1985; North and Reilly 1986). It may be extraordinarily difficult to tell that the system is underreading the true ICP; this is because an apparent fall in mean ICP can precede the eventual reduction in CSF pulse pressure that is the recognisable sign of damping and blockage of the subdural catheter system.

Implanting the transducer itself solves the problem of blockage of the system, but introduces a number of other limitations including inability to calibrate and rezero in situ in most systems, gain stability and reliability over long periods, and expense (Ostrup et al. 1987). The same applies if the transducer is inserted into the brain (Sundbärg et al. 1987). If spectral analysis of the ICP waveform is to be performed, the flat response of the transducer system must be adequate for the task. A range from DC to 30 Hz is suitable for this purpose. An ideal system has yet to emerge.

Monitoring of arterial pressure should be considered in every patient in whom ICP is measured. The cerebral perfusion pressure (CPP), estimated as the difference between arterial and intracranial pressure, needs in many cases to be considerably higher than the lower threshold of 40 mm Hg required to assure adequate brain tissue perfusion in normal subjects. This is because the local cerebrovascular resistance is high in a number of focal brain disorders, such as head injury, perifocal brain oedema and cerebral vasospasm following sub-arachnoid haemorrhage.

6

Cerebral perfusion pressure is only one of the factors that control the energy supply to the brain. Monitoring of ICP provides a means of identifying when dangerous, energy-limiting episodes are occurring, or are about to ensue. The status of blood or tissue oxygenation should also be known. Measurements of arterial blood gases provide accurate data, but only at a moment in time, and energy loss lasting longer than a minute constitutes a further brain insult. A continuous method is, therefore, of enormous added value to the brain monitoring armamentarium. Continuous transcutaneous pulse oximetry seems likely to be valuable in head injury patients.

To complement measurements of CPP and systemic oxygenation in paralysed ventilated patients, some measure of brain electrical function is of considerable value. These are not straightforward measurements. There are many possible sources of artefact.

Careful logging of important concomitant events is crucial to the informed interpretation of the clinical ICP recordings. Nursing manoeuvres, changes in body temperature, alterations in body or head position, ventilatory status and administration of drugs are examples of events that must be recorded.

The Incidence of Raised Intracranial Pressure

Intracranial hypertension is common in comatose patients. In a consecutive series of 215 comatose head injured patients, ICP levels in excess of 20 mm Hg were recorded in 53% (Miller et al. 1981). The reported incidence of intracranial hypertension will, however, depend upon the zero reference point, the accuracy of the system and the threshold pressure used to define the upper limit of normality. In most head injury series the level of 20 mm Hg is accepted, but persistent levels above 15 mm Hg are abnormal, and in the very young the upper limit of normal is much lower, 5 mm Hg in the first year of life (Welch 1980).

It is more important to define the pressure threshold above which action is to be taken. Arguments have been advanced for thresholds of 12, 15, 20, 25 and 30 mm Hg. Too low a threshold means that therapy may be employed too often; too high a threshold may mean that a further brain insult can occur before treatment is applied. In head injured patients, our current practice is to treat when ICP exceeds 25 mm Hg during the first 48 hours, and when ICP is above 30 mm Hg thereafter. Our measurements relate to zero reference at the external auditory meatus and 10 to 15 degrees of head-up tilt.

The first action to be taken is to check the accuracy of the pressure recording, then to correct any situations or abnormalities likely to lead to intracranial hypertension (Miller 1978; Dearden 1986). These include elevation of body temperature, poor neck position, inadequate analgesia, sedation or relaxation, hypercarbia or hypoxaemia. Other factors are arterial hypotension, hyponatraemia (serum Na^+ <120 mEq/L), and epileptic seizures. If these potential causes are assiduously treated or corrected, the requirement for specific therapy to treat raised intracranial pressure will be greatly reduced. Mannitol and/or hypnotic therapy has been employed in only 57% of the 208 comatose head injury patients

Table.1. ICP monitoring and therapy – Edinburgh 1986/87

Group	Outcome			
No ICP Monitor	Good/Mod	Severe/Veg	Dead	Total
No mannitol	32 (64%)	2 (4%)	16 (32%)	50
Mannitol given	10 (29%)	2 (6%)	23 (65%)	35
Subtotal	42 (49%)	4 (5%)	39 (46%)	85
ICP Monitor				
No mannitol	23 (79%)	4 (14%)	2 (7%)	29
One early bolus	5 (56%)	3 (33%)	1 (11%)	9
Repeat mannitol in ICU	22 (42%)	6 (12%)	24 (46%)	52
Hypnotics[a] ± mannitol	12 (36%)	8 (24%)	13 (39%)	33
Subtotal	62 (50%)	21 (17%)	40 (33%)	123
Total	104 (50%)	25 (12%)	79 (38%)	208

[a] A single patient had hypnotics only – good outcome.

treated in Edinburgh over the past two years, and in 69% of the 123 patients in whom continuous monitoring of ICP was utilised (Table 1).

Determining the Cause of Raised Intracranial Pressure

In settling upon the most suitable specific therapy for intracranial hypertension, the treatment most likely to reduce ICP without also reducing cerebral perfusion pressure, it appears logical to consider the predominating cause for the elevation of ICP in that particular patient at that particular time. A treatment that is appropriate to the cause is more likely to be successful, and less likely to be detrimental. In the time taken to reveal by trial and error that one form of therapy is not helpful, the ICP may have been elevated to a critical level for long enough to cause secondary ischaemic brain damage.

In practical terms, the causes for raised ICP can be divided into vascular and non-vascular causes. The vascular causes include active cerebral arterial vasodilatation, passive arterial distension due to a combination of increased arterial pressure and impaired autoregulation, and venous engorgement due to an obstruction in the venous outflow pathway. The non-vascular causes include all forms of oedema and factors that increase the outflow resistance of the cerebrospinal fluid pathways.

Determination of CSF outflow resistance remains a subject of controversy. The infusion of perfusion methods with pressure measurement from the lumbar sac or lateral ventricle remain the most widely accepted methods in cases of hydrocephalus (Ekstedt 1977; Børgesen and Gjerris 1982; Børgesen and Gjerris 1987), while the bolus method, described by Marmarou, finds most use in cases of head injury, subarachnoid haemorrhage and other situations where prolonged stability is difficult to obtain (Marmarou et al. 1975). The bolus method appears to underestimate the Ro measurement obtained by infusion under some circumstances, but in conditions where craniospinal compliance is reduced the discrepancy between the two measurements is much reduced (Takizawa et al. 1985).

The methods used to estimate craniospinal compliance or elastance also remain topics for vigorous discussion. The volume-pressure response, the rise in ICP that results from the introduction of 1 ml of fluid in one second into the CSF, varies according to the baseline ICP and when plotted against it produces a regression line, the slope of which is a measure of intracranial elastance (Miller et al. 1973). If the regression line intersects the baseline ICP scale at a pressure above zero, this is a way of estimating the "constant term" that Avezaat and van Eijndhoven (1979) and Tans and Poortvliet (1982) have used to improve upon the reliability and validity of the pressure-volume index. The PVI described by Marmarou, is derived from the quotient obtained from the volume of a bolus injection or withdrawal divided by the difference between the logarithms of baseline and peak pressures. It represents the notional volume in mls required to raise or reduce ICP tenfold. The relationships only hold over a range of ICP values. Nevertheless, a low PVI is predictive of raised ICP in patients with severe head injury (Maset et al. 1987).

Compliance/elastance is changed by alterations in blood pressure (but only when ICP is increased), by intracranial mass lesions and other factors that produce a mass effect, including cerebral oedema (Miller 1975).

Examples of most known forms of cerebral oedema can be seen in neurosurgical and head injured patients (Fishman 1975; Miller 1979 a). *Vasogenic oedema* is seen in the form of perifocal oedema, around brain tumours, abscesses, contusions and infarcts. The oedema fluid is protein-rich, emerges from cerebral blood vessels and accumulates in the white matter, where tissue compliance is greater than in the more densely-packed grey matter. *Cytotoxic oedema* is intracellular, due to failure of membrane pump mechanisms, and therefore occurs in relation to focal or generalised brain ischaemia or hypoxia. It is most commonly represented by the swelling within an infarct of the brain. (Vasogenic oedema also occurs around the margin of the infarct). *Hydrostatic oedema* often follows congestive brain swelling caused by passive distension of cerebral arteries produced by a combination of arterial hypertension and impaired pressure autoregulation. The fluid that emerges from the vessels to fill the extracellular space is protein poor, thus contrasting with vasogenic oedema (Schutta et al. 1968). *Osmotic oedema* occurs when serum sodium concentration falls below a critical threshold, around 120 mEq/L. The fluid accumulation is intracellular. *Interstitial oedema* occurs in the periventricular zone, related to high pressure hydrocephalus. While it can be easily seen on CT, similar appearances, not due to oedema, can be seen in other cases, so that the CT diagnosis may be inaccurate.

At present there is no certain means of distinguishing which of the two main classes of causes of raised intracranial pressure, vascular or non-vascular, is predominant, but evidence can be built up that favours one or the other. Elsewhere in this volume we describe one approach to this problem, using a combination of clinical features, CT findings and data on the relationship between the arterial and the respiratory-related pulsation of the ICP waveform. A more rigorous approach is that used by Marmarou, based upon the "Davson Equation" which states that steady state ICP is derived from the product of CSF formation and outflow resistance plus the cerebral venous outflow pressure. Marmarou calculates separately the rate of CSF formation and the CSF outflow resistance, then by withdrawing CSF at the rate of formation obtains the estimated venous pressure. It is then possible to calculate the proportion of the ICP that is related to CSF outflow resistance and that related to "vascular factors". In head injury the vascular component appears to account for about 75% of increased ICP (Marmarou et al. 1987).

Another approach is to measure cerebral blood flow: the defect with this is that cerebral blood volume may be increased and ICP elevated, yet volume flow in the cerebral circulation is low, while in another case the blood volume may be similarly increased but cerebral blood flow is high. In the first example the cerebral arteriovenous oxygen content difference will be above the normal value of 6 ml/100 ml, while in the latter example the cerebral a-v oxygen difference will be low. This can be measured if a catheter is inserted into the jugular bulb, but assumes that the blood sampled from that jugular vein is representative of the total cerebral venous drainage. In practice, most a-VO$_2$ measurements fall within the "normal" range of 4–9 ml/100 ml. Measurements of CBF or flow velocity are of considerable value, however, to establish the status of pressure autoregulation and CO$_2$ reactivity; reduction of ICP by mannitol appears to depend on the preservation of the former, and by barbiturates depends on the latter mechanism (Muizelaar et al. 1983; Messeter et al. 1986; Nordström et al. 1988).

A systems analysis approach has been suggested by Chopp and Portnoy (1980) taking the arterial pressure as the input and the ICP as the output of the system. By resolving the 2 waveforms into a series of harmonics and measuring the transfer functions for each harmonic it has been hoped to discriminate between vascular and other factors that affect pulse transmission across the cerebrovascular bed. Opinions remain divided as to the practical utility of such analysis which require high fidelity recording of arterial and intracranial pressure and complex analysis (Szewczykowski et al. 1980; Portnoy et al. 1982; Takizawa et al. 1986; Takizawa et al. 1987).

The Concept of Targeted Therapy for Raised Intracranial Pressure

The purpose in trying to determine the cause of raised ICP is to try to apply the treatment that is most appropriate to the cause. Broadly speaking, it can be proposed that when raised ICP is predominantly due to vascular factors the first line of therapy should be hyperventilation with reduction of arterial PCO$_2$. If that is unsuccessful hypnotic agents (e.g. barbiturates, gammahydroxybutyrate) can next be used, in the form of barbiturates or similar agents. When the increase in ICP is due mainly to non-vascular causes related to brain oedema formation, the best form of therapy is likely to be osmotherapy, usually employing mannitol. If an obstruction in the CSF pathway is the main cause, and hydrocephalus is present, CSF drainage is the preferred treatment. While it can be argued that it is just as practical to try one treatment first, then if that does not work, try another, this is open to the criticism that if the first therapy is unsuccessful it exposes the patient to a period of uncontrolled intracranial hypertension that might have been avoided if the first therapy had been better chosen.

At present, we are constrained in our choice of therapy for raised intracranial pressure, not only by difficulty in determining the predominating patho-physiological mechanism but also by incomplete knowledge of the mode of action of the agents that we use to control intracranial hypertension.

Steroid therapy is best employed for cases of chronic perifocal oedema, exemplified by peritumoral oedema. When successful, steroid therapy improves clinical status within 24 hours and reduces brain elastance in the same time frame. The frequency of ICP waves is also reduced early, while a reduction in the mean level of ICP does not occur for two or even three days (Miller and Leech 1975). Brain oedema does not seem to be reduced in patients at the time when clinical benefit is already manifest, as shown on CT and in studies using magnetic resonance scanning. Although the clinical benefits of steroid therapy in suitable cases are not to be doubted, the mechanisms of effect remain far from clear. What is abundantly clear, however, is that steroid therapy for acute brain swelling following head injury is entirely without benefit, reducing neither the mortality nor the incidence or severity of raised intracranial pressure (Braakman et al. 1983; Dearden et al. 1986).

The actions of the osmotic agent mannitol seemed clear for a number of years, withdrawing fluid from swollen brain along an osmotic gradient. It was argued that the osmotic effects of mannitol would be exerted most in areas of the brain where the blood brain barrier remained intact; in damaged areas it was considered that mannitol would soon diffuse into the brain, abolishing and even reversing the osmotic gradient, and perhaps explaining the phenomenon of rebound intracranial hypertension. Recent studies in Edinburgh, using regional T1 values obtained from magnetic resonance imaging compared with actual brain water measurements in vitro, now suggest that the first view of the effect of mannitol was probably correct. Mannitol causes withdrawal of water mainly from brain areas where the barrier is impaired, at least in patients with peritumoral oedema. If mannitol withdraws water across intact capillary walls, this is 30 times more likely to occur in capillaries in the gut wall or in muscle, where there is much greater conductance of water (Bell et al. 1987).

Muizelaar and his colleagues (1983) have proposed that the rapid effect of mannitol upon ICP is mediated, initially at least, by a reactive cerebral vasoconstriction in response to a reduction in blood viscosity, acting as a form of autoregulation to retain a normal level of cerebral blood flow. This effect depends upon retention of autoregulatory capacity in most of the brain. In cases where autoregulation is badly impaired, mannitol will not reduce ICP, but cerebral blood flow is likely to be increased. Finally, Takagi et al. (1983) has proposed that mannitol also causes withdrawal of water from the brain into the lateral ventricles.

Hypnotic drugs reduce the energy metabolism of the brain, reduce cerebral blood flow and volume, so that they not only lower ICP but may also provide brain protection. Unfortunately these drugs also depress the cardiovascular system so that arterial hypotension can occur. This is a most serious problem. If raised intracranial pressure is an insult to the injured brain, then low arterial pressure is an even greater insult (Miller 1979 b; Schwartz et al. 1984; Miller 1985; Ward et al. 1985; Leggate et al. 1986). Barbiturates also appear to have an immunosuppressive action, resulting in an increased risk of infective complications in the intensive unit. Brain electrical activity and CO_2 reactivity must be retained if hypnotic drugs are to be effective in reducing ICP; we must therefore add these to the indication list used to decide the most effective therapy for raised intracranial pressure (Nordström et al. 1988).

Many patients with raised ICP in the ICU do not require specific therapy because ICP settles when simple causative factors have been rigorously eliminated or ameliorated. Mannitol is effective in reducing ICP, without adversely affecting brain perfusion in the majority of cases in which specific therapy is required; hypnotic therapy must be applied with great care but in selected cases can safely reduce ICP when other methods are ineffective. We find some apparent inconsistency in our therapeutic strategy. Raised ICP of vascular cause should respond best to hyperventilation and hypnotic drugs, and vascular causes predominate in the intracranial hypertension that follows severe head trauma. However, we find that mannitol is more often effective in controlling ICP after head injury than hypnotics. This may be because in many cases hypnotic therapy is being used only when hyperventilation has been found ineffective, circumstances in which Messeter and his colleagues have found barbiturates to be less effective.

The Future Form of ICP Monitoring

What can we expect from patient monitoring systems in future? We will continue to require continuous and accurate data on ICP and arterial pressure, presented in a form that allows review of trends in pressure or pressure waves, and entry of clinical events that are relevant to the interpretation of the record. Systemic tissue oxygenation should also be displayed continuously and some measure of brain electrical function should be recorded in all patients who are paralysed and artificially ventilated.

The system should incorporate a means of providing early warning of increased ICP, should indicate a probable cause of intracranial hypertension and should therefore be used not only to indicate when treatment is required but which particular therapy to use. The safety of the treatment in improving or at least preserving brain perfusion and function should also be assessed by the monitoring system.

An informative and succinct summary of the pathophysiological events of the previous 12 or 24 hours should be provided, with the measures that were employed in treatment and their effectiveness. This summary should be both in printed form that can be inserted into the patient's clinical chart, and be stored.

Finally, to return to the simple question posed at the outset – does continuous monitoring of intracranial pressure result in a reduction in the mortality and morbidity of patients with head injury? This may be an impossible question to answer. In Edinburgh, as in many other departments, we do not monitor ICP in all head injured patients. Our current indications for monitoring ICP are that the patient be in coma due to a haematoma requiring surgical evacuation, or, if there is no haematoma, coma with abnormal motor responses, or a CT scan appearance predictive of raised ICP. This CT appearance consists of loss of the third ventricle and perimesecephalic cisterns (Teasdale et al. 1984). The final group of head injured patients in whom monitoring is carried are those with multiple injuries that require artificial ventilation, usually severe chest injuries. Among the non-monitored group of patients, there are therefore two distinct groups. There are patients whose head injury is not sufficiently severe to warrant monitoring; most of these will have a good prognosis. There is also a group of patients in whom the injury is so overwhelmingly severe and the patient so aged or infirm prior to the head injury that a decision is made against active therapy. Understandably mortality in this group is extremely high. It is not useful for us to compare outcome data from monitored and nonmonitored patients.

Others have adopted a non-monitoring policy in larger groups of head injured patients and have pointed out that the outcome is similar to that reported by groups utilising ICP monitoring (Stuart et al. 1983). This does not prove that monitoring is unnecessary. ICP monitoring is part of a programme of care in which the emphasis is on prevention or early detection and amelioration of secondary insults to the brain. Other management protocols that do not use ICP monitoring still have the same overall strategy. Therapy suitable to treat most forms of raised ICP may be provided empirically even if ICP is not measured. Our comparison studies of the relative efficacy of mannitol and hypnotic agents suggest that in the majority of cases of raised ICP following head injury mannitol is, in fact, the preferred agent. In this way, regimens that utilise regular doses of mannitol given by the clock rather than on the basis of demonstration of raised ICP, may in most instances be providing perfectly adequate and appropriate therapy, albeit on an empirical basis (Smith et al. 1986). It is likely, therefore, that only a small subset of head injured patients will prove to have problems detectable and treatable with the aid of ICP monitoring and by no other method. A difference in outcome in this small number of patients is unlikely to be detectable when broad categories of outcome in entire groups of patients are compared (Miller and Teasdale 1985).

The argument in favour of ICP monitoring probably has to be intellectual rather than practical. Only by continuing the practice of intracranial pressure monitoring can we continue to learn about the pathophysiology of the conditions we are trying to treat, and how changes in intracranial pressure interrelate to alterations in cerebral energy supply, brain electrical status and the processes of therapy and recovery in our patients.

References

Avezaat CJJ, van Eijndhoven JHM, Wyper DJ (1979) Cerebrospinal fluid pulse pressure and intracranial volume – pressure relationships. J Neurol Neurosurg Psychiatry 42:687 – 700
Barlow P, Mendelow AD, Lawrence AE, Barlow M, Rowan JD (1985) Clinical evaluation of two methods of subdural pressure monitoring. J Neurosurg 63:578 – 582

Bell BA, Smith MA, Kean DM, McGhee CNJ, MacDonald HL, Miller JD, Barnett GH, Tocher JL, Douglas RHB, Best JJK (1987) Brain water measured by magnetic resonance imaging: correlation with direct estimation and change following mannitol and dexamethasone. Lancet I: 66–69

Børgesen SE, Gjerris F (1982) The predictive value of conductance to outflow of CSF in normal pressure hydrocephalus. Brain 105: 65–86

Børgesen SE, Gjerris F (1987) Relationship between intracranial pressure, ventricular size and resistance to CSF outflow. J Neurosurg 67: 535–539

Braakman R, Schouten HJA, Blaauw-van Dishoeck M, Minderhoud JM (1983) Megadose steroids in severe head injury: Results of a prospective double-blind clinical trial. J Neurosurg 58: 326–330

Chopp M, Portnoy HD (1980) Systems analysis of intracranial pressure. Comparison of volume-pressure test and CSF pulse amplitude analysis. J Neurosurg 53: 516–527

Dearden NM (1986) Management of raised intracranial pressure after severe head injury. Br J Hosp Med 36: 94–103

Dearden NM, Gibson JS, McDowall DG, Gibson RM, Cameron MM (1986) Effect of high dose dexamethasone on outcome from severe head injury. J Neurosurg 64: 81–88

Ekstedt J (1977) CSF hydrodynamic studies in man. 1: Method of constant pressure CSF infusion. J Neurol Neurosurg Psychiatry 40: 105–119

Fishman RA (1975) Brain edema. N Engl J Med 293: 706–711

Guillaume J, Janny P (1951) Manometrie intracranienne continue: interêt de la methode et premiers resultats. Rev Neurol (Paris) 84: 131–142

Leggate JRS, Dearden NM, Miller JD (1986) The effects of gammahydroxybutyrate and thiopentone on intracranial pressure in severe head injury. In: Miller JD et al. (eds) ICP VI. Springer, Berlin Heidelberg New York Tokyo, pp 754–759

Leggate JRS, Baxter P, Minns RA, Steers AJW, Brown JK, Shaw JF, Elton RA. The role of a separate subcutaneous cerebrospinal fluid reservoir in the management of hydrocephalus. Br J Neurosurg (in press)

Lundberg N (1960) Continuous recording and control of ventricular fluid pressure in neurosurgical practice. Acta Psychiatr Scand [Suppl 149] 36: 1–193

Marmarou A, Shulman K, Lamorgese J (1975) Compartmental analysis of compliance and outflow resistance of the cerebrospinal fluid outflow system. J Neurosurg 43: 523–534

Marmarou A, Maset AL, Ward JD, Choi S, Brooks D, Lutz HA, Moulton RJ, Muizelaar JP, Desalles A, Young HF (1987) Contribution of CSF and vascular factors to elevation of ICP in severely head-injured patients. J Neurosurg 66: 883–890

Maset AL, Marmarou A, Ward JD, Choi SC, Lutz HA, Brooks D, Moulton RJ, Desalles A, Muizelaar JP, Turner H, Young HF (1987) Pressure-volume index in head injury. J Neurosurg 67: 832–840

Messeter K, Nordström C-H, Sundbärg G, Algotsson L, Ryding E (1986) Cerebral haemodynamics in patients with acute severe head trauma. J Neurosurg 64: 231–237

Miller JD (1975) Volume and pressure in the craniospinal axis. Clin Neurosurg 22: 76–105

Miller JD (1978) Intracranial pressure monitoring. Br J Hosp Med 19: 497–503

Miller JD (1979a) Clinical management of cerebral oedema. Br J Hosp Med 20: 152–166

Miller JD (1979b) Barbiturates and raised intracranial pressure. Ann Neurol 6: 189–193

Miller JD (1985) Head injury and brain ischaemia – implications for therapy. Br J Anaesth 57: 120–129

Miller JD, Leech PJ (1975) Effects of mannitol and steroid therapy on intracranial volume-pressure relationships in patients. J Neurosurg 42: 274–281

Miller JD, Teasdale GM (1985) Clinical trials for assessing treatment. In: Becker DP, Povlishock JT (eds) Central Nervous System Trauma Status Report – 1985. Byrd Press., Richmond, pp 17–32

Miller JD, Garibi J, Pickard JD (1973) Induced changes of cerebrospinal fluid volume: Effects during continuous monitoring of ventricular fluid pressure. Arch Neurol 28: 265–269

Miller JD, Butterworth JF, Gudeman SK, Faulkner JE, Choi SC, Selhorst JB, Harbison JW, Lutz H, Young HF, Becker DP (1981) Further experience in the management of severe head injury. J Neurosurg 54: 289–299

14

Muizelaar JP, Wei EP, Kontos HA, Becker DP (1983) Mannitol causes compensatory cerebral vasoconstriction and vasodilatation to blood viscosity changes. J Neurosurg 59:822–828

Nordström CH, Messeter K, Sundbärg G, Schalen W, Werner M, Ryding E (1988) Cerebral blood flow, vasoreactivity and oxygen consumption during barbiturate therapy in severe traumatic brain lesions. J Neurosurg 68:424–431

North B, Reilly P (1986) Comparison among three methods of intracranial pressure recording. Neurosurgery 18:730–732

Ostrup RC, Luersson TG, Marshall LF, Zornow MH (1987) Continuous monitoring of intracranial pressure with a miniaturised fiberoptic device. J Neurosurg 62:206–209

Portnoy HD, Chopp M, Branch C, Shannon MB (1982) Cerebrospinal fluid waveform as an indicator of cerebral autoregulation. J Neurosurg 56:666–678

Schutta HS, Kassell NF, Langfitt TW (1968) Brain swelling produced by injury and aggravated by arterial hypertension – A light and electron microscopic study. Brain 91:281–294

Schwartz ML, Tator CH, Rowed DW, Reid SR, Megura K, Andrews DF (1984) The University of Toronto Head Injury Treatment Study: A prospective randomised comparison of pentobarbital and mannitol. Can J Neurol Sci 11:434–440

Shulman K, Marmarou A (1971) Pressure volume considerations in infantile hydrocephalus. Dev Med Child Neurol [Suppl 25] 13:90–95

Smith HP, Kelly DL, McWhorter JM, Armstrong D, Johnston R, Transou C, Howard G (1986) Comparison of mannitol regimes in patients with severe head injury undergoing intracranial pressure monitoring. J Neurosurg 65:820–824

Stuart G, Merry G, Smith JA, Yelland JDM (1983) Severe head injury managed without intracranial pressure monitoring. J Neurosurg 59:601–605

Sundbärg G, Nordström C-H, Messeter K, Söderström S (1987) A comparison of intraparenchymatous and intraventricular pressure recording in clinical practice. J Neurosurg 67:841–845

Szewczykowski J, Korsak-Sliwka J, Kunicki A, Sliwka S, Dziduszko J, Dytko P (1980) Spectral analysis of the ICP signal – practical application in computer-assisted long-term patient care. In: Marmarou A et al. (eds) Intracranial Pressure IV. Springer, Berlin Heidelberg, pp 419–422

Takagi H, Saito T, Kitahara T, Morii S, Ohwada T, Yada K (1983) The mechanism of the ICP reducing effect of mannitol. In: Ishii S, Nagai H, Brock M (eds) Intracranial pressure V. Springer, Berlin Heidelberg New York, pp 729–733

Takizawa H, Gabra-Sanders T, Miller JD (1985) Validity of measurements of CSF outflow resistance estimated by the bolus injection method. Neurosurgery 17:63–66

Takizawa H, Gabra-Sanders T, Miller JD (1986) Spectral analysis of the CSF pulse-wave at different locations in the craniospinal axis. J Neurol Neurosurg Psychiatry 49:1135–1141

Takizawa H, Gabra-Sanders T, Miller JD (1987) Changes in the CSF pulse wave spectrum associated with raised intracranial pressure. Neurosurgery 20:355–361

Tans JTJ, Poortvliet DCJ (1982) Intracranial volume–pressure relationship in man. Part 1: Calculation of the pressure-volume index. J Neurosurg 56:524–528

Teasdale E, Cardoso E, Galbraith S, Teasdale G (1984) A new CT scan appearance with raised intracranial pressure in severe diffuse head injury. J Neurol Neurosurg Psychiatry 46:600–603

Ward JD, Becker DP, Miller JD, Choi SC, Marmarou A, Wood C, Newlon P, Keenan R (1985) Failure of prophylactic barbiturate coma in the treatment of severe head injury. J Neurosurg 62:383–388

Welch K (1980) The intracranial pressure in infants. J Neurosurg 52:693–699

15

Physical Characteristics of Various Methods for Measuring ICP

M.R. Gaab, H.E. Heissler, and K. Ehrhardt

Neurosurgical Department, Hanover Medical School, Konstanty-Gutschow-Str. 8, D-3000 Hannover 61 (FRG)

Introduction

Many data have been published on different methods for measuring "ICP" via ventricular, epidural, subdural or parenchymal record. Also during this meeting, several new devices are presented. However, most investigations only consider the *static* criteria of the methods, like linearity, zero point stability and hysteresis (Gaab and Heissler 1984, 1988). Little attention has been paid to the *dynamic properties* of the devices. Such data on frequency resolution (band width) and phase, however, are especially important for computerized evaluation of ICP dynamics including waveform analysis (Chopp and Portnoy 1980; Gaab et al. 1983; Gaab and Heissler 1984, 1988; Portnoy et al. 1983; Varju 1977). ICP pulse waves and the transfer characteristics from arterial blood pressure (SAP) to ICP contain continuous information on intracranial elastance, vasoregulation and CSF dynamics (Branch et al. 1988; Chopp and Portnoy 1980; Portnoy et al. 1983). Dynamic analysis could therefore replace invasive methods like bolus and infusion tests (Anile et al. 1988; Branch et al. 1988; Chopp and Portnoy 1980; Portnoy et al. 1983). However, the waveform investigation e.g., with Fourier transformation up to the 5th harmonic of the ICP pulsation (Piper et al. 1988) requires a bandwidth for recording of > 40 Hz (Gaab and Heissler 1984, 1988). We therefore investigated the frequency resolution and the phase lag of current methods used for measuring ICP and blood pressures.

Methods

Transducers and, if applicable, the complete measuring chain for clinical pressure record (e.g., needle, catheter, transducer, monitor) were investigated in vitro. In a pressure chamber, the response to test excitation was examined using a *DIRAC delta* (impulse) function (Table 1, Fig. 1 a). By switching a magnetic valve from atmospheric pressure to a reservoir of 20 mm Hg, an almost ideal DIRAC impulse was produced (transformation to the La Place level $= 1$, FFT $= 1$; Fig. 1 a). The dP by far exceeds the bandwidth of any of the devices under test (> 500 Hz, Fig. 1). The analogous response of the devices (Table 1) was averaged from 200 pseudo-randomized impulse functions and evaluated using discrete Fourier

Intracranial Pressure VII
Eds.: J.T. Hoff and A.L. Betz
© Springer-Verlag Berlin Heidelberg 1989

Table 1. Analysis of dynamic properties of devices for measuring pressures with the <u>DIRAC</u> <u>delta</u> function

Theoretical and mathematical approach

$$\text{E (s)} \longrightarrow \boxed{\text{H (s)}} \longrightarrow \text{R (s)}$$

excitation   device   response

$$\text{H (s)} = \frac{\text{R (s)}}{\text{E (s)}}$$

if   E (s) = α {Dirac delta (impulse) function}

then E (s) = 1

for   s →jω

H (jω) = R (jω)

H (jω) = frequency response of the device

s   = Laplace operator

jω   = complex frequency

transformation and further complex data manipulation according to the principles of digital signal analysis (Achilles 1978; Burrus and Parks 1985) on a HP series 9000, model 320 computer. For comparison with the device under test, a technical reference transducer with a bandwidth of >200 Hz (Sensodyne, Fig. 1 a) was used. The frequency resolution (log normalized amplitude = log ΔP normalized to first harmonic = damping) and the phase were investigated in a bandwidth of 100 Hz (Fig. 2).

Results

Characteristics of Transducers

All "fast" transducers (strain gauges, piezoresistors, resonant circuits) give an *accurate response* within a band width of at least 20 Hz (Fig. 1 b, Fig. 2 a, b) sufficient for an analysis of first to 4th/5th harmonic of pulse waves. Within this frequency range all standard external pressure transducers for measuring fluid pressures (Statham P23dB, P37, P50; Medex, Fig. 1 b, Hewlett-Packard) as well as the new, cheap sensors for single use (e.g., PVB Dispo-Sense, strain gauge) give a proportional response. Also the *microtransducers (MTCs) for intracranial implantation* on strain gauge technology (GAELTEC ICTb, PPG-Epidyn) have an optimal damping at least up to 20 Hz (Fig. 2 a). The band width of the new resonant circuit sensors suited for telemetric record (Rotterdam Teletransducer, Hellige Episensor, Fig. 2 b) also give an accurate response within 20 Hz bandwidth. Some minor fluctuations only result from digitalizing (D to A transfer, Fig. 1 b). The CAMINO system based on the measurement of light intensity via fiberoptics even has a bandwidth of >100 Hz (Piper et al. 1988).

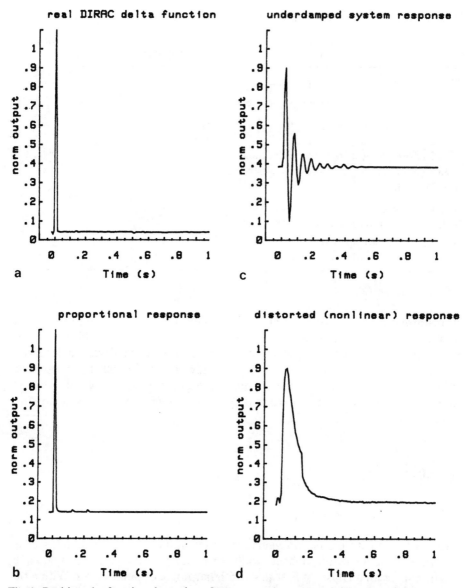

Fig. 1. Real impulse function shown by reference transducer (**a**), good response from a strain gauge transducer, Medex (**b**); oscillation due to resonance with silicone ventricle catheter, "ringing" (**c**), overdamping and nonlinearity with microcatheter (**d**)

Fiberoptic transducers using a pneumatic balance system for adjusting a mirror membrane (Ladd, Meadox), however, have a small frequency resolution of 0.1–2 Hz and allow only recording of mean ICP (Gaab and Heissler 1984, 1988). With all transducers, a considerable *phase lag* occurs at frequency > 2 Hz (Fig. 2).

Whereas most sensors would allow a sufficient waveform analysis of physiological pressures, *any system using fluid transmission* of the pressure to an external transducer considerably distorts any waveform in the range of SAP and ICP pulse wave frequency: The fluid filled needles and tubes come into resonance (Fig. 1c, *underdamped distortion*) or the *overdamp* (Fig. 1d).

For measuring SAP, the use of a Seldinger catheter attached to a Medex (or any other) transducer (Fig. 1c) gives a proportional response up to −8 Hz. At higher frequencies, the amplitude response rises by resonance, followed by damping with >20 Hz. A combination of a transducer with a longer needle, e.g., with a 19 g cannula for lumbar puncture (Fig. 2d) is even worse: resonance starts at 2 Hz with a maximal distortion at 7–10 Hz followed by considerable damping >20 Hz. Using *soft catheters* with diameters of >1 mm like silicone ventricle catheters (e.g., from Codman, Fig. 2e) or simple extension lines for monitoring blood pressure, an initially slightly overdamped waveform is seen within 1–6 Hz followed by underdamping with a maximum around 20 Hz, then again turning to overdamping at higher frequencies. *Microcatheters* for measuring ventricular or lumbar CSF pressure like the PORTEX syst. 4 microcatheter (Fig. 2f) severely *overdamp* at all frequencies >1 Hz with a 90% reduction in amplitude response already at 10 Hz. With all catheter/needle-transducer systems, too, a *phase lag* occurs which, however, is mainly defined by the properties of the transducer (Fig. 2).

Discussion

According to these results, the investigation of waveform characterists of ICP and blood pressure is *problematic:* For a proper analysis of frequency spectra and of transfer function at least the 5th harmonic of the pulse wave should be included (Branch et al. 1988; Piper et al. 1988), that means a bandwidth of >20 Hz in adults and even >40 Hz in infants. The bandwidth of all systems using fluid filled lines is far below, and even most transducers overdamp at >20 Hz.

Devices which measure ICP or blood pressure with an external transducer via fluid transmission are not even accurate in analyzing the first harmonic of pulsation. Tubes with larger diameters (>1 mm, ventricle catheters, extension lines) and stiff cannulas *underdamp due to resonance;* small catheters (microcatheters) do *overdamp*. The exact damping characteristics depend on stiffness of catheter material (hard = resonance, soft-damping) and on the diameter and length of the line. This *excludes* an absolute analysis of dynamic behavior of pressures with these devices, at least without an exact correction for the damping characteristics. If damping errors are not considered, the signal response may even be opposite real phenomena: The decrease in slope of the pulse amplitude described by Foltz and Aine (1981), for example, is probably caused by damping with the catheter system used for measuring ICP. The slope of ΔP even increases in active hydrocephalus using implanted pressure transducers with more accurate bandwidth (Gaab et al. 1983).

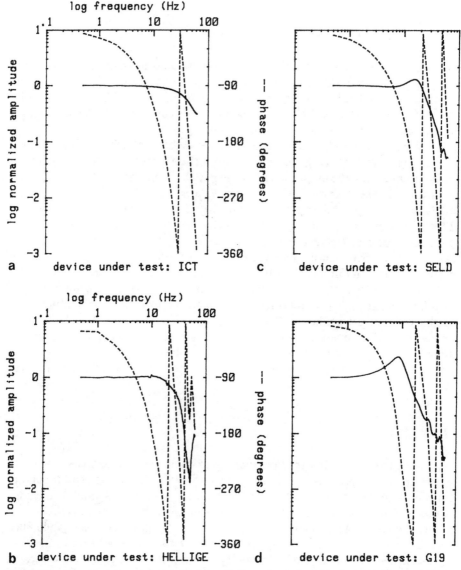

Fig. 2. Damping (— log. norm. amplitude) and phase lag (- -) within 0.1–100 Hz bandwidth: good response > 20 Hz with transducers, Gaeltec ICTb (**a**), Hellige Episensor (**b**) underdamping and slight overdamping with Seldinger catheter (**c**) needle G19 (**d**) and silicone ventricle catheter (**e**) Overdamping with microcatheter (**f**)

The use of implanted microtransducers with a higher bandwidth does not guarantee an accurate frequency resolution, however. Artifacts from the *operative approach* must be considered, like damping by the dura, small hemorrhages and lacerations around the transducer tip, etc. Again, this gives evidence that no simple "ICP" exists. There are different "ICP's" defined by the anatomical position of the device used for recording and by its dynamic properties. For any investigation of waveforms, frequency spectra, and transfer functions of pressures, the exact dynamic response of the systems used must be known, and data

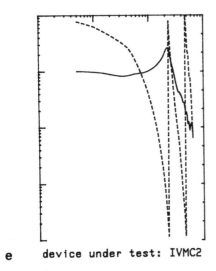 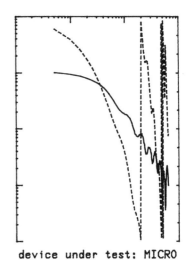

e   device under test: IVMC2   f   device under test: MICRO

Fig. 2 e, f

should be provided in the publications. For evaluation of the systems characteristics, we recommend the impulse function. Quantitative values (natural frequency, damping ratio, phase lag) can be approximated by assuming a second-order system (Achilles 1978; Gaab and Heissler 1988).

References

Achilles D (1978) Die Fouriertransformation in der Signalverarbeitung. Springer, Berlin Heidelberg New York

Anile C, Mangiola A, Andreasi F, Branch CA, Portnoy HD (1988) CSF pulse waveform morphology as an indicator of intracranial system impedance: an experimental study. This volume, pp 193–195

Branch CA, Chopp M, Portnoy HD (1988) Fourier analysis of intracranial pressures during experimental intracranial hypertension. This volume, pp 175–180

Burrus ChS, Parks TW (1985) DFT/FFT and convolution algorithms. J Wiley and Sons, New York Toronto

Chopp M, Portnoy HD (1980) Systems analysis of intracranial pressure. Comparison between the volume pressure test and CSF pulse amplitude analysis. J Neurosurg 53:516–527

Foltz EL, Aine C (1981) Diagnosis of hydrocephalus by CSF pulse wave analysis. A clinical study. Surg Neurol 15:283–293

Gaab MR, Heissler HE (1984) ICP Monitoring. CRC Crit Rev Biomed Engin 11:189–250

Gaab MR, Heissler HE (1988) Monitoring Intracranial Pressure. In: Webster JG (ed) Encyclopedia of Medical Devices and Instrumentation. J Wiley and Sons, New York Chichester Brisbane Toronto

Gaab MR, Haubitz I, Brawanski A et al. (1983) Pressure-volume diagram, pulse amplitude and intracranial pulse volume. Analysis and significance. In: Ishii S, Nagai H, Brock M (eds) Intracranial Pressure V. Springer, Berlin Heidelberg New York, pp 261–268

Piper IR, Dearden NM, Miller JD (1988) Can waveform analysis of ICP separate vascular from non-vascular causes of intracranial hypertension? This volume, pp 157–163

Portnoy HD, Chopp M, Branch C et al. (1983) CSF pulse wave, ICP and autoregulation. In: Ishii S, Nagai H, Brock M (eds) Intracranial Pressure V. Springer, Berlin Heidelberg New York, pp 180–185

Varju D (1977) Systemtheorie für Biologen und Mediziner. Springer, Berlin Heidelberg New York

An Approach to Noninvasive Analysis of Intracranial Pressure (ICP) Using an Ultrasonic Probe

H. Kuchiwaki, J. Itoh, H. Ishiguri, K. Andoh, S. Ogura, N. Sakuma, and T. Takishita

Department of Neurosurgery, Nagoya University, School of Medicine, 65 Tsurumai-Cho, Showa-Ku, Nagoya 466 (Japan)

Introduction

Several approaches using ultrasonic (UT) waves to study changes in intracranial pressure (ICP) have been previously reported. However, the studies were not successful in obtaining information throughout the range of the pathological variations in ICP levels (Oka et al. 1971). Additionally, operative procedures were necessary to open a hole in the skull (Itoh et al. 1986) or to install a spring coil (Numoto et al. 1983). The aim of our study was to procure noninvasively continuous wave forms and levels of ICP by using a UT probe on the scalp. The following is a report of experimental results including some clinical examples with our method.

Our method is based on the fact that, when UT waves are transmitted in order through mediums 1, 2, and 3 each of which has a different acoustic impedance (Z_1, Z_2, Z_3), and medium 2 is thin enough to produce interfering reflected UT-waves, the relative strength ($|\mathrm{re}|$) is expressed as follows:

$$|\mathrm{re}| = \sqrt{1 - \frac{4\dfrac{Z_1}{Z_3}}{\left(\dfrac{Z_1}{Z_3}+1\right)^2 \cos^2\left(\dfrac{2\pi l}{\lambda}\right) + \left(\dfrac{Z_1}{Z_2}+\dfrac{Z_2}{Z_3}\right)^2 \sin^2\left(\dfrac{2\pi l}{\lambda}\right)}} \qquad (1)$$

In this study we assumed that medium 1 is skull bone, medium 2 is the dura mater, and medium 3 is the brain tissue including the subarachnoid space.

Materials and Methods

Seven adult mongrel dogs (body weight; 8–14 kg) under enough intramuscular or intravenous Ketamine anesthesia for surgical procedures, were intubated and breathed spontaneously. Expiratory gases were monitored with a gas analyzer (IH 21A NEC Sanei Co. Ltd, Tokyo) and systemic blood pressure (BP) was measured through a catheter in the femoral artery. A venous catheter was introduced into the femoral vein for the continuous injection of saline solution during these experiments. Then the animal was fixed in a stereotaxic operation table and

Intracranial Pressure VII
Eds.: J.T. Hoff and A.L. Betz
© Springer-Verlag Berlin Heidelberg 1989

the skull was exposed. An epidural pressure (EDP) transducer (Toyota Cent. Res. Inst., Aichi) was inserted through one side of the skull and a UT probe was placed on the skull on the other side. Intracranial pressure was raised by inflation of an epidural balloon, infusion of lactate Ringer solution through the cisterna magna, neck compressions, hyperventilation, and 10%-CO_2 gas inhalation. Wave forms of BP, EDP, and UT-wave were simultaneously recorded. In clinical practice, three patients and several healthy adult persons were examined several times per person with our UT probe. We used a thin disk-type UT probe with a diameter of 25 mm (3.5, 5 MHz, less than 1 mW/cm^2). The patients had falx meningioma, fibrosarcoma occupying the orbit as well as frontal space showing increased ICP, and ventricular dilation. The last patient underwent ICP measurements in which case we were simultaneously studying ICP with UT methods.

Our UT apparatus consists of a UT wave transmission/receiver system, a peak detector and recording system, and a signal processing and recording system. In the UT wave transmisison/receiver system, a spike/burst pulser transmits UT waves to a probe (3.5 and 5 MHz, less than 1 mW/cm^2) which is attached to the skull or the temple. UT echoes from the receiver are simultaneously sent the other systems. We can observe the echoes on a synchroscope that is connected to the peak detector. From these echoes, those originating from the thin layers were selected by a gate circuit according to the delay time of the echo arrival on the synchroscope. The UT echo through the gate was searched for the maximum value of relative strength by the peak detector. This signal, amplified through a differencial DC amplifier, was continuously recorded as a UT wave form of ICP. On the other hand, UT-signals into the digitizer were processed with Fast Fourier

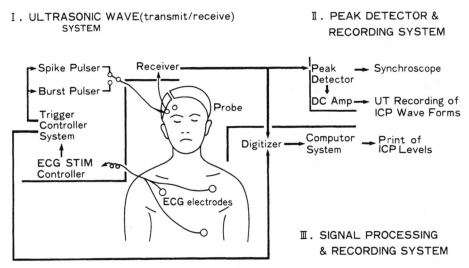

Fig. 1. Summary of our UT (ultrasonic) probe method of ICP measurements. This system consists of three main parts of I, II, and III. Operators can observe echoes on the time scale in a synchroscope and select the echoes originating from the dura mater with a gate circuit. Continuous recordings are made through a DC amplifier. Acquisition of FFT/Cepstrum analysis can be started by a signal from an ECG. The ratio of the thickness change indicates ICP levels. Both results are needed for our measurement

Transformation (FFT)/Cepstrum analysis resulting in a print of estimated ICP values. As this layer (medium 2) changes its thickness according to the cycle of the heart beat, the acquisition by FFT/cepstrum analysis was initiated by a trigger signal of R in the electrocardiogram. These systems are summarized in Fig. 1. The velocity of sound used was, 3360 (m/s) for bone, 1600 for dura mater, 1400–1500 for soft tissue and fat.

Results

As shown in Fig. 2a, UT wave forms changed during the gradual rise of ICP by an infusion into the cisterna magna in this experiment. Compared to the wave forms of an EDP transducer in a relatively lower level of ICP, the wave form by UT method showed a steep rise and fall within a short duration, while an EDP wave form was triangular. However, with greater increasing of ICP, UT wave forms became similar to those of EDP. UT waves increased their amplitudes up to 700 mm H_2O of ICP and their patterns became higher with sharper peaks. The reverse phenomenon was also observed by a decreasing of ICP. During ICP changes the phase of the UT wave was reversed at about 200–400 mm H_2O and the amplitude became smaller and smaller above the level of 800–1000 mm H_2O. The results by both balloon inflation and infusion methods were quite similar.

In Fig. 2b results of FFT/Cepstrum in one experiment with an infusion method are expressed as the rate of $D_p - D_p/D_0 =$ (epsilon) on the y axis and ICP on the x axis, here D_p is the thickness of the thin layers at pressure P and D_0 is the thickness at basal levels of pressure (prior to infusion). The thickness was calculated from the differences of Quefrency (n sec) between an echo-peak from the inner table of the skull and that from a thin layer (medium 2) which is changeable by ICP levels:

The Quefrency (n sec) $\times$ 1600 (m/s)/2 $\times 10^{-3} =$ (alpha) μm

From these, the rates of the change in thickness showed a near linear correlation with the level of ICP read by the EDP transducer. These pressure values ranged from 0 to 700 mm H_2O. In clinical practice, we also received echoes from the thin layers which were selected by the gate circuit of the peak detector. One example of a UT wave form of ICP from a 16 year-old patient with a bone defect invaded by a fibrosarcoma is shown in Fig. 2c. The UT probe was used on the scalp, so the echo signals included echoes from vessels in the scalp, intradiploic venous flow, and thin layers. Therefore, the time delay to catch interfering echoes of the layers by the gate circuit ranged from 8 to 12 μs. By continuous recordings, hyperventilation reduced the amplitude of a wave form of UT, while stopping breathing induced spiky rises of amplitudes of UT waves. UT wave changes correlated well with those of ICP in a patient with a ventricular dilation.

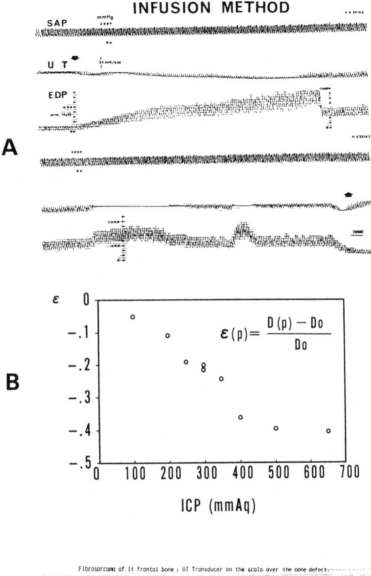

INFUSION METHOD

$$\varepsilon(p) = \frac{D(p) - Do}{Do}$$

ICP (mmAq)

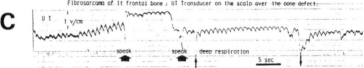

Fibrosarcoma of lt frontal bone ; UT Transducer on the scalp over the bone defect.

Fig. 2. A Recording showing UT wave changes during rises of ICP by infusion method. Systemic arterial pressure (SAP), UT wave form, and epidural pressure (EDP) are recorded. The bottom three waveforms are the continuation of the three wave forms at the top. Characteristic changes are explained in the text. **B** Graph showing a linear correlation between ratios of the thickness changes and ICP levels: Experimental data. **C** Clinical recordings of UT wave forms of ICP. A 16 year-old patient with increased ICP. An increased amplitude seems to be due to rise of ICP. Note the amplitude decreasing during hyperventilation

Discussion

The excellent correlation between values from a thickness gauge using a thin oil-membrane and a reflection coefficient of an interfering UT echo have been proved (Itoh et al. 1987). A noninvasive method is an ideal as a diagnositc procedure of ICP measurement. Our method with UT wave is noninvasive and free from painful stimulations. An important point is whether the probe can be closely attached to the skin for a long time without pain or disagreeable sensations. Our UT probe can be attached closely to the scalp with painless procedure. We used probes of 3.5 MHz and 5 MHz, each of which transmits and receives transcranial echoes well. However, from our data in operative monitorings, UT waves did not pass through 7–8 mm thickness of the skull. A UT probe should be placed on the temple or forehead regions. But in this area the echoes of the superficial temporal artery and its branches complicated the echoes from the thin layers.

It is important to select the echoes from the thin layers by using a gate circuit. From our results, change in the rate of relative strength of interfering thin-layer-echoes showed a linear correlation to ICP levels. It remains undetermined whether the thin layers (medium 2) are the dura mater or the dura mater including the subarachnoid space to the surface of the brain. By a balloon inflation method, shifting of the brain is supposed to be greater than by an infusion method. However, UT wave forms were very similar by the two methods. Therefore, the authors presumed that the thin layer is more likely the dura mater. Further studies are needed for the determination of the origin of interfering echoes. The phase reversal of UT waves at the level of ICP 200–400 mm H_2O indicated the decreasing power of the interfering echoes, according to the curve of the equation because the curve alternates periodically according to the value of l/lambda (l: thickness of the thin layer, lambda: wave length of UT wave). A remarkable decreasing of the echoes from the layers was observed above 1000 mm H_2O and is assumed to show a limitation in the theoretical ability to detect changes in the power of reflection rate.

Acknowledgements. This study was performed under a grant-in-aid for Japanese Ministry of Education from 1985 to 1987.

References

Itoh J, Kuchiwaki H, Nagasaka M, Kinomoto T, Takada S, Ishiguri H, Kageyama N (1986) A study of continuous recording of pulsatile movements of dura using a miniture ultrasonic probe. Igakunoayumi 138:529–530

Itoh J, Kuchiwaki H, Nagasaka M, Ishiguri H, Kageyama N, Sakuma N, Ogura S (1987) A basic study of continuous monitoring of intracranial pressure using ultrasonic probe. – A preliminary report from experimental model. Jpn J Med Ultrasonics 14:111–118

Numoto M, Hara M, Yokota M, Kadowaki C, Maeda T, Takeuchi K (1983) A simple clinical ICP meter. In: Ishii S, Nagai H, Brock M (eds) Intracranial Pressure V. Springer, Berlin Heidelberg New York Tokyo, pp 106–109

Oka M, Nishii T, Marusasa Y, Hazawa A, Horiwaki H, Arimoto T (1971) Intracranial echo pulsation in brain death, brain tumor and intracranial hypertension. Jpn J Surg 1:146–154

Clinical Evaluation of the Catheter Tipped Camino Transducer Inserted via a Subdural Screw

I.R. Chambers, A.D. Mendelow, J. Sinar, and P. Modha

Regional Medical Physics Department and Department of Neurosurgery,
University of Newcastle upon Tyne, Newcastle General Hospital, NE4 6BE (UK)

Introduction

Intracranial pressure (ICP) monitoring has become routine in many neurosurgical units. However, the procedure of ventriculostomy is invasive and carries risks. A search for alternative techniques of ICP monitoring has shown that some alternatives are less reliable than fluid-filled ventricular catheters: subdural screws and fluid-filled catheters under-read ICP, especially when it is high (Mendelow et al. 1983; Barlow et al. 1985); by contrast, subdural catheter-tipped transducers are accurate when compared to fluid-filled ventricular catheters (Barlow et al. 1985). The aim of this study was to compare pressure readings from a ventricular catheter with those from a Camino catheter tipped transducer.

We have compared the recordings from these two different methods in patients over extended periods of monitoring to determine the reliability of such a device in clinical practice.

Materials and Methods

Ten patients were selected with recent head injury who required ICP monitoring as part of their routine care. A ventricular catheter was inserted through a burr hole on one side of the head and a solid, narrow-bore catheter tipped transducer was inserted on the opposite side via a narrow gauge screw. The ventricular catheter was connected to an externally mounted pressure transducer fixed at the level of the patient's ear by a 0.5 m length of tubing. Both transducers were calibrated at regular intervals during the monitoring period.

In each patient the external transducer and the Camino transducer were connected to pressure modules on a Simonsen and Weel (S and W) Triscope monitoring system and a permanent recording of both traces made on a Gould two-channel pen recorder. For precise analysis the pressure modules were modified to extract the systolic, diastolic and mean values of the pressure waveforms in digital format. This information was fed into a custom built interface which sampled the readings from each transducer every 30 seconds and was then stored on a floppy disk using a Data Grabber (Mutek Ltd.). The Data Grabber is a digital buffer which can store incoming data on a 3.5 inch floppy disk in a similar fashion to a tape recorder. The data can subsequently be recovered for analysis. Each sampled value is thus identical to that displayed on the S and W pressure modules.

The mean pressure value from each device was recorded every 30 seconds and then 10 of these readings were averaged to obtain a mean pressure recording for each transducer for each five minute recording period. Additionally the difference between each recorded value was calculated and a frequency histogram derived from this data.

Results

Ten patients were studied over periods from 4.7 to 76.7 hours. In one patient the Camino failed three hours after insertion, the tracing becoming essentially flat with little pulsatile variation, having initially functioned correctly. In one other case the Camino failed early, prior to the completion of monitoring due to the optical fibre rupturing. The probable cause of this was excessive stress inadvertantly placed on the catheter. This was the first catheter used in the study and this problem did not occur again once staff became familiar with the equipment. The initial analysis of grouped data from eight patients revealed a correlation coeffi-

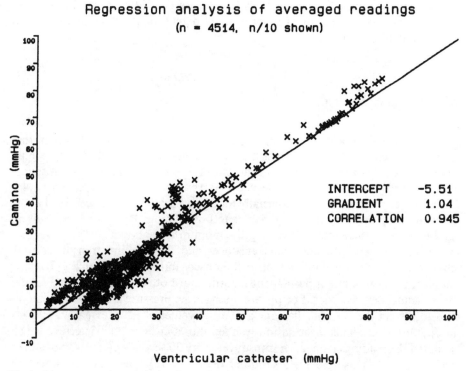

Fig. 1. Linear regression analysis of complete data set

28

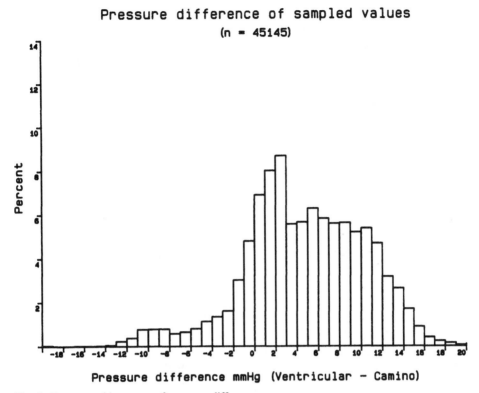

Pressure difference of sampled values
(n = 45145)

Percent

Pressure difference mmHg (Ventricular — Camino)

Fig. 2. Frequency histogram of pressure differences

cient of 0.81, a gradient of 0.78 and an intercept of −1.38. A further patient (number 9) with very high ICP was subsequently studied and in those nine patients data was available for analysis for a total length of 369.5 hours (average 41.0 hours per patient; maximum 76.7 hours, minimum 4.7). Pressure readings were averaged over a period of five minutes (10 half minute values) and linear regression analysis performed on the resultant data. The correlation coefficient from each transducer varied from 0.391–0.978, the gradient ranged between 0.41 and 1.06 and an intercept ranged from −4.39 to 9.35. On the complete data set the correlation coefficient was 0.945; gradient 1.04 and intercept −5.51 (Fig. 1). Figure 2 shows a histogram of the difference between the ventricular catheter and the Camino transducer. The Camino pressure was 5 mm Hg lower than the ventricular pressure on average, with 95% of the readings within 14 mm Hg of each other, and 99% of the readings within 16 mm Hg.

Discussion

Although a fluid-filled ventricular catheter gives the most reliable recording of intracranial pressure, it has several disadvantages which include the risk of infection, haemorrhage and epilepsy. Many of the techniques of subdural pressure monitoring have proved inaccurate (Mendelow et al. 1983; Barlow et al. 1985), and in certain circumstances potentially dangerous (Miller et al. 1986). By contrast, a catheter tipped transducer in the subdural space is accurate (Barlow et al. 1986) but practical problems have been encountered with inflating the membrane covered catheter tipped transducers. Firstly, they require an open burr hole operation. If a catheter malfunction occurs then a second operation is required. Secondly, the calibration procedure requires the inflation of a diaphragm: during inflation, any leak in the diaphragm may allow the pressurised escape of air into the patient's subdural space (Gentleman and Mendelow 1986). Alternative types of catheter tipped transducers are available that do not require inflation of a diaphragm for calibration, although in situ calibration is then not possible. Such catheters must therefore be shown to be inherently stable over prolonged periods.

In the present study we have demonstrated that the recordings from the Camino catheter tipped-transducer correlate well with the recordings from a contralateral fluid filled ventricular catheter over a wide range of ICP, and over long periods of monitoring.

Technical problems developed in one case, but it was clear from the outset that the optical fibre had been damaged with insertion. One of the advantages of the system evaluated was that a new transducer could be inserted without the need for re-operation. The fact that the Camino under read by 5 mm Hg may be accounted for by the position of the transducer in the frontal region (approximately 5 mm Hg above the centre of the head) which was used as the reference point for calibration and zeroing of the ventricular catheter. This 5 mm Hg (6.5 cm of water) difference should be taken into consideration when interpreting recording from the Camino subdural transducer.

References

Barlow P, Mendelow AD, Lawrence AE, Barlow M, Rowan JO (1985) Clinical evaluation of two methods of subdural pressure monitoring. J Neurosurg 63:578–582
Barlow P, Mendelow AD, Rowan JO, Barlow M (1986) Clinical evaluation of the Gealtec ICT/b Pressure Transducer placed subdurally. ICP VI, Springer, Berlin Heidelberg New York, pp 181–183
Gentleman D, Mendelow AD (1986) Intracranial rupture of a pressure monitoring transducer, technical note. Neurosurgery 19:91
Mendelow AD, Rowan JO, Murray L, Kerr AE (1983) A clinical comparison of subdural screw pressure measurements with ventricular pressure. J Neurosurg 57:45–50
Miller JD, Bobo H, Kapp JP (1986) Inaccurate pressure readings from subarachnoid bolts. Neurosurgery 19:253–255

Clinical and Laboratory Evaluation of the Camino Intracranial Pressure Monitoring System

J.R.S. Leggate, I.R. Piper, I. Robertson, A. Lawson, and J.D. Miller

Department of Clinical Neurosciences, Western General Hospital, University of Edinburgh (UK)

Introduction

It is common practice in head injured patients to measure intracranial pressure (ICP) using subdural screws or catheters with fluid filled linkages to external transducers. Problems of under-reading at ICP levels above 30 mm Hg and over-damping of the ICP waveform are well documented (Mendelow et al. 1983). Performance of the subdural catheter system can be improved by the use of the Accudynamic[2] device which enables optimal damping of the waveform to be achieved without altering the natural frequency response (Allan et al. 1988) but the disadvantages of under-reading the true ICP remains. The advantages of an intracranial transducer are: avoidance of over-damping of the waveform with a fast reaction time and a flat frequency response of up to 40 Hertz. Many such devices however, cannot be zeroed or calibrated in situ. One such device, the Camino[1] fibro-optic intracranial pressure transducer, has been used initially for measuring the intracranial pressure from brain parenchyma in children and after subsequent modification, can now be used to measure ICP when placed either in the ventricles, in the subdural space or through a subarachnoid bolt. Comparison has been carried out between the Camino 110-4G fibro-optic intracranial transducer placed subdurally with pressure recordings obtained from a subdural catheter, our most usual method, in 15 head injured patients.

Method

Fifteen severely head injured patients (GCS ≤ 8 on admission), undergoing ICP monitoring as part of their management, had a subdural catheter inserted and a Camino 110-4G transducer placed alongside for comparative recordings. The subdural catheter was linked via an Accudynamic tap to a Medex[3] transducer

---

[1] Camino fibre optic catheter-tip transducers, Camino Laboratories, San Diego, California (USA).
[2] Accudynamic adjustable damping devices. Abbott Critical Care Systems, Chicago, Illinois (USA).
[3] Medex Noratrans transducers. Medix Inc., Hilliard, Ohio (USA).

Table 1. Values obtained on bench testing of camino transducer system

	Max.	Min.
Zero drift	7 mm Hg/day	1 mm Hg/day
Calibration drift	6 mm Hg	2 mm Hg
Temperature drift (33 °C–39 °C) 8 mV = 1 mm Hg	47 mV	0 mV
Linearity slope	1.05	0.81
Y intercept	−11.4	0
Hysteresis	6 mm Hg	1.5 mm Hg

mounted on the side of the head at the level of the foramen of Monro. The Camino system was zeroed prior to insertion using the adjustment screw on the device. Both devices were then linked via amplifiers to a four channel chart recorder for continuous ICP monitoring. An IBM PC XT linked to a Teac MR10 cassette tape recorder sampled onto the tape five minute periods of ICP recordings which were taken at half hourly intervals throughout the period of ICP monitoring. Subsequent analysis of these tapes enabled comparative data to be obtained of absolute pressure values and also for waveform analysis. When a management decision was taken to stop ICP recording, the Camino device was removed from the patient and the zero drift checked immediately. The catheter device was then cleaned and sent for laboratory evaluation. Ten catheters from the 15 inserted were evaluated for zero drift and calibration drift over a five day period. Twelve of the 15 catheters were evaluated for the linearity of their response over a pressure range of 0–90 cm of water and the hysteresis (maximum difference between linearity up and linearity down) was determined from this. In addition, temperature drift over a 6° C range (33–39° C) was evaluated (Table 1).

Results

Of the 15 patients, 1 device failed at the outset although subsequent laboratory evaluation showed normal function. This failure was a step change of 40 mm Hg after insertion of the device and a period of stable recording whilst the patient was being transferred from the operating room to the Intensive Care Unit. Recordings from 2 other catheters deteriorated after three days due to the device migrating from the head into the subgaleal tissues subsequent to handling of the patient. Both these devices performed well on laboratory evaluation. In 5 patients, there was good correlation (correlation co-efficient equal to or greater than 0.9) between the two devices throughout a three day recording period. In the remaining 9 patients, there was poor correlation between the two devices. In these, the Camino consistently under-read the subdural catheter when the pressure was 10 mm Hg or less, whilst at higher pressures, in those patients with poor correlation, the subdural catheter under-read the Camino ICP by as much as 60% or more if the ICP was greater than 25 mm Hg. Persistent re-zeroing of the fluid-filled subdural catheter and flushing of the device restored good correlation of the ICP recordings, but this was short lived. In 1 patient, in whom subdural catheter-subdural Camino comparison showed poor correlation, a ventricular catheter connected to a subcutaneous reservoir was inserted and comparison made between the Camino and intraventricular ICP. This showed excellent correlation between the two recordings (R = 0.987, slope 1.05, intercept −1.1).

Discussion

This comparison between a subdurally placed Camino transducer and a subdural catheter has shown no correlation between ICP measurements, in 9 out of 14 patients in whom comparative recordings were obtained. This poor correlation would appear to be due to the poor performance of the subdural catheter as noted in the consistent under-reading of the Camino ICP values by as much as 62% when ICP was evaluated (Table 2). The example of excellent correlation between subdural Camino ICP recordings with those recorded from the lateral ventricle would suggest that when placed subdurally, the Camino catheter is a more reliable method of recording ICP than the subdural catheter which is at present widely used in head injured patients.

The laboratory data showed good linearity of response with minimal zero drift or calibration drift over the expected pressure ranges and with negligible drift over the commonly encountered temperature ranges for patients in a Neuro-Intensive Care Unit. The catheter that failed shortly after placement but yet still produced good laboratory data is disturbing in that a step wise change in pressure measurements of 40 mm Hg was seen in a clinical situation. Whilst this was not repeated during recording periods, observations have been made of similar step changes with slow decay back to the previous ICP levels in the Neuro-Intensive Care Unit. During laboratory testing of 1 catheter for temperature drift measurements, a single step wise change of 47 millivolts (approximately 6 mm Hg) has been recorded.

Table 2. Mean percentage difference between subdural catheter and subdural camino transducer recordings of ICP at different pressure levels

Pressure (mm Hg)	Subdural/Camino ICP (%)
0 – 10	+ 33
10 – 20	+ 13
20 – 30	− 38
30 – 40	− 27
> 40	− 62

Conclusions

The Camino 110-4G fibro-optic intracranial transducer is a safe method of recording intracranial pressure from the subdural space and appears superior to the frequently used method of inserting a fluid filled catheter into the subdural space. The previously described problems of fluid-filled catheter measurements from the subdural space have been confirmed. The Camino 110-4G placed subdurally appears to show a good correlation with pressure measurements from the ventricles. Further comparisons with intraventricular catheters would be needed to determine the reliability and accuracy of the Camino 110-4G.

References

Allan MWB, Gray WM, Asbury AJ (1988) Measurement of arterial pressure using catheter transducer systems. Improvement using the Accudynamic. Br J Anaesth 60:413–418
Mendelow AD, Rowan JO, Murray L et al. (1983) A clinical comparison of subdural screw pressure measurements with ventricular pressure. J Neurosurg 58:45–50

Clinical Experience with a Fiber Optic Brain Parenchymal Pressure Monitor

T.G. Luerssen [1,2], P.F. Shields [1], H.R. Vos [3], and L.F. Marshall [1]

Division of Neurosurgery [1], Department of Pediatrics [2], Neurosurgical Intensive Care Unit [3], UCSD Medical Center, San Diego, California (USA)

Introduction

Many devices have been developed for the clinical monitoring of intracranial pressure (ICP). Each system has its advantages, and each device has its limitations and complications. In 1985, we participated in the development of a system which can accurately measure ICP from several intracranial sites, including the brain parenchyma. Initial laboratory evaluations of the accuracy of this system, along with the results of an initial clinical trial, have now been reported (Ostrup et al. 1987). After this trial, we began using this device routinely and have accumulated over three years of further experience using this system in a variety of clinical situations.

Characteristics of the Monitor

This device utilizes a disposable four french catheter with a tip transducer that was initially developed for intravascular pressure measurements. It contains one sending and one receiving optical fiber and is entirely electronic and, therefore, completely closed to fluid or air. The technical information about this device is provided in Table 1*.

After initial laboratory experimentation indicated that ICP could be measured accurately, a housing device was developed for the catheter that is 3.5 mm in diameter at the point of insertion. This device is screwed into the skull and the probe is passed through it and secured in position by a compression ring mechanism. A sterile sheath covers these connections. The entire apparatus is shown as Fig. 1.

To insert the monitor, a small stab wound is made over the selected area of the cranium after sterile preparation of the skin. A 2.7 mm drill hole is made through the cranial bone. The housing device is secured and the dura is perforated with a stilette. The probe is then zeroed to atmosphere and inserted directly into the brain parenchyma. The compression ring is tightened, and the sterile sheath is secured.

---

* The Camino 420 OLM Intracranial Pressure System. Camino Laboratories, 5955 Pacific Center Blvd., San Diego, California, 92121 (USA).

Intracranial Pressure VII
Eds.: J.T. Hoff and A.L. Betz
© Springer-Verlag Berlin Heidelberg 1989

Table 1. Summary of technical information for the brain parenchymal pressure monitor

Catheter size	4 French
Frequency response of system	$-3\,\text{dB}$ @ 33 Hz
Pressure range	-10 to 250 mm Hg
Zero drift	≤ 3 mm Hg per 24 h
Temperature coefficient	≤ 3 mm Hg over temperature range of 22 °C – 38 °C
Linearity/Hysteresis	
-10 to 50 mm Hg	± 2 mm Hg or better
51–200 mm Hg	$\pm 6\%$ of reading or better
Reference pressure	Atmosphere
Overpressure	-700 to 1250 mm Hg

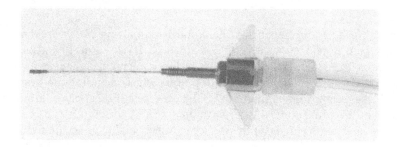

Fig. 1. The fiberoptic pressure monitor described in the text. The transducer tipped catheter is 4 French in diameter. The housing device is 3.5 mm in diameter at point of insertion into skull. The probe is secured by compression ring and covered by an additional sterile sheath

Results

Prior laboratory and clinical testing of this device had indicated that the intraparenchymal pressures obtained by the fiber optic monitor correlated extremely well with those pressures concurrently obtained by a well functioning ventricular cannula (Ostrup et al. 1987; Hollingsworth-Fridlund et al. 1988). Furthermore, the intraparenchymal pressures obtained were seen to be 2–5 mm Hg higher than simultaneously obtained ventricular fluid pressures. These pressure differences were not significant. Over the course of the past three years this monitor has been used in over 150 adult and 50 pediatric patients. It has been used either as an additional monitor of intracranial pressure in patients who are undergoing continuous ventricular drainage, or as the only monitor of intracranial pressure for patients whose ventricles cannot be cannulated or where measurements of intracranial pressure using ventricular cannulas is unwarranted or contraindicated.

No complications of placement or extended use have been observed to date. There have been no cases of intracerebral hemorrhage, although placement of this device is avoided in patients with a known bleeding diathesis. There have been no infections directly attributable to this device, even during extended placement. The longest period of continuous monitoring has been sixteen days.

Early in this series there were problems related to catheter breakage which required the placement of a new monitor. As physician and nursing experience was gained, accompanied by the company's development of more durable optical fibers, breakage now rarely occurs. The laboratory and clinical testing of this monitor demonstrated the tendency of the ICP monitor to drift, and drift has been noted consistently throughout this clinical series. It has always been upward in direction but has never exceeded 2 mm Hg per day.

Discussion

Despite the various devices available for the clinical monitoring of intracranial pressure, we continue to favor the ventricular catheter as the preferable monitor for the management of traumatic brain injury because it is a simple and accurate means of measuring intracranial pressure and adds the therapeutic avenue of CSF drainage as well. For most other situations, and as an adjunct to a ventricular catheter that is requiring frequent drainage, or when there is a question of malfunction, we have used this fiber optic probe placed directly into the brain parenchyma. It has proved to be a safe reliable means of measuring intracranial pressure.

This device seems ideally suited for use in the pediatric age group. Its small size and ease of insertion are a major advantage. The housing device can be secured even in a very thin skull. For infants, we have been able to pass the probe through a needle placed through the suture and simply secure the probe to the scalp.

References

Hollingsworth-Fridlund P, Vos H, Daily EK (1988) Use of fiberoptic pressure transducer for intracranial pressure measurements: A preliminary report. Heart Lung 17:111–120
Ostrup RC, Luerssen TG, Marshall LF, Zornow MH (1987) Continuous monitoring of intracranial pressure with a miniturized fiberoptic device. J Neurosurg 67:206–209

Test of a Non-invasive PVI Measure with a Fiber-optic Pressure Monitoring Device in Head Injured Patients

A. Wachi and A. Marmarou

Richard Reynolds Neurosurgical Research Laboratories, Division of Neurosurgery,
Medical College of Virginia, Richmond, Virginia 23298 (USA)

Introduction

Measurement of brain compliance has proven a valuable tool for understanding the biomechanics of intracranial pressure. More recently, we have shown that the pressure volume index, assessed within 24 h of injury, is a prognostic value in identifying those patients who subsequently develop raised intracranial pressure (Maset et al. 1987). However, methods for determining the pressure volume status in head injured patients, must be obtained via analysis of the pressure response to bolus injections or the removal of CSF through ventricular catheter systems. There are practical restrictions on the number of times PVI can be measured using these volume manipulation techniques. The concept, introduced by Bray at the Glasgow meeting, of extracting PVI measurements from analysis of the pulse pressure centroid, represents a less invasive technique and has the potential for providing PVI data continuously (Bray et al. 1986).

The objectives of this study were to confirm whether the centroid of the frequency power spectrum of ICP waves reflects brain compliance as assessed by manual techniques and to compare if VFP or tissue pressure (TP) could be used as a pressure source for this analysis.

Methods

We evaluated these comparative measures in 16 head injured patients admitted to the neurosurgical ICU. All patients had a ventricular catheter in place and 10 patients had a fiberoptic pressure sensing unit inserted. Six of the fiberoptic devices were positioned in the subarachnoid space, as determined by skull film, and four were positioned in brain tissue. The pressure volume index, obtained either by bolus injection or CSF removal, was considered the reference. We alternated routing the ventricular waveform and the fiberoptic (Camino Model 110-4B) waveform into the automated PVI system (Neurotrak, Neuro International Inc.) in order to compare the system operation with the two different pressure sources.

Results

Early in our studies, our bedside monitoring equipment had built-in digital filters with a bandwith of 8 Hz. This filter cutoff was inserted in the bedside monitor. It was necessary for the manufacturer to modify the equipment to extend the bandwidth to 15 Hz. With the appropriate bandwidth, the correlation between the centroid of the power spectrum and bolus PVI in all patients was statistically significant (34 studies, $r = 0.77$, $p < .01$). However, when pressure gradients between VFP and fiberoptic device exceeded 10% of baseline, the PVI and the centroid relationship was poor. When the data was grouped to select those cases when pressures were equal or gradients were less than 10%, correlation between the manual PVI and the centroid improved ($r = 0.77$, $p < .01$); Table 1.

Table 1. Linear regression of the centroid to manual PVI

Groups	Number	Correlation coefficient	Equation
All cases	34	0.77**	$PVI = -6.1\,C + 66.7$
with VFP	17	0.69**	$PVI = -6.2\,C + 68.0$
with FOD	17	0.79**	$PVI = -6.0\,C + 66.1$
ICP < 15 mm Hg	16	0.61*	$PVI = -4.4\,C + 53.1$
ICP > 15 mm Hg	18	0.87**	$PVI = -7.3\,C + 76.9$

FOD = fiberoptic device; C = the centroid (Hz); $* = p < 0.05$; $** = p < 0.01$.

Comparison of VFP and TP as pressure sources indicated that automated PVI using the tissue transducer correlated well ($r = 0.79$, $p < .01$). A linear correlation was also observed using ventricular fluid pressure ($r = 0.69$, $p < .05$). We found no significant differences between the regression slopes of PVI vs. centroid using either device.

Summary

Excluding equipment problems, we found that the reliability of automated PVI, using the Camino device as a pressure source, was poor when brain tissue and ventricular fluid pressure differed by more than 10%. However, in the absence of those gradients, either the ventricular fluid pressure or the Camino device could be used as a pressure source for automated PVI. Finally, taking these above factors into consideration, we obtained good correlation of manual PVI and centroid, confirming the earlier findings of Bray et al. In conclusion, our preliminary data show that the automated method of Bray, has potential as a less invasive method for PVI determination. We believe, with further refinement of the computer algorithm to improve the accuracy, that this approach could provide a reliable estimate of PVI continuously and automatically.

Acknowledgements. This research was supported in part by Grants NS-12587 and RO1-NS-19235 from the National Institutes of Health. Additional facilities and support were provided in part by the Richard Roland Reynolds Neurosurgical Research Laboratories.

References

Bray RS, Sherwood AM, Halter JA, Robertson C, Grossman RG (1986) Development of a clinical monitoring system by means of ICP waveform analysis. In: Miller JD, Teasdale GM, Rowan JO (eds) Intracranial Pressure VI. Springer, Berlin Heidelberg New York Tokyo, pp 260–264

Maset AL, Marmarou A, Work JD, Young HF (1987) Pressure-volume index in head injury. J Neurosurg 67:832–840

Differential Intracranial Pressure Recordings in Patients with Dual Ipsilateral Monitors

W.C. Broaddus, G.A. Pendleton, J.B. Delashaw, R.V. Short, N.F. Kassell, M.S. Grady, and J.A. Jane

Department of Neurosurgery, University of Virginia, Charlottesville, Virginia 22908 (USA)

Introduction

Intracranial pressure monitoring is a useful adjunct in the management of head injury patients, patients with spontaneous intracerebal hemorrhage, and post-operative patients at risk for intracranial complications (Narayan et al. 1982; Winn et al. 1977). Diagnostic inferences drawn from ICP-monitoring devices frequently make the assumption that intracranial pressure is uniform throughout contiguous subarachnoid spaces, although the relevant pathology can often be seen on CT or MR imaging to be asymmetrical. On the other hand, considerable experimental work has shown that pressure differentials can occur among any of the subarachnoid or parenchymal compartments of the central nervous system (Langfitt et al. 1964). The clinical importance of differential subarachnoid pressure measurements was pointed out by Weaver et al. (1982), who documented markedly asymmetric pressures between hemispheres in patients with unilateral mass lesions.

We suspected that in addition to bilateral asymmetry of ICP in patients with mass lesions, that pressure differentials might also develop between subarachnoid regions within the same hemicranium. We posed two questions: first, can differential pressures be demonstrated between *dual ipsilateral* ICP monitors, and second, are there clinical correlates of differential pressures, when present? We report here the results of monitoring fifteen patients using dual ipsilateral ICP monitors.

Methods

All patients during a four month period who required emergent placement of an ICP monitor had both frontal and parietal subarachnoid bolts placed (Winn et al. 1977). Both bolts were placed on the side of apparent major pathology seen on admission CT. Our criteria for emergent placement of ICP monitors include: all head injury patients with Glasgow Coma Score (GCS; Teasdale and Jennett 1974)) less than 13; minor head injury patients (GCS 13–15) with disorientation, increasing severe headache, or persistent vomiting; and spontaneous intracerebral hematomas with marked ventricular effacement, or greater than three millimeters midline shift.

Table 1. Summary of admission GCS, outcome, and distribution of CT pathology by patient groups

Patient group	N	Admission GCS		Predominant CT pathology			Outcome	
		Mean	SEM	Parietal	Frontal	Diffuse	Good/ fair	Poor/ expired
All patients	15	7.2	0.8	11	2	2	10	5
Equal ICP	8	9.0*	1.0	6	1	1	7	1
Unequal ICP	7	5.6*	0.9	5	1	1	3	4
Parietal > frontal	5	4.4**	0.7	5	0	0	1	4
Frontal > parietal	2	8.5**	1.1	0	1	1	2	0

* $p = 0.03$ comparing unequal ICP and equal ICP groups by t-test; ** $p = 0.04$ comparing parietal > frontal and frontal > parietal groups.

Patients had continuous ICP monitoring in an intensive care setting, where each bolt apparatus was routinely zeroed and calibrated on an hourly basis. Following this procedure, hourly readings of both ICP values were recorded on a clinical flow sheet. On retrospective analysis, maximal ICP values from the two bolts, and their differences were noted. Differential pressures arising from a single elevated reading from one bolt, or from readings in which one of the monitors exhibited dampening of the pressure tracing were not accepted. Treatment for elevated ICP was based on the higher ICP value, and involved sequential addition of hyperventilation for ICP greater than 15 mm Hg, intravenous mannitol and sedation (when indicated) for ICP greater than 20 mm Hg, and intravenous barbiturates for ICP greater than 40 mm Hg.

CT scans were reviewed to determine the regional distribution of pathologic changes, and were categorized as showing predominantly *frontal,* predominantly *parietal,* or *diffuse* pathology. Functional status of the patients at the time of discharge was also reviewed and graded (Table 1). *Good* outcome implies independence in most or all daily activities, with mild or no cognitive impairment. *Fair* outcome implies moderate functional or cognitive impairment, and *Poor* implies severe impairment, including vegetative state. Three patients expired due to their head injuries.

Results and Discussion

Of fifteen patients studied, thirteen (87%) required ICP monitoring for problems secondary to head injury, and two (13%) after spontaneous intracerebral hemorrhage. Among the head injuries were two acute subdural hematomas and one epidural hematoma which were monitored after surgical evacuation. The group was comprised of nine males and six females. The majority of patients were in the eighteen to thirty year-old range (10 or 15; 67%), with three patients in their seventies (20%), and two of intermediate ages (38 and 43). There were nine patients (60%) in the severe head injury group (GCS 3–8), five (33%) in the moderate group (GCS 9–12), and one in the mild group (GCS 13).

When ICP differences between frontal and parietal bolts were examined, a wide range of pressure differentials was found, with a suggestion of a bimodal distribution. Eight patients exhibited differentials of 7 mm Hg or less (53%), while the remaining seven (47%) had differentials of 10 mm Hg or greater. A minimum differential pressure of 10 mm Hg was thus felt to represent a conservative criterion for establishing the presence of a significant ICP differential within the same hemicranium. Patients meeting this criterion are grouped under the Unequal ICP designation, and the other eight patients comprise the Equal ICP group.

Comparison of other clinical characteristics between these two groups revealed a significant association between unequal ICP values and poorer admission GCS (Table 1). Although a trend toward poorer outcome in the Unequal ICP group was also noted, this did not attain statistical significance (Table 1). The two groups were statistically similar with respect to age and sex distribution, and mechanism of injury (data not shown). When the Unequal ICP group was subdivided into those with greater frontal ICP, and those with greater parietal ICP, the latter group was again noted to be associated with poorer admission GCS (Table 1).

In the Unequal ICP group, the regional distribution of CT pathology correlated well with location of greater pressure (Table 1). Patients with greater parietal pressures had parietally based lesions, and of the two patients with greater frontal pressures, one had bifrontal mixed-density lesions, and the other had diffuse CT pathology. In the Equal ICP group, most patients had parietally based lesions. Of the two that did not, one had frontal and the other diffuse CT pathology.

The reasons for such frequent differential subarachnoid pressures are not yet clear. Compromise of the subarachnoid space over the convexity of the brain seems likely to play a role. The correlation of differential pressures with increased severity of injury further suggests that specific sequelae of parenchymal injury may be involved, such as brain swelling due to edema or to altered vascular autoregulation. Furthermore, such regional elevations in ICP must have consequences with respect to local cerebral perfusion pressure, and thus could play a role in secondary brain injury.

Conclusions

We have found that significant differences in ICP frequently exist between frontal and parietal monitors placed ipsilateral to the major pathology seen on CT. The location of higher pressure is predicted by the region of major pathology, suggesting that placement of single ICP monitors should be guided by findings on admission CT. A correlation between unequal ICP values and poorer admission GCS suggests a role for mechanisms involved in parenchmyal injury in the development of differential pressures.

References

Langfitt TW, Weinstein JD, Kassell NF et al. (1964) Transmission of increased intracranial pressure. II. Within the supratentorial space. J Neurosurg 21:998–1005

Narayan RK, Kishore PRS, Becker DP et al. (1982) Intracranial pressure: to monitor or not to monitor? J Neurosurg 56:650–659

Teasdale G, Jennett B (1974) Assessment of coma and impaired consciousness: A practical scale. Lancet II:81–83

Weaver DD, Winn HR, Jane JA (1982) Differential intracranial pressure in patients with unilateral mass lesions. J Neurosurg 56:660–665

Winn HR, Dacey RG, Jane JA (1977) Intracranial subarachnoid pressure recording: experience with 650 patients. Surg Neurol 8:41–47

A New Fiberoptic Monitoring Device: Development of the Ventricular Bolt

R.S. Bray, R.G. Chodroff, R.K. Narayan, and R.G. Grossman

Department of Neurosurgery, Baylor College of Medicine, 6501 Fannin, Suite A404, Houston, Texas 77030 (USA)

The use of a new FOD (Fiberoptic device) pressure transducer, for recording of intracranial pressure, was evaluated initially in 22 comatose patients over 94 days of recording time and has been in routine use since that time. Fiberoptic technology has allowed the development of a 4 French fiberoptic transducer tipped catheter that can be placed at any location inside the dura for accurate ICP monitoring (Hollingsworth et al. 1988). The FOD was tested in subdural, intraparenchymal and intraventricular locations.

Results show it to be superior to other methods tested. Noise was evaluated by comparative analysis of 24 hour trend recordings. The percentage of ICP waveforms rejected by the computer analysis of waveform validity documented an average noise of the subarachnoid bolt at 40%, in a fluid filled ventriculostomy at 15%, and in the fiberoptic at <2%. Drift from a zero calibrated ventriculostomy was measured each 8 hour shift. The FOD was found most stable with a range of 2 mm Hg and a mean of 0.75. The ventriculostomy showed a range of 11 mm Hg with a mean of 5 and the subarachnoid bolt a range of 17 mm Hg with a mean of 11 (Narayan et al. 1981). The 24 hour trend recordings showed accurate tracking of the FOD to intraventricular pressures. The waveform on the FOD demonstrated increased fidelity with greater detail, and was less prone to patient movement artifact (Fig. 1).

The parenchymal placed FOD did demonstrate transient peaks that exceed the intraventricular fluid pressure. This was noted on rapid peaks in the ICP with up to 12–15 mm Hg higher recordings in the tissue compartments. This has been confirmed in other observations (Ostrup et al. 1981) and indicates the need for further research into compartmental tissue pressures.

As the standard for ICP measurement has remained intraventricular placement, and to facilitate CSF drainage, a kit was developed for FOD intraventricular placement. The kit combines the ease of bolt placement with the clinical advantage of an intraventricular catheter, and the accuracy of the FOD for measurement of ICP.

The bolt was designed to allow self tapping with a pipe thread seal to the skull. The characteristics of the internal diameters of the bolt align the catheter toward the ventricle as it is passed. The ventricular catheter secures with an O-ring, twist lock seal to the bolt, to provide a water tight seal to reduce infection risk. A sterile guard allows repositioning of the ventricular catheter after placement and protects the FOD from accidental breakage. The system allows the simultaneous drainage of CSF and the recording of intraventricular pressure. The FOD calibra-

Eds.: J. T. Hoff and A. L. Betz

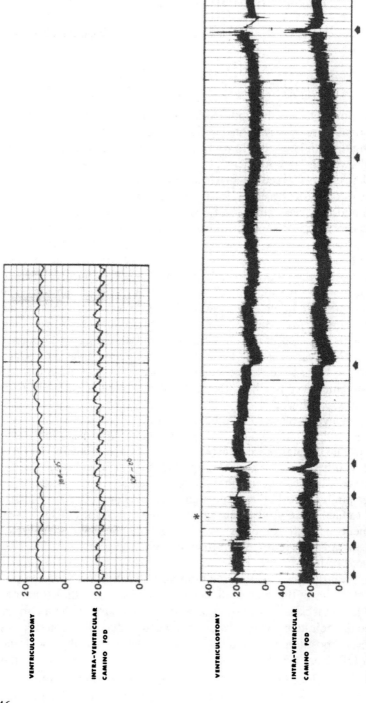

Fig. 1. Strip chart recorder shows increased detail of the FOD trace over the ventriculostomy. 24 hour recording shows tracking with intraventricular fluid pressure, *arrows* denote periods of noise or inaccurate recording on the fluid ventriculostomy

tion can be verified by comparison to the height of the fluid drain column on the marked scale. The kit contains a disposable drill for skull penetration with an adjustable safety depth guard. The components of the kit have gone through many modifications based on clinical use to assure ease of use and reliable function.

Initial problems with the Fiberoptic device included catheter tip corrosion with subsequent malfunction. This has been eliminated by redesign of the metal tip to exclude metals setting up an electric dipole which resulted in salt deposition. Fiber fragility has remained a problem. The protective guards on the new kits reduced fiber fracture. There remains a learning curve for nursing personnel in handling of the FOD. Inservice education has dramatically reduced the breakage rate. The overall acceptance by ICU staff remains very high as the FOD decreases nursing time in dealing with problems or calibration.

The FOD, fiberoptic device, represents an accurate and reliable method for ICP monitoring that exceeds the standards of the other modalities tested. New kits allow rapid bedside placement for intraventricular use.

References

Hollingsworth-Fridlund P, Voss H, Daily EK (1988) Use of fiberoptic pressure transducer for intracranial pressure measurements: A preliminary report. Heart Lung, J Cr Care 17:111 –118

Narayan R, Bray R, Robertson C, Gokaslan Z, Grossman R (1987) Experience with a new fiberoptic device for intracranial pressure monitoring. Presented AANS Dallas, May 3

Ostrup RC, Luerssen TG, Marshall LF (1987) A miniaturized fiberoptic device for continuous monitoring of intracranial pressure. J Neurosurg 67:206–209

Development of a Fully Implantable Epidural Pressure (EDP) Sensor

T. Ohta, H. Miyake, M. Yamashita, S. Tsuzawa, H. Tanabe, L. Sakaguchi, and S. Yokoyama

Department of Neurosurgery, Osaka Medical School, 2–7 Daigaku-echo, Takatsuki City, Osaka 569 (Japan)

Introduction

In order to avoid infection and inconvenience to patients, telemetric measurement of the extradural pressure (EDP) is the ideal method of monitoring intracranial pressure (ICP). We have developed a new telemetric EDP sensor in cooperation with Nagano Keiki Seisakusyo Co., Ltd.

Principle of Measurement and Structure

This is a passive resonant circuit transducer, 13 mm in diameter, 15 mm in height, and about 6 g in weight (Fig. 1). This EDP sensor is reliable and inexpensive, because of a simple counter scale design. The EDP on the pressure disc is transmitted to the ferrite core through a pair of leaf springs. The movement of the ferrite core changes the resonant frequency of the coil in the EDP sensory. Telemetric measurement of this change is done by a grid-dip of an external antenna coil (probe). This probe, 5.2 cm in diameter, is connected to the meter by a fine, flexible cable, 3 mm in diameter. The block diagram of this system is shown in Fig. 2.

Accuracy and Errors of this System

The zero point and sensitivity drifts are the most serious problems of this EDP sensor because this cannot be calibrated after implantation. These drifts have proved negligible for at least three months under a load of 60 mm Hg. Specifications of this system are shown in Table 1. Errors from misapplication are negligible within the 1 cm distance vertically and horizontally, and 15° inclination between the EDP sensor and the probe.

Animal Experiments

In acute experiments, the EDP values obtained by this EDP sensor well correlated with the intraventricular pressure (IVP) values obtained by the Statham P50

Eds.: J. T. Hoff and A. L. Betz

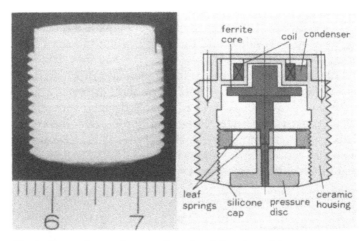

ferrite core — coil — condenser

leaf springs — silicone cap — pressure disc — ceramic housing

Fig. 1. External appearance and sectional drawing of the EDP sensor (measurement in mm)

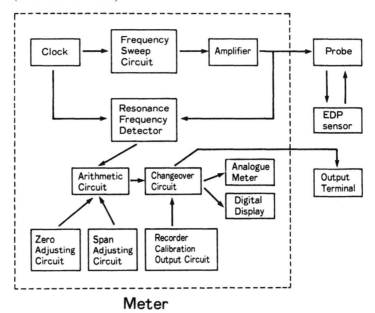

Meter

Fig. 2. Block diagram of this system

Table 1. Specifications of this system

1. Range	$1 \sim 110$ mm Hg
2. Accuracy	within 2% F.S.
3. Temperature coefficient	within 0.2% F.S./10 °C
4. Linearity	within 1% F.S.
5. Hysteresis	within 1% F.S.
6. Repeatability	within 0.5% F.S.
7. Sensitivity	0.1 mm Hg
8. Disinfection	Ethylene oxide gas

transducer. Triphasic pulse waves also could be detected. With low ICP levels, the EDP values were lower than the IVP values. As ICP rose, the EDP values became higher than IVP values and their difference also became wider. Their crossing point was about 10 mm Hg.

In chronic experiments of the implantation for one month, sensitivity drift was negligible in all five sensors. Zero point drift was also negligible except for EDP sensor No. 2. Only this sensor showed a large zero point drift toward minus, which proved to be due to fluid infiltration into the condenser because of a defective ceramic housing. In clinical use, faulty sensors can be identified by running a test for three months in a water bath after assembly. Histologically, a slight foreign body reaction occurred in the underlying dura.

Clinical Application

We have experience with two cases of ruptured cerebral aneurysm in which the EDP sensor was implanted postoperatively. In low ICP levels, the EDP values were nearly equal to the cisternal pressure, of which baseline was set at the level of the patient's external auditory meatus.

EDP recordings were done safely for 35 days and 15 days respectively. Pulse waves could be detected in both cases.

Discussion

Previously developed telemetric EDP sensors are divided into four groups. Generally speaking, EDP sensors of the battery type (Brock et al. 1972) and induction power type (Barbaro et al. 1979; Heppner et al. 1976; Ream et al. 1979; Rylander et al. 1982) have the disadvantages of being large and complicated. The EDP sensors in which the EDP is transmitted by bellows, like that of Rylander (1982) and Gücer (1979), have a high risk of zero point drift due to gas leak, because the bellows must be in a vacuum or filled with known gas in order to avoid thermal drift according to the Boyle-Charles law. The Rotterdam transducer (Jong et al. 1982) detects pressure change by the capacitance change of a condenser. This has a large inherent thermal error. Also the smallness of the pressure disc span increases the mgnidude of the errors. The miniature transensor of Olsen et al. (1967) also has a thermal drift. The pressure-balanced radio-telemetry system of Zervas et al. (1977) can be recalibrated to zero after implantation. This is done by resetting the sensor to the equilibrium state by the cuff between the scalp and the probe, but this maneuver is difficult especially when the scalp is edematous or when there is surgical scar. So, the accuracy of the measurement is questionable. The nuclear intracranial pressure sensory of Meyer et al. (1978) is not suitable for continuous ICP monitoring because of the large extracranial detector (gamma probe) and cannot detect pulse waves. Further investigation is also needed regarding the implantation of radioisotopes in human.

Compared to these sensors, our telemetric EDP sensor has many advantages as follows: (1) There is no zero point drift due to gas leak, because a leaf spring is used instead of bellows. (2) The pressure disc and ferrite core do not tilt because of paired leaf springs. A lateralized force on the pressure disc can be avoided. (3) There is no complicated system for atmospheric correction because of no vacuum space. (4) Pulse waves can be detected by sampling 50 times per second. (5) Thermal and chronological drifts are negligible. (6) The implantation is easy and constant. (7) The measurement is easy by applying the probe to the scalp, and the inconvenience to patients is slight.

Conclusion

This EDP sensor is safe and accurate enough to be used clinically. We will continue our clinical investigations, and we hope to make it possible to measure the intracranial compliance.

References

Barbaro V, Macellari V (1979) Intracranial pressure monitoring by means of a passive radio-sonde. Med Biol Eng Comput 17:81–86

Brock M, Difenthaler K (1972) A modified equipment for the continuous telemetric monitoring of epidural or subdural pressure. In: Brock M, Dietz H (eds) Intracranial pressure. Experimental and clinical aspects. Springer-Verlag, Berlin Heidelberg New York, pp 21–26

Gücer G, Viernstein LJ et al. (1979) Clinical evaluation of long-term epidural monitoring of intracranial pressure. Surg Neurol 12:373–377

Heppner F, Lanner G et al. (1976) Telemetry of intracranial pressure. Acta Neurochir (Wien) 33:37–43

Jong de DA, Maas AIR et al. (1982) The Rotterdam teletransducer-A telemetric device for measuring epidural pressure. Biotelemetry Patient Monitg 9:154–165

Meyer GA, Millis RM et al. (1978) Validation of a new technique for measurement of intracranial pressure with a scintillation counter. Neurosurgery 2:35–38

Olsen ER, Colins CC et al. (1967) Intracranial pressure measurement with a miniature passive implanted pressure transensor. Am J Surg 113:727–729

Ream AK, Silverberg GD et al. (1979) Epidural measurement of intracrtanial pressure. Neurosurgery 6:36–43

Rylander HG, Story JL, et al. (1982) Performance of chronically implanted induction-powered oscillator epidural pressure transducers. J Neurosurg 57:642–645

Zervas NT, Cosman ER et al. (1977) A pressure-balanced radiotelemetry system for the measurement of intracranial pressure. A preliminary design report. J Neurosurg 47:888–911

Evaluation of a Fibre-optic System for Monitoring Ventricular Pressure

D.J. Price, P.T. van Hille, and J. Mason

Department of Neurosurgery, Pinderfields Hospital, Wakefield WF1 4DG (UK)

Introduction

Although fluid-filled pressure systems have been widely used for ICP monitoring, we are all aware of their limitations. The search for a perfect system has continued over the last 2 decades.

More sophisticated methods of signal analysis had demanded a higher fidelity waveform with no damping (Price 1987). A fluid-linked external transducer inevitably has some intrinsic errors due to movement artefact and levelling although in ventilated patients these may be reduced to the minimum. When pulse wave analysis is used as a component of a treatment support system (Mason 1987), distortion due to air bubbles or partial obstruction becomes intolerable. We consider that the "perfect" solution to the increasing demands for a high fidelity system is a catheter tip transducer and it also has the advantage of measuring interstitial pressure if required.

Catheter Tip Transducers

Earlier experience with strain gauge transducers mounted at the tip of catheters was disappointing as zero drift was unauditable and incorrectable. Although the signal from these transducers was of excellent quality, the drift prevented their use for periods of more than a few hours (Price 1975). When Gaeltek transducers were introduced, their in-vivo zero capability was heralded with enthusiasm (Roberts et al. 1983; Barlow et al. 1985). Despite this, their fragility in the hands of neurosurgeons not involved in their evaluation has jeopardised their widespread acceptance.

Camino Fibreoptic Device

The more recent development of the Camino Transducer has aroused much interest and, although in vivo calibration is not possible, the manufacturers have claimed the zero drift to be acceptable for long-term monitoring. The disposable

Eds.: J.T. Hoff and A.L. Betz
© Springer-Verlag Berlin Heidelberg 1989

transducer at the end of its catheter has a protected diaphragm and this is illuminated through a fibre-optic pathway. The reflective modifications are transmitted through a second fibre-optic fibre to an Opto-transducer.

Evaluation of a Camino System

Short-term Monitoring

During the course of 20 infusion tests used to help discriminate between hydrocephalus due to atrophy and that due to CSF absorption defect, a Camino catheter was inserted into the ventricle through the same burr hole as the infusion and monitoring catheters. A comparison was then made between the mean ICP derived from the Fibre-optic System with that from an external Gould P60 transducer. Two Camino catheters proved to be faulty. One could not be zeroed before insertion and the other had a fracture of the transmission optic fibre. Each infusion test lasted an average of 1.5 hours and this provided an opportunity to compare the averages of simultaneous 3 second periods every 30 seconds. The external transducer was calibrated for zero and 50 mm Hg hydrostatically every half hour. The linear regressions using an average of 150 data pairs showed slopes from 0.95 to 1.17 and 16 of the 18 were within the 0.95–1.05 range. The off-sets ranged from −0.88 mm to +6.7 mm Hg with 13 of the 18 less than 2.5 mm Hg deviation from zero. The Camino system read higher values in all but 5 of the

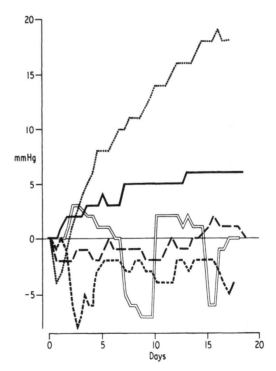

Fig. 1. Over longer periods of time, many of the catheters produced unacceptable drifting

studies. When strip-chart records of the signals were compared, we noted the higher fidelity of the signal transmitted from the Camino system. Its waveform resolution appeared superior and at high pressures, 10 of the 18 studies showed consistently higher pulse wave amplitudes at mean ICPs above 30 mm Hg.

Long-term Monitoring

The same fibre-optic catheters were then tested for longer term stability. Each catheter was immersed in a column of fluid at a constant depth for between 18 and 21 days. The initial pressure was between 20 and 30 mm Hg and any drift up or down was recorded twice daily. For 5 catheters, the drift during the period never exceeded 5 mm Hg but in the others, the pressures varied considerably and, at times, fluctuations were quite erratic. A fair representation of these is shown in Fig. 1.

Conclusion

The Camino fibre-optic system provides a high fidelity ICP waveform with freedom from artefacts. With the increasing availability of computer systems providing either peak to trough or Fourier Transform analysis, this system is superior.

When compared with conventional external transducers, the mean pressures correlated well for short periods of time. Unfortunately, we have found most catheters with unacceptable drifts over periods of several days. Without in-vivo calibration, reliability for long term monitoring is poor.

References

Barlow P, Mendelow AD, Lawrence AE, Barlow M, Rowan JO (1985) Clinical evaluation of two methods of subdural pressure monitoring. J Neurosurg 63:578–582
Mason J (1987) Intracranial pressure regulation by feedback. In: Singh MG (ed) Systems and control encylopedia. Pergamon Press, pp 2580–2583
Price DJ (1975) The clinical application and in-vivo calibration of implanted catheter-tip microtransducers in neurosurgical practice. Proceedings of Biocapt, 75. International Conference on Biomedical Transducers, Paris
Price DJ (1987) The use of computers in neurosurgical intensive care. In: Jewkes D (ed) Bailliere's Clinical Anaesthesiology. Bailliere, London
Roberts PA, Fullenwider C, Stevens FA (1983) Experimental and clinical experience with a new solid state intracranial pressure monitor with in vivo zero capability. In: Ishii S, Nagai H, Brock M (eds) Intracranial Pressure V. Springer, Berlin Heidelberg New York, pp 104–105

Clinical Evaluation of a Fiberoptic Device for Measuring PVI

A. Wachi and A. Marmarou

Richard Reynolds Neurosurgical Research Laboratories, Division of Neurosurgery,
Medical College of Virginia, Richmond, Virginia 23298 (USA)

Introduction

There is considerable evidence that CSF pressures at equilibrium are equal in magnitude to a pulse throughout the cerebrospinal fluid space (Marmarou et al. 1976). However, there is little data to show if transmission of CSF pressures are evenly distributed throughout the brain tissue. Moreover, if equilibrium is challenged by volume manipulation, it is not clear if the viscoelastic properties of brain are able to prevent uniform pressure gradients. Previous efforts to monitor rapid changes in brain tissue pressure using wick catheters were limited, due to poor frequency response. The purpose of this study was to determine to degree to which brain tissue pressure, as measured by a fiberoptic device (FOD), follows dynamic changes in CSF pressure induced by CSF volume manipulation.

Methods

We compared brain tissue pressure (TP) and ventricular fluid pressure (VFP) in 15 severely head injured patients. All subdural and epidural hematomas were surgically removed prior to this study. The VFP was monitored by a conventional fluid catheter connected to a strain gauge transducer. The FOD (Camino Model 110-4B) was placed 3 cm in brain tissue and the position confirmed by skull films. Both VFP and TP were routed to bedside monitors which in turn routed ICP signals to a stripchart recorder. Following stabilization of pressure, a standardized protocol was followed which assessed CSF derived PVI, Ro, and CSF formation at 12 h intervals as described in previous reports. All PVI data were obtained by averaging the pressure response to 3 or 4 bolus injections per study. PVI was computed without a constant term. The VFP pressure reference was established at the level of the external auditory canal and the TP device was zeroed to atmosphere prior to insertion.

Results

The time course of brain tissue pressure in response to CSF volume manipulation followed the CSF pressure response closely. Calculation of the Pressure Volume

Table 1

Pressure source	PVI (ml) (n = 60)	Ro (mm Hg/ml/min) (n = 22)	If (ml/min) (n = 24)
VFP	20.1 ± 5.9	6.9 ± 4.1	0.39 ± 0.15
TP (FOD)	19.8 ± 6.3	6.0 ± 3.8	0.38 ± 0.18

Ro: resistance to outflow of CSF; If: rate of CSF formation, VFP: ventricular fluid pressure; TP: tissue pressure; FOD: fiber-optic device

Index (PVI), resistance to outflow of CSF (Ro), and rate of CSF formation (If) assessed from the VFP and FOD pressure were similar (Table 1). This suggests that the viscoelastic properties of human brain did not alter pressure responses within the dynamic time frame produced by CSF column manipulation. We compared initial pressure and PVI data obtained from TP and VFP in patients with ICP less or greater than 15 mm Hg. We found that the initial pressure (Po) of VFP was slightly higher than TP ($p < 0.05$). We suspect this difference might be due to differences in pulsatile levels. A comparison of ICP waveforms from the two pressure devices indicated that VFP pulsations were greater in amplitude than those measured in tissue by the fiberoptic transducer. Upon closer inspection, the peak pressure of the VFP was greater than FOD by an average of 3.8 mm Hg (VFP 18.7 ± 8.6, FOD 14.9 ± 8.2). The minimum pressure levels were closer and only differed by 1.6 mm Hg (VFP 11.2 ± 6.8, FOD 9.6 ± 7.0). Nevertheless, both peak and minimum pressure levels were statistically different ($p < .01$).

Discussion

These studies showed that the relatively slow dynamic changes of VFP induced by bolus addition or removal of CSF volume are transmitted equally to the brain tissue. Calculation of PVI, Ro, and CSF formation from brain tissue pressure responses are similar to those from CSF pressure responses. This indicates that, although brain tissue exhibits viscoelastic properties, the characteristics are such that the dynamic pressure changes in tissue are not different from those measured in the CSF space. However, pulsatile transmission from the ventricle to the brain tissue surface does not appear to be equal. These data suggest there is a small but significant gradient from the ventricle radiating outward to the cortical tissue (on the order of 2.5 mm Hg). The existence of this outward gradient depends greatly on the reliability of the fiberoptic device to reproduce brain tissue pressure with no damping at the sensing surface.

In summary, simultaneous measurement of VFP and TP in brain injured patients shows that CSF pressure changes produced by volume manipulation are transmitted evenly throughout the brain tissue. However, brain tissue pressure pulsations, as measured by the FOD, are attenuated suggesting that an outward pressure gradient from ventricle to cortex of approximately 2.5 mm Hg exists. Further study is necessary to determine if the gradient is caused by a damping effect of the transducer element when positioned in brain tissue.

Acknowledgements. This research was supported in part by Grants NS-12587 and RO1-NS-19235 from the National Institutes of Health. Additional facilities and support were provided in part by the Richard Roland Reynolds Neurosurgical Research Laboratories.

Reference

Marmarou A, Shulman K, Shapiro K, Poll W (1976) The time course of brain tissue pressure and local CBF in vasogenic odema. In: Pappius HM, Feindel W (eds) Brain edema. Springer, Berlin Heidelberg New York, pp 113–121

Microprocessor-driven ICP Fiber Optic Monitor

A. Martinez-Coll, M. Dujovny, C. Wasserman, and A. Perlin

Henry Ford Neurosurgical Institute, 2799 West Grand Boulevard, Detroit, Michigan 48202 (USA)

Introduction

A study was designed to test the performance characteristics of an intracranial pressure (ICP) monitor composed of a Fiber Optic Transducer (FOT). The evaluation protocol was divided into two portions: in vitro and in vivo. Frequency response, time constant and other instrument specifications data were determined by the in vitro data. The response time, accuracy, and time needed to return to baseline pressure following pulse changes were evaluated in the in vivo portion of the experiment.

Materials and Methods

The FOT monitor is a microprocessor-driven non-electrical sensor. A source in the monitor sends light down the optic fiber which terminates in an Elgiloy sensing membrane tip. This membrane, when perpendicular to the fiber (zero pressure) reflects the same amount of incoming light. The existence of pressure causes the membrane to be deflected and; therefore, the amount of light reflected to be different from that emitted. The amount of light reflected is then passed onto photosensitive cells which in turn pass the information to the microprocessor. The program in the microprocessor calculates the existing pressure and it is displayed numerically (Perlin et al. 1988). An "OUTPUT" jack allows for connection to an oscilloscope or physiograph in order to view the characteristic ICP waveforms (Fig. 1).

In Vitro Model. On a sealed acrylic skull filled with water, two pressure monitors were placed on the frontal region. A pulsative pump was connected to the skull to allow for pulse generation. The two monitors used were: 1-Camino 420 ICP monitor (Camino Laboratories, San Diego, California, USA), and 2-FOT ICP monitor (Metatech Corp., Wheeling, Illinois, USA).

Pulse changes were recorded, compared, and analyzed. A total of ten runs of the experiment were obtained.

In Vivo Model. The in vivo portion of the evaluation involved the development of a canine model. ICP was varied in the dog via the use of drugs (mannitol,

Eds.: J. T. Hoff and A. L. Betz

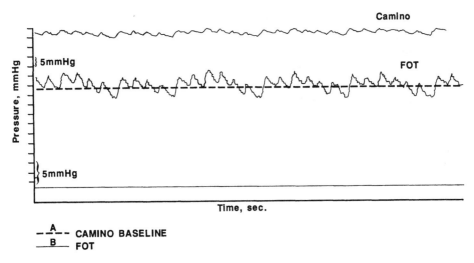

Pressure, mmHg

5mmHg

FOT

5mmHg

Time, sec.

- - A - - CAMINO BASELINE
___ B ___ FOT

Fig. 1. Characteristic ICP waveforms of the Camino monitor (*A*) and the FOT monitor (*B*)

thiopental), hyperventilation, and global cerebral ischemia. These affected the animal's ICP, with the changes monitored by the two systems simultaneously.

Results

Under general anesthesia physiological conditions which increased or decreased ICP were simulated and the results (total of nine dogs) subjected to repeated measures analysis of variance (Morrison 1976). Fifty random readings were tested in each of ten sets of data (in vitro), and for each of the nine dogs (in vivo). Means $\pm$ SD are presented for the two fiber optic monitors:

In vitro:
Camino = 31.8 mm Hg $\pm$ 2.9
FOT   = 25.6 mm Hg $\pm$ 3.1

In vivo:
Camino = 26.8 mm Hg $\pm$ 8.79
FOT   = 26.2 mm Hg $\pm$ 8.68

The statistical analysis concluded that the difference in behavior between the two fiber optic monitors over time was not significant (p 0.41). Also a difference between the 50 levels of time was not significant (p 0.08).

Discussion

The FOT monitor offers several advantages over the Camino monitor. These include: flat transducer (does not become obstructed with tissue), quick, accurate display of changes in ICP (either in mm Hg or mm H_2O), more flexible, less fragile transducer fiber, self-calibration every hour, "last 25-hours of ICP monitoring" memory bank, monitor automatically switches to "battery operation" in case of AC outlet failure.

As shown by the in vivo data (in vitro data is a little different since the FOT's sensitivity had not been assessed) the two monitors perform quite similarly. Of special interest is the fact that the Camino monitor did not seem to have good wave reproducibility at low pressures. Calibration procedures were the same for both monitors (column of water), as well as the amplification settings on the physiograph. Therefore, we conclude that the FOT is more sensitive than the Camino at low pressures. An appreciable advantage of the FOT is the tip of the instrument. By making the transducers flat, the life of these is increased while the possibility for higher than normal readings is decreased.

References

Morrison DF (1976) Multivaried statistical methods, 2nd ed. McGraw-Hill, New York
Perlin A et al. (1988) Microprocessor-driven ICP monitor: Instrumentation. Proceedings: Seventh International Symposium on Intracranial Pressure and Brain Injury. Ann Arbor, Michigan

Microprocessor-driven ICP Monitor: Instrumentation

A. Perlin, M. Dujovny, A. Martinez-Coll, and J.I. Ausman

Henry Ford Neurosurgical Institute, 2799 West Grand Boulevard, Detroit, Michigan 48202 (USA)

Introduction

The Fiber Optic Transducer (FOT) ICP monitor is an electrically safe microprocessor driven system which employs a non-electrical pressure sensor. It monitors ICP in a range of -6 to 250 mm Hg, with a frequency response of 100 Hz or higher. The FOT device is based on a breakthrough in fiberoptic technology which allows information to be transmitted through a single optical fiber of about 50 μm in diameter. The sensing unit, which gives a direct readout of pressure, can be made small enough to pass through a 17 gauge needle (1.5 mm diameter).

Instrumentation

The pressure transducer consists of a single optical fiber which has, at one end, a transducer head containing an Elgiloy membrane with a mirrored surface. This membrane deflects as pressure is applied to it. A source at the other end of the fiber sends light towards the tip. When the light reaches the mirrored surface it is reflected back towards the monitor. If the Elgiloy membrane is perpendicular to the emitted light, then it reflects the same amount of light and the pressure is zero.

The Elgiloy membrane's deflection is a function of the pressure applied to it. This deflection changes the amount of light reflected up the optical fiber (Fig. 1). Photosensitive cells inside the monitor measure the change in reflected light. This information is then passed to the microprocessor which correlates the amount of reflected light into pressure.

The microprocessor is an 8 bit device, such as the Intel 8051 with a 10 bit A/D converter with multiplexer. This device accommodates two analog inputs one from the FOT and one from a Standard Pressure Transducer (SPT). The output from the microprocessor (0–5 V) is handled by a 10 bit D/A converter. OFFSET is adjusted to zero voltage, while the GAIN is set to proximity of maximum voltage (5 volts).

The monitor offers a continuous numerical display of ICP. The small size of the optic fiber allows for a variety of ICP recording sites: intraventricular, epidurally, subarachnoid, and intraparenchymally.

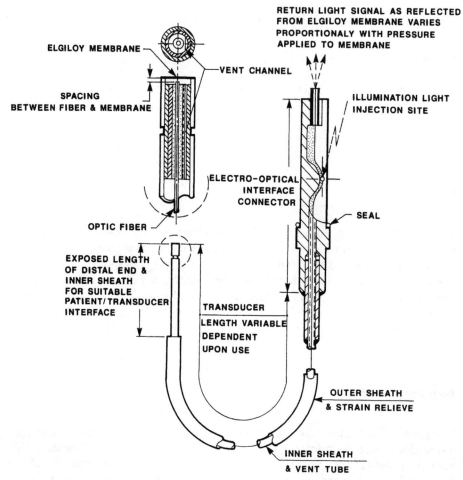

Fig. 1. Schematic diagram showing principle of operation of the FOT-ICP monitor

Specifications

Driving Unit:	Microprocessor-driven.
Transducer Type:	Fiber optic distal-end sensor: single glass fiber inside vinyl tubing, no electrical contact with patient.
Transducer Diameter:	2.5 mm
Transducer Length:	0.3 mm
In vivo Duration:	15 days
Glass Fiber:	50 μm diameter
Frequency Response:	100 Hz
Accuracy:	± 1 mm Hg
Sensitivity:	TBD
Over Pressure:	-700 to $+1500$ mm Hg

Reference Pressure:	Atmospheric
Linearity and Hysteresis:	TBD
Zero Drift (Temp);	TBD
Operating Temp:	20 °C to 45 °C

Advantages

The FOT (Metatech Corp., Wheeling, Illinois, USA) has proven to be reliable, fast, and accurate. One of the most important aspects of biomedical instrumentation is the electrical safety of the device. The FOT is extremely safe since there are no electrical connections to the body. Another feature which makes the FOT very appealing is its self-calibrating capabilities, along with a "last 25-hour of monitoring" memory bank. An important consideration to the buyer is the life time of the product. The FOT transducers are very flexible and durable. A numerical display of ICP in either mm Hg or mm H_2O is available along with an OUTPUT jack to an external unit for wave reproduction.

Comparison of Intracranial Pressure Transducers

A.P. Rosiello, E.L. McCleary, and P.R. Cooper

Department of Neurosurgery, Boston University, 720 Harrison Ave., Suite 710, Boston, Massachusets 02118 (USA)

Initial experience with intracranial pressure depended on a catheter which was volume-coupled to an external strain gauge transducer. Lundberg (1960), Lundberg et al. (1965) demonstrated the safety and efficacy of intraventricular catheters. Vries et al. (1973) subsequently devised a skull bolt which communicated with the subarachnoid space. Both systems required free communication with an intracranial fluid space, and failure of the recording system was associated with obliteration of these fluid spaces or obstruction of the catheters. Volume-coupled systems were also limited by noise due to movement of the fluid path and difficulties in maintaining consistent calibration. The frequency response of volume-coupled systems is also poor, restricting its use with certain mathematical techniques. A technique utilizing cotton wicks for measuring brain tissue pressure has also been described (Marmarou et al. 1975), but this method was the least reliable of all volume-coupled approaches.

Technical improvements leading to decreased transducer size allowed direct placement of electrical strain gauge transducers on intracranial catheters (McCleary and Cooper 1983). However, catheter size, price, and fragility limited widespread use. Catheter tip transducers must be calibrated before insertion. Those catheters that connect directly to standard hospital pressure amplifiers cannot be reliably recalibrated if the patient is moved to another location and/or pressure amplifier.

Fiber-optic technology was initially employed in an epidural monitor utilizing its own amplifier. A numeric display of ICP was presented, but lack of an analog waveform display prevented visual assessment of the catheter's reliability. The new disposable fiber-optic catheter tip transducer has resolved many of the previous limitations. Its small size allows great flexibility in insertion and site of placement. Both fluid and tissue pressures are reliably measured with the same catheter. Although the catheter can be easily damaged, it is designed and priced for use in a single patient. The catheter requires a dedicated microprocessor amplifier which provides a numeric display, but the microprocessor amplifier can also be connected to a standard pressure amplifier for presentation of the ICP waveform. Calibration requires only the catheter and microprocessor amplifier, and is maintained by the catheter's own integral microprocessor. Therefore, monitoring is not compromised by a change in amplifier or patient location.

Over a period of four years, 14 patients have been monitored with ventricular catheters, subarachnoid bolts, electrical catheter tip transducers, and fiber-optic catheter tip transducers. ICP is best registered by catheter tip transducers. When they are functioning well, there is no significant difference between electrical and fiber-optic designs. Volume-coupled devices are the least expensive, least reliable, and most sensitive to noise.

References

Lundberg N (1960) Continuous recording and control of ventricular fluid pressure in neurosurgical practice. Acta Psychiatr Neurol Scand (Suppl 149) 36:1–193

Lundberg N, Troupp H, Lorin H (1965) Continuous recording of the ventricular fluid pressure in patients with severe acute traumatic brain injury. A preliminary report. J Neurosurg 22:581–590

Marmarou A, Shulman K, Erlich S (1975) An evaluation of static and dynamic properties of tissue pressure catheters. In: Lundberg N, Ponten U, Brock M (eds) Intracranial Pressure II. Springer, Berlin Heidelberg New York, pp 211–214

McCleary EL, Cooper PR (1983) Characteristics of a new ICP monitoring device. In: Ishii S, Nagai H, Brock M (eds) Intracranial Pressure V. Springer, Berlin Heidelberg New York, pp 122–123

Vries JK, Becker DP, Young HF (1973) A subarachnoid screw for monitoring intracranial pressure. Technical note. J Neurosurg 39:416–419

Intraparenchymal Brain Pressure – Clinical Evaluation

T. Bergenheim, E. Bålfors, and L. Rabow

Departments of Neurosurgery and Anesthesiology, Umeå University Hospital, Umeå (Sweden)

ICP-monitoring by means of an intraventricular indwelling catheter was introduced for routine clinical work by Lundberg (1960). This technique seems to have comparatively few complications, as shown by Sundbärg (1988) and it is still the "gold standard" with which other methods are compared.

In head injury cases, with collapsed or severely shifted ventricles, the IVC-technique has, however, some obvious drawbacks. For this reason, other methods to measure ICP have been developed, e.g. devices for subdural or extradural pressure monitoring (Sundbärg et al. 1985).

Materials and Methods

Intraparenchymal cerebral pressure was measured with a fiberoptic probe (Camino 420 OLM intracranial pressure system) in a series of 12 consecutive patients with severe head injury, i.e. not reacting to verbal stimuli and with their eyes continuously closed. (Glasgow coma score 8 or less.) All patients had a CT-scan carried out and any localized mass evacuated before starting ICP-monitoring. The probe with the pressure transducer was introduced 1.5 cm into the parenchyma through a burr hole with a diameter of 2.7 mm after the dura had been opened with diathermy. Calibration was carried out before insertion of the probe and checked after its removal, when possible. The probe was usually placed in the nondominant frontal lobe, but in some cases with a strictly left-sided lesion, it was inserted on that side. We tried not to keep the probe in place for more than 7 days. The tip of the probe was sent for bacterial culturing after its removal in 6 cases.

All patients were treated, according to a protocol, to keep ICP below 20 mm Hg. It included: 1. slightly elevating the head end of bed. 2. maintaining unobstructed venous outflow from the head. 3. artificial hyperventilation to $PaCO_2$ 3.5–4.2 kPa, and maintaining $PaO_2 > 10$ kPa. If ICP stayed at a level of > 20 mm Hg for fifteen minutes, Mannitol, 0.5 g/kg bodyweight, was administered and a control CT-scan was performed to exclude a mass or hydrocephalus. If these measures did not lower ICP, barbiturate treatment was instituted with a bolus dose of 3–5 mg/kg bodyweight of Thiopental and continuous infusion of 2–5 mg/kg/hr for 2–3 days. The dose was then tapered off over two days. Serum levels were checked once a day. Arterial blood pressure was monitored and inotropic drugs used when needed.

Table 1

Pat. no.	Age	Diagnosis	Operation	Monitoring duration (days)	Maximal pressure (mm Hg)	>20 mm Hg (hours)	>25 mm Hg (hours)	>30 mm Hg (hours)	Pharmacol. treatment duration days	Early outcome, GCS
1	16	Subdural hematoma Contusion	Craniotomy	8	23	3	–	–	Mannitol 5	14
2	76	Contusion	–	2	24	1	–	–	–	14
3	28	Contusion	–	6	42	11	4	0.5	Mannitol 5 Thiopental 9	15
4	15	Subdural hematoma Contusion	Craniotomy	11	40	25	0.5	–	Mannitol 3 Thiopental 6	15
5	19	Contusion	–	5	36	5	4	0.5	Mannitol 4	15
6	20	Contusion	–	1	19	–	–	–	Mannitol 1	15
7	6	Contusion Fracture	Craniotomy	4	33	8	2	–	Mannitol 2 Thiopental 5	15
8	39	Epidural hematoma Contusion	Craniotomy	10	35	12	4	0.5	Mannitol 2	15
9	61	Subdural hematoma Intracerebral hematoma	Craniotomy	14	60	139	58	22	Mannitol 4 Thiopental 4	11
10	21	Contusion	–	10	37	11	6	2	Mannitol 7 Thiopental 6	14
11	14	Contusion	–	6	26	6	0.5	–	Mannitol 5 Thiopental 5	14
12	28	Subdural hematoma Contusion	Craniotomy	11	33	20	4	0.5	Mannitol 3 Thiopental 5	11 (aphasic)

Results

The pressure transducer seemed to give accurate information on ICP, as judged from the effects of treatment and handling of the patients. Mean monitoring time was 7.3 days (range 1–14 days). The function was good over the whole monitoring period in all patients, although the probe did inadvertently fall out in one patient. Breakage or kinking occurred in 3 cases. In these patients as well as in the one where the probe fell out, a new one was installed. The zero drift was between 0 and 2 mm Hg (after 14 days). There were no mortalities in this series. When discharged, the patients' status was improved (Table 1). It is still too early to determine their final outcome.

There was no bacterial growth in the 6 probe tips sent for culture and no signs of infection from the probe in any of the patients. There were no hematomata or other complications referable to the pressure transducer in this series.

Discussion

Although this series is small, it can be concluded that the fiberoptic pressure device is reliable over a clinically relevant period, and that the information it gives about intraparenchymal pressure seems accurate. Two patients who showed a late rise of ICP turned out to have a progress of an intracerebral hematoma and a subacute subdural hematoma respectively. The ICP returned to acceptable levels after surgery in both cases. It has been shown earlier (Ostrup et al. 1987) that intraparenchymal pressure correlates well with ventricular pressure.

So far this technique appears safe, since there have been no complications attributable to the probe or its use. The main disadvantage is, of course, that the intraparenchymal probe does not give access to the CSF for pressure reduction or biochemical analysis. At the same time, the risk of infection is probably lower than with an intraventricular catheter and some of the problems related to fluid-filled systems are reduced.

References

Lundberg N (1960) Continuous recording and control of ventricular fluid pressure in neurosurgical practice. Munksgaard, Copenhagen

Ostrup RC, Luerssen TG, Marshall LF, Zornow MH (1987) Continuous monitoring of intracranial pressure with a miniaturized fiberoptic device. J Neurosurg 67:206–209

Rabow L (1987) On intracranial pressure monitoring in the treatment of severe head injury. J Clin Monit 3:324–326

Rowan JO, Galbraith SL, Mendelow AD (eds) Intracranial Pressure VI. Springer, Berlin Heidelberg New York Tokyo

Sundbärg G, Messeter K, Nordström C-H, Söderström S (1985) Intracerebral versus intraventricular pressure recording. In: Miller JD, Teasdale GM (eds) Intracranial Pressure VI. Springer, Berlin Heidelberg New York Tokyo, pp 187–192

Sundbärg G (1988) Neurosurgerical intensive care and the management of severe head injuries. Student literature, Lund

Lumbar Pressure Monitoring
with a New Fiberoptic Catheter

H.G. Bolander

Department of Neurosurgery, University Hospital, S-751 85 Uppsala (Sweden)

Introduction

The syndrome of progressive dementia, gait disturbance, hydrocephalus and normal intracranial pressure is usually termed normal-pressure hydrocephalus (NPH). Since the initial reports of good results of shunting cerebrospinal fluid (CSF) in these patients, interest has been aimed at selection of patients for shunting. Continuous pressure recording in the investigation of hydrocephalus has gained increasing attention and especially the occurrence of B-waves can be of interest (Børgesen and Gjerris, 1982). Long-term pressure monitoring has so far been restricted to techniques for intracranial pressure-monitoring, usually involving some minor surgical procedure.

A new fiberoptic catheter with a tip transducer, initially developed by Camino laboratories for intravascular pressure recordings, makes it possible to monitor cerebro-spinal pressure in the spinal canal. This system has been adapted for intracranial pressure monitoring and clinical experience has proved it to be accurate and easy-to-handle (Ostrup et al. 1987).

Technique and Results

The catheter is introduced into the spinal canal through a large-bore needle with an inner diameter permitting the passage of the catheter (outer diameter 1.3 mm) by lumbar puncture. The needle is pointed upwards as much as possible to minimize the angulation needed in entering the spinal canal. After the needle is withdrawn, the catheter is fixed to the skin in smooth curves to avoid breakage of the optic fibers. The part of the catheter not fixed to the skin was protected with an outer plastic tube thread over it (split i.v. line). The patient is restricted to bed rest and kept horizontal during the time of registration. Ten patients with suspected NPH were monitored in this way for 2–70 hours (mean 24 hours). Chart recordings were analyzed by inspection and the mean pressure and patterns of pressure variations were noted. Between 70–100% of the recordings were judged as satisfactory and the occurrence of B-waves could be noted (Fig. 1). Three recordings were terminated prematurely due to breakage of the optic fiber without damage to the outer catheter and one other recording terminated when the patient went out of bed and pulled out the catheter in a disoriented state.

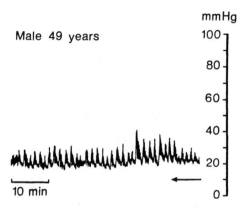

Male 49 years

mmHg

Fig. 1. Part of lumbar pressure recording from a patient with posttraumatic hydrocephalus with elevated resting pressure and B-wave pattern

In 3 patients simultaneous registration of pressure with an external transducer and a second lumbar needle during a lumbar infusion test was possible. Comparison of the registrations showed good linear correlation but deviations up to 4 mmHg was noted. The cause of these deviations are not clear, but there were no systematic deviations that could be explained. In one patient leakage of CSF along the catheter was noted after 40 hours monitoring. No sign of internal leakage of CSF through the dura into the epidural space was found in 4 patients when checked by controlling that pressure level was equal before and after setting the patient upright for 10–15 minutes. No complications occurred during these measurements.

Conclusion

More experience is needed before one could say that this will be a clinically useful technique, but these preliminary results show that it is technically possible to use the fiberoptic catheter to monitor CSF-pressure and warrants further investigations. In the future, one could also hope that newer and thinner catheters will be developed that would make this application even easier.

References

Børgesen SE, Gjerris F (1982) The predictive value of conductance to outflow of CSF in normal pressure hydrocephalus. Brain 105:65–86

Ostrup RC, Luerssen TG, Marshall LF, Zornow MH (1987) Continuous monitoring of intracranial pressure with a miniaturized fiberoptic device. J Neurosurg 67:206–209

Evaluation of Continuous Lumbar Subarachnoid Pressure Monitoring

O. Hirai[1], H. Handa[1], H. Kikuchi[2], M. Ishikawa[2], and Y. Kinuta[2]

[1] Department of Neurosurgery, Hamamatsu Rosai Hospital, 25-Shogencho, Hamamatsu-430 (Japan)
[2] Department of Neurosurgery, Faculty of Medicine, Kyoto University (Japan)

Introduction

Continuous intracranial pressure (ICP) monitoring has been regarded as useful in predicting shunt response in communicating hydrocephalus (Symon and Dorsch 1975). However, burrhole making may be sometimes so uncomfortable for patients for diagnostic purpose only that the lumbar subarachnoid pressure (LSP) was substituted by some authors (Hartmann and Alberti 1977; Ishikawa et al. 1985). This less invasive method without perforating the skull, however, has a problem whether it accurately represents net ICP. In this communication, a combined experimental and clinical study was designed to validate continuous LSP monitoring.

Materials and Methods

Using twelve cats, the LSP was recorded simultaneously with epidural pressure (EDP) during steady state cisternal infusion. A polyethylene catheter of 0.5 mm I.D. was introduced in the lumbar subarachnoid space, which was connected to a transducer referenced to the level of the right atrium. Rapid pressure change by cisternal bolus injection was also determined, and expressed in compliance (Co) using Marmarou's formula (Marmarou et al. 1975). Co was separately calculated from the LSP and the EDP. In three other cats, an epidural balloon was inflated.

Clinical assessment of the LSP was carried out in 54 hydrocephalic patients in terms of selection of candidates for shunt operation. The way of measurement was the same as in animals. Overnight recording was done for 12 to 15 hours, placing patients in the horizontal position.

Results

In steady state infusion, the LSP correlated well with the EDP up to 50 mm Hg. Despite slight underestimation or pressure, the LSP was more than 90% of the EDP at any pressure (Fig. 1 a). Rapid pressure change by bolus injection could

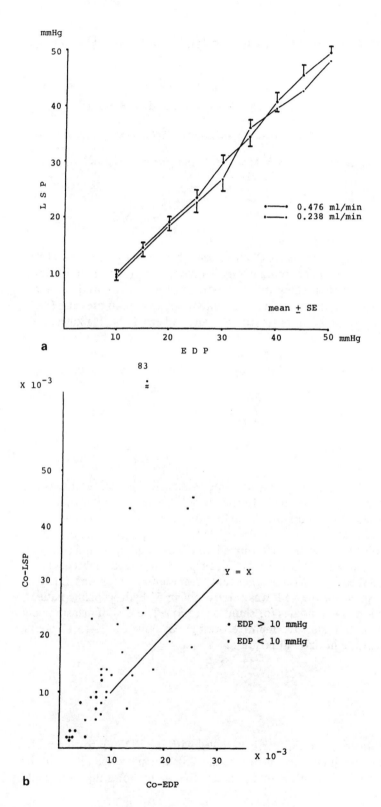

83

72

also be demonstrated in the LSP tracing. Although Co calculated from the LSP was slightly greater than that from the EDP at resting pressure, these values became the same above 10 mm Hg of the EDP (Fig. 1b). However, the LSP was not elevated during epidural balloon inflation.

Shunt operation was effective in 32 patients (group E), ineffective in 8 patients (group N) and 14 cases were not shunted (group NS). Subsequent observation revealed no clinical deterioration in group NS. The mean values of resting and peak pressures were 13.2 and 27.1 mm Hg in group E, 11.8 and 22.6 mm Hg in group N, and 9.1 and 17.6 mm Hg in group NS, respectively. Statistically significant difference was noted between group E and group NS. Complication related to this method was negligible except for a case of meningitis which was easily treated by antibiotics.

Discussion

Although the LSP has been reported to exactly parallel ICP by several authors (Hartmann and Alberti 1977; Lofgren et al. 1973; Marmarou et al. 1975), slight dampening of the pressure can occur under the use of a thin and long spinal tube. In addition, the spinal subarachnoid space plays an important role in compensating an increase of intracranial volume at a relatively lower pressure (Lofgren et al. 1973; Marmarou 1975). Slight underestimation of pressure in the LSP, within clinical permission, may be partly due to this compensatory capacity of the spinal axis. This capacity, however, becomes exhausted even by a small increment of CSF volume (Takizawa et al. 1986). In the present study also, Co values calculated from the cranial and the spinal compartments did not differ from each other above 10 mm Hg, where the resting LSP in hydrocephalic patients was around this range.

Results in hydrocephalic patients substantiated the clinical usefulness of the LSP, especially in eliminating unnecessary shunt. The patients with peak pressure of more than about 25 mm Hg will benefit from shunting. This practical and less invasive method of estimating ICP can be applied in clinical practice, as long as any intracranial mass lesion which can impede CSF circulation with the risk of cerebral herniation is excluded with the aid of a CT scan.

Fig. 1. During steady state cisternal infusion, the LSP correlated well with the EDP, although slight underestimation of the pressure was noted (**a**). Co calculated from the LSP was greater than that from the EDP, at resting pressure, however, these values became almost identical at above 10 mm Hg (**b**)

References

Hartmann A, Alberti E (1977) Differentiation of communicating hydrocephalus and presenile dementia by continuous recordings of cerebrospinal fluid pressure. J Neurol Neurosurg Psychiatry 40:630–640

Ishikawa M, Handa H, Hirai O (1985) CSF pressure changes in case of non-developing normal pressure hydrocephalus after subarachnoid hemorrhage. Jpn J Stroke 7:15–21

Lofgren J, Zwentnow N (1973) Cranial and spinal components of the cerebrospinal fluid pressure-volume curve. Acta Neurol Scand 49:575–585

Marmarou A, Shulman K, LaMorgese J (1975) Compartmental analysis of compliance and outflow resistance of the cerebrospinal fluid system. J Neurosurg 43:332–344

Symon L, Dorsch NWC (1975) Use of long-term intracranial pressure measurement to assess hydrocephalic patients prior to shunt surgery. J Neurosurg 42:258–273

Takizawa H, Gabra-Sanders T, Miller JD (1986) Variations in pressure-volume index and CSF outflow resistance at different locations in the feline craniospinal axis. J Neurosurg 64:298–303

Intracranial Pressure Monitoring After Elective Surgery: A Study of 514 Consecutive Patients

S. Constantini, S. Cotev, Z.H. Rappaport, S. Pomeranz, and M. N. Shalit

ICU and Department of Neurosurgery, Hadassah University Hospital and Hebrew University-Hadassah Medical School, P.O.B 12000, 91120 Jerusalem (Israel)

In this retrospective study we try to resolve the controversy relating to the indications for ICP monitoring after *elective* intracranial surgery (Johnston and Jennett 1973; Kaye and Brownbill 1981; Langfitt 1976; Nakagawa et al. 1975; Narayan et al. 1982, Takagi et al. 1986). We ask the following questions that pertain to benefits and risks of ICP monitoring: Which are the procedures and subpopulations that are most likely to be associated with raised postoperative ICP? What are the sensitivity and specificity of ICP elevations in detecting clinical deterioration? Which are the changes in patient management following ICP elevations? What is the risk of infection associated with ICP monitoring? Based on answers to these questions we attempt to formulate an optimal policy for ICP monitoring after elective surgery.

Material and Methods

Included in the study were 514 consecutive patients who underwent elective intracranial surgery between 1980–1986. ICP was monitored postoperatively via a 5F "feeding" tube left at the end of surgery in the ipsilateral subdural space. It was exteriorized via a separate scalp incision. A purse-string suture was used to tighten the incision when the catheter was pulled out to prevent CSF leakage. After June 1982, a single IV dose of vancomycin (10 mg/kg) and gentamicin (2 mg/kg) was administered to all patients intraoperatively. ICP was continuously monitored postoperatively for an overall mean of 1.3 d (range 1–9 d). All catheter tips were cultured after removal. ICP elevation is defined as >20 mm Hg, sustained for >2 h.

Results

Table 1 lists the intracranial findings with the relative incidence of ICP elevation for each finding. The overall incidence of postoperative ICP elevation was 89/514 (17.3%). There was no statistically significant difference between this incidence after supra- or infratentorial surgery. Surgery for malignant glioma, as compared to the rest of the patients, was associated with significantly ($p < 0.05$) higher

Table 1. Incidence of postoperative ICP elevation in the various histological tumor types

	No.	% of total		No.	% of total
Supratentorial:			*Infratentorial:*		
Meningioma	29/166	17.5	Acoustic neurinoma	4/35	11.4
Glioblastoma M.	28/103	27.2*	Meningioma	1/18	5.6
Low grade astrocytoma	6/28	21.4	Astrocytoma	3/15	20.0
Others	13/115	11.3	Medulloblastoma	1/9	11.1
			Others	4/25	16.0
Total:	76/412	18/4		13/102	12.7

* $p < 0.01$ as compared to the rest of the group.

Table 2. The relationship between ICP elevation and clinical deterioration (CD)

	Supratentor.	Infratentor.	Total	%
No. CD:	35	7	42	47
Associated CD:				
ICP before CD:	18	1	19*	21
CD before ICP:	8	0	8**	9
Simultaneous:	15	5	20	23
Total:	76	13	89	100

* Mean time gap 5.2 ± 4.0 h; ** mean time gap 2.4 ± 1.2 h.

incidence of ICP elevation (27.2% vs. 15.5%, respectively). Two additional, significant ($p < 0.001$) risk factors were identified: Re-do surgery was associated with ICP elevation in 15/35 pts (42,9%), and prolonged (i.e., >6 h) surgery in 20/48 pts (41.7%).

Age of the patients and location of surgery was not associated with increased risk of elevated ICP.

Table 2 shows the relationship between ICP elevation and clinical deterioration in patients in whom ICP was elevated postoperatively. Clinical deterioration was observed in 47/89 pts (53%) with elevated ICP. In 19 pts, elevated ICP preceeded clinical deterioration by a mean of 5.2 ± 4.0 h, while in 8 pts deterioration was noted 2.4 ± 1.2 h before ICP elevation. The higher the ICP elevation peak, the more likely it was to be associated with clinical deterioration.

In 21/514 pts (4.1%), clinically relevant deterioration was not accompanied by ICP elevation. Thus, as many as 30.9% of patients (21/68) deteriorated without ICP elevation.

We recorded response by the treating physicians in 30% of patients who experienced ICP elevations *without* associated changes in neurological status. The response rate, however, was 95% when ICP elevation was associated with neurological manifestations. In all the latter patients, CT scan was performed, and resulted in surgical evacuation of tumor-bed (7 pts), epidural (2 pts) and subdural

76

(1 pt) hematomata, as well as frontal lobectomy, ventriculostomy and V/P shunt, in 1 pt each. Non-surgical treatments included: reintubation, augmented hyperventilation, mannitol and pentothal.

Cranial infection occurred in 6/514 (1.2%) patients. Of these, 4 had isolated wound infection. Meningitis occurred in 2 pts, but in only one of them was the organism identical to that cultured from the catheter-tip.

Discussion

Previous reports on ICP monitoring after elective intracranial surgery failed to define risk factors for the occurrence of intracranial hypertension. Nor did these studies describe the clinical course, or therapeutic modalities used following raised ICP.

In this study we identified several risk factors for the occurrence of postoperative intracranial hypertension. Elevated ICP after glioblastoma surgery is probably related to the invasiveness of the tumor and its tendency, together with surrounding tissues, to swell postoperatively. Repeat and protracted surgery is likely to be associated with difficult excision and hemostasis, as well as prolonged and difficult retraction, with subsequent brain edema and/or residual bleeding.

Postoperative intracranial hypertension was found to be a rather sensitive and specific indicator of neurological deterioration. In 19 patients, elevated ICP preceeded clinical signs of deterioration and enabled timely performance of CT scanning, followed by the appropriate therapeutic modality. Deterioration which was not accompanied by ICP elevation might have been due to either technical failure, or to functional alterations not associated with pressure elevations at the site of ICP measurement (i.e., intracranial pressure gradients).

The risk of infection associated with ICP monitoring in this study was negligible, and may be related to our protocol for ICP monitoring and antibiotic prophylaxis.

Conclusions

ICP measurement after elective surgery is advantageous and is almost risk-free. It is especially indicated when risk factors (i.e., glioblastoma, re-do or protracted surgery) can be identified, but can never replace vigilant clinical monitoring; rather, it complements it. ICP monitoring is especially useful when clinical evaluation is difficult (e.g., residual anaesthetic or sedative effects), and to study the effectiveness of therapeutic modalities. Attention must be drawn, however, to the danger of a false sense of security when ICP measurements are normal.

References

Johnston IH, Jennett B (1973) The place of continuous intracranial pressure monitoring in neurosurgical practice. Acta Neurochir (Wien) 29:53–56

Kaye AH, Brownbill D (1981) Postoperative intracranial pressure in patients operated for cerebral aneurysms following subarachnoid bleeding. J Neurosurg 52:726–732

Langfitt TW (1976) Incidence and importance of intracranial pressure monitoring in head-injured patients. In: Beks JWF, Bosh DA, Brock M (eds) Intracranial Pressure III. Springer, Berlin Heidelberg New York, pp 67–72

Nakagawa Y et al. (1975) Clinical significance of ICP measurement following intracranial surgery. In: Lundberg N, Ponten U, Brock M (eds) Intracranial Pressure II. Springer, Berlin Heidelberg New York, pp 350–354

Narayan PK, Kishore PRS, Becker DP (1982) Intracranial pressure: to monitor or not to monitor? A review of our experience with severe head injury. Neurosurg 56:650–659

Tagaki H et al. (1986) Clinical experience of 780 cases of postoperative ICP monitoring. In: Miller JD, Teasdale GM, Rowan JO, Galbraith SL, Mendelow AD (eds) Intracranial Pressure VI. Springer, Berlin Heidelberg New York Tokyo, pp 695–700

Intracranial Compliance Monitoring with Computerized ICP Waveform Analysis in 55 Comatose Patients

Z.L. Gokaslan, R.K. Narayan, C.S. Robertson, R.S. Bray, C.F. Contant, and R.G. Grossman

Department of Neurosurgery, Baylor College of Medicine, 6501 Fannin, Suite A-404, Houston 77030, Texas (USA)

Introduction

A computerized system that estimated the intracranial compliance (ICC) from an analysis of the frequency content of the intracranial pressure (ICP) waveform has been previously described as a means of monitoring ICC continuously and avoiding the volumetric manipulations of the cerebrospinal fluid (CSF) system (Bray et al. 1976). We have reported earlier that shifts within the frequency range of 4 to 15 Hz were related to changes in the compliance of the brain (Bray et al. 1976). The power weighted mean frequency within this range was defined as the High Frequency Centroid (HFC = C_2 centroid) and was shown to have an excellent inverse relationship to the pressure volume index (PVI). A HFC of 6.5 – 7.0 Hz was normal, and a HFC of 9.0 Hz corresponded to a critical reduction in the PVI to approximately 13 ml (Bray et al. 1976).

The purpose of this study was to evaluate the prognostic value of changes in the HFC and to assess the clinical usefulness of this system as an indicator of impending neurological deterioration.

Material and Methods

Between July 1984 and October 1987, trend recordings of mean ICP and the HFC were obtained in head injured patients who were admitted to the NICU and required ICP monitoring. Trend recordings were begun soon after placement of the ICP monitor (usually within 6 hours) and continued for as long as the monitor was in place.

All patients were treated by a standard protocol that emphasized early surgical evacuation of intracranial hematomas, controlled ventilation, and monitoring of ICP. Routine medications included phenytoin, morphine for sedation, and antibiotics. ICP greater than 20 mm Hg were treated with hyperventilation (pCO_2 25 – 30 mm Hg), CSF drainage, sedation, paralysis, mannitol and, if necessary, barbiturates.

Clinical information, including age, sex, initial Glasgow Coma Score (GCS), type of injury, and Glasgow Outcome Score (GOS) at 3 months post injury were obtained. Detailed information regarding episodes of neurological emergencies were kept for comparison to the trend recordings. A neurological emergency was

defined as either uncontrollable intracranial hyperension without clinical neurological changes, or dilation of one or both pupils.

The mean ± standard deviation of the ICP, HFC and the percent of time that
HFC was ≥ 9.0 Hz were calculated for each patients.

Results

A total of 55 patients, who were comatose on admission or deteriorated to coma,
were studied for an average of 5 days per patient. Coma was defined as an
inability to follow even simple commands after successful cardiopulmonary stabilization.

The majority of the injuries were closed head trauma, including: 12 (22%)
diffuse brain injuries, 4 (7%) epidural hematomas, 17 (31%) subdural hematomas, and 10 (18%) intracerebral hematomas. Twelve (22%) of the patients had
gun shot wounds or other penetrating head injuries. The patients were predominantly male (76%) and young (median age of 30).

The mortality rate was 26%, and 36 (66%) had a poor neurological outcome,
defined as Glasgow Outcome Score of severe disability, persistent vegetative
state, or dead at 3 months post injury. Five patients had a good recovery, and
14 (26%) recovered with moderate disability.

The risk of dying in the first 3 months after a severe head injury was related
to alterations in the HFC. As shown in Fig. 1, the mortality rate increased directly
with the mean HFC, from 7% when the HFC was < 7.5 Hz, to 46% when the
HFC was ≥ 8.5 Hz. The longer the period of time that the HFC was ≥ 9.0 Hz also

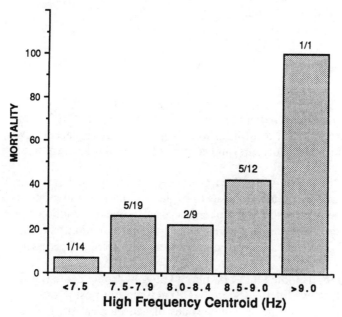

Fig. 1. Mean high frequency centroid (HFC) vs. mortality

increased the mortality rate. If the HFC was never ≥ 9.0 Hz, the mortality rate was 16%. However, if the HFC was ≥ 9.0 Hz for more than 6 hours, the mortality rate increased to 42%, and if the HFC was ≥ 9.0 Hz for more than 12 hours, the mortality rate was 60%.

Quality of neurological recovery also appeared to be related to changes in the HFC. Only 1 of 13 patients (8%) who had a mean HFC ≥ 8.5 Hz, recovered with moderate disability at 3 months post injury: the remainder were severely disabled, in a persistent vegetative state, or dead. Forty-three percent of the patients, who had a mean HFC < 7.5 Hz had a good or moderate recovery at 3 months (Fig. 2). If HFC was never ≥ 9.0 Hz or transiently elevated, 45% of the patients had a good or moderate recovery, while only 2 (17%) of the patients who had the HFC ≥ 9.0 Hz for more than 12 hours, recovered with moderate disability.

Patients with uncomplicated courses typically had HFC that was only moderately elevated (7.5–8.0 Hz), or was elevated above 8.5–9.0 Hz only transiently during the first 24 hours after injury.

A total of 12 patients developed neurosurgical emergencies during the time of trend recordings. When the trend recordings of the ICP and HFC were examined in relation to clinical neurological deterioration, three different patterns were noted, namely, abrupt increase in HFC, gradual increase in HFC and no significant alteration in HFC in association with neurological decompensation. In 4 patients, neurological deterioration was found to be due to an intracranial hematoma by CT scan. In all of these cases, an abrupt increase in HFC preceded the emergency with a mean time interval of 3 hours. Five patients developed neurological emergency due to cerebral edema. In these patients, a gradual increase in HFC over several hours was the typical pattern.

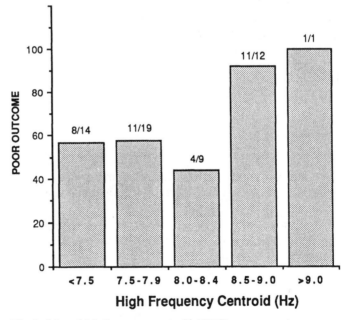

Fig. 2. Mean high frequency centroid (HFC) vs. poor outcome

Three patients developed a neurological emergency due to diffuse swelling, requiring barbiturates to control intracranial hypertension. In all of these cases, the HFC remained 7.5–8.0 Hz before and after the episode of intracranial hypertension. CBF measurements obtained during that time period demonstrated normal or elevated values.

From these observations it has been suggested that an abrupt increase in HFC is usually associated with a surgical intracranial mass lesion. More gradual increase in HFC over several hours is probably indicative of a slowly progressive process such as cerebral edema. Diffuse swelling may be associated with elevated CBF, and in these patients, neurological emergency may occur without a considerable change in HFC.

Discussion

Clinical and experimental studies, using volume pressure response (VPR) or PVI to express ICC, have demonstrated a relationship between reduced compliance and intracranial hypertension. Several investigators studied the temporal relationship between changes in VPR, ICP, and clinical neurological signs during progressive inflation of an epidural balloon (Sullivan et al. 1977; Leech and Miller 1974; Lofgren and Zwetnow 1973). The VPR became abnormal prior to a marked increase in ICP, and at a balloon volume that was approximately 60% of that at which signs of uncal herniation first appeared.

In patients with head injury, a reduced PVI has been an accurate predictor of impending intracranial hypertension (Shapiro et al. 1980; Maset et al. 1987). During the first 24 hours after injury, a PVI of 15–20 ml predicted significant ICP elevations which could usually be controlled with medical treatment. The greater the reduction in PVI below 15 ml, the higher the risk of developing uncontrollable intracranial hypertension (Maset et al. 1987). A change in VPR has been reported to precede clinical signs of a delayed intracranial hematoma (Miller and Pickard 1974).

Conclusions

Decreased compliance estimated by a computerized system from analysis of the frequency content of the ICP waveform is associated with increased mortality and morbidity.

Continuous monitoring of compliance from computerized ICP wave analysis may be used as an early warning system for impending neurological emergencies in head injury patients.

References

Bray RS, Sherwood AM, Halter JA, Robertson C, Grossman RG (1976) Development of a clinical monitoring system by means of ICP waveform analysis. In: Miller JD, Teasdale GM, Rowan JO, Galbraith SL, Mendelow AD (eds) Intracranial Pressure VI. Springer, Berlin Heidelberg New York Tokyo, pp 260–264

Leech P, Miller JD (1974) Intracranial volume–pressure relationships during experimental brain compression in primates. I. Pressure responses to changes in ventricular volume. J Neurol Neurosurg Psychiatry 37:1093–1098

Lofgren J, Zwetnow NN (1973) Influence of a supratentorial expanding mass on intracranial pressure–volume relationships. Acta Neurol Scand 48:599–612

Maset AL, Marmarou A, Ward JD, Choi S, Lutz HA, Brooks D, Moulton RJ, DeSalles A, Muizelaar JP, Turner H, Young HF (1987) Pressure-volume index in head injury. J Neurosurg 67:832–840

Miller JD, Pickard JD (1974) Intracranial volume-pressure studies in patients with head injury. Injury 5:265–269

Shapiro K, Marmarou A, Schulman K (1980) Characterization of clinical CSF dynamics and neurol axis compliance using the pressure-volume index. Ann Neurol 7:508–514

Sullivan HG, Miller JD, Becker DP, Flora RE, Allen GA (1977) The physiological basis of intracranial pressure change with progressive epidural brain compression. J Neurosurg 47:532–539

Software for Neurosurgery Intensive Care

M. Czosnyka [1], D. Wollk-Laniewski [2], P. Darwaj [1], M. Duda [1], L. Batorski [3], and W. Zaworski [1]

Institute of Electronics Fundamentals, Warsaw University of Technology [1],
Department of Anesthesiology and Intensive Care, Child's Health [2],
Clinic of Neurosurgery, Child's Health Centre [3], Warsaw (Poland)

Neurosurgical intensive care and diagnostics have specific needs for the analysis and interpretation of intracranial pressure (ICP) (Gaab et al. 1982). The cost of most monitoring hardware is very high, constituting the most important barrier in popularization of ICP analysis. During the Symposium on Intracranial Hypertension in Clinical Practice (Warsaw 1985), Professor M. Brock presented a solution based on a personal home microcomputer. Our own programs are similar in concept, the software pack is based on at least 5 years of clinical experience using a personal computer (IBM-PC). Advantages of this approach are obvious: to exchange scientific information stored on diskettes, to reduce cost, and to open new propositions and programs. We present programs already prepared at the Warsaw University of Technology and clinically tested in the Child's Health Centre and Warsaw Medical University.

Continuous Neurosurgical Intensive Care Monitoring

This program is designed for intracranial pressure (ICP) monitoring and other signals analysis in intensive care units and neurosurgical departments. It is recommended for prolonged patient monitoring. The program is helpful in monitoring reaction to drugs or $PaCO_2$ reactivity testing. Intracranial Pressure (ICP), Cerebral Perfusion Pressure (CPP), Temperature (Temp) and partial pressure of CO_2 in arterial blood ($PaCO_2$ – end-tidal or transcutaneous) can be measured, registered and analyzed simultaneously. The general concept of the ICP analysis is based upon on-line examination of cerebrospinal compensatory mechanisms.

The linear relationship between the amplitude of the pulse wave of the ICP signal and the mean pressure is of important clinical significance (Marmarou 1976; Chop and Portnoy 1980; Avezaat and Eijndhoven 1984). On the basis of our recent work, we introduced the RAP – the correlation coefficient between the amplitude of the pulse wave and the mean pressure level. This index involved time-dependent amplitude-pressure characteristics. Moreover, it reflects the state of the cerebrospinal space vascular bed – especially in states near the limits of autoregulation reserve.

The ICP signal is processed by a spectral analysis algorithm – all its components can be detected and measured separately (slow, respiratory and pulse waves). The heart rate can be calculated on the basis of the ICP waveform. Hence,

Intracranial Pressure VII
Eds.: J. T. Hoff and A. L. Betz
© Springer-Verlag Berlin Heidelberg 1989

the correlation coefficient between ICP and HR (RHP) can be calculated. It provides information on central responses to pressure level variations such as the early signs of the Cushing reflex.

The regression relationship between a chosen pair of registered trends can also be evaluated graphically. It helps in a better understanding of interdependences between the monitored parameters.

All the monitoring data, including physician notes, are automatically stored on disks, forming a library suitable for reviews or follow-up studies. The program is also protected from power failure.

ICP Analysis in Infusion Tests

This program is designed for ICP analysis of infusion tests in the diagnosis of hydrocephalic patients. The aim of constant rate infusion tests is an estimation of cerebrospinal space compensatory mechanisms. The model of these mechanisms, introduced by A. Marmarou and verified in many clinical and experimental works (Avezaat and Eijndhoven 1984; Sliwka 1986; Ekstedt and Frieden 1983) describes the cerebrospinal system capacity for production, absorption and storing of cerebrospinal fluid (CSF). Some disorders commonly observed in hydrocephalus, can be expressed as loss of equilibrium between these three factors.

We have assembled all the calculated parameters of clinical value into one package, prepared for use with the IBM-PC, XT, or AT microcomputer.

Static analysis enables the calculation of resorption resistance to CSF, baseline pressure, elasticity and CSF formation rate. The non-linear regression of ICP during the infusion delivers information on the same parameters, even if a new equilibrium state is not reached. It also allows for neglect of artifacts following infusion tests (B waves for example), that normally disturb static analysis. The minimization of standard deviation of the pressure-volume index (PVI) in the observed pressure range allows for not only the calculation of the model parameters but also the choice of its optimal form. Full analysis of the amplitude/pressure characteristic can also be made. All the calculated parameters are presented in the summarized final protocol, helpful in the review of already examined patients, Fig. 1 a.

Analysis of the Shape of Pulse Wave

The program is designed for continuous monitoring of ICP and automatic recognition of the shape of its pulse wave. The following parameters of the pulse wave are registered in the form of time-trends: amplitudes and delays with respect to the onset of pulse evolution, in subsequent peaks commonly observed in the pulse wave (if they exist), its period and the mean pressure level. Their trends are automatically stored on disk, and can be reviewed in the off-line mode. The program is based on the advanced and efficient pattern-recognition algorithm. It

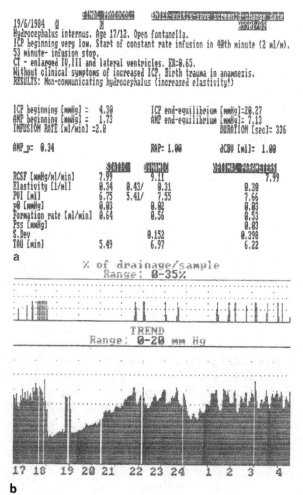

19/6/1984
Hydrocephalus internus. Age 17/12. Open fontanella.
ICP beginning very low. Start of constant rate infusion in 40th minute (2 ml/w).
53 minute- infusion stop.
CT - enlarged IV,III and lateral ventricles. ER=0.65.
Without clinical symptoms of increased ICP. Birth trauma in anamnezis.
RESULTS: Non-communicating hydrocephalus (increased elasticity!)

ICP beginning [mmHg] =   4.30   ICP end-equilibrium [mmHg]=20.27
AMP beginning [mmHg] =   1.73   AMP end-equilibrium [mmHg]= 7.13
INFUSION RATE [ml/min] =2.0   DURATION [sec]= 336

AMP_p= 0.34   RAP= 1.00   dCBV [ml]= 1.00

RCSF [mmHg/ml/min]	7.99	9.11	7.99
Elasticity [1/ml]	0.34	0.43/ 0.31	0.30
PVI [ml]	6.75	5.41/ 7.55	7.66
p0 [mmHg]	0.03	0.02	0.03
Formation rate [ml/min]	0.64	0.56	0.53
Pss [mmHg]			0.03
S.Dev		0.152	0.390
TAU [min]	5.49	6.97	6.22

a

% of drainage/sample
Range: 0-35%

TREND
Range: 0-20 mm Hg

17 18   19 20 21   22 23 24   1   2   3   4

b

Fig. 1. a The final protocol obtained after infusion test. Patient's identification and physician notes are placed in the *top. Below* the pressure and amplitude levels are shown. The next field contains amplitude/pressure characteristic analysis. *Below,* the calculated data from static, dynamic (nonlinear regression of ascending slope of ICP) and minimization of standard deviation of PVI from the same period are presented. **b** 24 hour trend of ICP recorded in case after operation of tumor of fossa posterior, with the controlled drainage of CSF in closed loop. Fluid was drained above the level of 15 mm Hg. *Above* the trend – the percentage of draining time in subsequent periods. *Abscissa* – time in hours, *ordinate:* ICP in mm Hg

is recommended for use in the diagnosis of hydrocephalus, where the shape of the pulse wave; observed during volume (infusion or bolus) excitation is important.

Because the pulse wave contains synthetized information, both on the features of CBF autoregulation and compensatory mechanisms, the program is useful in intensive care long-term monitoring.

External Drainage of CSF Under Pressure Control (Closed Loop System)

This program supports external drainage of CSF in a closed loop system. The loop consists of a special electromagnetic clamp which opens or closes an external drain connected to an intraventricular or lumbar-space catheter, according to the ICP level pre-programmed. The system maintains the pressure level within the desired range, chosen on the basis of clinical needs. External drainage occurs whenever ICP exceeds the upper pressure limit and lasts until it reaches the lower limit. If the chosen range is narrow enough, ICP can be maintained at a constant level. The program turns on an alarm signal whenever drainage is insufficient (i.e., it cannot decrease the current ICP level) or the ICP level is too low. It also has a built-in artifacts-recognition routine, which helps to avoid draining during movement artifacts. It is secured against power failure and produces a full documentation of monitoring and draining in the form of trends of the mean ICP level and effective time of drainage (Fig. 1 b).

References

Avezaat CJ, Eijndhoven JHM (1984) Cerebrospinal fluid pulse pressure and craniospinal system. Doctor's Thesis. Erasmus University, Jongbloed en Zoon Publishers, The Hague

Chopp M, Portnoy HD (1980) System analysis of intracranial pressure – comparison with volume-pressure test and CSF pulse amplitude analysis. J Neurosurg 53:516–527

Gaab MR, Ottens M, Busche F, Möller G, Trost HA (1986) Routine computerized neuromonitoring. In: Miller JD, Teasdale GM, Rowan JO, Galbraith SL, Mendelow AD (eds) Intracranial Pressure VI. Springer, Berlin Heidelberg New York Tokyo, pp 240–247

Frieden HG, Ekstedt J (1983) Volume pressure relationship of the cerebrospinal space in human. Neurosurgery 13:351–366

Marmarou A (1976) A theoretical and experimental evaluation of the cerebrospinal fluid system. PhD Thesis, Drexel University, Philadelphia

Sliwka S (1986) Static and dynamic cerebrospinal elastance–clinical verification. In: Miller JD, Teasdale GM, Rowan JO, Galbraith SL, Mendelow AD (eds) Intracranial Pressure VI. Springer, Berlin Heidelberg New York Tokyo, pp 84–88

The Best Dichotomous Parameters for Predicting Mortality and a Good Outcome Following 48 Hours of ICP Monitoring

C.P. McGraw, D.G. Changaris, J.E.S. Parker, and R.A. Greenberg

University of Louisville, School of Medicine, Louisville, Kentucky 40492 (USA)

Introduction

Simple clinical measures of Intracranial Pressure (ICP), Mean Arterial Pressures (MAP), Cerebral Perfusion Pressure (CPP-MAP-ICP) and the Highest Glasgow Coma Scale (HGCS) are potentially useful parameters to guide therapy and predict outcome. We reviewed an initial grouping of 136 consecutive head injured patients, monitored 6 parameters and identified 17 critical points in predicting mortality or morbidity. We then applied these critical points to another group of 44 patients. Sixteen of seventeen points were confirmed ($p < 0.05$).

Methods

All 180 consecutive closed head injury patients from the University of Louisville trauma population had a Glasgow Coma Score (GCS) of seven or less at the time ICP monitoring was initiated. Each patient had a Glasgow Outcome Scale (GOS) done at least one year following admission.

In the first 136 patients (Group I), we defined patterns of intracranial and arterial pressure and clinical status during the first 48 hours after admission based upon the one year follow-up. This was done by constructing plots of the percent mortality (GOS = 1) and percent good outcomes (GOS = 4 or 5) for the first two 24 hour periods of monitoring versus the CPP, ICP, Mean Arterial Blood Pressure (MABP) and Highest Glasgow Coma Score (HGCS). From these plots of outcome information we observed critical points in the parameters monitored during the first 48 hours that were significant by the Fisher exact test. We then tested these observations on an additional 44 patients (Group II). From these observations and subsequent verification on a second group of patients not used in the initial observations, it was possible to calculate specific odds ratios.

Results

We observed 17 critical points in the parameters monitored during the first 48 hours by the Fisher exact test and they are displayed in Table 1.

Intracranial Pressure VII
Eds.: J.T. Hoff and A.L. Betz
© Springer-Verlag Berlin Heidelberg 1989

Table 1. Critical points in ICP monitoring parameters by Fisher exact test

Critical point	Outcome	Group I p value	Group II p value
1) Day 2 ACPP < 60	Expire	< 0.0001	< 0.0001
2) ACPP < 80	Increased mortality	< 0.0001	0.0051
3) ACPP > 80	Increased good outcome	< 0.0001	0.0142
4) Day 2 AICP > 25	No good outcome	< 0.0001	0.0074
5) AICP > 25	Increased mortality	< 0.0001	0.0019
6) AICP < 25	Increased good outcome	< 0.0001	0.0172
7) Day 2 HICP > 50	Expire	< 0.0001	0.0001
8) HICP > 40	Increased mortality	< 0.0001	0.0106
9) HICP < 40	Increased good outcome	< 0.0001	0.0381
10) Day 1 HGCS = 3	Expire	< 0.0001	0.0303
11) Day 2 HGCS < = 5	Expire	< 0.0001	0.0080
12) HGCS < = 5	Increased mortality	< 0.0001	0.0497
13) HGCS > = 5	Increased good outcome	< 0.0001	0.0164
14) AMAP < 90	Increased mortality	< 0.0001	0.0006
15) AMAP > 90	Increased good outcome	< 0.0001	0.0281
16) LMAP < 70	Increased mortality	0.0003	0.0015
17) LMAP > 70	Increased good outcome	0.0006	0.0592

Expire = 100% mortality
Increased mortality = increased incidence of mortality (GOS of 1)
Increased good outcome = increased incidence of good outcome (GOS of 4 or 5)

The resulting odds ratios provide suggestive evidence that the following parameters should be valuable in the prediction of outcome. Average Cerebral Perfusion Pressure (ACPP), Lowest hourly Cerebral Perfusion Pressure (LCPP), Highest Glasgow Coma Scale (HGCS), Highest Hourly Intracranial Pressure (HICP), and Average Mean Arterial Blood Pressure (AMABP) over the first 48 hours can predict both good and poor outcome at one year ($p < 0.0005$). Utilizing dichotomous groupings of these data, death has occurred in all patients ($n = 47$ in Group I; $n = 17$ in Group II) when ACPP < 60 mm Hg, day 2 HGCS < 5, or AMABP < 90 mm Hg and the odds of expiring were 43, 20, and 19 fold respectively. Similarly the dichotomous grouping for the surviving end of the patient population is equally suggestive. When the AMABP > 90 mm Hg, HICP < 40 mm Hg, LCPP > 40 mm Hg, HGCS > 6 the odds of not requiring nursing care are improved 18, 14, 10, and 9 fold respectively. Of the 180 patients screened with a one year follow-up in producing these results 81 were alive (45%), 59 required no further nursing care (32% GOS = 4 or 5), 37 had full function recovery (20.6% GOS = 5), and only seven (4%) required total nursing care.

Discussion

This study has delineated how patients who do not have a HGCS greater than 3 for 0–24 hours or patients who HGCS is less than 5 for 24–48 hours expire 100%

of the time. Similarly patients whose ACPP is below 60 mm Hg or HICP is above 50 mm Hg for 24–48 hours expire 100% of the time.

During the first 48 hours of ICP monitoring patients who have an ACPP less than 80 mm Hg, an HGCS less than 5, an AICP above 25 mm Hg, a HICP above 40 mm Hg, an AMABP less than 90 mm Hg or an hourly Lowest MABP (LMABP) below 70 mm Hg have an increased incidence of mortality. During the first 48 hours of ICP monitoring patients who have an ACPP greater than 80 mm Hg, an HGCS greater than 5, an AICP less than 25 mm Hg, a HICP less than 40 mm Hg, and AMABP greater than 90 mm Hg or an LMABP above 70 mm Hg have an increased incidence of a good outcome.

With respect to the odds ratio data, we believe that this evidence suggests that whether the ACPP is above 60 mm Hg, HGCS is above 6, or AMABP is above 90 mm Hg, and LCPP is above 40 mm Hg, are important levels in predicting outcome. These should be incorporated into any trauma severity data bank for the prediction of outcome.

Non-invasive Monitoring of ICP in Infants

W.C.G. Plandsoen [1,2], D.A. de Jong [1], C.J.J. Avezaat [3], J.H.M. van Eijndhoven [4], M.C.B. Loonen [1], and P.G.H. Mulder [5]

Departments of (Child) Neurology [1,2], Neurosurgery [3], Automation Informatics [4] and Biostatistics [5], University Hospital of Amsterdam [2] and Rotterdam (The Netherlands)

Introduction

The anterior fontanelle in infants affords a natural access to the intracranial compartment. Various techniques have been attempted to measure intracranial pressure (ICP) in infants accurately (Gaab et al. 1980; Menke et al. 1982, Vidyasagar and Raju 1977; Wealthall and Smallwood 1974). Problems in interpreting results may be encountered due to the externally exerted pressure when applying a transducer to the fontanelle. The Rotterdam Teletransducer (RIT) is a passive telemetric device which has proven to be reliable, for measuring epidural pressure in patients with closed sutures (de Jong et al. 1982; Maas and de Jong 1986). Also it has proven to be reliable for the purpose of AFP monitoring (de Jong et al. 1984; Plandsoen et al. 1986). The main difference between epidural and fontanelle pressure measurements is that in the latter case only the skin is interposed between the dura and the transducer. Accurate depth positioning of the RTT in the fontanelle by means of a special skull adaptor avoids the fact that externally exerted pressure may interfere with the actual recording of ICP (Plandsoen et al. 1987). The aim of this study was to define normal values of AFP with the RTT.

Material and Methods

We used the Rotterdam Teletransducer for monitoring of AFP. The principles of operation have been described extensively by de Jong et al. (1982, 1984). For the purpose of AFP monitoring the RTT has been mounted in a special light weight perspex adaptor which rests on the skin overlaying the bony structures adjacent to the fontanelle. The adaptor is maintained in place by means of a light weight frame consisting of a loading spring connected to soft silicone tubing around the chin and occiput of the child. Proper depth setting of the transducer in the fontanelle is done by manual rotation of the piston (containing the RTT) in its thread (Fig. 1). As long as the position of the transducer is maintained the pressure to be measured, exerted to the diaphragm is continuously balanced by naturally generated reaction forces (Fig. 1). Surplus of application forces runs off to the skull. As a result of this method aplanation pressure does not interfere with the recording of ICP.

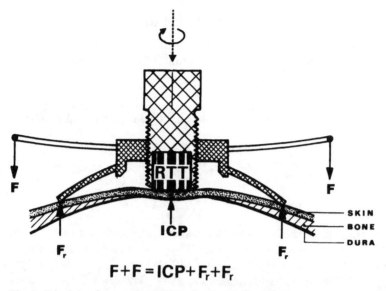

$$F + F = ICP + F_r + F_r$$

Fig. 1. Principle of measuring ICP in the fontanelle with the Rotterdam Teletransducer in the perspex adaptor. Note the balance of forces: Aplanation forces (F) do not interfere with ICP monitoring as surplus of application force ($F_r + F_r$) runs off to the skull by means of the special adaptor and fixation frame

The technique for proper depth setting resembles the technique for epidural pressure measurement, which had been described extensively by Schettini et al. (1974). Proper depth setting of the RTT is done according to the appearance of the characteristic pressure depth curve. The RTT measures pulse pulsations. Just prior to the point at which the transducer touches the skin zero set point for pressure and insertion depth are established on the chart. As the insertion depth is uniformely increased the pressure rises where after a plateau is reached at which cardiac pulsations remain constant. On further insertion the transducer traverses the subarachnoid space and does not encounter extra opposing forces. The plateau pressure thus recorded is equal to ICP. On further increasing its depth, the transducer contacts brain tissue. As a result of this the pressure sharply rises. On subsequent withdrawal the pressure depth curve is recorded in a reversed way. Using the above described technique AFP was recorded in 82 normal infants. Group I consisted of 30 normal newborn babies (aged 1–9) days in the University Hospital of Rotterdam. Group II consisted of 52 normal infants (aged 1–12) months) in the buro for neonatal care.

Results

Successful AFP recordings in 82 normal infants were performed. Mean AFP in group I was 8.9 mm Hg ± SD 2.9. Mean AFP overall in group II was 11 mm Hg ± SD 1.9. In group II there was no relation between value of AFP and age. The difference in mean AFP value between group I and II is statistically significant ($p \leq 0.01$).

Discussion

Measuring AFP with the RTT in the special light weight skull adaptor has proven to be a reliable technique, since the transducer is maintained at accurate depth in the fontanelle. Therefore according to the balance of forces (Fig. 1) recording of ICP is not influenced by aplanation pressure, as surplus of application forces runs off to the skull by means of the special skull adaptor. Accurate positioning of the RTT is performed according to the technique to perform epidural pressure measurements. The pressure depth curve is used for defining the proper depth of the transducer and for the recording of true ICP. Normal values of AFP with the RTT correspond well with those found in literature (Gaab et al. 1980, Robinson et al. 1977; Salmon et al. 1977). Also the difference in AFP value between the group of newborns (I) and the group of infants (II) is a fact which has also been noted by other authors (Bromme et al. 1985; Philip et al. 1981). The exact mechanism of the difference in pressure between newborns and older infants is still not well understood; therefore it can be considered to be an interesting field for research activities.

References

Bromme W, Baun WF, Hirsch W, Schaps P, Schobess A (1985) Methode zur nicht-invasiven Messung und Registrierung des intrakraniellen Druckes (ICP) über die offene Fontanelle des Säuglings. Zentralbl Neurochir 46:159–170

Gaab MR, Sörensen N, Hufenbeck B (1980/1981) Fontanometrie zur nicht-invasiven Registrierung des Intrakraniellen Druckes. Paediat Prax 24:631–644

Jong DA de, Maas AIR, Berfelo MW, Ouden AH den, Lange SA de (1982) The Rotterdam Teletransducer. A telemetric device for measuring epidural pressure. Biotelemetry Patient Monitg 9:154–165

Jong DA de, Maas AIR, Ouden AH den, Lange SA de (1984) Long-term intracranial pressure monitoring. Med Prog Technol 10:89–96

Jong DA de, Maas AIR, Voort E van de (1984) Non-invasive intracranial pressure monitoring. A technique for reproducible fontanelle pressure measurements. Z Kinderchir 39:274–276

Maas AIR, Jong DA de (1986) The Rotterdam Teletransducer: state of the device. Acta Neurochir (Wien) 79:5–12

Menke JA, Miles R, McIlhany M, Bashiru M, Chua C, Schwied E, Menten ThG, Khanna NN (1982) The fontanelle tonometer: A non-invasive method for measurement of intracranial pressure. J Pediatr 100:960–963

Philip AGS, Long JG, Donn SM (1981) Intracranial pressure. Sequential measurements in full-term and preterm infants. Am J Dis Child 135:521–524

Plandsoen WCG, Jong DA de, Maas AIR, Stroink H, Eijdhoven JHM van (1986) The pressure depth curve in anterior fontanelle pressure monitoring. In: Miller JD, Teasdale GM, Rowan JO, Galbraith SL, Mendelow AD (eds) Intracranial Pressure, Vol VI. Springer, Berlin Heidelberg New York Tokyo, pp 193–196

Plandsoen WCG, Jong DA de, Maas AIR, Stroink H, Avezaat CJJ (1987) Fontanelle pressure monitoring in infants with the Rotterdam Teletransducer: A reliable technique. Med Prog Technol 13:21–27

Robinson RO, Rolfe P, Sutton P (1977) Non-invasive method for measuring intracranial pressure in normal newborn infants. Dev Med Child Neurol 19:305–308

Salmon JH, Hajjar W, Bada H (1977) The Fontogram: A non-invasive intracranial pressure monitor. Pediatrics 60:721–725

Schettini A, Walsh EK (1974) Experimental identification of the subarachnoid and subpial compartments by intracranial pressure measurements. J Neurosurg 40:609–616

Vidyasagar D, Raju TNK (1977) A simple non-invasive technique of measuring intracranial pressure in the newborn. Pediatrics 59:957–961

Wealthall SR, Smallwood R (1970) Methods of measuring intracranial pressure in the fontanelle without puncture. J Neurol Neurosurg Psychiatry 37:88–96

The Human Factor in the Accuracy
of Intracranial Pressure (ICP)
Monitoring Using Extradurally Placed Microtransducers

W. Poon, J.R. South, and C. Poon

Neurosurgical Unit, Department of Surgery, Chinese University of Hong Kong,
Prince of Wales Hospital, Shatiu (Hong Kong)

Introduction

Most neurosurgeons are sceptical about the accuracy of extradurally placed microtransducers for routine ICP monitoring, despite the excellent bench accuracy of these transducers (Powell 1985; Richard 1979). However, as early as 1977, in reporting his extensive experience in monitoring ICP in 140 patients using the Ladd fiberoptic transducer placed extradurally, Levin (Levin 1977) concluded that it was easy to insert, reliable and free of complications.

We have carried out a systematic comparison of ICP using the extradural Ladd fiberoptic transducer with the intraventricular pressure (IVP) in 16 consecutive head injured patients.

Methods

The ventricular catheter and the microtransducer were inserted via the same pre-coronal frontal burr hole by the first author. A 3 cm dural pocket was created frontally for the transducer, which measured 1 cm in diameter. Simultaneous dual recordings were obtained hourly in the pen-recorder chart running at a paper speed of 6 cm per hour for analysis. The mean ICP (averaged over 1 minute) = diastolic pressure + ⅓ pulse pressure.

Results

Corresponding rate with IVP in 10 mm Hg ranges was worked out in four sets of four patients in chronological order:

In the first set of 4 patients, the corresponding rate was 15.5% (23/148), 84.5% read high (Fig. 1a); in the second set of 4 patients, 35% corresponded (42/120), 60% read high (72/120), 5% read low (6/120) (Fig. 1b); in the third set of 4 patients, 43% corresponded (47/109), 47% read high (51/109), 10% read low (11/109) (Fig. 1c); in the last set of 4 patients, 73% corresponded (101/139), 17% read high (24/139), 10% read low (14/139) (Fig. 1d).

Intracranial Pressure VII
Eds.: J. T. Hoff and A. L. Betz
© Springer-Verlag Berlin Heidelberg 1989

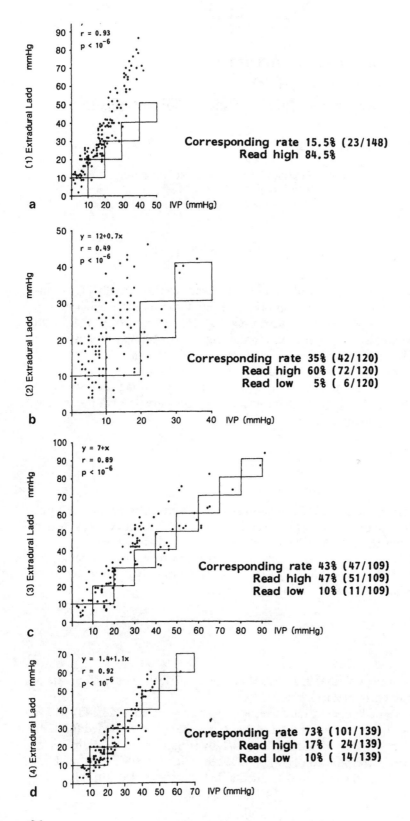

(1) Extradural Ladd mmHg

r = 0.93
p < 10^{-6}

Corresponding rate 15.5% (23/148)
Read high 84.5%

a IVP (mmHg)

(2) Extradural Ladd mmHg

y = 12+0.7x
r = 0.49
p < 10^{-6}

Corresponding rate 35% (42/120)
Read high 60% (72/120)
Read low 5% (6/120)

b IVP (mmHg)

(3) Extradural Ladd mmHg

y = 7+x
r = 0.89
p < 10^{-6}

Corresponding rate 43% (47/109)
Read high 47% (51/109)
Read low 10% (11/109)

c IVP (mmHg)

(4) Extradural Ladd mmHg

y = 1.4+1.1x
r = 0.92
p < 10^{-6}

Corresponding rate 73% (101/139)
Read high 17% (24/139)
Read low 10% (14/139)

d IVP (mmHg)

Discussion and Conclusion

ICP monitoring in acute head injury using extradurally placed Ladd fiberoptic transducers achieved a poor corresponding rate with IVP in 12 consecutive patients. With experience, corresponding rate improved to 73% in the last set of 4 patients, an acceptable accuracy for the management of acute head injury. This definite learning curve appeared to be due to inadequate stripping of the dura. We therefore suggest that although most commercially available microtransducers are bench-accurate and reliable, before extradural monitoring can be employed on its own, an initial comparison with IVP has to be performed.

References

Levin AB (1977) The use of a fiberoptic intracranial pressure monitor in clinical practice. Neurosurgery 1:266–271

Powell MP, Crockard HA (1985) Behaviour of an extradural pressure monitor in clinical use. J Neurosurg 63:745–749

Richard KE, Frowein RA (1979) Long-term measurement of ICP, technical problems and indications. Neurosurgery 2:143–151

Fig. 1. a Scatter diagram of simultaneous ICP measurements using the extradural Ladd fiberoptic transducer and ventricular catheter in the first set of 4 patients. **b** Scatter diagram in the second set of 4 patients. **c** Scatter diagram in the third set of 4 patients. **d** Scatter diagram in the fourth set of 4 patients. Hypothetical straight line if 100% accurate; □ *Square* if corresponded within 10 mmHg ranges

Rate of Infection and Cost Containment in Intracranial Pressure Recording

N. Stocchetti, T. Serioli, M. Mergoni, M.G. Menozzi, P. Paini, and P. Zuccoli

First Department of Anesthesia and Intensive Care, USL, Department of Neurosurgery, USL, Department of Microbiology, First Laboratory University of Parma, 43100 Parma (Italy)

Introduction

The monitoring of intracranial pressure (ICP) is associated with a high risk of meningitis (Mayhall et al. 1984). We performed a prospective epidemiologic study in 118 consecutive patients to assess the infection rate during ICP recording and to compare the safety of a cheap device assembled in our intensive care unit with the more expensive monitoring equipment currently available.

Patients and Methods

From January 1984 until March 1987, 118 consecutive patients in coma caused by head injury or subarachnoid hemorrhage and submitted to ICP monitoring were reviewed prospectively. No patients received steroids or prophylactic antibiotics; trauma patients with cerebrospinal fluid leaks were included. A silicon catheter (Cordis Intraventricular Pressure Monitoring Catheter with Stopcock 910-127) was tunneled for about 5 cm under the scalp then inserted into the lateral ventricle or, if it was difficult, into the subdural space (Sugiura et al. 1985). The equipment for ICP monitoring was kept closed until the end of the measurement. We compared 3 ICP recording systems: Cordis External Ventricular Monitoring and Drainage Set (Cordis Corporation, Florida Mod. 910-118), Becker External Drainage and Monitoring System (Pudenz Schulte Medical, California), and a selfmade system assembled in our ICU using stopcocks, a plastic bag for blood conservation, two vascular lines to link the catheter and dome and an infusion set to connect the drainage bag. The choice of the system depended on the availability from the hospital stockroom. Cerebrospinal fluid (CSF) samples were aspirated from the catheters just before their removal or if the duration of the monitoring exceeded 72 hours, on the fourth day and thereafter, every two days. All specimens were examined with Gram stain and CSF formulas; they were also cultured daily. If, after the removal of the catheters, the patient had fever, samples of CSF were obtained by lumbar puncture and submitted to the same examinations. The recording equipment was changed after a week of monitoring or in the case of meningitis. Patients did not receive prophylactic antibiotics but, during the ICP measurement, they were treated with antibiotics for other infections such as pneumonia. The CSF specimen with a positive culture obtained from patients without signs and symptoms of meningitis was considered infected. Ventriculitis

Eds.: J.T. Hoff and A.L. Betz

or meningitis was defined using the following criteria (McGee 1985): fever (>38), leukocytosis ($>11\,000$ cells/mm^3 blood), neck stiffness, abnormal CSF formula (>1000 cells/CSF ml, protein concentration >150 mg/CSF dl, CSF glucose concentration less than 30 mg/dl), positive culture of CSF. The outcome was evaluated six months after admission to the intensive care unit (ICU). Statistical analysis was performed using the chi square test.

Results

This study was carried out on 118 patients, 82 males and 36 females (mean age 43.8 years, Standard Deviation [SD] 20.4); 79 had head injuries and 39 subarachnoid hemorrhages. The trauma patients included 13 extradural hematomas, 21 subdural hematomas, 16 intraparenchymal hematomas, 22 cerebral contusions, 7 diffuse brain damage cases, 11 had CSF leaks. The monitoring of ICP was provided by 84 ventricular catheters and 36 subdural catheters (two patients had

Table 1. Monitoring duration

(Hours)	Min/Max	Avg	SD
With ventricular catheter	20–524	124	80.70
With subdural catheter	24–456	99	94.78
Home-made equipment	20–374	112	81.51
Pudenz-Schulte equipment	24–360	136	99.85
Cordis equipment	24–408	126	56.14

Table 2. CSF samples with positive culture (obtained from patients without signs and symptoms of meningitis)

N. of samples obtained from:	
Ventricular catheter	10
Lumbar puncture	5
Subdural catheter	1
N. of samples obtained from:	
Home-made set	6
Podenz-Schulte set	5
Cordis set	4
(NS)	

Bacteria (in brackets the number of samples with culture positive for the species) – Often several species grew in the same culture

Enterococcus	(2)
Staphylococcus epidermidis	(5)
Staphylococcus aureus	(1)
Klebsiella	(2)
Escherichia coli	(1)
Proteus mirabilis	(1)
Bacillus cereus	(1)
Streptococcus non haemolyticus	(1)

a subdural at the beginning and a ventricular later). We used 66 apparatuses assembled in our ICU, 38 Pudenz-Schulte and 41 Cordis devices. The mean duration of recording in this group of patients was high, averaging more than four days and exceeding a week in 23 cases (Table 1). We obtained 244 CSF samples directly from the catheters and 71 specimens from lumbar punctures after the withdrawal of the monitoring system; 230 and 64 samples respectively, did not show any bacterial growth. Table 2 summarizes data about the samples with positive cultures. Five patients had signs and symptoms of meningitis associated with positive cultures. Two patients in this group had a CSF leak; the chi square analysis was significant ($p < 0.05$) when this variable was tested. Four patients were head injured and one had a subarachnoid hemorrhage.

Discussion

Infection is a significant risk of all invasive monitoring and particularly of ICP recording (Mayhall et al. 1984; McGee and Kaiser 1985). Many authors (Levin et al. 1982) assess this risk in rates ranging from less than 3% up to 100%. Several risk factors are reported: surgical technique during the insertion of the catheter (Mayhall et al. 1984), – the type of intracranial pressure monitor, previous neurologic surgery, revealed irrigation of the system and other causes of opening the system, and – the duration of recording (Levin et al. 1982; Mayhall et al. 1984). The rate of contamination and infection in our series was low. Meningitis developed in patients after almost one week of monitoring, with a mean duration exceeding 12 days. The presence of a CSF leak was associated with a higher incidence of infection ($p < 0.05$). Ventricular catheterization is a greater risk than subdural. Statistical analysis does not show any difference in the rate of infection or contamination between the three pieces of equipment examined. Thus, it is of interest to compare the costs of products that seem to offer comparable safety. The cost of our selfmade system in June, 1987 was half that of the Cordis device and one-third that of the Pudenz-Schulte system. Infection is an important risk in ICP monitoring but in our group of patients the rate of infection was low and all the patients recovered from their meningitis; therefore, this risk seems to be acceptable. Our data suggests that, from a bacteriologic point of view, low-cost equipment, self assembled in the intensive unit, is as safe as the more expensive systems on the market.

References

Levin AB, Braun SR, Grossman JE (1982) Physiological monitoring of the head injured patient. In: Weiss MH (ed) Clinical Neurosurgery, vol 29,14. Baltimore, Williams and Wilkins, pp 240–287
Mayhall CG, Archer NH, Lamb VA, Spadora AC, Bagget JW, Ward JD, Narayan RK (1984) Ventriculostomy-related infections. N Engl J Med 311:553–559
McGee ZA, Kaiser AB (1985) Acute meningitis. In: Mandell GL, Douglas RG, Bennet JE (eds) Principles and practice of infectious diseases. J. Wiley and Sons, New York, pp 561–573
Sugiura K, Hayama N, Tachisawa T, Baba M, Takizawa H (1985) Intracranial pressure monitoring by a subdurally placed silicone catheter: technical note. Neurosurgery 16:241–244

Continuous Monitoring of Middle Cerebral Arterial Blood Velocity and Cerebral Perfusion Pressure

T. Lundar, K.-F. Lindegaard, and H. Nornes

Department of Neurosurgery, Rikshospitalet, The National Hospital, University of Oslo, N-0027 Oslo (Norway)

Introduction

Intracranial pressure (ICP) monitoring has been used clinically for over 30 years, providing an understanding of the ICP dynamics in clinical situations. With the addition of systemic artery blood pressure (BP) recordings, continuous monitoring of the cerebral perfusion pressure (CPP), which is estimated by subtracting the ICP from the BP, is now a standard method in the management of critically ill neurosurgical patients. In the individual patient, CPP monitoring yields prognostic information and may be helpful when evaluating different treatment modalities.

When the transcranial Doppler (TCD) technique was introduced (Aaslid et al. 1982) it became evident that recordings of blood velocity in the basal cerebral arteries contains clinically relevant information on cerebral hemodynamics. Serial blood velocity measurements are useful in the assessment of patients with recent subarachnoid hemorrhage, providing atraumatic means for monitoring the occurrence and the course of cerebral vasospasm (Seiler et al. 1986). In such patients TCD is employed to detect narrowing of the proximal brain arteries on a day to day basis. In the short term, however, the diameter of the cerebral artery mainstems remain remarkably constant. Simultaneous and continuous recordings of middle cerebral artery (MCA) blood velocity and ipsilateral internal carotid artery (ICA) flow have shown that relative changes in MCA blood velocity reflect changes in volume flow with an accuracy that is adequate for clinical purposes (Lindegaard et al. 1987).

The main purpose of CPP monitoring is to provide a basis for assessing the impact of an elevated ICP on brain perfusion. When combined with CPP monitoring, MCA blood velocity recording could give additional information on the relation between changes in CPP and changes in brain perfusion. The aim of the present study was to investigate the value of continuous MCA blood velocity monitoring to assess changes in brain perfusion in patients with increased ICP.

Clinical Material and Methods

A total of 24 patients underwent ICP monitoring via the ventricular or epidural route. Indications for monitoring included head injury (10 patients), brain tumor

(2 patients), pseudotumor (4 patients), Reye's syndrome (1 patient), and hydro-cephalus (7 patients). The BP and the intraventricular pressure were recorded by means of standard fluid pressure transducers (AME 840, made by AME, Horten, Norway), and the intracranial epidural pressure was assessed using an epidural pressure transducer (AME 832, made by AME, Horten, Norway). The pressure reference point was at the mid-cranial level. The MCA blood velocity was mea-sured with a 2 MHz range-gated pulsed Doppler instrument with on-line spec-trum analysis and a self-retaining ultrasound probe (TC64-2, made by EME, Überlingen, FRG), as shown in Fig. 1. Following identification of the MCA as previously described (Aaslid et al. 1982), the probe was fixed in the position providing the best MCA blood velocity signal. This was obtained using sampling depths between 40 and 50 mm. The blood velocity spectrum was shown continu-ously on the TCD display. Moreover, analog tracings of the spectrum outline (Lindegaard et al. 1987) and of BP and ICP were stored on tape and on a multi-channel pen recorder.

Repeated samples were drawn from the BP monitoring cannula for arterial CO_2 partial pressure (P_aCO_2) analysis.

Results

Monitoring the MCA blood velocity was feasible and useful in these 24 patients. The MCA blood velocity monitoring period ranged from 1 to 10 days. The probe fixture proved adequate for monitoring over several hours (Fig. 1). Transporta-tion of the patient to CT-scanning required temporary probe removal. Moreover, patient movement sometimes displaced the probe and the MCA blood velocity signal became lost. Nevertheless, whenever the probe had to be repositioned, the MCA signal was retrieved using the same probe position and sampling depth as before. Thus, using the best MCA signal as the reference point for these adjust-ments seemed to be adequate when performed by the same examiner and when repeated by different examiners, provided that they had some experience with the TCD method.

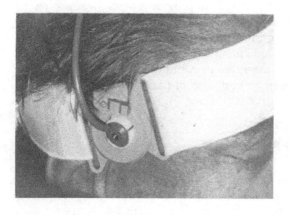

Fig. 1. Self-retaining ultrasound probe positioned for continuous monitoring of MCA blood velocity on the right side. The MCA is insonated through the relatively thin bone above the zygomatic arch

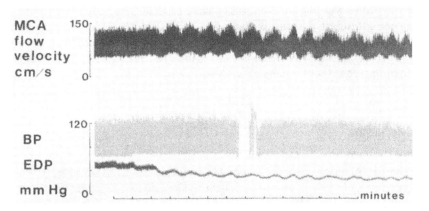

Fig. 2. Continuous recording of MCA flow velocity, systemic artery blood pressure (*BP*), and epidural intracranial pressure (*EDP*). Note the occurrence of B-waves in the EDP recording with concomitant MCA blood velocity fluctuations

In this series of 24 patients, the absolute MCA blood velocity was between 24 and 110 cm/s at the start of monitoring. The following relationships were emphasized when comparing the blood velocity and the CPP data. *a)* Blood velocity responses to changes in P_aCO_2. *b)* Changes in blood velocity and CPP at constant P_aCO_2. *c)* Blood velocity changes during ICP waves.

a) The CO_2 reactivity (the percentage blood velocity change divided by the P_aCO_2 change in mm Hg) was tested at least once in 18 of the 24 patients. A P_aCO_2 step was induced in the patients on artificial ventilation by bagging for about 30 s. Patients being awake were instructed to hyperventilate. All but two patients with severe head trauma showed CO_2 reactivity between 3 and 5%/mm Hg. The blood velocity drop was easily seen from the TCD display provided that the P_aCO_2 step was more than 5 mm Hg.

b) During rapid CPP changes with a constant P_aCO_2, the mean MCA blood velocity did not change significantly unless CPP was reduced to below 40–45 mm Hg. Below this threshold blood velocity changed passively with CPP. Exceptions to this were five head injury patients who demonstrated pressure-passive blood velocity fluctuations throughout the observed CPP range (up to 120 mm Hg). The blood velocity waveform also revealed information of clinical interest. In severe intracranial hypertension, CPP becomes critically low. Under such circumstances there is an increased systolic blood velocity while diastolic blood velocity becomes typically reduced (Lindegaard et al. 1980). Such waveforms were observed in patients with a CPP reduction to below 40 mm Hg. When mean CPP was reduced to 10–20 mm Hg, diastolic CPP and diastolic blood velocity approach zero. In two patients with severe head injury the intracranial hypertension progressed to brain tamponade as demonstrated by zero CPP, a reverberating MCA blood velocity pattern (inflow in systolic with diastolic outflow resulting in flow over the cardiac cycle being zero); and cerebral circulatory arrest documented by 4 vessel cerebral arteriography.

c) Pressure waves were commonly seen, especially in patients with head trauma or pseudotumor. During B waves (1–2 per minute), blood velocity fluctuations occurred (Fig. 2). During A waves (plateau waves) mean MCA blood velocity was sometimes reduced, but the amplitude of the pulsatile blood velocity waveform increased with decreasing CPP.

Discussion

The MCA blood velocity in normal resting persons is between 35 and 90 cm/s (Aaslid et al. 1982), probably reflecting individual variation in vessel diameter and cerebral blood flow. In view of this wide normal range, comparing absolute blood velocity (in cm/s) in different persons is not feasible. Nonetheless, relative variations in blood velocity permits estimating relative variations in volume flow. These estimations seem to be sufficiently accurate for clinical purposes (Lindegaard et al. 1987). Further support is gained from the fact that the CO_2 reactivity determined from blood velocity recordings in healthy volunteers (Markwalder et al. 1984) and during open-heart surgery (Lundar et al. 1986) is very close to the CO_2 reactivity demonstrated using the well known tracer methods (Olesen et al. 1971). For long term monitoring it is emphasized, however, that the lumen of the MCA could change considerably, due to vasospasm following subarachnoid hemorrhage, and in patients with severe head trauma. This fact should be remembered when comparing observations on absolute MCA blood velocity obtained days apart.

The present data on MCA blood velocity responses in face of rapid changes in CPP were limited by the fact that the CPP remained within a narrow range in many patients. Five patients demonstrated MCA blood velocity fluctuating passively with the variations in CPP. The other patients showed MCA blood velocity remaining nearly constant as long as the CPP level remained above 40–45 mm Hg. This suggests that the blood velocity in basal cerebral arteries is autoregulated with a lower regulatory limit of 40–45 mm Hg (Greenfield and Tindall 1965). Thus, it seems that the lumen diameter of the MCA remains remarkably constant on a short time basis even under these extreme conditions. Moreover, continuous recording of blood velocity lends itself to investigating acute effects of therapeutic intervention and of different anesthetic regimens (Lundar et al. 1987).

References

Aaslid R, Markwalder T-M, Nornes H (1982) Noninvasive transcranial Doppler ultrasound recording of flow velocity in basal cerebral arteries. J Neurosurg 57:769–774

Greenfield JC, Tindall GT (1965) Effect of acute increase in intracranial pressure on blood flow in internal carotid artery of man. J Clin Invest 44:1343–1351

Lindegaard K-F, Grip A, Nornes H (1980) Precerebral hemodynamics in brain tamponade. Part 2: Experimental studies. Neurochirurgia (Stuttg) 23:187–196

Lindegaard K-F, Lundar T, Wiberg J, Sjøberg D, Aaslid R, Nornes H (1987) Variations in middle cerebral artery blood flow investigated with noninvasive transcranial blood velocity measurements. Stroke 18:1025–1030

Lundar T, Lindegaard K-F, Frøysaker T, Grip A, Bergman M, Am-Holen E, Nornes H (1986) Cerebral carbon dioxide reactivity during nonpulsatile cardiopulmonary bypass. Ann Thorac Surg 41:525–530

Lundar T, Lindegaard K-F, Refsum L, Rian R, Nornes H (1987) Cerebral effects of isoflurane in humans: Intracranial pressure and middle cerebral artery flow velocity. Br J Anaesth 59:1208–1213

Markwalder TM, Grolimund P, Seiler RW, Roth F, Aaslid R (1984) Dependency of blood flow velocity in the middle cerebral artery on end-tidal carbon dioxide partial pressure: A transcranial Doppler study. J Cereb Blood Flow Metab 4:368–372

Olesen J, Paulson OB, Lassen NA (1971) Regional cerebral blood flow in man determined by the initial slope of the clearance of intra-arterially injected [133]Xe. Theory of the method, normal values, error of measurement, correction for remaining radioactivity, relation to other flow parameters, and response to P_aCO_2 changes. Stroke 2:519–540

Seiler RW, Grolimund P, Aaslid R, Huber P, Nornes H (1986) Cerebral vasospasm evaluated by transcranial ultrasound correlated with clinical grade and CT-visualized subarachnoid hemorrhage. J Neurosurg 64:594–600

Analysis of Frequency Spectrum
of the Intracranial Pulse Wave in Cerebral Vasospasm

E.R. Cardoso and D. Bose [1]

Cerebral Hydrodynamics Laboratory, [1] Departments of Surgery, Pharmacology and
Therapeutics, and Internal Medicine, University of Manitoba, R3A 1R9 Winnipeg (Canada)

Introduction

It is frequently assumed that the systemic arterial pulse wave (SAPW) is the main
determinant of the configuration of the intracranial pulse wave (ICPW) (Cardoso
1983). Thus, cerebral arterial vasospasm, which causes secondary decrease of
arterial pulsations, should narrow the amplitude of the ICPW. We tested this
hypothesis by producing cerebral vasospasm through cisternal injections of blood
(SAH) or 5-hydroxytryptamine (5-HT, serotonin) (Mayberg et al. 1978). Furthermore, we compared two methods of measurement of the ICPW, namely, magnitude of the frequency components of the Fast Fourier Transformed (FFT) and
ICPW amplitude in the time domain.

Method

Experiments were performed on 30 anesthetized adult cats with controlled respiration and body temperature. SAPW was monitored from the descending aorta.
ICPW was monitored with a metallic needle inserted stereotactically into the third
cerebral ventricle. Injections of 2 ml of artificial CSF, autologous blood, or
10^{-4} M solution of 5-HT into the subarachnoid space were performed through
a cannula inserted into the cisterna magna. ICPW and SAPW signals were stored
with an instrumentation recorder (TEAC) and later digitized for measurements of
total amplitude of ICPW and SAPW in the time domain as well as the magnitude
of their frequency components obtained by FFT. For spectral analysis of the
ICPW and SAPW, the data was sampled at a rate of 2 kHz for a total of 4,096
points and analysed by a Fast Fourier Transform algorithm with the help of a
Data 6000 wave form analyser (Data Precision). Low frequency components
related to cyclic respiratory waves were excluded from the analysis. The magnitudes of the fundamental wave (F) and the three first harmonics were correlated
with the ICPW and SAPW, as measured on time domain.

    Thirteen animals underwent angiography of the vertebro-basilar system be-
fore and after subarachnoid injections. Alterations of amplitudes of the ICPW,
the SAPW and their spectral components obtained by FFT were compared to
changes of the mean angiographically determined vessel diameter, as calculated

      Eds.: J. T. Hoff and A. L. Betz
      © Springer-Verlag Berlin Heidelberg 1989

by the ratio between area of the vessel obtained by planimetry with a graphics tablet and its length. The difference between values obtained before and after each subarachnoid injection was calculated as percent of control.

Results

Subarachnoid injections of artificial CSF in 34 experiments increased the total ICPW amplitude, with a mean increase of $20.47 \pm 3.88\%$ from baseline. There was a close correlation between total wave amplitude changes in the time domain and alterations in the magnitude of the fundamental wave seen with FFT

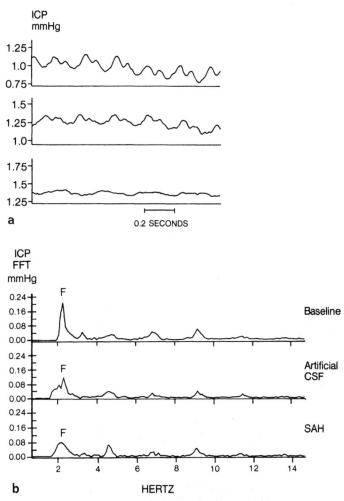

Fig. 1. Simultaneous recordings of ICPW on time (**a**) and frequency (**b**) domains during baseline conditions (*top*), following subarachnoid injection of artificial CSF (*middle*) and SAH (*bottom*). Note narrowing of the entire ICPW as well as decrease in amplitude of the fundamental (*F*) wave on FFT

($r=0.86$). However, no correlation was found with any of the harmonics measured after FFT analysis.

Subarachnoid injection of blood in 14 experiments lowered the total amplitude of the ICPW by $25.21 \pm 7.94\%$. The amplitude of the SAPW increased by $5.11 \pm 10.49\%$. The drop in ICPW amplitude was significantly different from the changes observed in the SAPW amplitude ($r=0.98$, $P<0.03$), indicating that vasospasm and not alterations in SAPW amplitude, was responsible for the observed narrowing of the ICPW amplitude. ICPW narrowing in the time domain, showed high correlation with narrowing of the fundamental wave on FFT analysis ($r=0.92$) (Fig. 1). There was no correlation with other harmonics. Cerebral vasospasm caused by subarachnoid injection of 5-HT in 8 experiments produced narrowing of the ICPW of $21.37 \pm 7.9\%$ which also correlated with the magnitude of the fundamental wave on FFT ($r=0.9$).

Angiographically measured vasospasm of the vertebro-basilar arteries correlated well with the decrease of ICPW amplitude ($r=0.96$, $p<0.001$) and fundamental wave after FFT ($r=0.93$, $p<0.001$).

Discussion

The results can be explained by the model devised by Klassen et al. (1988) for the origin of the ICPW. Cerebral arterial spasm alters the thickness of the arterial wall as well as its elastic properties, thus, interfering with the transmission of the intraluminal pulsations across the vascular wall.

Our findings suggest that diffuse cerebral vasospasm, as observed after subarachnoid injections of blood and 5-HT in cats, can be diagnosed and continuously monitored by measurement of ICPW amplitude. Furthermore, the results also indicate that the degree of vasospasm can be estimated by measurement of the narrowing of the fundamental wave on FFT (Takizawa et al. 1981).

Acknowledgements. We wish to thank the St. Boniface General Hospital Research Foundation for financial support as well as Miss. Raquel Baert and Dr. Kesh Reddy for expert technical assistance.

References

Cardoso ER, Rowan JO, Galbraith S (1983) Analysis of the cerebrospinal pulse wave in intracranial pressure. J Neurosurg 59:817–821

Klassen PA, Shwedyk E, Cardoso ER (1988) Mathematical modelling of the contribution of arterial diameter pulse to the configuration of the intracranial pulse wave. ICP VII

Mayberg MR, Houser DW, Sundt TM Jr (1978) Ultrastructural changes in feline arterial endothelium following subarachnoid hemorrhage. J Neurosurg 48:49–55

Takizawa H, Gabra-Sanders T, Miller JD (1987) Changes in the cerebrospinal fluid pulse wave spectrum associated with raised intracranial pressure. Neurosurgery 20:355–361

Intracranial Volume and Pressure Load Tolerance Evaluated by Continuous Measurement of Doppler Flow Velocity in Intracranial Vessels in Cats

S. Nakatani, K. Ozaki, K. Hara[1], and H. Mogami

Department of Neurosurgery, Osaka University Medical School, 1-1-50 Fukushima, Osaka, and [1] Sharp Corp., Osaka 533 (Japan)

Introduction

In order to study the noninvasive evaluation of intracranial hemodynamics during intracranial hypertension a technique employing pulsed Doppler ultrasound (MF-20 microvascular Doppler, EME) was developed to measure blood flow velocity in the basal arteries of cats. Flow tolerance to volume and pressure loading was assessed by changes in the Doppler flow velocity and wave form.

Material and Method

Intraocular contents were evacuated to expose the optic nerve and the optic foramen. A 20 MHz probe positioned just before the optic foramen was maintained in a fixed position throughout each experiment. Doppler ultrasound signals were analyzed by an ECHOSPEC real-time spectrum analyzer. Instantaneous changes of mean flow velocity (MFV), systolic (S), diastolic (D), mode frequency (MD), S/D ratio and Pourcelot's resistance index were assessed in 14 anesthetized cats under controlled respiration, monitoring EEG and BSR, during 1) control, 2) epidural balloon inflation at a rate of 2 ml/hr, and 3) hydrostatic pressure loading of the CSF space.

Results

Epidural Balloon Inflation (Fig. 1 a–c)

In seven cats the supratentorially placed epidural balloon was inflated at a rate of 2 ml/hr simulating an expanding mass lesion. The flow velocity started to decrease, the systolic peak became rounded and lower and the diastolic component became lower at high ICP ($> 70-80$ mm Hg). At CPP below 80.42 ± 38.43 mm Hg no diastolic flow was seen, making the flow pattern a single systolic peak. The systolic peak started to decrease soon after initiation of balloon

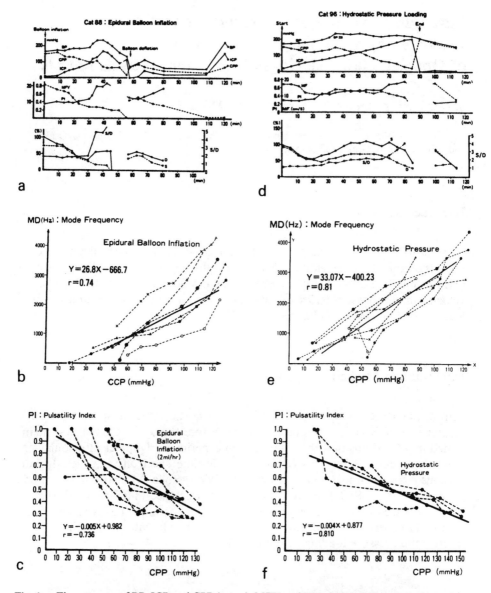

Fig. 1. a Time courses of BP, ICP and CPP (*upper*), MFV and PI (*middle*), S/D ratio and percent changes in S and D (*lower*) during and after inflation of the epidural balloon. **b** Relation between MF and CPP. **c** Relation between PI and CPP. **d** Time courses of BP, ICP and CPP (*upper*), MFV and PI (*middle*), S/D ratio and percent changes in S and D (*lower*) during and after hydrostatic pressure loading. **e** Relation between MF and CPP. **f** Relation between PI and CPP

inflation. No systolic or diastolic flow was found at CPP of zero. Correlation was found between CPP and MD and between CPP and PI.

Hydrostatic Pressure Loading (Fig. 1 d–f)

In seven cats hydrostatic pressure was changed in the cerebrospinal fluid space through a needle inserted into the cisterna magna to study the effect of pressure per se on flow velocity and wave form. Flow velocity was relatively undisturbed until CPP was less than 60 mm Hg (in comparison with balloon inflation). At CPP below 26.57 ± 10.83 mm Hg a systolic peak without a diastolic component was found. No systolic and diastolic flow was found at CPP zero. Correlations between CPP and MD and between CPP and PI were found.

Blood pressure elevation elicited by the Cushing response was mandatory for the flow velocity wave to be maintained in both groups.

Discussion

By using the transorbital approach, exposure of the arteries and enlargement of the optic foramen are not required. The intracranial environment remains totally undisturbed with maintenance of the integrity of the cranium and the dural sac, leaving the basal arteries intact. The absence of CSF leakage was also an advantage. Although Doppler flow velocity does not provide quantitative data, changes in flow velocity correlate well with changes in cerebral blood flow (Batton et al. 1983). This new transorbital technique allows a noninvasive determination of the flow velocity in order to assess instantaneous changes of CBF and provide continuous monitoring of intracranial hemodynamics during experimentally induced intracranial hypertensive states.

Our present study confirms the report that the correlation between basal ICP and cerebral blood flow is variable, depending on the pathological state which caused elevated ICP. In cats under controlled respiration epidural balloon loading was less tolerated than hydrostatic pressure loading in relation to CPP in contrast to previous reports (Zwetnow et al. 1985; Nakatani and Ommaya, 1972). This finding may be attributed to species differences and different respiratory conditions. The importance of blood pressure in maintaining the cerebral blood flow (Schrader et al. 1985) was confirmed.

Summary and Conclusion

Doppler ultrasound of intracranial vessel was obtained by a transorbital method in cats to study the flow tolerance to volume loading and pressure loading. The latter was less tolerated than the former in relation to CPP. Hypertension associated with an elicited Cushing response was essential to maintain critical flow in both groups.

References

Batton DG, Hellmann J, Hernandez MJ et al. (1983) Regional cerebral blood flow, cerebral blood velocity, and pulsatility index in newborn dogs. Pediatr Res 17:908–912
Nakatani S, Ommaya AK (1972) A critical rate of cerebral compression. In: Brock M, Dietz H (eds) Intracranial Pressure. Springer, Berlin Heidelberg New York, pp 144–148
Schrader H, Lofgren J, Zwetnow NN (1985) Influence of blood pressure on tolerance to an intracranial expanding mass. Acta Neurol Scand 71:114–126
Zwetnow NN, Lofgren J, Schrader H (1986) Intracranial volume load tolerance. In: Miller JD, Teasedale GM, Rowan JO, Galbraith SL, Medelow AD (eds) Intracranial Pressure VI. Springer, Berlin Heidelberg New York, pp 404–408

Simultaneous Monitoring of ICP and Transcranial Doppler Sonogram on the Middle Cerebral Artery

S. Nakatani, K. Ozaki, K. Hara [1], and H. Mogami

Department of Neurosurgery, Osaka University Medical School, 1-1-50 Fukushima, Osaka, and [1] Sharp Corp., Osaka 533 (Japan)

Introduction

It has been pointed out that an absolute value of ICP alone, although important, does not provide enough information about the on-going critical changes of intracranial hemodynamics. Using transcranial Doppler it is possible to record blood flow velocities (FV) of basal arteries of the brain allowing us to monitor the hemodynamic changes instantaneously (Aaslid et al. 1982). We assessed the correlation between ICP and FV to investigate a noninvasive measure of intracranial pathology.

Clinical Material and Methods

The study involved 30 patients who underwent neurosurgical intervention. ICP was measured with a Camino transducer tipped catheter connected to a 420 digital pressure monitor (San Diego, California, USA). FVs were recorded at the depth of 4 to 5.5 cm from the temporal scalp with the FP2 probe attached to a transcranial Doppler (TC2-64 EME, Überlingen, FRG). Data were recorded with a polygraph and data recorder, analyzed by an Echospec spectrum analyzer. The resistance index by Pourcelot (PI) was calculated from the Doppler sonogram. A minicomputer analyzed ICP and BP data.

Results

In certain conditions and at a constant $PaCO_2$ the correlation between ICP and FV (Fig. 1 a) and between ICP and PI (Fig. 1 b) was good, and statistically significant. However, the correlation between either ICP and FV or IVP and PI was not significant, depending on the basic pathological state which caused an elevated ICP.

With increasing ICP above a critical level (30–40 mm Hg) FV started to decrease while PI increased. When CPP decreased below the critical level of 40 mm Hg, the diastolic component of the Doppler sonogram decreased, finally leaving only a sharp systolic peak with impending brain death. In brain tampo-

Intracranial Pressure VII
Eds.: J. T. Hoff and A. L. Betz
© Springer-Verlag Berlin Heidelberg 1989

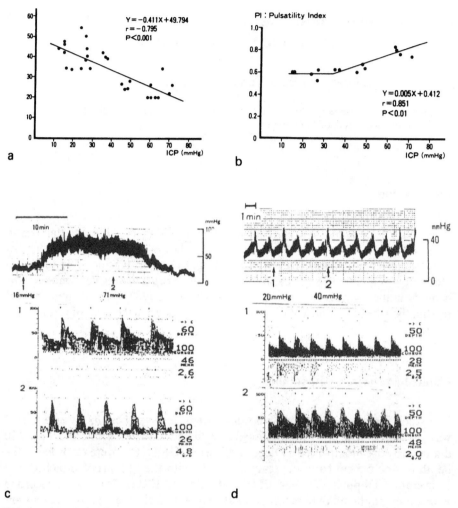

Fig. 1. a Correlation between ICP and FV. **b** Correlation between ICP and PI showing significance after ICP reach 40 mm Hg. **c** Recording showing an A-wave (*upper*) and transcranial Doppler sonogram before (*1*) and during (*2*) an A-wave. At the plateau diastolic flow was minimal. **d** Recording showing B-waves and transcranial Doppler sonogram at the peak (*1*) and trough (*2*) of a B-wave which revealed different sonogram patterns

nade a sharp single systolic peak was accompanied by reverberating flow in the diastolic phase. During the B wave trough FV decreased (Fig. 1c). During a plateau wave FV decreased and PI increased with a sharp systolic peak and minimum diastolic flow (Fig. 1d).

Discussion

ICP monitoring provides information on CPP as well as intracranial compliance. However, they are indirect measures of intracranial hemodynamics. Changes in

FVs measured by TCD correlated well with the findings obtained by standard methods of CBF measurement (Greisen et al. 1984). However, FVs in normal subjects may have a wide range due to individual variation that may occur from differences in heart rate, blood pressure, blood viscosity, vascular tone, vascular caliber and arterial pCO_2. In pathological states many factors influence FV. Effects of drugs, for example, are significant. It may be possible to correlate ICP with FV only when factors influencing FV are kept constant, a circumstance not possible in clinical conditions. Only when CPP decreases below a critical level does a decreasing diastolic component indicate a critical state of intracranial hemodynamics (Kirkham et al. 1987; Klingelhofer et al. 1987; Nakatani et al. 1988).

Summary and Conclusion

While ICP or FV alone fall short of providing useful information about the on-going critical changes of intracranial hemodynamics, a continuous recording of FV together with ICP proved to be very useful as an indicator of impending intracranial crisis.

References

Aaslid R, Markwalder T-M, Nornes H (1982) Noninvasive transcranial Doppler ultrasound recording of flow velocity in basal arteries. J Neurosurg 57:769–774
Greisen G, Johnasen K, Ellison PH et al. (1984) Cerebral blood flow in the new born infant: comparison of Doppler ultrasound and xenon clearance. J Pediatr 104:411–418
Kirkham FJ, Levin SD, Padayachee TS et al. (1987) Transcranial pulsed Doppler ultrasound findings in brain stem death. J Neurol Neurosurg Psychiatry 50:1504–1513
Klingelhofer J, Conrad B, Benecke R et al. (1987) Intracranial flow patterns at increasing intracranial pressure. Klin Wochenschr 65:542–545
Nakatani S, Ozaki K, Wakayama A et al. (1988) Intracranial pressure and pressure waves evaluated by transcranial Doppler sonography. In: Fieschi C, Aaslid R (eds) First International Conference on Transcranial Doppler. Springer, Berlin Heidelberg New York Tokyo

Effect of Jugular Bulb Catheterization on Intracranial Pressure

M.G. Goetting and G. Preston

Department of Pediatrics, Henry Ford Hospital, 2799 West Grand Boulevard, Detroit, Michigan 48202 (USA)

Cerebral blood volume is one determinant of intracranial pressure (ICP) and is directly proportional to venous outflow resistance. Most cerebral venous blood drains through the internal jugular veins and the vertebral venous plexus. Obstruction to venous drainage by jugular vein compression, especially on the right side, is known to elevate ICP. Some clinicians are reluctant to catheterize the internal jugular vein (IJ) in patients with elevated ICP for fear of exacerbating intracranial hypertension. Yet it is these patients who could benefit most from jugular bulb catheterization (JBC).

We evaluated the effect of JBC and maintenance on patient's in whom ICP was monitored.

Methods

Patients undergoing both ICP and JBC were eligible for the study. All data were recorded prospectively. If the ICP monitoring device was inserted first, the change in ICP was noted during JBC. The pressure reading was recorded immediately before venous puncture and after catheter insertion. Any elevation in ICP during the procedure was noted.

Once daily we compressed the ipsilateral, contralateral and bilateral jugular veins near the thyroid cartilage. Firm digital pressure was applied slightly laterally to the carotid impulse. Compression was maintained until a new ICP stabilized, the ICP increased by 5 mm Hg, or 30 seconds elapsed without change in ICP. During compression testing the patient's head was in a neutral position, the patient was calm and no nursing procedures were being performed. All catheters were placed in the right IJ. Results were compared using a paired t-test or Wilcoxon rank-sum test.

Results

Twenty-six patients underwent simultaneous JBC and ICP monitoring. The mean age was 9.19 yrs $\pm$ 6.1 with a range of 1 month to 19 years. ICP monitoring devices included the subarachnoid bolt (13), ventriculostomy (9), and intraparenchymal

Eds.: J. T. Hoff and A. L. Betz

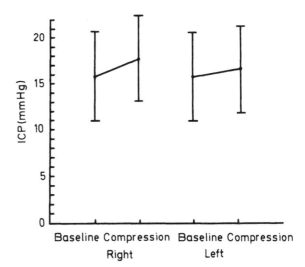

Fig. 1. Effect of jugular venous compression on ICP

fiberoptic device (4). Diagnoses were as follows: head trauma, 19; brain infarction, 2; hypoxic-ischemic encephalopathy, 1; intracerebral hemorrhage, 1; encephalitis, 1; meningitis, 1; acute toxic encephalopathy, 1. The duration of simultaneous monitoring was 1 to 6 days (median = 3 d). The peak ICP sustained for at least 5 minutes not during compression was 12–58 mm Hg (mean = 28.31 ± 11.3).

Eighteen patients had ICP monitoring during JBC. The mean ICP prior to insertion was 17.00 mm Hg $\pm$ 5.30. After insertion the pressure was 17.06 mm Hg $\pm$ 5.49 ($p = 0.8162$). The maximum increase occurred in 1 patient and was 2 mm Hg. A total of 72 venous compression tests were performed. Right jugular vein compression increased the ICP from 15.85 mm Hg $\pm$ 4.89 to 17.82 mm Hg $\pm$ 4.69. The left compression elevated the ICP from 15.74 mm Hg $\pm$ 4.84 to 16.55 mm Hg $\pm$ 4.86. The ICP rose 1.97 mm Hg with right-sided compression ($p = 0.001$) and with left-sided compression, 0.81 mm Hg ($p = 0.0137$). We separated patients into 2 groups, those whose mean ICP during all tests was ≤ 15 mm Hg and those whose mean ICP was ≥ 15 mm Hg. There was no difference between the groups in the degree of elevation with venous compression.

Bilateral venous compression always resulted in an ICP elevation of at least 5 mm Hg. Unilateral compression never caused a 5 mm Hg rise.

In tests where the ICP rose, it did so instantly and equilibrated in 30 seconds. When compression ceased the ICP fell immediately in all cases. There were no apparent adverse effects from jugular venous compression (Fig. 1).

Discussion

There are several mechanisms by which ICP could be elevated by JBC placement: 1) hematoma at puncture site; 2) venous spasm; 3) venous thrombosis. Compres-

117

sion of the contralateral vein (left side) eliminates this route of venous drainage, placing more dependence on the right internal jugular. ICP would likely increase markedly if there were a significant increase in right sided venous resistance. Additionally there would be no significant increase in ICP with ipsilateral compression. Thus we found no evidence for embarrassment of cerebral venous drainage due to JBC placement. The degree of ICP elevation with unilateral and bilateral venous compression, and the greater dependence on the right IJ for venous drainage is in agreement with previous studies in awake children without intracranial hypertension (Emery and Peabody, 1983; Grady et al. 1986).

The magnitude of ICP elevation during compression was not greater in those with intracranial hypertension compared to those without. This may be due to a lower cerebral blood flow and decreased venous drainage.

Conclusion

Jugular bulb catheterization and maintenance does not affect ICP.

References

Emery JR, Peabody JL (1983) Head position affects intracranial pressure in newborn infants. J Pediatr 103:950–953
Grady MS, Bedford RF, Park TS (1986) Changes in superior sagittal sinus pressure in children with head elevation, jugular venous compression, and PEEP. J Neurosurg 65:199–202

Jugular Bulb Catheterization in Children

M.G. Goetting and G. Preston

Department of Pediatrics, Henry Ford Hospital, 2799 West Grand Boulevard, Detroit, Michigan 48202 (USA)

The use of jugular bulb catheterization (JBC) in neurologically injured patients to monitor adequacy of cerebral blood flow and metabolism is increasing. However little is written about the technique, success rate and complications. We describe our method and the results of JBC in 60 consecutive children.

Methods

The patient is placed supine with the neck in a neutral position and the head slightly extended. The area from the mandible to below the clavicle is scrubbed with iodophor. The patient is draped leaving a window over one side of the neck. Local anesthetic is infiltrated into the proposed puncture site. For older children and adults the puncture site is at the level of the inferior border of the thyroid cartilage and slightly lateral to the common carotid artery. For small infants the puncture site is somewhat lower.

A 21 g needle is advanced at a 30 degree angle to the skin, aiming medial to the mastoid process. Gentle suction is applied to an attached syringe as the needle is advanced and withdrawn. A guidewire is inserted through the needle into the vein until resistance is met. The needle is withdrawn and the catheter is advanced over the guidewire cephalad until resistance is met. This should be approximately the distance from the mastoid process to the puncture site. The catheter is kept patent by a constant infusion of 2–3 cc per hour heparinized saline (1 unit/ml). The hub is sutured to the patient. Radiographic confirmation is obtained.

Data sheets were filled out prospectively on 60 consecutive patients. The insertion time is defined as beginning when the patient is prepped and draped and ending when the catheter has been secured with sutures.

Results

The median age was 6 years (range; 1 day to 21 years). All patients were successfully catheterized. Two patients failed the first attempt because of hypovolemic shock with jugular venous collapse and severe subcutaneous emphysema. Following volume resuscitation the first patient was easily catheterized two hours later.

The second patient was catheterized six hours later after some resolution of his emphysema.

The median number of skin punctures for successful JBC was 2 (range; 1 to 6). The median insertion time was 14 minutes (range; 6 to 35 min). Accidental arterial puncture occurred twice without sequelae. The catheter looped in the internal jugular vein or was in a venous branch in three patients, requiring catheter repositioning. The catheter was left in place for a mean duration of 57 hours range; 6 to 240 h). No catheter-related infections occurred.

Forty-four of the 66 patients survived their hospital course. None of the survivors showed evidence of injury to the phrenic or recurrent laryngeal nerves. There were no cases of Horner's syndrome.

Discussion

JBC in children has been previously reported. Swedlow et al. described their method in which the head is turned to the left and the direction of puncture is from the puncture site at mid-neck slightly lateral to the carotid artery toward the foramen magnum (Swedlow et al. 1981). They were successful in an older age group in 17 of 19 children. The carotid artery was punctured in three of 19. They reported no other complications. Our larger experience with a different method suggests our technique is superior, yielding a higher success and lower complication rate.

JBC insertion using our method is safer and has a higher success rate than internal jugular catheterization for central venous pressure (CVP) monitoring (English et al. 1969; Prince et al. 1976). Carotid artery puncture during CVP placement occurred in up to 23% of attempts. The success rate ranged between 77 and 91%.

Conclusion

JBC in children is a safe, rapid, and technically easy procedure.

References

English ICW, Frew RM, Pigott JF (1969) Percutaneous catheterization of the internal jugular vein. Anaesthesia 24:521–531
Prince SR, Sullivan RL, Hackel A (1976) Percutaneous catheterization of internal jugular vein in infants and children. Anesthesiology 44:170–174
Swedlow DB, Kettrick RG, Raphaely RC (1981) Crit Care Med 9:287

Transcardiac Method of Jugular Bulb Catheterization

M.G. Goetting and G. Preston

Department of Pediatrics, Henry Ford Hospital, 2799 West Grand Boulevard, Detroit, Michigan 48202 (USA)

The measurement of cerebral venous oxygen content obtained by jugular bulb catheterization (JBC) allows bedside assessment of adequacy of cerebral blood flow. The usual technique for JBC is by direct internal jugular vein (IJ) puncture and cannulation. Neck swelling from soft tissue injury, subcutaneous emphysema, burns or infection, spine trauma, and severe coagulopathy all are relative contraindications to direct IJ cannulation. Direct IJ puncture may prove difficult for the inexperienced operator in very small infants. We devised the transcardiac method via the femoral vein (FV) for the JBC (TCJBC) for the above conditions.

Materials and Methods

Twelve pediatric intensive care unit (PICU) patients aged 3 weeks to 14 months (Table 1) were selected for TCJBC during a 12 month period based on the need for JBC and the presence of contraindications to the direct route. Informed consent was obtained. An insertion protocol was followed and data concerning the technique was collected at the time of TCJBC on a specially formulated data sheet. The procedure time starts with skin preparation and concludes with suturing the catheter into position. Fluoroscopy time is the total time of exposure.

Table 1

Patient	Age	Diagnosis	Procedure time	Fluoroscopy time
1	3 wk	Encephalitis	18 min	0
2	3 wk	Meningitis	30 min	0
3	3 wk	Meningitis	22 min	0.3 min
4	1 mo	Encephalitis	28 min	2.0 min [a]
5	1 mo	Meningitis	30 min	1.5 min [a]
6	1 mo	Toxic encephalopathy	25 min	2.8 min
7	1 mo	Hypoxia/Ischemia	35 min	0
8	2 mo	Status epilepticus	26 min	0
9	3 mo	Meningitis	18 min	2.0 min [b]
10	3 mo	Hypoxia/Ischemia	20 min	0
11	8 mo	Hypoxia/Ischemia	20 min	0
12	14 mo	Head trauma	20 min	0

[a] failed without fluoroscopy; [b] first operator failed.

Protocol

The patient is monitored by continuous 3 lead electrocardiogram. The urinary bladder is catheterized. Sedation or neuromuscular blockade is administered if necessary. The child is supine with the hip externally rotated and the knee flexed. The inguinal area is scrubbed with iodophor and the patient is draped with sterile towels from the mastoid process to the knees. A 0.018 inch diameter, J-tipped, soft, stainless steel guidewire (Cook, Inc., Bloomington, IN, USA) is placed over the patient from the mastoid to the insertion site. A small hemostat clamped to the wire approximates the length of insertion. A 3 F polyethylene catheter (Cook, Inc., Bloomington, IN, USA) is likewise marked by lightly crimping the catheter with a hemostat.

A 21 g stainless steel needle is introduced into the FV percutaneously and the guidewire is threaded into the vein through the needle. The guidewire is advanced the estimated length and an additional 2–3 centimeters until resistance is met unless a cardiac arrhythmia is detected or premature resistance is met. If either arrhythmia or premature resistance occurs the wire is withdrawn into the FV and advanced again. Fluoroscopy is used following three failures of the blind technique.

The catheter is advanced over the guidewire to the point of the crimp and a small additional distance until resistance is met. The guidewire is withdrawn, blood is aspirated from the catheter hub, and the catheter is flushed with heparinized saline. If no blood can be aspirated the catheter is withdrawn 2–3 millimeters at a time until free flow occurs. The catheter is sutured in place and a continuous flush (1 unit heparin/ml 0.9 NS) of 3 ml/hour is delivered to maintain patency.

A single film cassette is placed under the patient extending from the groin to the ear, the head is rotated away from the side of insertion and a single X-ray will confirm proper placement. If head or neck injury precludes head rotation a cross-table lateral x-ray of the skull will adequately demonstrate catheter position.

Results

Twelve patients underwent TCJBC. Blind attempts were successful in 7/9 cases; two failed the blind technique due to repeated premature resistance. The two failures were cannulated using fluoroscopy. Three additional patients were cannulated under fluoroscopy following fluoroscopy guided pulmonary artery or right atrial catheterization. The blind approach was not attempted due to the potential difficulty of passing a second catheter over the existing one in the central circulation and the immediate availability of fluoroscopy.

No arrhythmias occurred during the procedure. All catheters remained patent (28.5 patient days). There were no other complications.

Discussion

Percutaneous cannulation of the central circulation via the FV is a common PICU procedure performed without fluoroscopy. Advantages of using the FV route include ease of stabilization and the ability to control hematoma formation by direct pressure. The catheter-related infection rate is the same as or lower than for other sites. Vascular complications are uncommon in children at this as well as other site (Kanter et al. 1986; Stenzel et al. 1987).

When we began performing JBC the transcardiac approach was chosen frequently. Our technical skills have improved to the point that very small patients, poor landmarks, and coagulopathy do not preclude direct JBC.

Conclusion

Candidates for TCJBC include patients with neck, trauma, subcutaneous emphysema, severe coagulopathy, and those who have failed the direct approach. TCJBC appears to be a safe, practical alternative to direct JBC.

References

Kanter RK, Zimmerman JJ et al. (1986) Central venous catheter insertion by femoral vein: Safety and effectiveness for the pediatric patient. Pediatrics 77:842–847
Stenzel JP, Carlson PE et al. (1987) Complications of femoral venous catheters in a pediatric population: Prospective study. Crit Care Med 15:359

Dynamic Pressure Volume Index via ICP Waveform Analysis

Z. Gokaslan, R.S. Bray, A.M. Sherwood, C.S. Robertson, R.K. Narayan, C.F. Contant, and R.G. Grossman

Department of Neurosurgery, Baylor College of Medicine, 6501 Fannin, Suite A-404, Houston 77030, Texas (USA)

Introduction

Intracranial pressure (ICP) monitoring is used as an early sign of neurological deterioration in the management of patients with a variety of neurosurgical conditions. Mean ICP is the most commonly used for this purpose; however, mean ICP is a relatively late indicator of many secondary injury processes, and neurological deterioration may occur in the presence of normal ICP.

Intracranial compliance (ICC) has been proposed to be an earlier and more sensitive indicator than ICP of impending neurological deterioration due to cerebral edema or mass lesions (Sullivan et al. 1977). Volume Pressure Response (VPR) and Pressure Volume Index (PVI) are the two commonly used methods for the expression of ICC. PVI is the volume that would have to be added to the intracranial contents to raise the mean ICP tenfold.

In clinical practice, however, the risk of infection and fear of inducing dangerous increases in ICP have prevented widespread use of VPR or PVI, since both require volumetric manipulation of the closed CSF system. In addition, the intermittent nature of the measurements limit the ability to detect rapidly changing processes early.

A system has been developed (Trinity Computing, Houston, Texas, USA) for on-line continuous monitoring of intracranial compliance by a computerized analysis of the ICP waveform (Bray et al. 1976). The system is based on the hypothesis that with each cardiac cycle, blood flows through the brain in a pulsatile fashion, creating the ICP waveform (Cardoso et al. 1983). Much like any other physical system, when struck by an input force, the brain "rings" with a characteristic vibrational pattern that is represented in the ICP waveform. As the brain becomes less compliant because of edema or a mass lesion, these characteristic vibrations occur at a higher frequency.

The purpose of this study was to determine if computerized ICP waveform analysis could accurately estimate the PVI and if it could have a clinical applicability to monitor cerebral compliance continuously.

Method

Between July 1984 and June 1985, PVI measurements and computerized analyses of the ICP waveform were obtained from 22 patients admitted to the NICU who required continuous ICP monitoring.

The ICP and waveform analysis recordings were begun as soon after placement of the ICP monitor as possible, often within six hours, and continued for as long as the ICP monitor was in place. The ICP monitor was calibrated according to the usual NICU routine by the bedside nurse. The ICP computer was calibrated every eight hours. Proper calibration of the computerized ICP trend recordings was confirmed by comparing the pressures to the ICP recorded hourly by the bedside nurse. Segments of the recordings in which there was a discrepancy between the pressure values were not included in the final analysis.

The ICP was recorded from a ventriculostomy or a Camino fiberoptic catheter on a Space Labs patient monitor. The EKG and ICP analog signals from the monitor were directed to the analog-to-digital converter of an IBM PC-XT computer. The EKG was used for timing purposes. The ICP and EKG data were acquired beginning with the QRS complex at 100 samples per second per channel for 256 points. The ICP waveform was analyzed for artifact and for drift of the baseline.

To quantitate subtle changes in the brain's vibrational characteristics, each satisfactory ICP waveform acquired by the computer was analyzed individually by the discrete Fourier transform (DFT) (Fig. 1). Over 1.5 million DFT waveform analyses were performed. For purposes of this analysis, the ICP waveform was assumed to result from the summation of a large number of sinusoidal waves, each with a different power. The ICP waveform, as it is acquired by the computer, represents the intracranial pressure as a function of time. The Fourier transform converts the time axis, or domain, to a frequency axis, so that the function is now one of the frequency, or pitch, of the pressure wave. The ordinate becomes the

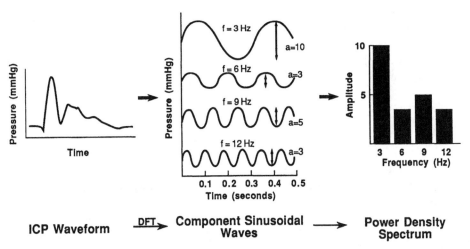

Fig. 1. ICP waveform analysis

power of the pressure wave at a particular frequency. That is, the ordinate indicates the contribution of the frequency indicated on the abscissa to the total waveform.

The goal of the Fourier transform analysis is to detect shifts in the power spectrum of the ICP waveform which would indicate changes in the physical characteristics of the brain.

It was found in earlier studies that shifts within the frequency range of 4 to 15 Hz reflected changes in the vibrational characteristics of the brain (Bray et al. 1976). To describe these frequency shifts, the center of balance of the power within the 4 to 15 Hz range was calculated; this value is the High Frequency Centroid (HFC).

PVI measurements were obtained by injecting or withdrawing a known volume of fluid into the CSF system and recording the changes in mean ICP. The PVI was calculated as:

$$PVI\ (ml) = \frac{\Delta V}{\log \frac{PI}{PF}}$$

where ΔV = the volume of fluid injected or withdrawn, PI = the initial mean ICP, and PF = the final mean ICP. By this method, the normal PVI value is 26 ± 4 ml. Although a PVI of 18 or less is considered pathological, 13 is the critical value, indicating near exhaustion of the volumetric compensatory mechanism (Shapiro et al. 1980).

All patients were treated by a standard protocol that emphasized early surgical evacuation of intracranial hematomas, controlled ventilation, and monitoring of intracranial pressure. Routine medications included phenytoin, morphine for sedation, and antibiotics. Intracranial pressures greater than 20 mm Hg were treated with hyperventilation, CSF drainage, sedation and paralysis, mannitol, and if necessary, barbiturates.

Clinical data, including age, sex, initial Glasgow Coma Score (GCS), type of injury, and Glasgow Outcome Score (GOS) at three months following the injury, were obtained on all patients.

Two measurements of intracranial compliance, the PVI and HFC values, were compared by regression analysis. Samples of the ICP waveform were stored to demonstrate if changes in compliance correlated to alterations of the HFC and to the overall shape of the ICP wave.

Results

Ninety (90) PVI values were available for correlation with the HFC values. The HFC values demonstrated an excellent inverse relationship to the PVI values ($r = 0.94$, $p < 0.01$).

Patients with uncomplicated courses typically had HFC values that were only moderately elevated (7.5–8.0 Hz), or elevated above 8.5–9.0 Hz only transiently during the first 24 hours following injury.

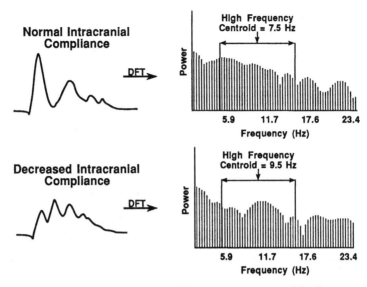

Fig. 2. Intracranial compliance and high frequency centroid values

Alterations in HFC were noted to start either in the form of abrupt elevations or gradual increases from the baseline prior to neurosurgical emergencies such as intracranial hematomas or cerebral edema. Especially with the abrupt HFC changes, neurological deterioration followed within a few hours. Thus, continuous monitoring of compliance appears to have potential as an early warning system for identifying neurosurgical emergencies. ICP waveform samples collected during the recording and corresponding HFC values were compared to determine if the changes in ICC as measured by the PVI would indeed cause alterations in the HFC and ICP waveform.

In a patient with normal compliance (Fig. 2), the ICP wave had prominent early and more subtle late components. These are reflected in the relatively low HFC value of 7.4 Hz. In the waveform of a patient with decreased cerebral compliance, there is a loss of prominent early components, and a correspondingly higher HFC value of 9.5 Hz. This confirms that subtle and rapid changes in the ICP waveform and PVI can be detected instantly with on-line continuous monitoring of intracranial compliance by computerized analysis of the ICP waveform. Detection of these changes would be delayed with intermittent measurements of the PVI.

Conclusions

ICP waveforms can be broken down into their frequency components by computerized fast Fourier transform analysis; the center of balance of the power within the 4–15 Hz range (the HFC) shows an excellent relationship to the PVI.

Computerized ICP waveform analysis may provide a means of monitoring intracranial compliance continuously without the risk of infection or sudden alterations in the ICP due to manipulation of the closed CSF system.

References

Bray RS, Sherwood AM, Halter JA, Robertson C, Grossman RG (1976) Development of a clinical monitoring system by means of ICP waveform analysis. In: Miller JD, Teasdale GM, Rowan JO, Galbraith SL, Mendelow AD (eds) Intracranial pressure VI. Springer, Berlin Heidelberg New York Tokyo, pp 260–264

Cardoso ER, Rowan JO, Galbraith S (1983) Analysis of the cerebrospinal fluid pulse wave in intracranial pressure. J Neurosurg 59:817–821

Shapiro ER, Marmarou A, Schulman K (1980) Characterization of clinical CSF dynamics and neurol axis compliance using the pressure-volume index. Ann Neurol 7:508–514

Sullivan HG, Miller JD, Becker DP, Flora RE, Allen GA (1977) The physiological basis of intracranial pressure change with progressive epidural brain compression. J Neurosurg 47:532–539

Single Pulse Pressure Wave Analysis by Fast Fourier Transformation

L. Christensen [1] and S.E. Børgesen [2]

[1] Department of Neurosurgery, University Hospital, and [2] University Clinic of Neurosurgery, DK-2100 Copenhagen (Denmark)

The Fast Fourier Transformation (FFT) is a useful tool in analyzing waveforms (Bracewell 1965).

The PPW is a periodic function of time $f(t)$, and as such can be transformed according to the Fourier theorem (Fig. 1).

$$f(t) = \frac{1}{2} a_0 + \sum_{n=1}^{\infty} (a_n \times \cos(nwt) + b_n \times \sin(nwt))$$

$$A_n = SQRT(a_n^2 + b_n^2)$$

a_n and b_n:	Fourier coefficients for $n=1$ to ∞
A_n:	Amplitude of the nth harmony
T:	Period of the function $f(t)$
w:	Angular frequency
a_0:	Mean of the original wave

Fig. 1

Materials and Method

114 pressure recordings of different pressure levels were obtained from 20 patients during tests for measurement of CSF dynamics. A sequence of about 20 to 70 pulse pressure waves (PPW) at stable pressure levels was analyzed by a computer program developed for Fast Fourier Transformation (FFT) (Cooley and Tukey, 1965; Stanley and Peterson, 1978). Mean ICP (MICP), Pulse Amplitude (PA), and Rise Time coefficient (RT).

Sampling frequency was adjusted automatically by the pulse rate to yield approximately 256 values per pulse pressure wave, as the FFT required 2^n values per wave.

MICP was computed as the mean of these 256 values, and therefore represents the true Mean ICP.

PA is the difference between the systolic and diastolic pressure level.

Pearson correlation was performed on the data from the rising part of the pulse pressure wave to calculate the RT equal to the slope of the regression line.

For each sequence the means of the Fourier coefficients, MICP, PA and RT were computed.

Results

The aim of this investigation was to find possible parallel changes in the Fourier spectrum and PA, RT and ICP as the ICP was elevated.

With a sampling frequency of 256/PPW, it can be shown that only the first half of these, i.e., 128 are meaningful. The second half of the harmonies are exactly equal to the first.

In the actual analysis of the PPW we found that only harmonies No. 1 to 9 were of significant size (Fig. 2).

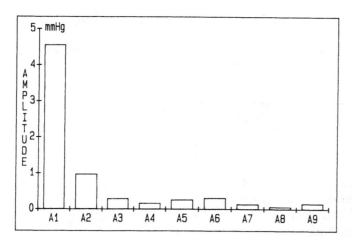

Fig. 2. The amplitude of the 9 most significant harmonies (A1 to A9) from the Fourier transformation

The correlation between the a_0 of the FFT and the MICP was highly significant ($r=0.99$, $p<0.001$).

There was also significant correlation between the amplitude A_1 of the 1. harmony and the PA ($r=0.99$, $p<0.001$).

The RT increased with both MICP ($r=0.70$, $p<0.001$) and PA ($r=0.81$, $p<0.001$). RT also increased with amplitudes of the 5th, a_5 ($r=0.73$, $p<0.001$) and the 6th harmony a_6 ($r=0.78$, $p<0.001$).

Discussion

We found a good correlation between the a_0 and MICP. The Fourier theorem defines a_0 as the mean of the function under investigation. This finding, per se, is therefore a confirmation of the assumption that the PPW is in fact suitable for the FFT. The close correlation between the amplitude of the 1st harmony and the PA indicates that PPW is mainly composed of low frequency components, because the amplitude of the 1st harmony is the most significant in the Fourier spectrum of the PPW.

The amplitude of the higher harmonies increased with increasing RT of the PPW because waves with abrupt changes are composed of more high frequency components than waves with slower changes.

In our investigation RT increased by increasing PA. This explains why the amplitudes of the lower harmonies also increases by increasing RT.

There is a correlation between low frequency components and cerebral blood flow and high frequency components and pressure volume index (PVI) (Bray et al. 1986).

Others found that Fourier transformation of PPW might identify a critical point of ICP and cerebral perfusion pressure (Takizawa et al. 1987).

The conclusions of our investigations are that the PPW is suitable for FFT. The PPW is mostly composed of low-frequency, slowly changing waves, but with increasing ICP and RT more high-frequency components are present.

We think that further investigations are needed to show if the FFT is a powerful tool for investigations of the compliance of the brain, either in traumatic, hydrocephalic, or other high-pressure states.

Acknowledgements. Supported by the Danish "Foundation for Experimental Research in Neurology", and "Foundation of Managing Director Jacob Madsen and Olga Madsen".

References

Bracewell R (1965) The Fourier transform and its applications. McGraw-Hill, New York
Bray RS et al. (1986) Development of a clinical monitoring system by means of ICP waveform analysis. Intracranial pressure VI. Springer, Berlin Heidelberg New York Tokyo, pp 260–264
Cooley JW, Tukey JW (1965) An algorithm for the machine calculation of complex Fourier series. Math Computation 19:297–301
Stanley WD, Peterson SJ (1978) Fast Fourier Transforms on your home computer. Byte 12:14–25
Takizawa H et al. (1987) Changes in the cerebrospinal fluid pulse wave spectrum associated with raised intracranial pressure. Neurosurgery 20:355–361

A Minicomputer System for Analysis and Display of ICP Related Data

K. Hara, S. Nakatani, K. Ozaki, and H. Mogami

Department of Neurosurgery, Osaka University Medical School, 1-1-50 Fukushima, Osaka and Sharp Corp., Osaka 533 (Japan)

Introduction

It has been suggested that analog data recording of ICP on paper does not provide enough information on the real condition of the patient, making further data processing impossible. Several microcomputer systems have been reported recently, that deal only with fragmental portions of the intracranial pressure dynamics. With a minicomputer we developed a total system of comprehensible color graphic display and digital printing of ICP related data, creating a new technique and improving the algorithms of sampling and analysis already reported.

Methods

ICP was measured in patients and cats through a catheter inserted into the lumbar subarachnoid space, connected to a pressure transducer (Statham-Gould Db 23) and recorded with a polygraph (Nihon Kohden RM-6000) and a data recorder (TEAC-30). Transcranial Doppler (TCD) ultrasound of the middle cerebral artery was detected with an EME TC2-64. The ICP and TCD data were processed by a minicomputer (Data General Desktop Generation, Model 30) with a software program we developed. The results were displayed on a color graphic terminal (Hask CGX-4).

Results and Discussion

Using fast Fourier transform (FFT) this system achieved the following:

1. Continuous display of BP (systolic, diastolic, mean), ICP (systolic, diastolic, mean) and CPP (Gaab et al. 1986).
2. Histogram display and digital printing for every 30 minutes of data of BP, ICP, CPP.
3. Display and printing of the power spectrum of ICP, using FFT for detection of B-waves. ICP including B-waves was sampled every 8 seconds. Results of

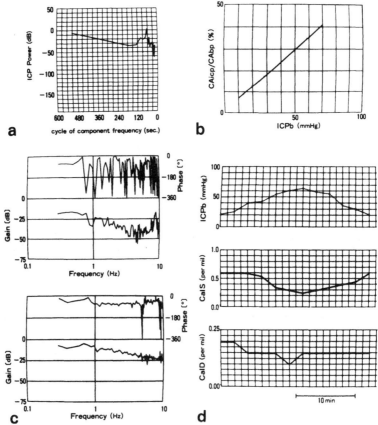

Fig. 1. a Graphic display of the power spectrum of B-waves. *Ordinate:* ICP power in dB. *Abscissa:* Time in seconds. **b** Relationship between the quotient cardiac induced component of ICP (CAicp)/cardiac induced component of BP (CAbp) (*Ordinate* in%) and the basic level of ICP (ICPb) (*Abscissa* in mm Hg). **c** Transfer function (XFR). (*Ordinate:* gain in dB and phase in 0. *Abscissa:* frequency in Hz). *Upper panel:* XFR during baseline ICP. *Lower panel:* XFR during increased ICP. **d** Trendgraph of ICP (*upper panel*), CaIs (*middle*) and CaID (*lower panel*). (*Upper ordinate* in mm Hg, *middle* and *lower ordinates* in per mil, *Abscissa* in min)

FFT are shown in Fig. 1 a as a graphic display. The power spectrum shows a peak exceeding dB at around 60 sec which corresponds to the B-wave frequency. Analysis of various recordings of ICP with or without B-waves revealed that a B-wave peak was identified in the power spectrum whenever ICP included B-waves, and never without B-waves, indicating that a power spectral peak above dB, between 30 and 120 sec is the criterion for B-wave detection.

4. Detection of A waves to distinguish them from steadily rising ICP.
5. A measure of intracranial compliance (Cic). Using FFT analysis Cic could be monitored continuously in real time including: (a) Display of the relationship between the standard deviation of the ICP amplitude and the mean value of ICP (Szewczykowski et al. 1977); (b) Display of the relationship between

CAicp, RAicp and ICPb (Brawanski et al. 1983); (c) Trendgraph of CAicp and RAicp; (d) Display of the quotients CAicp/CAbp and RAicp/RAbp and their relationships to ICPb. (CAicp/CAbp increased until CPb reached around 70 mm Hg, whereas RAicp/RAbp decreased at ICPb higher than 40 mm Hg in a cat during hydrostatic pressure loading (Fig. 1 b); and (e) Calculation of the transfer function (XFR) Chopp et al. (1980) defining BP as an input and ICP as an output by FFT. The phase shifts between 1 and 10 Hz were widely distributed and the gain was about -40 dB during baseline ICP (Fig. 1 c, upper panel). The distribution of the phase shift between 1 and 10 Hz was narrow and the gain was about -16 dB during increased ICP (Fig. 1 c, lower panel). Transmission of pressure from within the blood vessels to the intracranial cavity increased with a rising ICPb.

6. A measure of arterial compliance (Ca): Trendgraph of CaIS ($=$ HFpp/2 MHz) and CaID (LFpp/2 MHz).

Doppler signals were analyzed by FFT and the frequencies with maximum power in peal systolic (HFpp) and in end-diastolic (LFpp) were extracted from a power spectrum array of a single ultrasound velocity wave. 2 MHz was the oscillation frequency of the ultrasound transmitter.

During initiation of the A wave, CAIS decreased when ICP reached about 40 mm Hg and increased as the ICP decreased (Fig. 1 d, middle). CaID decreased from a lower level of ICP than CaIS, with more sensitivity than that of CaIS and remained low even when ICP decreased (Fig. 1 d, lower panel).

These results indicate that the trendgraph of CaIS and caID may be useful in estimating arterial compliance.

Summary

This presentation of ICP related data, processed with a minicomputer, provides the basis for studying intracranial pathophysiology and seeking objective evaluations of better treatment modalities.

References

Brawanski A, Gaab MR, Heissler HE (1983) Computer-Analysis of ICP-Modulations. In: Ishii S, Nagai H, Brock M (eds) Intracranial pressure V. Springer, Berlin Heidelberg New York Tokyo, pp 186–190

Chopp M, Portnoy HD (1980) System analysis of intracranial pressure. J Neurosurg 53:516 –527

Gaab MR, Ottens M, Busche F et al. (1986) Routine computerized neuromonitoring. In: Miller JD, Teasdale GM, Rowan JO, Galbraith SL, Mendelow AD (eds) Intracranial pressure VI. Springer, Berlin Heidelberg New York Tokyo, pp 240–247

Szewczykowski J, Sliwka S, Kunicki A et al. (1977) A fast method of estimating the elastance of the intracranial system. J Neurosurg 47:19–26

Modified Auditory Brainstem Responses (MABR) in Patients with Intracranial Lesions

J.L. Stone, R.F. Ghaly, K.S. Subramanian, and P. Roccaforte

Division of Neurosurgery, Departments of Surgery and Anesthesiology, Cook County and University of Illinois Hospitals, 1835 W. Harrison Street, Chicago, Illinois 60612 (USA)

The standard auditory brainstem response (ABR) has not been reported as useful in detecting patients with intracranial lesions and mild or moderately increased intracranial pressure (ICP) within the ranges frequently encountered clinically (Goitein et al. 1983; Stone et al. 1988). The present investigation was designed to enhance the sensitivity of ABR testing in this patient population.

Methods

A standard ABR at two intensities (75 and 110 dB pe SPL) and a modified ABR (MABR) were performed in 106 consecutive patients with CT scan suspected (67) or surgically recorded (39) of increased ICP. MABR is a rapid rate (70/sec) binaural ABR performed at four different stimulus intensities (85, 75, 72, and 65 dB). Latency and amplitude, versus stimulus intensity function of wave V of the MABR were studied as were various latency (3SD) and amplitude (2SD) parameters of the ABR and MABR. Instrumentation and technical parameters were identical for pathologic and non-pathologic groups. The patient population was classified according to the etiology of elevated ICP into two groups; head trauma (56 patients, 53%), and non-trauma (50 patients, 47%). The non-trauma etiology was brain tumor in 22 cases, spontaneous hemorrhage in 13 cases, hydrocephalus in 11, and pseudotumor in 4.

Results

Most patients had mental status changes and 29% had a Glasgow Coma Score of 8 or less. Recorded ICP was predominately in the 16–25 mm Hg range. The MABR was abnormal in 88% (93 patients), whereas ABR was abnormal in less than one-half (49%) of patients. The standard ABR was normal in 45% of patients with an abnormal MABR. No case was noted to have a normal MABR and an abnormal ABR. Abnormality of MABR wave V latency/intensity function was the commonest finding (75% of cases). Diminished wave V amplitude was seen in 62% of cases and prolonged latency in 42%. Twenty one percent with an abnormal MABR had only a latency/intensity abnormality without significant latency or amplitude changes. Analysis of variance with repeated measures (ANOVA) demonstrated a significant difference ($p < 0.05$) between the normative group and patient population (trauma and non-trauma) regarding MABR wave V latency/intensity and amplitude/intensity functions. Twenty-six of forty patients (65%) showed clear improvement or normalization of the MABR following surgical and/or medical treatment. Since MABR testing requires about 10 minutes to perform, in addition to the standard ABR, and improves the sensitivity of ABR in patients with intracranial lesions and mild to moderately increased ICP further investigation of this non-invasive approach is warranted.

References

Goitein KJ, Fainmesse P, Sohmer H (1983) The relationship between cerebral perfusion pressure and auditory nerve brainstem evoked responses – diagnostic and prognostic implications. In: Ishii S, Nagai H, Brock M (eds) Intracranial pressure V. Springer, Berlin Heidelberg New York Tokyo, pp 468–473
Stone JL, Ghaly RF, Hughes JR (1988) Evoked potentials in head injury and states of increased intracranial pressure. J Clin Neurophysiol 5:135–160

Detection of the Site of V-P Shunt Malfunction Using a Telemetric IVP Sensor

T. Ohta, M. Yamashita, H. Miyake, S. Tsuzawa, H. Tanabe, M. Shiguma, K. Osaka, I. Sakaguchi, and S. Yokoyama

Department of Neurosurgery, Osaka Medical School, 2-7 Daigaku-cho, Takatsuki City, Osaka 569 (Japan)

Introduction

We have already reported the clinical applicability of our implantable IVP sensor at the 5th ICP Symposium (Osaka et al. 1980; 1983). Since then, the instrument has been improved and we have gained much clinical experience. We report a brief outline of our new sensor, meter, standard operative procedure, and some clinical applications.

Outline of the Sensory and Meter

Our IVP sensor (Fig. 1) is small, 13 mm high, 14 mm in diameter, and 7 g in weight, and can be used in the line up of a V-P shunt system. Table 1 shows the specifications of the sensor and meter. IVP is transmitted to the ferrite core placed on the bellows and the movement of the ferrite core changes the resonant frequency of the L-C circuit (coil and capacitor) in the sensory. This change is measured telemetrically by a grid dip of the probe 50 times per second, so pulse waves can

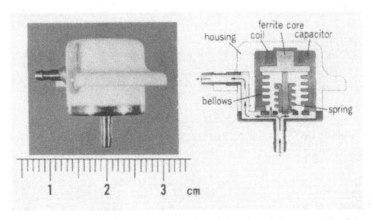

Fig. 1. The IVP sensor, an outside appearance and a sectioned drawing. It is easy and painless to measure IVP at the bedside (measurement in mm)

Table 1. Specifications of the IVP sensor and meter

Pressure range	$-25 \sim +75$ mm Hg (gauge pressure)
Accuracy	$\pm 1.5\%$ F.S.
Temperature error	$\pm 0.2\%$ F.S./deg.
Linearity	$\pm 0.5\%$ F.S. $(0 \sim +75$ mm Hg)
	$\pm 1.0\%$ F.S. $(-25-0$ mm Hg)
Repeatability	$\pm 0.5\%$ F.S.
Hysteresis	0.3% F.S.
Sensitivity	0.2 mm Hg
Limit of atmospheric pressure (Sensor)	$964 \sim 1072$ mb
Limit of atmospheric pressure	$850 \sim 1180$ mb
Limit of temperature	$5 \sim 40\,°C$
Weight (meter)	7 grams
Sampling frequency	50 times/second
Power	A C 100 V $\pm 10\%$, 50/60 Hz, 50 VA
Power output	D C $-0.25 \sim +0.75$ V or $-2.5 \sim +7.5$ V
	(F.S.; Full Scale)

be detected. The effect of atmospheric change on IVP is corrected by a built-in barometer, and this corrected value of IVP (gauge pressure) is displayed on a DC output terminal.

Clinical Applications

The V-P shunt should be done with a frontal horn puncture and an on-off flushing reservoir (on-off valve) on the chest. The outer table of the skull is drilled to inset the sensor and a groove is made for the peritoneal connector of the sensor to avoid tearing the peritoneal catheter. IVP is measured through the scalp by application of the probe over the implanted sensor.

In a well-functioning shunt, especially with tilting the body, IVP decreased to negative pressure and pulse pressure reduced after opening the valve (Fig. 2). This negative pressure is caused partly by the siphon effect. Some patients showed subdural fluid collection (SFC) after a V-P shunt all of whom had extreme negative IVP pressure in a sitting or upright position. The low intracranial pressure syndrome was present in them. Adjusting the fine on-off valve control and regulating body position based on IVP values were performed. The SFC disappeared after this procedure.

When the patient showed symptoms of shunt malfunction and ventricular dilatation on CT scan, recordings of the IVP and reactions to on-off valve pumpings showed three types of malfunctions.

Case Y.N. (Fig. 3A): This is a case of ventricular catheter obstruction. Pulse waves are not seen because ventricular fluid pressure is not conducted to the sensor. Among well functioning cases, however, slit ventricles may show no pulse wave as the catheter is caught between tiny ventricular walls and pulse waves cannot be conducted directly through the catheter. In slit ventricle cases, pulse waves appear and the IVP value increases gradually after the valve is turned off. This IVP

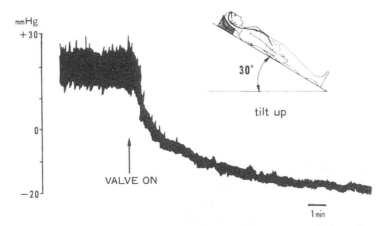

Fig. 2. A case of well functioning V-P shunt; IVP decreased to negative pressure and also pulse pressure reduced after opening the valve, with tilting up position

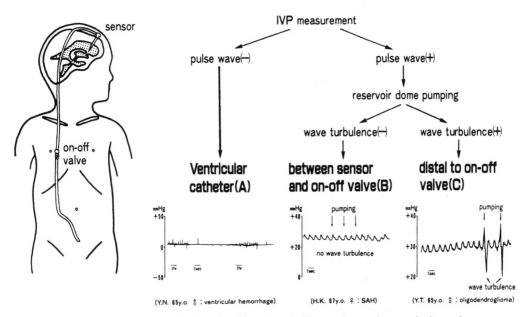

Fig. 3. Flow chart detecting the site of malfunction. **A** Obstruction at the ventricular catheter; pulse wave cannot be seen. **B** Trouble between the sensory and on-off valve; pulse waves are seen but without "wave turbulence". **C** Malfunction site is distal to the on-off valve; pulse waves and "wave turbulences" are seen

recording provides useful information about the slit ventricle syndrome to supplement the clinical situation and the CT scan.

Case H.K. (Fig. 3 B): This record shows malfunction between the IVP sensor and the on-off valve. Pumping the reservoir dome of the on-off valve makes no change of the wave form, because there is no conduction of pressure from the on-off valve to the sensor through the catheter. In these cases, trouble is mostly caused by either a disconnection or tearing peritoneal catheter.

Case Y.T. (Fig. 3 C): The third type shows a normal wave form which has pulse waves and "wave turbulence", a term we use for a marked biphasic wave seen during pumping of the reservoir dome. Presence of this wave suggests communication between the sensor and the on-off valve. Thus, in a case of shunt malfunction with both a normal wave form and "wave turbulence", the malfunction site is probably distal to the on-off valve. Trouble from the lower peritoneal catheter (the catheter distal to the on-off valve) may be due to disconnection or obstruction, especially at the distal end of the catheter.

Discussion

One clinical application of our IVP meter is prevention of some postoperative complications of a V-P shunt. Our sensor can reveal the chronological change of IVP and even negative pressure (Fig. 2). IVP, particularly negative, is influenced by both positional and siphon effects of the shunt (Chapman et al. 1986). IVP recordings show disappearance of the siphon effect by turning off the on-off valve. In some shunted patients, excessive reduction of IVP after shunt operation may cause a low intracranial pressure syndrome and subdural hematoma (Portnoy et al. 1973; McCullough et al. 1974). It is valuable to measure and adjust IVP by controlling the on-off valve and the patient's position to prevent such complications.

Another clinical application is the detection of the site of V-P shunt malfunction by following the flow chart (Fig. 3) as follows:

At first, IVP is measured. The absence of pulse waves suggests ventricular catheter obstruction (Case Y.N.). When pulse waves are present, the reservoir dome of the on-off valve is pumped next. If no "wave turbulence" is observed with this maneuver, the malfunction site is between the IVP sensory and on-off valve (Case H.K.), whereas the presence of "wave turbulence" indicates obstruction distal to the on-off valve (Case Y.T.). These procedures provide a non-invasive diagnosis and minimal operative revisions.

Conclusion

If the V-P shunt is overfunctioning, it should be regulated and the on-off valve and patient's position controlled on the basis of IVP values. This procedure prevents some complications of the V-P shunt.

When the V-P shunt is not functioning, we are able to diagnose the site of malfunction using the IVP sensor along the flow chart. Accurate and quick diagnosis is possible by this non-invasive way even in the outpatient clinic.

References

Chapman PH et al. (1986) The effect of position on ventricular pressure in shunted and unshunted individuals. A telemetric study. In: Miller JD, Teasdale GM, Rowan JO, Galbraith SL, Mendelow AD (eds) Intracranial pressure VI. Springer, Berlin Heidelberg New York Tokyo, pp 213–217

McCullough DC, Fox JL (1974) Negative intracranial pressure hydrocephalus in adults with shunts and its relationship to the production of subdural hematoma. J Neurosurg 40:372 −375

Osaka K, Ohta T (1980) Limits of various methods for evaluation of shunt function, and development of new intracranial pressure meter incorporated in the shunt system. Neurol Surg (Tokyo) 8:811−817

Osaka K et al. (1983) Experiences with a New Telemetric Pressure Meter. In: Ishii S, Nagai H, Brock M (eds) Intracranial pressure V. Springer, Berlin Heidelberg New York Tokyo, pp 131−134

Portnoy HD, Shulte RR, Fox JL et al. (1973) Anti-siphon and reversible occlusion valves for shunting in hydrocephalus and preventing post-shunt subdural hematomas. J Neurosurg 38:729−738

Relationship of Intracranial Pressure Changes to CT Changes in Children

S.S. Kasoff[1], A.S. Mednick[1], D. Leslie[2], M. Tenner[2], P. Sane[2], J. Mangiardi[1], and T.A. Lansen[1]

Departments of Neurosurgery[1], and Radiology[2], New York Medical College, Valhalla, New York 10595 (USA)

Several studies have been published that attempted to determine if any correlations exist between elevated intracranial pressure (ICP) (Lobato et al. 1979; Narayan et al. 1982), as occurs in acute head trauma, and morphological changes in the brain, as determined by examining computed tomography scans (CTs) (Sadhu et al. 1979; Fasol et al. 1980; Haar et al. 1980; Papo et al. 1980). These studies, however, examined primarily adult head trauma. Thus, the purpose of this study was to determine if such correlations exist between ICP and CT in pediatric head trauma. We sought to correlate changes on the initial CTs of children that could serve as reliable predictors of raised intracranial pressure.

We studied the CTs of 60 children who presented with evidence of cerebral dysfunction compelling enough to warrant monitoring with an epidural intracranial pressure monitor. Criteria for inclusion into the study were a Glasgow coma score of 8 or less and an ICP measurement obtained within 1 hr of the CT. Thirty five of the 60 children (17 mos. – 18 years of age; mean – 11.0 yrs.) examined fulfilled the criteria. All patients had sustained acute head trauma. The CT variables examined were focal and diffuse mass effect, hydrocephalus, midline shift, and bicaudate and ventricular distances and ratios.

Mass effect is considered to be diffuse when general sulcal effacement or ventricular compression were seen. Determination of mass effect can be difficult in children, in whom sulci and ventricles are normally quite small. Thus, mass effect has a subjective component, when unassociated with low attenuation changes, such as occurs with contusion or edema, or with focal hyperdensity, such as occurs with intra- or extra-axial hematoma.

The midline shift was determined by measuring the maximum width of the brain, between the inner tables, dividing this distance by 2, and determining the distance between this midline and structures in question, e.g., septum pellucidum. Clinical experience has taught us that midline shift in acute head trauma is abnormal only when it is greater than 3.5 mm.

Bicaudate and ventricular ratios were measured, seeking an objective criterion of ventricular deformity. The bicaudate ratio was determined by dividing the distance between the caudate nuclei at their midportions by the transverse width of the brain at that level between the inner tables. The ventricular ratio was determined by dividing the widest distance between the lateral tips of the frontal horns by the transverse width of the brain at that level.

In addition to these 35 patients, an additional 42 children served as age-matched controls; these children presented with CTs that showed no evidence of raised ICP (i.e., patients with psychiatric illness or seizure) and did not sustain acute head trauma. These children had normal CTs, never received ICP monitors, and are presumed to have normal ICP.

The CT variables were examined alone and in different combinations, using a 3×5 (patient group [Groups I, II; Controls] $\times$ CT variables [focal or diffuse mass effects; hydrocephalus; midline shift; bicaudate ratio; ventricular ratio] examined) two-way analysis of variance, with square-root transformation and tested for homogeneity of variance. Appropriate post-hoc comparisons were then made to determine the source of any significant findings. We also subjected the same data to a nonparametric test, the Wilcox rank sum test.

Eleven of the 35 patients died and had a mean ICP of 53.7 mm Hg (SE = 10.9). The surviving 24 patients had a significantly lower ($P < 0.05$) ICP (mean = 15.2 mm Hg; SE = 2.7). The results of all 35 patients were included in the data analysis.

One combination of abnormalities was found to be a significant predictor of raised ICP, allowing us to divide the patients into two logical study groups. Group I consisted of patients with a midline shift of less than 3.5 mm. Group II consisted of patients with a midline shift of greater than 3.5 mm. Predictably, all patients in this second group had evidence of focal or diffuse mass effect.

Our results indicate no significant difference ($P > 0.05$) in ICP comparing patients with and without hydrocephalus. Similarly, the bicaudate ratio and ventricular ratio failed to show a significant difference in ICP when comparing patients with ICP of greater than 20 mm Hg (upper limit of normal) to those with ICP of less than 20 mm Hg. Furthermore, there was no significant difference in the bicaudate and ventricular ratios in the study groups versus the controls. Hydrocephalus and the measurements of the lateral ventricles were not found to be significant indicators of raised ICP, even in combination with other factors. However, patients with focal or diffuse mass effect, associated with a midline shift of greater than 3.5 mm had significantly ($P < 0.01$) higher ICP than patients with neither mass effects nor midline shift.

These preliminary data suggest that the presence of both mass effect and midline shift is a statistically significant predictor of raised intracranial pressure. Neither hydrocephalus nor ventricular measurements are reliable predictors of intracranial hypertension. No patient with a normal CT had an ICP of greater than 20 mm Hg.

Our results, correlating ICP changes with CT changes, for pediatric patients who sustained acute head trauma, are consistent with those shown for adults (Eisenberg et al. 1988). CT scanning, already proven efficacious in the localization of intracranial mass lesions, may enjoy a role in predicting the need for ICP monitoring. This preliminary investigation addresses only decisions made at the time the children present. We are currently expanding this research to evaluate the entire spectrum of the acute phase of injury, to identify patients at risk for delayed deterioration and to seek reliable predictors of the ultimate outcome.

References

Eisenberg HM, Gary HE, Jane JA, Marmarou A, Marshall LF, Young H (1988) CT scan findings in a series of 595 patients with severe closed head injury: a report from the NIH Traumatic Coma Data Bank. Am Assoc Neurol Surgeons, April 24–28, 1988 Meeting, p 371

Fasol P, Binder H, Reisner T, Schedl R, Schmid L, Strickner M (1980) Correlations between intracranial pressure, neurologic deficit and computer tomographic findings in patients with acute severe head injury. In: Shulman K, Marmarou A, Miller JD et al. (eds) Intracranial pressure IV. Springer, Berlin Heidelberg New York, pp 70–72

Haar FL, Sadhu VK, Pinto RS, Gildenberg PL, Sampson JM (1980) Can CT scan findings predict intracranial pressure in closed head injury patients? In: Shulman K, Marmarou A, Miller JD et al. (eds) Intracranial pressure IV. Springer, Berlin Heidelberg New York, pp 48–53

Lobato RD, Rivas JJ, Portillo JM, Velasco L, Cordobes F, Esparza J, Lamas E (1979) Prognostic value of the intracranial pressure levels during the acute phase of severe head injuries. Acta Neurochir [Suppl] (Wien) 28:70–73

Narayan RK, Kishore PRS, Becker DP, Ward JD, Enas GG, Greenberg RP, Da Silva AD, Lipper MH, Choi SC, Mayhall CG, Lutz HA, Young HF (1982) Intracranial pressure: to monitor or not to monitor? J Neurosurg 56:650–659

Papo I, Caruselli G, Luongo A, Scarpelli M, Pasquini U (1980) Traumatic cerebral mass lesions: correlations between clinical, intracranial pressure, and computed tomographic data. Neurosurgery 7:337–346

Sadhu VK, Sampson J, Haar FL, Pinto RS, Handel SF (1979) Correlation between computed tomography and intracranial pressure monitoring in acute head trauma patients. Radiology 133:507–509

Noninvasive Measurement of Intracranial Pressure (ICP) as a Screening Method for Evaluation of Hydrocephalus in Newborn and Infants

B. Valjak

Department of Pediatrics, University Hospital Zagreb, Rebro, 41000 Zagreb, Kispaticeva 12 (Yugoslavia)

Cerebral lesions leading to hydrocephalus are relatively common in newborn children and infants. The methods of choice for diagnosis and follow-up of intracranial lesions is brain sonography. Not only does it allow a precise diagnosis but it lets us follow the dynamics of brain lesion development through repeated examinations. However, ultrasonographic follow-up of developing hydrocephalus, in our opinion, does not suffice, since it causes a marked delay in therapeutic drainage.

Noninvasive measurement of the ICP through the fontanelle compliments sonography by giving us more precise and timely insight into the development of the impairment. Diagnosis of the progress of the disease or its standstill may be done through continuous measurement of ICP. There is, of course, a certain difference in opinion regarding this method (Kaiser and Whitelaw 1987; Levine et al. 1987).

The only purpose of this report is to show our experience with the use of ICP measurements as criteria for surgery.

Methods and Patients

In the Department of Pediatrics, University Hospital Zagreb, real time ultrasound scans were performed with the Advanced Technology Laboratories unit, Mark 300 with a 5 and 7.5 mHz rotary scan head. ICP was measured noninvasively through the anterior fontanelle with the Ladd system. The procedures were performed on hospitalized children as well as on those directed to the Neurosurgical Policlinic and to Childrens Neurology.

Results and Discussion

A total of 43 children with hydrocephalus followed before, and for some, after surgery gave us the following information: some showed a standstill of the process (especially premature infants) while others indicated acute or chronic hydrocephalus development.

The postsurgical follow-up of these children called for shunt revision or implantation of another shunt in 12 of the cases. We noted that children with periodically elevated ICP later developed constantly elevated ICP. The obstruction of the distal part of the ventriculoperitoneal system was evident at surgery.

When we first started using this method, we waited for a permanent ICP elevation, or even according to the neurosurgeon's criterium, an enlargement of the ventricular system. These patients did not develop the desired ventricular shrinkage which proved to us that surgery was too late. We now perform surgery when ICP is only temporarily elevated. This procedure has proven justified because we found obstruction of the system in all reoperated children.

The long range ICP measurement of hospitalized neonates and prematures with an enlargement of the ventricular system after bleeding, anoxia or malformation, also showed, in some cases, a periodically elevated ICP. In some of these cases, there were occasional groups of high oscillating waves but in one case only there was an increase of the plateau form lasting about 5–10 min. Schwalbe et al. (1987), reported similar results. In five cases, this experience lead us to immediate surgery which resulted in total normalization of the ventricular system. However, the number of children diagnosed is not sufficient to state flatly how long and how often the ICP should be elevated periodically as an indication for surgery.

There is always a danger of not recognizing ventriculomegaly. In ambulatory patients, even a hypertensive hydrocephalus may be overlooked. Normal ICP values may be obtained after a minimal enlargement of the ventricular system (2 mm) that may not be recognizable sonographically and that may have been caused by a previous high ICP. Such cases require prolonged and more frequent ICP measurements (every 8–10 days).

In conclusion, it is our opinion that periodically elevated ICP justifies surgery. However, the time element still remains an unanswered question: how many minutes of repeatedly elevated ICP are really needed before surgery is indicated.

References

Kaiser AM, Whitelaw AGL (1987) Noninvasive monitoring of intracranial pressure – fact or fancy? Dev Med Child Neurol 29:320–326
Levene MI, Evans DH et al. (1987) Value of intracranial pressure monitoring of asphysiated newborn infants. Dev Med Child Neurol 29:311
Schwalbe J, Schobess A et al. (1987) Nicht progrediente Ventrikelerweiterung im Säuglingsalter – Was tun? Kinderarzt 12:1682–1690

Correlations Between CT Features and ICP in Patients with Intracranial Lesions

M. Hara, C. Kadowaki, T. Shiogai, M. Numoto, and K. Takeuchi

Department of Neurosurgery, Kyorin University School of Medicine, 6-20-2 Shinkawa, Mitaka, Tokyo 181 (Japan)

The correlations between intracranial pressure (ICP) and various CT parameters were studied in 79 patients with supratentorial lesions (head injury, 42; hypertensive intracerebral hemorrhage, 20; brain tumor, 12; and cerebral infarction, 5) admitted to our department during the past 5 years. The mean age was 48 years (range, 11 to 81 years). All patients were examined prior to surgery (external and/or internal decompression and ventricular drainage).

The following CT features were evaluated: 1) shift in midline structures (MLS); 2) maximum diameter of lesion; 3) Evans' ratio; 4) compression of ipsilateral ventricle and dilatation of contralateral ventricle; 5) disappearance of basal cisterns and cerebral sulci; and 6) ventricular hemorrhage.

ICP was measured for an average of 3 days by either the epidural or the intraventricular method. Patients were divided into 4 groups on the basis of ICP values: ≤ 20 mm Hg; 21 to 40 mm Hg; ≥ 41 mm Hg; and ≥ 41 mm Hg and uncontrollable.

Results

1) Correlation Between ICP and MLS

ICP and MLS were significantly correlated ($p < 0.01$) in patients with closed head injury and those with hypertensive intracerebral hemorrhage. However, there was no correlation in cases of brain tumor (Fig. 1).

2) Correlation Between ICP and Mass Size

A significant correlation was found in the closed head injury group ($p < 0.01$) but not in the intracerebral hemorrhage and brain tumor groups.

3) Correlation Between ICP and Evans' Ratio

ICP was not significantly related to Evans' ratio in patients with brain tumor or intracerebral hemorrhage. However, a rapid increase in Evans' ratio within several days of onset portended uncontrollable ICP of over 40 mm Hg.

Intracranial Pressure VII
Eds.: J. T. Hoff and A. L. Betz
© Springer-Verlag Berlin Heidelberg 1989

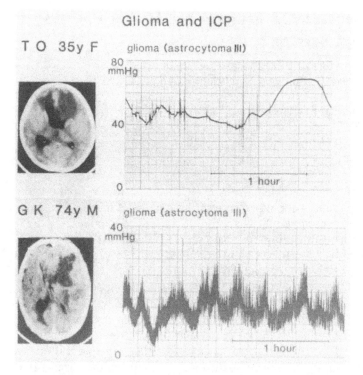

Glioma and ICP

T O 35y F glioma (astrocytoma III)

G K 74y M glioma (astrocytoma III)

Fig. 1. These two cases of glioma (astrocytoma grade III) each had a mass lesion of over 4 cm in diameter in the frontal lobe and MLS exceeding 1 cm. However, mean ICP in case *TO* (*top panel*) was over 40 mm Hg, and in case *GK* (*bottom panel*) under 20 mm Hg

4) Correlations between ICP and CT Findings of Ventricles, Basal Cisterns, Sulci and MLS

Of the thirty-five patients whose ICP was over 20 mm Hg, 28 had ipsilateral ventricular compression of over 50%, and 12 (43%) of these also had contralateral ventricular dilatation. Furthermore, 10 of these 12 patients had ICP of 30 to 40 mm Hg or even higher, a MLS of over 10 mm, and unclear or undetectable basal cisterns, including sulci.

Discussion

If increased ICP could be precisely determined on the basis of CT features alone, patient management could be focused on detection and prevention of secondary brain damage. Tabaddor et al. (1982) reported a correlation between ICP and CT findings in 40 closed head injury patients. They observed a relationship between the ICP level and intraventricular clot and ventricular compression. They also

148

reported that the size of the mass was related to ICP although not significantly, and that MLS and ICP were not correlated. Tabaddor et al. (1982) asserted that Evans' ratio is the best indicator of ICP level, barring rapid development of a unilateral mass lesion or acute obstructive hydrocephalus due to intraventricular hemorrhage.

In our 79 cases, there was a stastistically significant correlation between ICP and mass lesion size. However, this did not apply to patients with brain tumor, in whom age and the tumor growth rate may be influential factors. We found no correlation between Evans' ratio and ICP, perhaps because of diffuse brain swelling in cases of head injury and, in patients with lesions, because of variable pathology. Age may have been a factor as well. ICP was best correlated with Evans' ratio in patients with a third and/or fourth ventricular clot in whom the ratio increased.

Sadhu et al. (1982) reported that ICP had no relationship with asymmetrical ventricular compression, MLS, or obliteration of cisterns, fissures, and sulci. The greatest correlation in their 21 cases of head injury involved dilatation of the contralateral temporal horn. In our cases, ipsilateral ventricular obliteration and contralateral ventricular dilatation (10 of 12 cases) were acompanied by uncontrollable ICP of 30 to 40 mm Hg or higher.

Conclusion

In patients with intracranial lesions, it is possible to estimate ICP on the basis of CT findings concerning MLS, size of the lesion, contralateral ventricular dilatation, and Evans' ratio, provided the nature of the lesion and the patient's age are taken into account.

References

Sadhu VK, Sampson S, Haar FL, Pinto RS, Handel SF (1979) Correlation between computed tomography and intracranial pressure monitoring in acute head trauma patients. Radiology 113:507–509
Tabaddor K, Danziger A, Wisoff HS (1982) Estimation of intracranial pressure by CT scan in closed head trauma. Surg Neurol 18:212–215

EEG Spectrum Changes After the Bolus Injection of Thiopental

S. Kadoyama, K. Sugiura, H. Takizawa, M. Baba, T. Tachizawa, K. Kunimoto, and K. Mochimaru

Department of Neurosurgery and Department of Anesthesiology, Tokyo Rohsai Hospital, Ohmori Minami 4-13-21, Ohta-ku, Tokyo 143 (Japan)

Purpose

Barbiturate coma is accepted therapy in controlling intracranial hypertension (Marshall et al. 1979; Rockoff et al. 1974). One of the problems in applying this method is to maintain the serum barbiturate at an adequate level. The burst-suppression pattern of EEG is advocated as a guide to an appropriate concentration but it does not develop in all patients (Kassell et al. 1980; Ward et al. 1985; Yano et al. 1981).

We studied the feasibility of EEG spectral analysis in monitoring serum concentration of barbiturates.

Methods

The study was carried out in 18 patients during the induction of general anesthesia for various neurosurgical operations. Thiopental (5 mg/kg or 8 mg/kg) was intravenously injected as a bolus within 30 seconds and bifrontal EEG was recorded. The spectrum of EEG was estimated by the method of fast Fourier transform every 10 seconds. Blood was sampled sequentially for 20 minutes after the injection and the concentration of thiopental was measured by HPLC.

Results

The decline of the mean serum concentration of thiopental after the injection presented a biphasic pattern. The correlation between the serum concentration of thiopental and the percentage of each band of EEG is shown in Fig. 1. The correlation coefficient was significant except for the α band. Various other analyses to find a practical index were not rewarding.

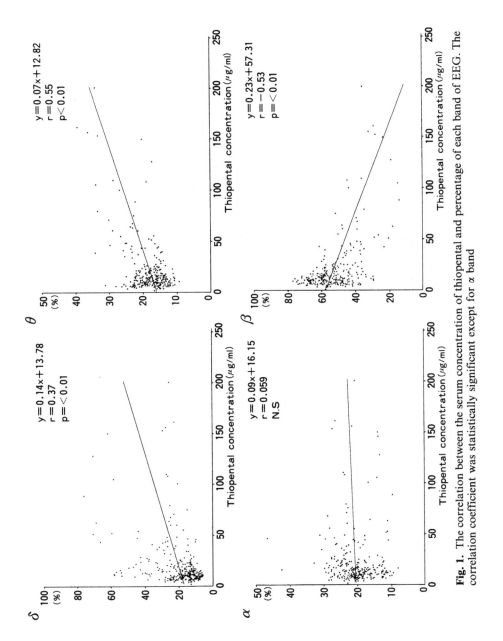

Fig. 1. The correlation between the serum concentration of thiopental and percentage of each band of EEG. The correlation coefficient was statistically significant except for α band

Discussion

This study revealed that the EEG spectrum and serum concentration of thiopental have a definite correlation. The data of each band, however, was scattered widely due to individual differences of EEG responsiveness to thiopental. Thus, an accurate one-to-one estimation of serum concentration proved to be difficult. Another limitation of this study, was that data acquisition was carried out only from patients with a bolus injection of drug. Further analysis using some form of evoked potentials or other spectral analysis during continuous administration may be worthwhile as a indicator of barbiturate concentration.

References

Kassell NF, Hitchon PW et al. (1980) Alternation in cerebral blood flow, oxygen metabolism and electrical activity produced by high dose sodium thiopental. Neurosurgery 7:598–603
Marshall LF, Smith RW et al. (1979) The outcome with aggressive treatment in severe head injuries. Part 2. Acute and chronic barbiturate administration in the management of head injury. J Neurosurg 50:26–30
Rockoff MA, Marshall LF et al. (1974) High-dose barbiturate therapy in humans; a clinical review of 60 patients. Ann Neurol 6:194–199
Ward JD, Becker DP et al. (1985) Failure of prophylactic barbiturate coma in the treatment of severe head injury. J Neurosurg 62:383–388
Yano M, Kobayashi S et al. (1981) Barbiturate overloading in 85 cases of severe head injury. Neurol Med Chir (Tokyo) 21:163–170

Session II: Biophysics Session

Chairmen: H.D. Portnoy and J. Rowan

Can Waveform Analysis of ICP Separate Vascular from Non-Vascular Causes
on Intracranial Hypertension?
I.R. Piper, N.M. Dearden, and J.D. Miller

The Origin of CSF Pulse Waves
C.M. Zee and K. Shapiro

Significance of Cortical Venous Pulse Pressure and Superior Sagittal Sinus
Pulse Pressure on ICP-Pulse Pressure
Y. Ueda, H. Nagai, K. Kamiya, and M. Mase

Mathematical Modelling of the Contribution of Arterial Volumetric Pulsation
to the Intracranial Pulse Wave
P.A. Klassen, E.R. Cardoso, and E. Shwedyk

Single Pulse Spectral Analysis of Intracranial Pressures
C.A. Branch, M. Chopp, and H.D. Portnoy

Fourier Analysis of Intracranial Pressures During Experimental
Intracranial Hypertension
C.A. Branch, M. Chopp, and H.D. Portnoy

Analysis of the Power Spectrum of the Pulse Pressure Wave During Induced
Intracranial Hypertension in Humans
S.E. Børgesen and L. Christensen

CSF Pulse Waves in a Model of Progressive Hydrocephalus:
An Effect Not a Cause of Ventricular Enlargement
C.M. Zee and K. Shapiro

Normal Pressure Hydrocephalus: A Retrospective Study on Clinico-
Radiological Data, CSF Dynamics and CSF Pulse Waveform Morphology
C. Anile, G. Maira, A. Mangiola, and G.F. Rossi

Application of Advanced Forms of Intracranial Pressure Analysis
in Craniosynostosis
L. Batorski, M. Czosnyka, P. Wollk-Laniewski, and W. Zaworski

CSF Pulse Waveform Morphology as an Indicator of Intracranial System
Impedance: An Experimental Study
C. Anile, A. Mangiola, F. Andreasi, C.A. Branch, and H.D. Portnoy

Can Waveform Analysis of ICP Separate Vascular from Non-Vascular Causes of Intracranial Hypertension?

I.R. Piper, N.M. Dearden, and J.D. Miller

Department of Clinical Neurosciences, Western General Hospital, University of Edinburgh (UK)

Introduction

Intracranial pressure (ICP) depends at least as much on pressure changes within the cerebrovascular bed (CVB) as on cerebrospinal fluid (CSF) formation, circulation and absorption mechanisms (Marmarou et. al. 1987). Chopp and Portnoy (1980) were the first to apply spectral analysis of the ICP waveform, in experimental models of intracranial hypertension, as the basis of a systems analysis approach whereby the arterial pressure (BP) waveform and the intracranial pressure (ICP) waveform were studied as measures of input and output functions respectively to the CVB. This analysis assumes that pressure pulse transmission through the CVB, as determined by the system transfer characteristics of the CVB, will provide insight into factors affecting ICP. It is our hypothesis that the system transfer characteristics of the CVB will be detectably different when ICP is increasing due to changes in cerebrovascular resistance, as compared to when ICP is increasing due to non-vascular causes detectable as alterations in compliance. This paper presents preliminary data in support of this hypothesis collected from three sources: a pilot animal study, a clinical study assessing Isoflurane neuroanaesthesia and data from our head injury intensive care unit (ICU).

Methods

ICP and BP waveforms were monitored using either Camino (Camino Laboratories, San Diego, CA, USA) fibre optic catheter-tip pressure transducers or fluid filled catheter-transducer systems that were optimally damped using Acudynamic (Abbott Critical Care Systems, Chicago, IL, USA) adjustable damping devices. Waveform segments were stored to FM magnetic tape for offline spectral analysis using a 32-bit microcomputer based waveform analysis system. The entire waveform analysis system, including pressure transducers, preamplifier, patient monitor, FM tape recorder and anti-aliasing low-pass filter, has a flat amplitude frequency response from DC to 70 Hz $\pm$ 2 db (DC to 20 Hz $\pm$ 2 db with the optimally damped fluid filled catheter-transducer system) and a linear phase shift of 0.09 radians/Hz. Phase shifts are corrected in the software for the linear phase shifts inherent in the waveform analysis system. Each waveform segment (4096 points) is digitized at a sampling rate of 400 Hz. A 4096 point fast Fourier transform (FFT) is calculated and the modulus of the transformed data is plotted against frequency as the amplitude spectrum. The system transfer characteristics of the CVB are determined from the ICP and BP amplitude spectra using a systems analysis approach. In systems analysis an attempt is made to define the physical characteristics of a system using only the system input and output signals. The assumption is made that the BP waveform is the chief input signal to the cerebrovascular system and the ICP waveform is the output signal emanating from the CVB. The system transfer function is defined as the relationship that describes how the stimulus signals are transformed by the system into response signals. The system transfer function consists of amplitude and phase components where both components are calculated from the Fourier transformed data by standard methods (Marmareliz and Marmareliz 1978). Harmonic components of both cardiac and respiratory origin are present in the amplitude spectrum, only the cardiac component harmonics present in the ICP and BP spectra are analysed for the purposes of calculating the system transfer function.

Pilot Experimental Studies

In an experimental model of intracranial hypertension in cats ($n=3$) ICP was raised, through intracisternal infusion of mock CSF, in increments of 10 mm Hg pressure from the postoperative baseline value (ICP 3–7 mm Hg) through to a maximum ICP of 60 mm Hg. ICP was monitored from the cisterna magna and BP from the thoracic aorta using Camino fibre optic catheter-tip transducers. In addition to waveform analysis, cerebral blood flow (CBF) was measured at six cortical sites by the hydrogen clearance technique and the volume pressure response (VPR), calculated as a measure of intracranial compliance, was determined from the pressure response resulting from rapid intracisternal injections of 0.05, 0.1, 0.15, 0.2, 0.25 and 0.3 ml of saline. The highest and lowest VPRs were discarded and the average of the remaining estimates was used as the measure of intracranial compliance. The cerebrovascular resistance (CVR), calculated as the cerebral perfusion pressure divided by the CBF, decreased steadily with increasing ICP. The VPR increased, indicating a reduced intracranial compliance, with increasing ICP and reached a plateau between an ICP of 30 and 40 mm Hg. Blood pressure remained steady throughout the experiment. As ICP increases, the amplitude transfer function increases at all frequencies (Fig. 1). However, the increase at each harmonic is not uniform but frequency dependent. In particular, the third harmonic component amplitude transfer function increases proportionally more than the lower or higher harmonics, suggesting the presence of a resonance within the cerebrovascular system. Resonance is a phenomenon determined by frequency dependent properties of the CVB of which cerebrovascular compliance is one such term. In one experiment, an increase in CVR associated with a decrease in the first harmonic component amplitude transfer function was noted at an ICP of 30 mm Hg compared to the CVR and amplitude transfer function response at 20 mm Hg. Thereafter, the CVR continued a downward trend coupled with an increasing first harmonic component amplitude transfer

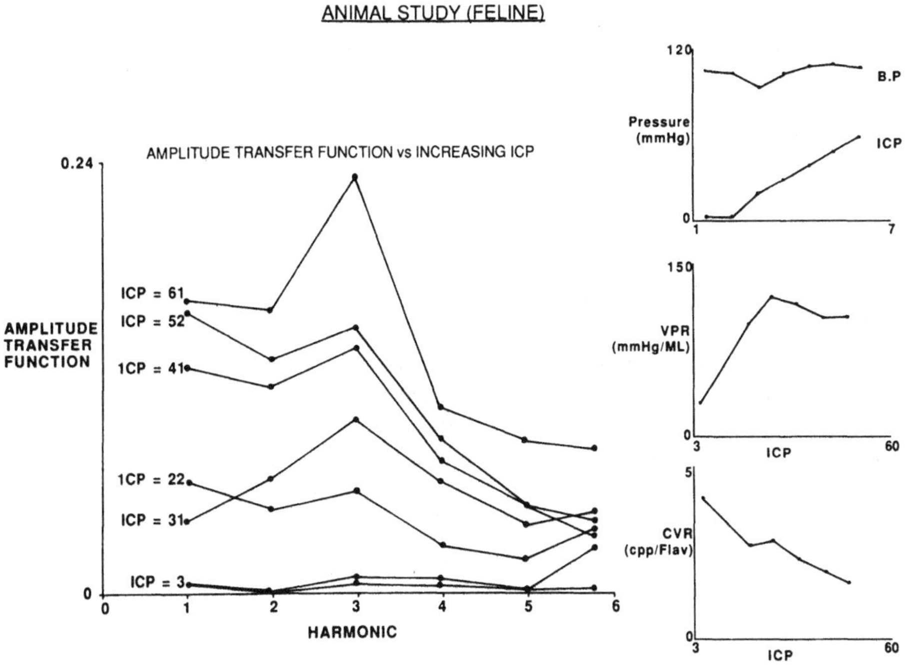

Fig. 1. The amplitude transfer function versus increasing ICP in a cat model of intracranial hypertension. The first cardiac component amplitude transfer function increases with ICP (except at 30 mm Hg where it increases from the value at 20 mm Hg) CVR decreases with increasing ICP (except at 30 mm Hg where it increases from the value at 20 mm Hg). The third cardiac component amplitude transfer function shows a frequency dependent increase more than the lower or higher harmonics. With increasing ICP, the VPR increased, indicating a reduced intracranial compliance, and reached a plateau between an ICP of 30 and 40 mm Hg. BP remained stable throughout the study

function as ICP increased above 30 mm Hg. These results suggest that the first harmonic component amplitude transfer function reflects changes in CVR and that there are also, associated with raised ICP, frequency dependent mechanisms that may include compliance, acting independently of CVR.

Isoflurane Neuroanaesthesia Study

Isoflurane induces hypotension by both peripheral vasodilation and myocardial depression and it is a mild cerebral vasodilator at low concentrations (less than 1%), an effect which is reversible with hypocapnia (Van Aken et al. 1986). This study was aimed at comparing the effects of Isoflurane and Ethrane neuroanaesthesia on ICP and cardiovascular parameters in patients whose ICP is already elevated. Patients were induced with Thiopentone (5 mg/kg) and narcotic Fentanyl (100 µg), paralysed with pancuronium (8 mg) and ventilated under positive pressure with 70%/30% N_2O/O_2. Ventilatory dead space was adjusted to main-

159

tain $PaCO_2$ between 4.5–5.0 kpa. Samples of ICP and BP waveforms were recorded simultaneously on to magnetic tape from five patients prior to removal of supratentorial tumours at three stages during the procedure: before administration of either 1.0% Isoflurane or 1.5% Ethrane anaesthesia, after 15 min administration of anaesthetic and finally after a further 5 min administration of anaesthetic coupled with hyperventilation (arterial pCO_2 3.5–4 kpa). In addition to waveform analysis, the volume pressure response (VPR), calculated as a measure of intracranial compliance, was determined from the pressure response resulting from rapid intraventricular injections of 0.5, 1.0, 2.0, and 4.0 ml of saline. The highest and lowest VPRs were discarded and the average of the remaining estimates was used as the measure of intracranial compliance. Waveform segments stored to tape underwent spectral analysis using a microcomputer based waveform analysis system. The amplitude transfer function of the first harmonic component was calculated as a measure of the low frequency response of the CVB and similarly the amplitude transfer function of the fourth harmonic as a measure of the high frequency response (Fig. 2). Both anaesthetic agents reduced systemic blood pressure (between 10% and 54%) in all cases and in four of five patients ICP increased (27%–80%). In association with these changes, in every case, both the low (100%–171%) and high (49%–913%) frequency response increased from control levels. Hyperventilation always returned the elevated ICP to control

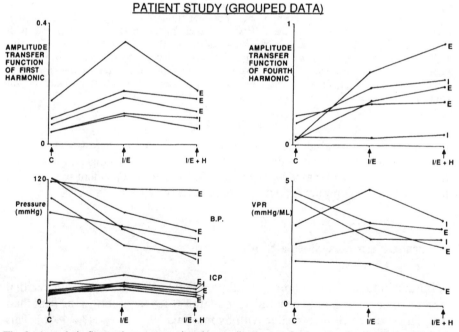

Fig. 2. A study in five patients comparing the amplitude transfer function for the first and fourth cardiac component harmonics prior to removal of supratentorial tumours at three stages during the procedure: before administration (*C*) of either 1.0% Isoflurane (*I*) or 1.5% Ethrane (*E*) anaesthesia, after 15 minutes' administration of anaesthetic and finally after a further 5 minutes' administration of anaesthetic coupled with hyperventilation (*I/E + H*). Volume pressure response (*VPR*), ICP and BP are also compared at each stage

levels and the reduced blood pressure remained unaltered. Furthermore, hyperventilation returned the low frequency response to or below control levels while the high frequency response remained elevated. The VPR in 4 out of 5 patients was lower at the completion of the study compared to control readings (indicating an increased compliance), although grouped analysis between patients did not reach statistical significance. These results suggest that the low frequency response of the CVB is directly related to alterations in cerebrovascular resistance while the high frequency response may be related to blood pressure dependent mechanisms that include compliance.

Head Injury ICU Study

Samples of ICP and BP waveforms were recorded simultaneously on to magnetic tape from two normotensive head injury patients with normal ICP (<15 mm Hg) ventilated to normocapnia ($PaCO_2$ 3.8–4.08 kpa). Waveform segments underwent spectral analysis using a microcomputer based waveform analysis system. The amplitude transfer function of the first harmonic component was calculated as a measure of the low frequency response of the intracranial compartment and similarly the amplitude transfer function of the fourth harmonic as a measure of the high frequency response. The amplitude transfer function of the first harmonic component in both patients was found to decrease markedly (32% and 42%) with progressive hypocapnia ($PaCO_2$ 3.02–3.5 kpa) whereas the amplitude transfer function of the fourth harmonic component in one patient decreased by only 14% and in the other patient there was no decrease. ICP decreased in both patients (28% and 47%) to progressive hypocapnia the BP remaining stable in one patient but in the other decreasing by 14%. These results indicate the first harmonic component amplitude transfer function of the CVB to be affected by alterations in cerebrovascular resistance whereas the fourth harmonic component amplitude transfer function showed little response to CO_2 induced changes in vascular resistance.

Discussion

The ability to detect when ICP is increasing from vascular causes (active arterial vasodilation, passive arterial distension due to a combination of arterial hypertension with impaired autoregulation) as opposed to non-vascular causes (all forms of brain oedema, factors increasing CSF outflow resistance) will have significant consequences for the management of raised ICP in severely head injured patients. Experimental investigations by Portnoy and Chopp (1981–1983) and later Hirai et al. (1984) and Takizawa et al. (1986) suggest that it is predominantly the first cardiac component harmonic in the ICP spectrum that reflects changes in cerebrovascular resistance. O'Rourke and Taylor (1966) in an experimental study of the vascular impedance of the femoral bed have shown that vasodilation and vasoconstriction affect predominantly the low frequency transmission characteristics of the femoral bed. Our results support the evidence that under conditions known to cause cerebral vasodilation or vasoconstriction it is the lower frequency transmission characteristics of the CVB that are chiefly affected. In a study of severely head injured patients, Bray et al. (1986) correlated the low frequency components present in the power-density spectrum of the ICP waveform to cerebral blood flow (CBF), and the high frequency components to the PVI as a measure of intracranial compliance. Kasugi et al. (1987), in an experimental study applying pressure pulse waves into the CVB, have shown resonance within the intracranial cavity and suggest that resonance is closely related to intracranial compliance. In a mathematical model of the femoral bed O'Rourke and Taylor (1966) have shown that under conditions of vasodilation, the femoral bed behaves in a purely resistive manner compared to control conditions or vasoconstriction where pressure pulse reflection phenomena occur resulting in significant frequency dependent changes in the amplitude and phase characteristics of the femoral bed. Furthermore, they suggest that it is the arterioles that are the major site for these reflection phenomena. In the CVB, the pressure pulse reflection sites may be different. The CVB is enclosed in a rigid container and it is likely, though not proven, that a major source of intracranial compliance is the large bore, thin walled, low pressure venous segment of the vascular bed. These compliant vessels are collapsible and as such are ideal sources for pressure pulse reflection phenomena. Our results suggest that non-vascular causes of ICP may be detectable by alterations in the pressure pulse reflection properties of the CVB which are dependent on intracranial compliance.

Conclusions

It is our hypothesis that the system transfer characteristics of the CVB will be detectably different when ICP is increasing due to changes in cerebrovascular resistance, from when ICP is increasing due to non-vascular causes detectable as alterations in compliance. Preliminary results from three sources support this hypothesis. The poor reproducibility of our measures of intracranial compliance and inability to directly measure CVR in the clinical setting, coupled with the difficulty in designing experimental models for separating vascular from non-vascular causes of raised ICP, detract from our results. Future studies must address these issues in order to test this hypothesis effectively.

Acknowledgement. This work has been supported by Action Research for the Crippled Child (Grant number A/8/1671).

References

Bray RS et al. (1986) Development of a clinical monitoring system by means of ICP waveform analysis. In: Miller JD et al. (eds) Intracranial pressure VI. Springer, Berlin Heidelberg New York Tokyo, pp 260–264

Chopp M, Portnoy H (1980) Systems analysis of intracranial pressure. J Neurosurg 53:516–527

Hirai O et al. (1984) Epidural pulse waveform as an indicator of intracranial pressure dynamics. Surg Neurol 21:67–74

Kasugi Y et al. (1987) Transmission characteristics of pulse waves in the intracranial cavity of dogs. J Neurosurg 66:907–914

Marmareliz PZ, Marmareliz VZ (1978) In: Analysis of physiological systems: The white-noise approach. Plenum, New York

Marmarou A et al. (1987) Contribution of CSF and vascular factors to elevation of ICP in severely head-injured patients. J Neurosurg 66:883–890

O'Rourke MF, Taylor MG (1966) Vascular impedance of the femoral bed. Res 18:126–139

Portnoy H, Chopp M (1981) Cerebrospinal fluid pulse wave form analysis during hypercapnia and hypoxia. Neurosurgery 9:14–27

Portnoy H et al. (1982) Cerebrospinal fluid pulse waveform as an indicator of cerebral autoregulation. J Neurosurg 56:666–678

Portnoy H et al. (1983) Hydraulic model of autoregulation and the cerebrovascular bed: The effects of altering systemic arterial pressure. Neurosurgery 13:482–497

Takizawa H et al. (1986) Spectral analysis of the CSF pulse wave at different locations in the craniospinal axis. J Neurol Neurosurg Psychiatry 49:1135–1141

Van Aken H, Fitch W et al. (1986) Cardiovascular and Cerebrovascular Effects of Isoflurane-Induced Hypotension in the Baboon. Anesth Analg 65:565–574

The Origin of CSF Pulse Waves

C.M. Zee and K. Shapiro

Humana Advanced Surgical Institutes, Humana Hospital Medical City Dallas,
7777 Forest Lane, Dallas, Texas 75230 (USA)

Introduction

Many researchers have looked at the CSF pulse wave and its response to conditions in the cranial vault (Guinane 1975, Avezaat et al. 1979). However, despite these studies the origin of the pulse wave is still unclear (Adolph et al. 1966). Two theories of where the CSF pulse wave originates are 1) it is generated in the choroid plexus and 2) it is a result of cerebral vascular pulsations. In this study the origin of the CSF pulse wave was investigated as well as its response to increases in intracranial pressure.

Methods

Six adult male cats (3 – 5 kg) were anesthetized with pentobarbital, paralyzed with gallamine, intubated, and mounted in a stereotactic frame. The animals were ventilated and arterial blood gases, temperature, EKG, and heart rate were monitored. Pulse waves were monitored in the lateral ventricle, cisterna magna, convexity subarachnoid space, the sagittal sinus and the lingual artery. All pressure signals were monitored through fluid filled microbore catheters (34 cm) coupled to Statham P23-ID pressure transducers, and output to a strip chart recorder. The pulse wave signals were then filtered, amplified and displayed on an oscilloscope. The pulse waves were sampled at 100 Hz and analyzed using a DEC PDP11-23 computer.

Table 1. Percent change in pulsewave height with increased ICP

	Bolus injection cisterna magna	Bolus injection lateral ventricle	Infusion cisterna magna	Infusion lateral ventricle
Cisterna magna	90.0%	104.0%	87.1%	142.8%
Lateral ventricle	NSD	128.1%	280.2%	300.0%
Sagittal sinus	NSD	83.5%	40.7%	NSD
Subarachnoid space	77.8%	67.5%	105.2%	147.1%

NSD: No significant difference; alpha $= 0.05$

Intracranial Pressure VII
Eds.: J.T. Hoff and A.L. Betz
© Springer-Verlag Berlin Heidelberg 1989

Baseline data were collected for 15 min then the following ICP manipulations were performed, pulse waves were sampled and the animal was allowed to recover after each manipulation: 1) an intracisternal bolus injection (0.15–0.20 ml); 2) an intraventricular bolus injection (0.15–0.20 ml); 3) infusion into the cisterna magna; 4) infusion into the lateral ventricle. Infusion rates were calculated to raise ICP 15 mm Hg above baseline pressure.

Results

Consistent and statistically significant differences ($p < 0.05$) in pulse wave size, as indicated by peak height and area, were observed between sites (Table 1). The largest pulse waves were observed in the cisterna magna (0.177 mm Hg ± 0.02 (SE)) with the ventricular (0.103 mm Hg ± 0.49 (SE)), sagittal sinus (0.087 mm Hg ± 0.037 (SE)) and subarachnoid space (0.048 mm Hg ± 0.011 (SE)) pulse waves decreasing in size, respectively. No significant differences between the latencies at each site referenced to the R wave of the EKG were observed. When ICP was raised via bolus injections and infusions, significant increases ($p < 0.05$) in pulse wave size occurred at most sites. The largest increases were observed in the ventricle where the pulse wave height increased 128–300%. In most cases, no increase was observed during the intracisternal bolus injection. The pulse waves in the cisterna magna and the subarachnoid space increased consistently from 67–147% in all cases. The method and site of the pressure manipulations did not affect the magnitude of these changes in pulse size. No changes in latencies with respect to the EKG were noted with increased ICP.

Discussion

No latencies were observed between sites with respect to the R wave of the EKG, indicating that the pulse wave is produced by cerebral vascular pulsations throughout the brain, as opposed to originating in the choroid plexus and being transmitted throughout the ventricular system. Also, pulse wave size changes were not affected by the method or site of the ICP manipulation. Pulse wave size seemed to be dependent on intracranial pressure only and the ventricular pulse waves were the most sensitive to increases in intracranial pressure.

References

Adolph RJ, Fukusuma H, Fowler N (1967) Origin of cerebrospinal fluid pulsations. Am J Physiol 212 (4):840–846

Avezaat CJ, Van Eijndhoven JHM, Wyper DJ (1979) CSF pulse pressure and the intracranial volume–pressure relationships. J Neurol Neurosurg Psychiatry 42:686–700

Guinane JE (1979) Cerebrospinal fluid pulse pressure and brain compliance in adult cats. Neurology 25:559–564 •

Significance of Cortical Venous Pulse Pressure and Superior Sagittal Sinus Pulse Pressure on ICP-Pulse Pressure

Y. Ueda, H. Nagai, K. Kamiya, and M. Mase

Department of Neurosurgery, Nagoya City University Medical School (Japan)

We have already reported that the pulse pressure (PP) of the intracranial epidural pressure (EDP) is altered by a change of the intracranial components and compliance of the craniospinal cavity (Matsumoto et al. 1986, Nagai et al. 1986). In order to clarify the correlation between cerebral cortical venous pressure (CoVP)-PP and superior sagittal sinus pressure (SSSP)-PP in relation to EDP-PP, an animal experiment was performed as follows.

Materials and Methods

Adult mongrel dogs were immobilized and ventilated mechanically under light anesthesia. Pressure in the carotid artery, CoV and SSS were measured via hard polyethylene catheters connected to pressure transducers (Statham P50). ICP was measured epidurally (Toyoda EDP Monitor BPM-01). After preparation, bone defects were filled with bone cement. Each pulse pressure was obtained during several seconds of respiratory cessation in order to exclude any influence of respiration and was calculated by computer after A-D converting. ICP was changed by four methods as follows. Group I (control group, 11 dogs); ICP was changed by gradual cisternal injection of saline up to 90 mm Hg. Group H (10 dogs); ICP was changed by hypercapnia. Group B (9 dogs); ICP was changed by obstructive hydrocephalus by inflation of a posterior fossa epidural balloon for about six hr. Group M (9 dogs); acute hydrocephalus with hypercapnia. Animals with arrhythmia and bradycardia (< 80/min) were excluded.

Results

The value of CoVP was almost the same as that of EDP up to 90 mm Hg in each group, but the change of SSSP associated with an increase of EDP was different in each group. SSSP reached higher levels in group I, group H and group M than in group B (Table 1). These results suggest that SSSP was less effected when ICP increased gradually.

There were no statistically significant differences in carotid arterial pressure and heart rate among the groups. There were linear correlations between CoVP

Intracranial Pressure VII
Eds.: J. T. Hoff and A. L. Betz
© Springer-Verlag Berlin Heidelberg 1989

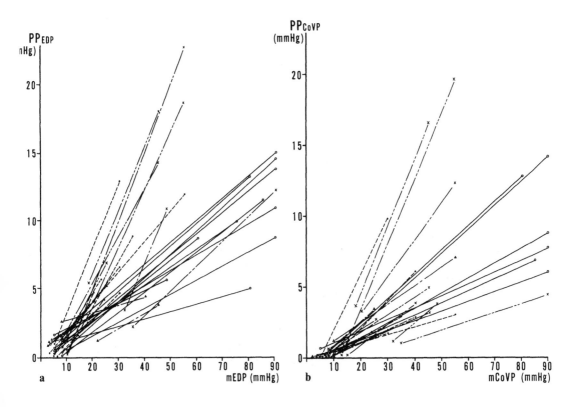

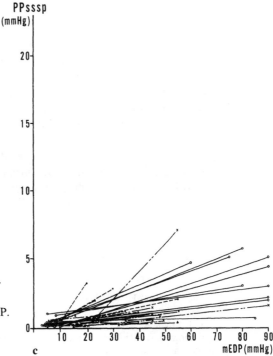

Fig. 1a–c. Relationships between pressure values and pulse pressures. Different characters showing different methods of increasing ICP.

○————○: *cisternal infusion,*
●-----●: *hypercapnia,*
▲—·—▲: *CSF pathway blockade,*
×----×: *CSF pathway blockade and hypercapnia.*

a Relationship between mean EDP and EDP-PP.
b Relationship between mean CoVP and CoVP-PP.
c Relationship between mean EDP and SSSP-PP

167

Table 1. Gradient of EDP-pulse pressure curve

Group	PP_{EDP}	PP_{CoUP}	PP_{SSSP}	mSSSP
I	$0.1305 + 0.0392$	0.1165 ± 0.0479	0.0412 ± 0.0269	0.5138 ± 0.2605
H	0.3261 ± 0.1020 **	0.1525 ± 0.1406	0.0708 ± 0.0861	0.6748 ± 0.3527
B	0.1360 ± 0.0817	0.1336 ± 0.0574	0.0039 ± 0.0075 **	0.1267 ± 0.2522 *
M	0.3839 ± 0.1004 ***	0.2134 ± 0.1561	0.0420 ± 0.0624	0.3485 ± 0.2044

I = cisternal infusion, H = hypercapnia, B = CSF pathway blockade by posterior fossa epidural balloon, M = mixture of B and H, EDP = epidural pressure, CoVP = cortical venous pressure, SSSP = superior sagittal sinus pressure, PP = pulse pressure, m = mean pressure.
* $p < 0.005$; ** $p < 0.002$; *** $p < 0.0005$.

and CoVP-PP and between SSSP and SSSP-PP as well as between EDP and EDP-PP. The gradient of the EDP-EDPPP curve was steeper in group H and group M than in group I with statistically significant difference (Fig. 1a and Table 1). The gradient of the CoVP-CoVPPP curve did not differ statistically among the groups, although some of the dogs in group H and group M had steeper ones than dogs in group I (Fig. 1b and Table 1). SSSP-PP was influenced by the value of the SSSP and the difference among groups in the gradient of the SSSP-SSSPPP curve was not clear (Fig. 1c and Table 1).

Discussion

The results showed that EDP-PP was affected by a change of the intracranial component, especially cerebral blood volume, CSF pathway blockage in conjuction with hypercapnia had a tendency to increase EDP-PP. However, pulse pressure differences among the groups are not clear concerning CoVP-PP and SSSPP-PP. The mechanism for the difference between EDP-PP and other PPs is uncertain but it might be explained by differences in the methods of pressure measurement. Venous pressure is measured intraluminally but EDP is done epidurally. A dampening effect of the blood vessel itself may make CoVP-PP uniform in all groups. This study suggests that the pulse pressure of the ICP is not regulated by the cerebral venous system, either the cortical vein or the superior sagittal sinus.

References

Matsumoto T, Nagai H, Kasuga Y, Kamiya K (1986) Changes in intracranial pressure (ICP) pulse wave following hydrocephalus. Acta Neurochir (Wien) 82:50–56
Nagai H, Kamiya K, Ohno M, Matsumoto T (1986) Importance of the pulse amplitude in ventriculomegaly. In: Ishii S (ed) Hydrocephalus. Excerpta Medica, Amsterdam Princeton Geneva Tokyo, pp 126–134

Mathematical Modelling of the Contribution of Arterial Volumetric Pulsation to the Intracranial Pulse Wave

P.A. Klassen, E.R. Cardoso, and E. Shwedyk

Department of Electrical Engineering, Department of Surgery, University of Manitoba, Winnipeg (Canada)

Summary

Previous studies have traditionally taken the systemic arterial and venous pulse waves as the input signals responsible for the generation of the intracranial pulse wave (ICPW) (Adolph et al. 1967, Chopp and Portnoy 1980, Dereymaeker et al. 1971). The ICPW, however, depends not only on the input pressure waves but also on the filtering effect of the vessel wall. Intraluminal to extravascular pressure pulse transmission was studied in a system which consisted of a single artery enclosed inside a fluid-filled elastic container. A mathematical model describing pulse transmission across the vessel wall was derived and experimentally verified. The results can be extrapolated to the cerebral circulation and the generation of the ICPW.

Mathematical Model

The mathematical model is based on a system consisting of a single vessel sealed inside a fluid-filled elastic container as shown in Fig. 1. Each intraluminal pressure pulse of amplitude ΔPi causes a volumetric change of the vessel segment within the container. The magnitude of the vessel volume pulse, ΔVi, depends on the intraluminal pressure pulse and the distensibility of the vessel. Since the vessel is sealed inside the container, the volume change experienced by the container is equal to the change in vessel volume, $\Delta Vo = \Delta Vi$. The change in container volume in turn causes a pressure pulse of amplitude ΔPo according to the pressure-volume characteristic of the container. A mathematical expression has been derived to describe these relationships. It is of the form:

$$\Delta Po = (-a \cdot (MPi - MPo) + b) \ (MPo + 1) \Delta Pi$$

where 'a' and 'b' are constants determined by the pressure-volume properties of the vessel and the container, ΔPo is the container pulse amplitude, ΔPi is the arterial pulse amplitude, MPi is the mean aterial pressure, and MPo is the mean container pressure. The form of the equation depends on the functions used to approximate the pressure-volume curves of the vessel and the container. Our

Eds.: J.T. Hoff and A.L. Betz
© Springer-Verlag Berlin Heidelberg 1989

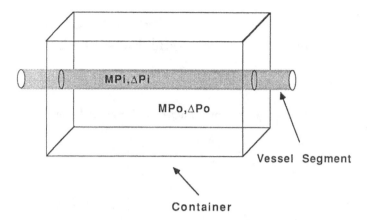

Fig. 1. The vessel-container system consisting of a single vessel sealed inside a fluid-filled elastic container. *MPi* and *ΔPi* are mean and pulse pressures inside the vessel. *MPo* and *ΔPo* are mean and pulse pressures in the container

equation assumes an exponential pressure-volume curve for the container and a quadratic expression for the vessel.

Model predictions can be examined by considering independent variations of the model variables. Increases of intraluminal pulse amplitude (ΔPi) result in proportional increases in container pulse amplitude (ΔPo). Changes of mean container pressure (MPo) also cause proportional changes in the container pulse (ΔPo) as expected from the exponential pressure-volume curve of the container. Increasing mean transmural pressure (MPi − MPo) results in decreasing container pulsation as the vessel becomes less distensible.

Experimental Verification

The mathematical expression was verified by means of experiments performed on an anatomical representation of the single vessel container system in cats. Upon removal of the large and small intestines, a 5 cm segment of abdominal aorta was exposed. A section of small bowel was prepared and then sutured around the vessel wall to provide a sealed biological chamber. A catheter was inserted into the container for fluid withdrawal and infusion as well as pressure measurement. Pressure was recorded in the aortic segment by a catheter inserted through the femoral artery.

Three procedures were used to vary system pressures. Mean intraluminal arterial pressure (MPi) was altered by Valsalva maneuvers in 19 trials. A range of arterial pulse amplitudes (ΔPi) were obtained by stepwise application of a proximal vascular clamp in 16 trials. Container pressure (MPo) was varied by fluid infusion or withdrawal from the container in 12 trials. The data were recorded on a video tape recorder and analyzed using a Data 6000 Waveform Analyzer.

The model constants 'a' and 'b' were defined by pressure-volume tests performed on the vessel and the container.

For each container pulse measured in the experimental system a corresponding value was calculated by the mathematical model. A correlation coefficient of 0.90 was obtained for 220 experimental and calculated data points. Thus, pressure pulse transmission predicted by the model was confirmed in the experiments.

Discussion

The concepts related to pressure pulse transmission in our mathematical model can be extrapolated to study the generation of the ICPW. The model has shown that the contribution of each intracranial vessel segment to the ICPW depends on: the global distensibility of the craniospinal cavity, the local distensibility of each vessel segment and the intraluminal pulse amplitude. The pressure-volume properties of the craniospinal cavity and the intracranial vessels are nonlinear and, therefore, their distensibilities depend on mean intracranial and mean transmural pressures respectively.

Considering the low distensibility of large cerebral arteries it is unlikely that they contribute greatly to the ICPW despite large intraluminal pressure pulsation. However, the more distensible veins may make a large contribution to the ICPW, despite relatively small intraluminal pressure pulsation.

Acknowledgement. This study has been supported by a Fellowship from the Department of Surgery Education and Research Fund, Winnipeg, Canada.

References

Adolph RJ, Fukusumi H, Fowler NO (1967) Origin of cerebropsinal fluid pulsations. Am J Physiol 212:840–846
Chopp M, Portnoy HD (1980) Systems analysis of intracranial pressure. J Neurosurg 53:516–527
Dereymaeker A, Stevens A, Rombouts JJ, Lacheron JM, Pierguin A (1971) Study on the influence of the arterial pressure upon the morphology of cisternal CSF pulsations. Eur Neurol 5:107–114

Single Pulse Spectral Analysis of Intracranial Pressures

C.A. Branch, M. Chopp, and H.D. Portnoy

Department of Neurology, Henry Ford Hospital, Detroit, Michigan 48202 (USA)

Introduction

A spectral analysis technique is described for the investigation of intracranial pressures. Spectral analysis has been used extensively for the study of vascular impedance (McDonald 1974), and more recently to study alterations in the transmission of cardiac pressure pulsations through the intracranial space (Branch 1988, Portnoy et al. 1982, 1983). The rigid encasement of the intracranial contents facilitates study of the cerebral vasculature by monitoring reflections of the cardiac pulsation in the cerebrospinal fluid (CSF).

Spectral analysis of individual pressure pulsations is achieved with the fast Fourier transform (FFT). Its uses and limitations in biological systems have been investigated (Attinger et al. 1955). These techniques provide a quantitative tool facilitating intra- and cross-comparisons of intracranial pressures.

Methods

Time series data are digitally acquired, stored, and transformed into the frequency domain with the FFT on computers. Analysis software was composed of home written routines in fortran and assembly languages. Selected DEC (Digital Equipment Corporation) subroutine software was employed for data acquisition. The program flow may be partitioned into four subdivisions: (1) analog to digital conversion of the waveform(s), (2) pulse isolation, (3) pulse preparation for the FFT, and (4) the FFT.

Waveform sampling was performed routinely at 200 Hz to avoid aliasing errors. The onset of a pulse is taken as the initial rise in pressure (called the foot) and is terminated by the next such rise. When two or more waveforms are considered, their individual pulsations are defined to lie within the same time interval to allow for determination of phase shifts between corresponding harmonics.

The FFT assumes the data to be periodic with period T, i.e., $f(t) = f(t+T)$. Thus, slow waves, such as respiratory waves, must be filtered to insure continuity of each pulse. Respiratory fluctuations are subtracted in an interpolatory manner while the pulse is digitally reconstructed. No slow wave effects or high frequency artifacts appear in the reconstructed waveforms.

Eds.: J.T. Hoff and A.L. Betz
© Springer-Verlag Berlin Heidelberg 1989

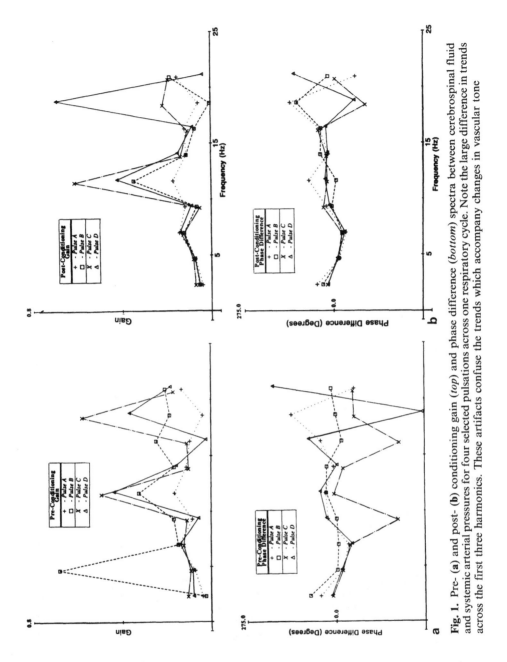

Fig. 1. Pre- (**a**) and post- (**b**) conditioning gain (*top*) and phase difference (*bottom*) spectra between cerebrospinal fluid and systemic arterial pressures for four selected pulsations across one respiratory cycle. Note the large difference in trends across the first three harmonics. These artifacts confuse the trends which accompany changes in vascular tone

Results

Four individual pulsations selected from different locations on a pulse train demonstrate the analysis. The CSF/arterial gain and phase difference, before and after conditioning, are illustrated in Fig. 1.

Amplitude and phase spectra from pulses A and D changed little with conditioning, while spectra from pulses B and C changed significantly. The relative

173

power of the lower harmonics varied considerably between pulsations and before conditioning due to significant discontinuities. These variations over the respiratory cycle are compounded in the gain and phase spectra illustrated for each pulse in Fig. 1. However, following conditioning the gain and phase difference spectra demonstrate a remarkable degree of similarity.

Discussion

The application of the FFT to pressure signals imposes three restrictions on those signals (Stearns 1975). First, the signals must satisfy the Dirichlet conditions. Second, the signals must be 'band limited' to avoid errors. Third, the signal must be periodic.

The Dirichlet requirements are easily satisfied for the duration of each cardiac pulsation. Intracranial signals are generally sufficiently band limited at 20 Hz or less. Finally, the periodicity of each waveform is assured by its separation into individual cardiac pulsations, with low frequency respiratory variations removed.

These techniques serve as an ideal probe of the state of the intracranial vasculature which is continuously responding to the naturally occurring arterial pulse wave. They are easily employed, requiring only pressure monitoring equipment through the vasculature. Accumulated evidence (Branch 1988, Portnoy et al. 1982, 1983) suggests that the status of myogenic autoregulatory mechanisms at the arterioles and the state of the compressible venous vasculature may be inferred from the gain and phase spectra of pulse waves acquired with these techniques as it transverses the cerebrovascular bed.

References

Attinger EO, Anne A, McDonald DA (1966) Use of fourier series for the analysis of biological systems. Biophys J 6:291–304
Branch CA (1988) An investigation into the relationship of cerebrovascular dynamics to intracranial pressures and pulsations. Ph. D. Dissertation, Oakland University, Rochester, Michigan
Mcdonald DA (1974) Blood flow in arteries, second edition. Williams and Wilkins
Portnoy HD, Chopp M, Branch CA et al. (1982) Cerebrospinal fluid pulse waveform as an indicator of cerebral autoregulation. J Neurosurg 56:666–678
Portnoy HD, Chopp M, Branch CA (1983) Hydraulic model of myogenic autoregulation and the cerebrovascular bed: The effects of altering systemic arterial pressure. Neurosurgery 13:482–498
Stearns SD (1975) Digital signal analysis, first edition. Hayden Book Company, New Jersey, pp 36–50

Fourier Analysis of Intracranial Pressures During Experimental Intracranial Hypertension

C.A. Branch, M. Chopp and H.D. Portnoy

Department of Neurology, Henry Ford Hospital, Detroit, Michigan 48202 (USA)

Introduction

Intracranial pulse transmission under three conditions of intracranial hypertension was investigated with single pulse spectral analysis in an effort to elucidate the effects of intracranial hypertension on the cerebrovasculature.

Methods

Systematic arterial (SA), cortical vein (CV), cerebrospinal fluid (CSF) and sagittal sinus (SS) pressures were investigated in eleven mongrel dogs (7 to 11 kg). Surgical preparation was identical to that reported previously (Portnoy et al. 1982). Additionally, CV pressure was measured in five dogs by inserting a 22 gauge catheter into a CV via the lateral lacuna, and in six dogs by cannulating the smaller of two joining cortical veins and advancing the catheter tip to their junction.

Spectral analysis was performed during a control condition (ventilation with 25% O_2, bal N_2) and during intracranial hypertension produced by 1) ventilation with 5% CO_2, 2) manual compression of the external jugular veins and 3) injection of 0.5 ml Ringer's lactate solution at 0.1 ml/sec. During jugular compression and volume infusion, spectral analysis commenced when mean CSF pressure reached the same level attained during 5% CO_2 ventilation.

Spectral analysis yielded amplitude and phase spectra of pressure pulse wave trains at each stage of the experiment. Gain spectra were calculated for CV/CSF, CSF/SA and SS/CSF (Branch 1988). All signals were analyzed over the same time interval. Changes in gain spectra were evaluated with ANOVA tests for repeated measures and Hotelling's T^2 statistic. The first three harmonics of gain spectra are treated statistically for each pulse train analyzed.

Results

Figure 1 illustrates analog data from a representative animal. Mean control CSF pressure (8.2 ± 1.5 mm Hg) was less ($p < 0.05$) than during 5% CO_2

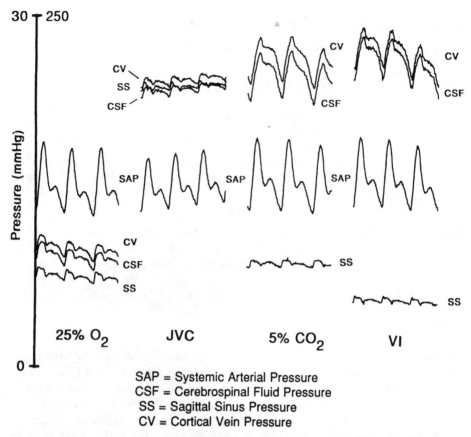

Fig. 1. SA, CSF, SS and CV pressure waveforms during control, 5% CO_2 ventilation, volume infusion and jugular vein compression. Note that CSF pressure reaches approximately the same level during all hypertensive conditions, but that waveform contour during jugular vein compression resembles that of control

(18.0±4.1 mm Hg), volume infusion (18.6±4.0 mm Hg) or jugular compression (17.4±4.3 mm Hg).

Spectral Comparison of CV and CSF. The CV/CSF gain spectra, illustrated in Figure 2, were reviewed for any difference from unity or across conditions. No interaction between conditions was observed, nor was the gain spectra different from unity across the first three harmonics.

Spectral Analysis Across Conditions. Figure 2 shows the CSF/SA and SS/CSF gain spectra for the control and hypertensive conditions.

Control Spectra. The CSF/SA gain spectra were unremarkable for differences between the first three harmonics. In general, amplitude of the first three harmonics were nearly equal.

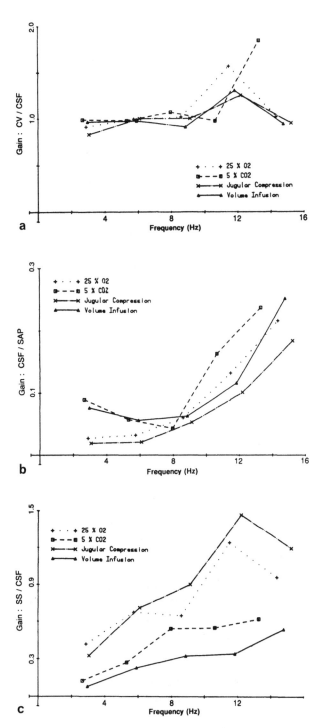

Fig. 2. CV/CSF (**a**), CSF/ SAP (**b**) and SS/CSF (**c**) gain spectra taken from the animal in Fig. 1. Note the change in trend between the first three harmonics of the CSF/SAP gain spectra during 5% CO_2 ventilation and the volume infusion test compared to the other conditions

The SS/CSF gain spectra demonstrated a positively sloping trend for the first three harmonics ($p < 0.05$), originating with a slightly suppressed fundamental frequency component (compared with higher frequency harmonics). This trend persisted throughout the hypertensive conditions.

Ventilation with 5% CO_2. The hypercapnic CSF/SA gain spectra indicate increased SA pulse wave transmission to the CSF (and CV) from control. The fundamental frequency component was elevated compared to the second harmonic ($p < 0.05$), and both harmonics exceeded the level achieved during the control condition ($p < 0.05$). These changes correlate with the increasing similarity in waveform contours observed at hypercapnic equilibrium and are consistent with data reported previously (Portnoy et al. 1982).

The SS/CSF gain spectra was statistically unchanged from the control condition. However, differing trends emerged between animals. In two animals the gain resembled the CSF/SA gain, in three animals the gain was flat, and in the remaining animals the gain was unchanged or decreased from control gain spectra.

Volume Infusion Test. The CSF/SA gain spectra exhibited a fundamental harmonic elevated above the second harmonic ($p < 0.05$) and both the fundamental and second harmonic were elevated above their respective control condition harmonics ($p < 0.05$).

The SS/CSF gain spectra was unchanged from control.

Jugular Vein Compression. The CSF/SA gain spectra during jugular vein compression resembled the control spectra in all respects. The fundamental and second harmonic were less than during 5% CO_2 and volume infusion ($p < 0.05$).

The mean level of the SS/CSF gain spectra was elevated from control, 5% CO_2, and volume infusion levels ($p < 0.05$).

Discussion

Cortical Vein and Cerebrospinal Fluid Pressure Similarities. The CV/CSF gain spectra demonstrated no statistical differences from unity and the spectra were similar across all experimental conditions studied, indicating a strong coupling mechanism. This coupling may be associated with a hydraulic feedback mechanism by which changes in cerebral venous pressures impart their effect on the pre-capillary vasculature through the CSF pressure to help maintain a constant cerebrovascular resistance.

5% CO_2 Inhalation. Increased CO_2 tension in the arterial blood leads to a loss in arteriolar vasomotor tone and a decrease in arteriolar resistance (Folkow 1964). These effects are evident from the increase in the CSF/SA gain spectra and result in the increased CSF pulse amplitude and rounding of the waveform characteristic of hypercapnia (Portnoy et al. 1981, 1982). Hence the arterial pulse wave is transmitted readily to the cerebral veins and through their walls to the CSF.

Volume Infusion Test. The volume infusion test produces compression of the cerebral venous bed. The result is a redistribution of cerebrovascular resistance from the pre- to post-capillary vasculature, facilitating a rise in intracranial pressures (Johnston and Rowan 1974). Following a volume infusion, the increase in the fundamental frequency component of the CSF/SA gain spectra reflects the decreased arteriolar impedance to arterial pulse wave and is similar to that observed during 5% CO_2 ventilation. However, as indicated in Fig. 2, the change in gain which occurs with volume infusion is slightly less than during 5% CO_2. During hypercapnia the gain increases due to increased pulse wave transmission through the arterioles, while during the volume infusion test, the same effect is achieved by compression the cerebral veins and increasing the efficiency of pulse wave transmission across their walls. Increased pulse wave impedance at the lateral lacuna immediately following the volume infusion test is reflected by an attenuated SS/CSF gain spectra. Thus, the volume infusion test has the same effect on the gain spectra as ventilation with 5% CO_2.

Jugular Compression and Its Relation to the Other Conditions. Mean cerebrospinal fluid pressure attained the same level examined during 5% CO_2 ventilation and volume infusion. The CSF/SA gain spectra indicate that cerebral arteriolar impedance during this condition is no different from control and it can thus be assumed that either minimal or no change in arterial vasomotor tone occurred with elevation of venous pressure by this technique.

The mean of the SS/CSF gain spectra during jugular vein compression was elevated over all the other conditions. This is compatible with distension of the venous vasculature. The increase in gain indicates that a 'barrier' at the junction between the lateral lacuna and SS (Nakagawa et al. 1974) is being forced open in a way which increases pulse transmission to the SS.

In summary, the data suggest that when jugular compression is performed, the increase in venous pressure is transmitted to the SS, lateral lacuna, and finally to the cerebral veins, and through the walls of the veins to the CSF. Essentially no change occurs in pulse transmission through the arterioles. The pulsation within the cortical veins is transmitted with less attenuation into the SS as a result of the forced dilatation of the junction between lateral lacuna and SS. While ventilation with 5% CO_2 produces an increase in CSF pressure secondary to impairment of myogenic autoregulation and volume infusion produces a primary increase in CSF pressure resulting in adjustment of cerebrovascular tone with results similar to ventilation with 5% CO_2, jugular vein compression produces a direct increase in CSF pressure without myogenic autoregulatory impairment.

Comparison of the CSF and CV pressures lead to the conclusion that the CSF pressure pulsation is, if not of venous origin, at least strongly coupled to venous pulsations under the conditions investigated. The importance of the relationship of CSF pressure to cerebral venous pressure in determining the status of cerebrovascular resistance is evident from these studies.

References

Branch CA (1988) An investigation into the relationship of cerebrovascular dynamics to intracranial pressures and pulsations. Ph. D. Dissertation, Oakland University, Rochester, Michigan

Folkow B (1964) Description of the myogenic hypothesis. Circ Res [Suppl 1] XIV:279–283

Johnston IH, Rowan JO (1974) Raised intracranial pressure and cerebral blood flow. 3. Venous outflow tract pressures and vascular resistances in experimental intracranial hypertension. J Neurol Neurosurg Psychiatry 37:392–402

Nakagawa Y, Tsuru M, Yada K (1974) Site and mechanism for compression of the venous system during experimental intracranial hypertension. J Neurosurg 41:427–434

Portnoy HD, Chopp M (1981) Cerebrospinal fluid pulse wave form analysis during hypercapnia and hypoxia. Neurosurgery 9:14–27

Portnoy HD, Chopp M, Branch CA et al. (1982) Cerebrospinal fluid pulse waveform as an indicator of cerebral autoregulation. J Neurosurg 56:666–678

Analysis of the Power Spectrum of the Pulse Pressure Wave During Induced Intracranial Hypertension in Humans

S.E. Børgesen[1] and L. Christensen[2]

[1] University Clinic of Neurosurgery, and [2] Department of Neurosurgery, University Hospital, Rigshospitalet, DK-2100 Copenhagen (Denmark)

During the lumbo-ventricular perfusion test for measurement of resistance to CSF outflow (Rout) the intracranial pressure level (ICP) is increased stepwise to several steady state pressure levels. When the pressure is increased (by elevating the outflow tube) the pulse pressure amplitude (PA), risetime (RT) and the power spectrum from the Fourier transformation and relating these parameters to mean ICP (MICP) and pressure volume index (PVI) gives a possibility for interpretation of their relation to the intracranial elastance.

Methods and Material

Lumbo-ventricular or ventricular perfusion were performed by the method described by Børgesen et al. (1978). When a steady ICP was reached, the system was closed (i.e. the outflow tube was closed at the 3-way stopcock) and the bolus injection for measurement of PVI was given at several pressure levels. The volume injected ranged from 1 to 4 ml, injected by hand in less than 2 sec. The mean intracranial pressure was never elevated above 40 mm Hg. The pulse waves at each steady-state pressure level were analyzed by the methods described by Christensen and Børgesen (1989).

PVI was measured 58 times at different pressure levels in 20 patients undergoing the perfusion study.

Results

In Figure 1, the course of PVI is shown in some of the perfusion studies. It is apparent that there is no meaningful change in PVI with the increasing pressure levels.

In Figure 2, PVI is shown to have no correlation with the PA. PVI could not be related to RT, or to any of the harmonics from the Fourier transformation.

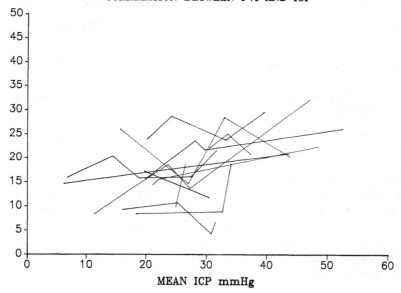

Fig. 1. Plot of PVI with the pulse amplitude. Increases in pulse amplitude are not reflected in changes in PVI

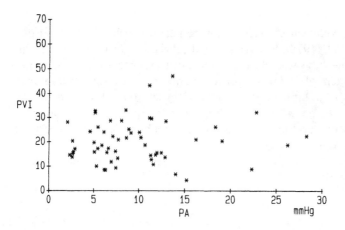

Fig. 2. Plot of PVI with pulse amplitude ($n = 58$). No correlation with the PA

Discussion

It was not possible to relate PVI to any parameters of the pulse pressure wave. Pulse amplitude (PA), risetime (RT) and the first and second harmonics correlated well with the mean intracranial pressure. The decrease in the higher harmonics described by Takizawa et al. (1987) to occur at high ICP levels was not observed. A possible explanation may be that the intracranial pressure was not raised sufficiently high for this phenomenon to occur. The PVI was not very

182

stable during the perfusion test, as is apparent in Fig. 2. No trend of PVI can be deducted, and it can not be postulated that the pressure volume curve tended to shift during the perfusion. There was a clear increase in PA and RT with increasing pressure levels. The study failed to show that the elasticity of the CSF compartment increased with increasing IMCP as evaluated by PVI. Concluding that the increase in PA and RT, therefore, must have another cause (e.g. changes in blood volume loading per pulse beat) is not correct, however, as the PVI measurements varied too much and were too inconsistent. The reason for this is probably purely technical, and refinement of the bolus technique may lead to better, useful results.

Acknowledgement. The study has received financial support from ESKOFOT A/S, Denmark.

References

Børgesen SE, Gjerris F, Sørensen SC (1978) The resistance to cerebrospinal fluid absorption in humans. Acta Neurol Scand 57:88–96
Christensen L, Børgesen SE (1988) Single pulse pressure wave analysis by Fourier transformation. ICP VII, Ann Arbor, Michigan
Takizawa H, Gabra-Sanders T, Miller JD (1987) Changes in the cerebrospinal fluid pulse wave spectrum associated with raised intracranial pressure. Neurosurgery 20:355–361

CSF Pulse Waves in a Model of Progressive Hydrocephalus: An Effect Not a Cause of Ventricular Enlargement

C.M. Zee and K. Shapiro

Humana Advanced Surgical Institutes, Humana Hospital Medical City Dallas, 7777 Forest Lane, Dallas, Texas 75230 (USA)

Introduction

Pulsations in the cerebropsinal fluid have long been identified by researchers (Bering 1955, Dunbar et al. 1966). The origin, configuration, and amplitude of these pulse waves and their response to conditions in the cranial vault have been of interest as well as their role in the pathogenesis of neurologic diseases (White et al. 1979, Foltz and Aine 1980). In this study CSF pulse wave changes are observed with progressive hydrocephalus and its role in the disease process is determined.

Methods

Six adult male cats (3–5 kg) were subjected to craniectomy and rendered hydrocephalic by an intracisternal injection of kaolin. These six cats and six intact animals were used in this study. All animals were anesthetized with pentobarbital, paralyzed with gallamine, intubated, and mounted in a sterotactic frame. The animals were ventilated and arterial blood gases, temperature, EKG, and heart rate were monitored. The pulse waves were monitored in the right lateral ventricle, cisterna magna, subarachnoid space, the sagittal sinus and the lingual artery. All pulse waves were monitored through fluid filled microbore catheters (34 cm) coupled to Gould Stathem P23-ID pressure transducers. All pressure signals were displayed on a Gould strip chart recorder. The pulse wave signals were then filtered and amplified. A DEC PDP11-23 computer was used to sample the signals at 100 Hz and analyze them. The pulse wave signals were continuously monitored on an oscilloscope.

Results

In hydrocephalus a dramatic decrease in pulse size was observed as compared to intact animals (Table 1). This was indicated by a decrease in pulse area and height of at least 85% at all sites ($p < 0.05$). An increase in pulse width of 26.9% ± 1.2,

Eds.: J.T. Hoff and A.L. Betz
© Springer-Verlag Berlin Heidelberg 1989

Table 1. Normal and hydrocephalic pulse wave data

	Site	Area	Height mm Hg	Width msec
Intact	Lateral ventricle	3.947	0.187	9.247
	Cisterna magna	5.839	0.251	8.588
	Subarachnoid space	1.283	0.056	9.080
	Sagittal sinus	2.067	0.093	9.970
Hydrocephalic	Lateral ventricle	0.279	0.012	11.879
	Cisterna magna	0.338	0.011	12.717
	Subarachnoid space	0.046	0.002	11.480
	Sagittal sinus	0.270	0.012	12.553

however, was observed in the ventricle, subarachnoid space, and sagittal sinus with a 48.1% increase in width occurring in the cisterna magna. Prior studies have shown significant differences in pulse wave height between most sites in intact animals. In this study, the hydrocephalic animals evidenced no significant differences in pulse wave height between the lateral ventricle, cisterna magna and the sagittal sinus. The pulse wave observed in the subarachnoid space, however, was significantly smaller. No significant latencies were noted between sites.

Discussion

In this study a dramatic decrease in pulse wave size, at all sites, was observed with hydrocephalus. This decrease in pulse size may be attributed to the higher brain compliance associated with hydrocephalus. The higher brain compliance causes increased damping in the ventricular system resulting in a decreased pulse size due to over damping. From these data, we conclude that the pulse waves themselves do not facilitate ventricular enlargement. Pulse size decreases result from alterations in the ventricular system during the hydrocephalic process.

References

Bering EA (1955) Choroid plexus arterial pulsations of cerebrospinal fluid. Arch Neurol Psychiatry 73:165–172
Dunbar HS, Guthrie TC, Karpell B (1966) A study of the cerebrospinal fluid pulse wave. Arch Neurol 14:624–630
Foltz EL, Aine C (1980) Diagnosis of hydrocephalus by CSF pulsewave analysis: A clinical study. Surg Neurol 15,4:283–293
White DN, Wilson KC, Curry GR, Stevenson RJ (1979) The limitation of pulsatile flow through the aqueduct of sylvius as a cause of hydrocephalus. J Neurol Sci 42:11–51

Normal Pressure Hydrocephalus:
A Retrospective Study on Clinico-Radiological Data, CSF Dynamics and CSF Pulse Waveform Morphology

C. Anile, G. Maira, A. Mangiola, and G.F. Rossi

Institute of Neurosurgery, Catholic University, Largo Gemelli 8, 00168 Rome (Italy)

Introduction

Many pathogenetic factors have been reported to be involved in the genesis and development of so-called normal pressure hydrocephalus (NPH). Among these, the most current are a defect in CSF absorptive capacity (Børgesen 1984) and an increase in the intraventricular CSF pulse amplitude (Di Rocco et al. 1976). However no recent paper has clarified the relationships between the disturbances in CSF and ICP dynamics, often observed in this pathology, with the severity of the clinical picture and/or the brain damage demonstrated by the ventricular enlargement.

Methods and Materials

To this aim we have retrospectively analyzed, in a series of 40 patients all regarded as affected by Hakim-Adams' syndrome and treated by CSF shunting, the following data:

1) *Severity of the symptomatology* dividing the patients in four groups on the basis of the occurrence of one or more symptoms of the triad (to the fourth group belong the patients with all three symptoms and confined to bed in a semivegetative state);
2) *Ventricular size* evaluated by utilizing the ventricular index (VI) of Sklar et al. (1980);
3) *CSF absorptive reserve* by infusing saline at a constant rate into the spinal subarachnoid space up to a plateau pressure;
4) *Intracranial elastance* by calculating the slope of the linear regression between CSF diastolic and pulse pressure values in resting conditions and during spontaneous (REM phase of sleep) or artificially induced (jugular compression, intraventricular infusion) ICP increases;
5) *CSF pulse wave (CSFPW) morphology* by Fourier's spectral analysis in resting and dynamic conditions as described above;
6) *Surgical outcome* by neurological and neuropsychological testing.

Medium pressure valves were employed in all the cases: the shunt patency was post-operatively verified by radiological and/or dynamic controls. No complications were observed after surgery.

Intracranial Pressure VII
Eds.: J.T. Hoff and A.L. Betz
© Springer-Verlag Berlin Heidelberg 1989

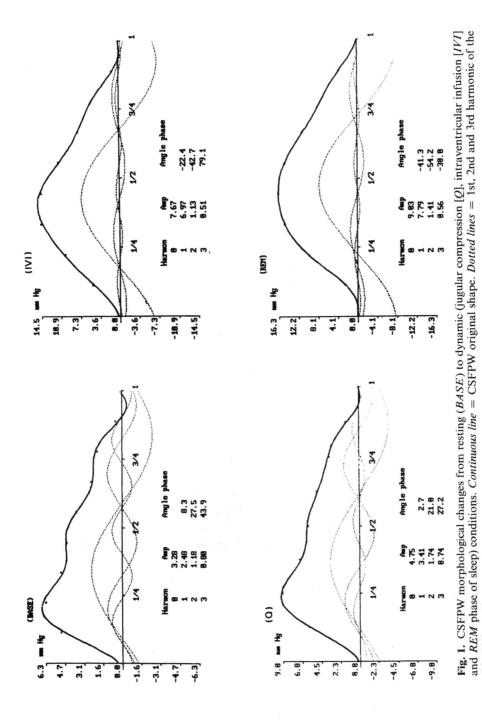

Fig. 1. CSFPW morphological changes from resting (*BASE*) to dynamic (jugular compression [*Q*], intraventricular infusion [*IVI*] and *REM* phase of sleep) conditions. *Continuous line* = CSFPW original shape. *Dotted lines* = 1st, 2nd and 3rd harmonic of the CSFPW spectrum

187

Results

In 30 patients, the result of surgery was regarded as positive, because of a significative improvement in the neurological and neuropsychological performances; in the remaining 10 patients the surgical treatment was clinically ineffective.

An improvement after surgery was seen in all the patients with a VI above 0.75, as well as with an intracranial elastance value more than 0.22, 0.25 and 0.42, during jugular compression, intraventricular infusion and REM sleep, respectively.

Intracranial elastance was, moreover, significatively correlated with the ventricular size; this correlation, represented by a parabolic line, increased from a $VI = 0.5$ to about 1 and then progressively decreased.

No correlation was found between surgical outcome, ventricular size and CSF absorptive reserve.

A particular feature of the CSFPW was noted in the improved patients: in these, in fact, the shape of the CSFPW became more rounded, with disappearance of the dicrotic notch, from resting to dynamic conditions. This phenomenon was particularly evident during the REM phase of sleep. The Fourier's spectral analysis shows that this change in the shape of the CSFPW was associated with a greater increase in amplitude of the fundamental harmonic and a negative phase-shift in respect to the second one (Fig. 1).

Conclusions

The results here presented confirm, in a larger series, those previously published (Rossi et al. 1987) on the reliability of the intracranial elastance compared with the CSF absorptive reserve in identifying, among the patients suspected to suffer from NPH, those with a positive post-shunting surgical outcome. Furthermore, looking at the findings on the correlation between intracranial elastance and ventricular size and on the CSFPW morphology, we can speculate that an impairment in the CSFPW transmission through the intracranial system due to an increase in intracranial elastance could represent an important pathogenetic factor in the genesis and development of NPH.

References

Børgesen SE (1984) Conductance to outflow of CSF in normal pressure hydrocephalus. Acta Neurochir 71:1–45

Di Rocco C, Maira G, Rossi GF, Vignati A (1976) Cerebrospinal fluid pressure studies in normal pressure hydrocephalus and cerebral atrophy. Eur Neurol 14:119–128

Rossi GF, Maira G, Anile C (1987) Intracranial pressure behaviour and its relation to the outcome of surgical CSF shunting in normotensive hydrocephalus. Neurol Res 9:183–187

Sklar FH, Diehl JT, Beyer CW, Clark WK (1980) Brain elasticity changes with ventriculomegaly. J Neurosurg 53:173–179

Application of Advanced Forms of Intracranial Pressure Analysis in Craniosynostosis

L. Batorski[1], M. Czosnyka[2], P. Wollk-Laniewski[3], and W. Zaworski[2]

[1] Clinic of Neurosurgery, Child's Health Centre, [2] Institute of Electronics Fundamentals,
[3] Department of Anesthesiology and Intensive Care, Child's Health Centre, Warsaw (Poland)

Craniosynostosis is a well known clinical syndrome, described in detail in many works. Most reports deal with studies of ICP in this clinical entity (Renier et al. 1982; Gobiet et al. 1976). There have been no reports of analysis of the intracranial pressure (ICP) signal in craniosynostosis using advanced techniques, which could enable one to obtain important information on compensatory mechanisms, and the state of volume-pressure balance of the cerebrospinal system.

It should be emphasized that the state of these mechanisms are, in general, correlated with the phase of craniosynostosis. In the initial and dynamic phases the permanent loss of compensatory reserve and cerebrospinal balance can be noticed. In the prolonged or ex-vacuo stages, advanced atrophic processes may result in a pathological recovery to an equilibrium state and good compensatory ability. It is also well documented that prolonged loss of compensatory ability need not to be followed by an increase in ICP, hence the correlation between the ICP and the period of disease is rather poor.

Therefore, in the present study, advanced forms of ICP processing were applied in signal analysis. The short-term spectral analysis of ICP, which proved to be helpful in the interpretation of the cerebrospinal processes in intensive care (Czosnyka et al. 1987) was applied in preoperative monitoring in craniostenotic patients.

Material and Method

ICP was monitored preoperatively in 11 cases of craniosynostosis of different types. The purpose was to decide on the character and strategy for surgery. Patients, aged from 1 to 9 years, were subjected to the insertion of an epidural Hirsch sensor, connected by stiff manometer line (1 m long) to a pressure transducer (HP 1280 c) and pressure monitor. ICP was monitored continuously for at least 12 hrs. Only slight sedation was maintained (Pentobarbital) to avoid frequent movement artifacts in recordings. It should be emphasized that monitoring during ICP was analyzed by means of a signal analyzer of our own design, prepared for the IBM-PC/XT microcomputer (Czosnyka et al. 1988, in press).

The following parameters were calculated periodically (the period could be chosen from 1 to 5 min): (1) mean ICP level; (2) amplitude of the pulse wave (AMP); (3) averaged power of the slow waves (SLOW); (4) amplitude of the respiratory wave (RESP); (5) heart rate (HR); (6) correlation coefficient between the amplitude of the pulse wave and the mean ICP level (RAP); (7) the slope of the short-term amplitude-pressure characteristic (A-P).

The above parameters are presented and stored on the disk as time trends with the full possibility of performing correlation analysis, zooming, smoothing, etc.

Results and Discussion

ICP remained in the range reported in other papers concerning craniosynostosis, with the mean ICP of about 12 mm Hg, and never exceeding a level of 30 mm Hg. Only slight differences in courses of the mean ICP between examined patients were noticed. No A waves were observed in the described material. Only medium intensity B waves were noticed. This suggests that the mean ICP level alone cannot be regarded as a significant factor for differentiation between patients. Mean amplitude of the pulse wave also did not differ from the range observed in other kinds of cerebrospinal pathologies (1–5 mm Hg).

The most important finding was the specific behavior of the short-term and averaged relationships between the amplitudes of the pulse wave and the mean pressure level. These relationships, according to many works and the authors' own experience, characterize mechano-elastic properties of the cerebrospinal system. Strong statistical relationships between pressure and pulse wave amplitude reveal poor compensatory ability commonly observed in this pathology. The short-term correlation coefficient (RAP) was very close to 1 even over relatively long periods, without evidence of external reasons for introducing uncompensated volume processes (Fig. 1 a). In some cases, the averaged amplitude-pressure relationship (AMP-P) was non-linear – its slope increasing with rising ICP level (Fig. 1 b). A positive and statistically significant correlation between the mean ICP level and the slope of the short-term AMP-P regression line (A-P) was detected (Fig. 1 c). According to our interpretation of the short-term correlation coefficient, RAP (Czosnyka et al. 1987), these findings indicate the presence of an uncompensated volume process.

From a typical illustration of the state of the cerebrospinal system on an amplitude-pressure plane, we conclude that, in craniosynostosis, where a positive regression coefficient between the amplitude and the pressure is observed, it remains permanently above the lower breakpoint of the AMP-P characteristic. The nonlinear (of an exponential shape) amplitude-pressure characteristic, as well as the positive correlation between the slope of the short-term AMP-P line and mean ICP, seems to be typical for the acute or dynamic stage of craniosynostosis with clinical evidence of permanent decompensation. The prolonged or ex-vacuo stage can be differentiated by taking into account the correlation (both short and long-term) between the ICP and the amplitude of the pulse wave. It differs significantly from 1 in long period and the slope of AMP-P line is much lower.

In conclusion it should be emphasized that both the AMP-P characteristic and the short-term correlation coefficient RAP are good indices of the level of cerebrospinal compensation, and can be applied effectively in monitoring patients with craniosynostosis.

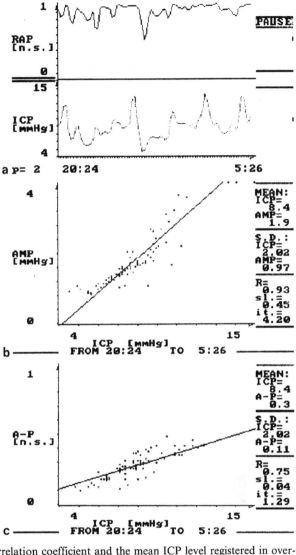

Fig. 1. a Trends of the RAP correlation coefficient and the mean ICP level registered in overnight monitoring. RAP remains close to 1 in all periods (*abscissa* – time; trends sampled every 7 min). **b** The amplitude (*AMP – ordinate*) – pressure (*ICP – abscissa*) characteristic calculated from the period presented above. Note non-linear character of the relationship. It can be considered as monoexponential due to positive and significant ($p < 0.01$) correlation coefficient between the slope of the short term AMP/p characteristic and mean pressure level. **c** *Ordinate* – slope of AMP/p, *abscissa* – mean ICP

References

Czosnyka M, Laniewski P, Batorski L (1987) Clinical application of system for intracranial pressure monitoring and processing in intensive care. Proc of VIIth Nordic Meeting on Medical and Biological Engineering, University of Trondheim, Norway

Czosnyka M, Laniewski P, Batorski L, Zaworski W (1988) A system for ICP processing and interpretation in intensive care. In: Advances in Biomedical Measurement, Plenum Publ Corp, pp 101–109

Gobiet W, Strahl EW, Bock WJ (1976) Direct measurement of ICP in cases of craniosynostosis as a diagnostic aid for operation. In: Beks JWF, Bosh DA, Brock M (eds) Intracranial Pressure III. Springer, Berlin Heidelberg New York, pp 336–339

Renier D, Saint-Rose C, Marchac D, Hirsch JF (1982) Intracranial pressure in craniostenosis. J Neurosurg 57:370–377

CSF Pulse Waveform Morphology as an Indicator of Intracranial System Impedance: An Experimental Study

C. Anile, A. Mangiola, F. Andreasi[1], C.A. Branch[2], and H.D. Portnoy[2]

Institute of Neurosurgery, [1] Institute of Physics, Catholic University, Rome (Italy), and [2] Department of Neurology, Henry Ford Hospital, Detroit, Michigan (USA)

Introduction

Our previous studies in dogs have demonstrated that the pressure-volume responses at a constant rate of 0.2 cc/sec and the slow ICP waves due to the respiratory cycle are dependent on the rigidity of the skull. They are significantly reduced by opening the intracranial system (ICS) to the atmosphere as previously described (Anile et al. 1987). In contrast, the amplitude of short perturbations, such as a very rapid bolus-injection and the ICP pulse waves remains unchanged.

We suggested that the capability of the ICS to compensate for variations in its volume depends on the length of time during which such variations occur, and introduced the concept of physical and physiological compliance, the former related to the physical structure of the skull and dura, and the latter probably related to the venous outflow resistance.

Other studies (Cardoso et al. 1983; Hirai et al. 1984) have suggested that variations in the various components of the CSF pulse waveform (CSFPW) could give precise information about the ICS. Portnoy et al. (1982), using Fourier spectral analysis noted a correlation between the harmonics of the carotid artery pulse wave and the CSFPW, particularly the fundamental harmonic.

Methods and Materials

In four animals using the previously described experimental model, we have analyzed the modifications in the CSF, arterial, sagittal sinus and bridging veins pulse wave morphology during the same experimental conditions of opening/ closing of the ICS at different ICP levels. We have analyzed both the shape of the different pulse pressure curves looking, in particular, at the area under the curve and the amplitude of the dicrotic peak and their spectral composition.

Results

No modifications of the shape of the systemic blood pulse pressure (SBP) was observed in the different experimental conditions. There was a linear correlation

Intracranial Pressure VII   193
Eds.: J. T. Hoff and A. L. Betz
© Springer-Verlag Berlin Heidelberg 1989

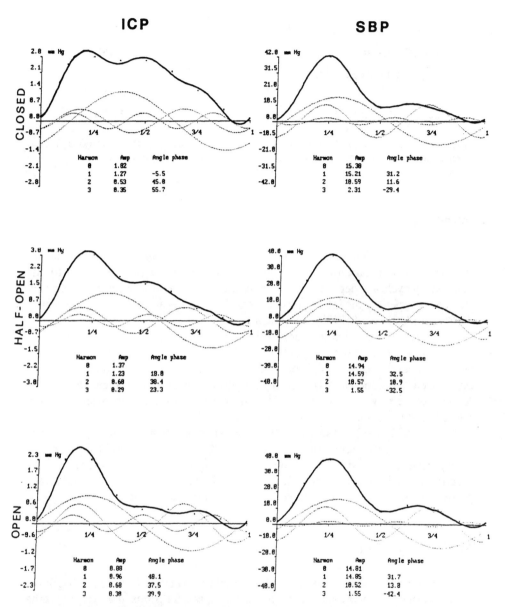

Fig. 1. Arterial (*SBP*) and CSF (*ICP*) pulse wave morphological changes induced by gradual ICS opening to the atmosphere. *Continuous line* = arterial and CSF pulse wave original shape. *Dotted lines* = 1st, 2nd and 3rd harmonic of the arterial and CSF pulse wave spectrum

found between the area under the total pulse wave curve and the amplitude of the dicrotic peak of the CSF pulse with diastolic ICP. The area under the curve and the dicrotic peak decrease as ICS is progressively opened to the atmosphere (Maira et al. 1987). The bridging vein pulse waveform is exactly the same as the CSF and has the same relationship to the dicrotic vein pressure. The morpholo-

194

gical changes of the sagittal sinus pulse waveform are independent of the diastolic ICP values. Furthermore, spectral analysis shows a decrease in the amplitude of the CSFPW fundamental frequency with a positive phase-shift in respect to the second harmonic as ICS becomes more open (Fig. 1).

Conclusions

Our findings support the proposal that the CSFPW analysis may give insight into the status of inflow (arterial) and outflow (laterales lacunae) impedances and, therefore, insight into the cerebral autoregulation. The period of the fundamental harmonic closely approximates the value of the "time-constant" of our model, as the ICS moves from a "physiological" to a "physical" status and vice versa. We believe that arterial and venous outflow impedances are affected by the physical compliance of the ICS, and CSFPW analysis may be of value in conditions where alterations in physical compliance of the ICS are a factor.

References

Anile C, Portnoy HD, Branch C (1987) Intracranial compliance is time-dependent. Neurosurgery 20:389–395

Cardoso ER, Rowan JO, Galbraith S (1983) Analysis of the cerebrospinal fluid pulse wave intracranial pressure. J Neurosurg 59:817–821

Hirai O, Handa H, Ishikawa M, Jim S-H (1984) Epidural pulse waveform as an indicator of intracranial pressure dynamics. Surg Neurol 21:67–74

Maira G, Anile C, Mangiola A, Proietti R, Zanghi F, Della Corte F (1987) Intracranial elastance and CSF pulse waveform. Experimental study and clinical applications in comatose patients. J Ped Neurosc 3:92–100

Portnoy HD, Chopp M, Branch C, Shannon M (1982) Cerebrospinal fluid pulse waveform as an indicator of cerebral autoregulation. J Neurosurg 56:666–678

Transmission Characteristics of Pulse Waves in the Intracranial Cavity of Dogs During Normal Intracranial Condition, Intracranial Hypertension, Hypercapnia, and Hydrocephalus

Y. Kasuga[1], H. Nagai[2], and Y. Hasegawa[3]

[1] Department of Neurosurgery, Meitetsu Hospital, and [2] Department of Neurosurgery, and [3] First Department of Physiology, Nagoya City University, Nagoya 451 (Japan)

Recently, some new mathematical analyses have been applied to the field of ICP, most of which use a computer to easily calculate the complex computations required. Systems analysis is one example of these mathematical approaches, first used by Chopp and Portnoy in ICP in 1980. They calculated power spectra of systemic arterial pressure pulse waves and ICP pulse waves by a fast-Fourier transformation (FFT) and transfer functions were made by the power spectra. Since then, investigations about the power spectra of ICP pulse waves have been successively reported, but have not been systems analyses but simple frequency analyses. While, we have continued to study, the intracranial physical characteristics by using systems analysis from 1979, we have also determined and reported transfer functions in continuous forms (Kasuga et al. 1987). In this paper we report transfer functions under some specific intracranial conditions, which include normal intracranial conditions, intracranial hypertension, hypercapnia, and kaolin-induced hydrocephalus.

Materials and Methods

The canine intracranial cavity was assumed to be a linear system to which we applied systems analysis. The carotid arterial pressure pulse waves were used as the input and the epidural pressure (EDP) pulse waves as the output. We determined the transfer functions, using the least squares method. The analytical method was fully described in a previously published paper (Kasuga et al. 1987).

Twenty adult mongrel dogs weighing about 10 kg each were used. The dogs were divided into five groups, each consisting of four dogs. Group 1 dogs had normal intracranial conditions, Group 2 dogs had elevated ICP caused by inflation of a small balloon in the epidural space, Group 3 dogs had elevated ICP caused by infusion of saline into the cisterna magna, Group 4 dogs had hypercapnia induced by decreasing their respiratory volumes and rates, and Group 5 dogs were subjected to infusion of 50 mg/kg of kaolin into the cisterna magna to induce hydrocephalus within 4 weeks.

Intracranial Pressure VII
Eds.: J. T. Hoff and A. L. Betz
© Springer-Verlag Berlin Heidelberg 1989

Each dog was anesthetized by intravenous administration of thiopental sodium. Endotracheal intubation was performed and controlled mechanical ventilation conducted. A No. 19 polyethylene catheter was inserted into the common carotid artery to record arterial pressure pulse waves, and a Cranomet EDP sensor (Nagai et al. 1980) was attached in the parietal region to record ICP pulse waves. The input information was randomized during recordings by a cardiac pacemaker electrode placed in the epicardium in order to accurately interpret the characteristics of a system as a continuous transfer function. The data of ICP pulse waves and arterial pressure pulse waves were recorded for 4 min on an analog data recorder and digitized every 5 msec on an analog-to-digital converter, followed by computer analysis. To eliminate changes due to respiration, data were collected after signals of 1 Hz or less were discarded by means of software processing. Up to 500 msec was the lag time.

Results

The Bode diagrams and step responses of the transfer functions for the representative cases of each group are illustrated in Fig. 1. Group 1 dogs showed a remarkable peak at about 10 to 15 Hz in the gain curve of the Bode diagram (Fig. 1 A). The finding indicates that resonance occurs in the system at that frequency. In Group 2 and 3 dogs, the peak of resonance became fairly obscure as ICP rose. This seemed to be caused by relatively increasing the gains at frequencies lower than 10 Hz (Fig. 1 B, C). There was almost no difference in the transfer functions between Group 2 and 3 dogs. Group 4 dogs showed that the peak of resonance was still clearly observed in spite of a relative increment of the gain at frequencies lower than 10 Hz (Fig. 3 D). In Group 5 dogs, however, the peak of resonance at about 10 to 15 Hz completely disappeared and the gains at frequencies lower than 10 Hz were remarkably increased (Fig. 1 E).

Discussion

The results showed that there was resonance in the intracranial cavity system of dogs under a normal intracranial environment. The resonance became fairly obscure as ICP rose. We interpret the disappearance or obscurity of resonance with rising ICP as being apparent rather than real, because the peak of resonance at the frequency clearly exists in spite of a relative increment of gains at frequencies lower than 10 Hz. The resonance did not disappear or become obscure in hypercapnic dogs. This finding indicates that the resonance is almost independent of intracranial vascular tonicity. Finally, the resonance completely disappeared in hydrocephalic dogs. It is difficult to understand what causes this loss of resonance. We assume, however, that the resonance is somehow related to the viscoelasticity of the brain parenchyma.

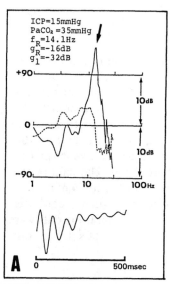

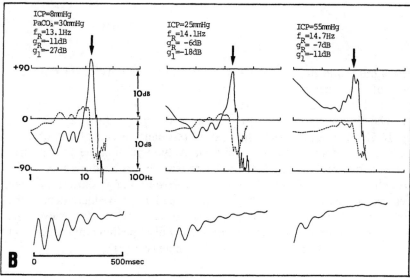

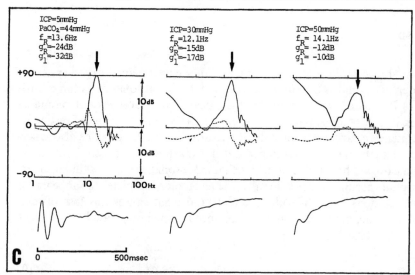

Fig. 1 A–C

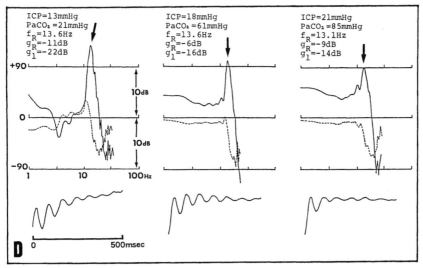

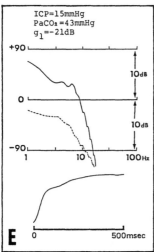

Fig. 1. Bode diagrams and step responses of representative dogs in Group 1 (**A**), Group 2 (**B**), Group 3 (**C**), Group 4 (**D**), and Group 5 (**E**). In the Bode diagrams, gain (*solid line*) and phase shift (*dotted line*) of the system are plotted against the logarithm of the frequency. Step response is equivalent to the system output, which is related to the system input of stepping signals. Note each gain curve except Group 5 forms a remarkable peak (*arrow*) that represents resonance. f_R: resonance frequency, g_1: absolute gain value at 1 Hz, g_R: absolute gain value at f_R

Considering the transfer functions, we noticed there were two different systems – a "first order system" and a "second order system" – in the intracranial cavity. The former is also called "first order lag element" and features a relationship between the input and output that can be expressed as a first order differential equation. Its Bode diagram and step response are shown in Fig. 2A. The results of our experiments indicate that the first order system mostly appeared in hydrocephalic dogs. The latter is also called "second order lag element" and features a relationship between the input and output that can be expressed as a second order differential equation. Its Bode diagram and step response are shown in Fig. 2B. Resonance sometimes occurs in this system. The second order system seemed to be clearly apparent in normal intracranial conditioned dogs and both

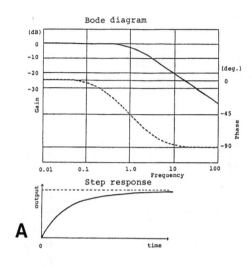

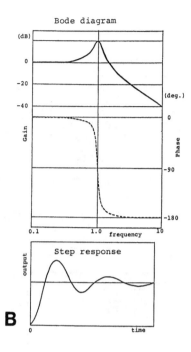

Fig. 2. Bode diagrams and step responses of a first order system (**A**) and a second order system (**B**). *Slid line* represents gain curve and *dotted line* represents phase shift curve

systems appeared at nearly half the rate in hypercapnic dogs. The first order system seemed to be stronger than the second order system in intracranial hypertensive dogs.

References

Chopp M, Portnoy HD (1980) Systems analysis of intracranial pressure. J Neurosurg 53:516–527

Kasuga Y, Nagai H, Hasegawa Y, Nitta M (1987) Transmission characteristics of pulse waves in the intracranial cavity of dogs. J Neurosurg 66:907–914

Nagai H, Kamiya I, Ikeyama J, Inagaki O (1980) A newly devised transducer for epidural pressure measurement and its clinical use. In: Shulman K, Marmarou A, Miller JD, Becker DP, Hochwald GM, Brock M (eds) Intracranial Pressure IV. Springer, Berlin Heidelberg New York, pp 417–418

Cerebral Pulse Amplitude in a Canine Model of "Slit" Ventricle Syndrome

J.S. Nichols and F.H. Sklar

Division of Neurological Surgery, University of Colorado, Health Sciences Center, P.O. Box C-307, 4200 East Ninth Avenue, Denver, Colorado 80262 (USA)

Introduction

Continuously draining shunts resulting in "slit" ventricles have been associated with symptoms mimicking shunt malfunction and increased intracranial pressure (ICP). However, when tested, the mean ICP is normal or low. Recent clinical investigations have suggested that patients with "slit" ventricles may have augmented cerebral pulse amplitude (CPA) at normal or low ICP (Foltz and Blanks 1988). This study investigates the relationship between CPA and mean ICP in a computer-controlled canine model simulating "slit" ventricle syndrome.

Methods

Four healthy mongrel dogs of either sex, weighing approximately 10 kilograms were used in this study. Animals were anesthetized with sodium pentobarbital, intubated, mechanically ventilated and positioned prone in a sterotaxic frame. A femoral arterial catheter was used to monitor blood pressure and obtain arterial blood gases. Blood pressure, blood gases and body temperature were maintained within normal physiological ranges. The lateral ventricle was cannulated with an 18 gauge spinal needle connected via high pressure tubing to a Statham pressure transducer and Sanborn polygraph.

ICP was controlled using a 18 gauge spinal needle placed in the opposite lateral ventricle. A servo-controlled infusion pump with a reciprocal syringe arrangement, a fluid reservoir and a solenoid valve switching device controlled the continuous infusion or withdrawal of normal saline over ICP ranges between negative 15 mm Hg and 35 mm Hg. A PDP 11/34 dual drive computer (Digital Equipment Corporation) activated the solenoid valve allowing constant artifact free infusion or withdrawal of fluid.

In addition to controlling ICP, the PDP 11/34 computer collected mean ICP at one second intervals and measured CPA at 10 msec intervals. Fast sampled data was displayed on a Textronix 4010 graphics terminal and visual identification was made of the diastole and systole to determine CPA.

Mean ICP and CPA were entered into a DEC-10 computer (Digital Equipment Corporation) for statistical analysis and curve fitting.

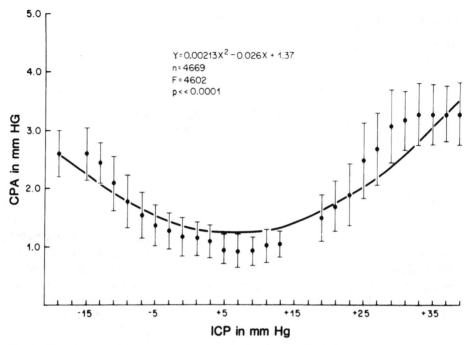

Fig. 1. Mean intracranial pressure versus cerebral pulse amplitude in a computer controlled canine model of "slit" ventricle syndrome

Results

Data from four dogs were averaged and represents 4600 data points (Fig. 1). Results comparing CPA and mean ICP fit a parabolic equation of $Y = ax^2 + bx + c$. The p value was significantly less than 0.001. CPA increased at both low and high value of mean ICP. The nadir or the parabolic curve approximates the resting intracranial pressure.

Conclusions

These data define a parabolic relationship between the CPA and mean ICP. CPA significantly increases at both low and high ICP. Likely, at low mean ICP's there is a decrease in the CSF buffering capacity to pressure changes resulting in an augmented CPA. Decreased CSF volume resulting in an augmented CPA may be responsible for the symptoms of "slit" ventricle syndrome. In addition the nadir of the parabolic relationship between mean ICP and CPA may define the ideal CSF volume for maximum buffering capacity.

Reference

Foltz EL, Blanks JP (1988) Symptomatic low intracranial pressure in shunted hydrocephalus. J Neurosurg 68:401–408

Intracranial and Venous Pressures
Part I: Intracranial Pulse Wave Changes During
Hemodynamic Maneuvers in Humans

E.R. Cardoso and D. Piatek

Cerebral Hydrodynamics Laboratory, Department of Surgery, University of Manitoba,
Winnipeg, Manitoba R3A 1R9 (Canada)

Introduction

The configuration of the intracranial pulse wave (ICPW) depends upon the temporal summation of pulsations traveling through the entire cerebral vascular tree (Cardoso et al. 1983). A correspondence between each segment of the cerebral circulation and different portions of the ICPW has not yet been established. Thus, we induced hemodynamic changes on the venous portion of the cerebral circulation in order to observe simultaneous changes on the ICPW.

Material and Methods

Continuous intracranial pressure monitoring was carried out on twelve consecutive patients for confirmation of the diagnosis of occult communicating hydrocephalus.
 Patients were subjected to the following sequential maneuvers:
1. Bilateral manual jugular compression
2. 15° elevation of the head of the bed
3. Bilateral manual jugular compression at 15° head elevation.

 ICP and ICPW data obtained during the maneuvers were digitized and analyzed by a microcomputer coupled to a wave analyzer (Data 6000 Wave Analyzer). The three main ICPW components P1, P2, and P3 were identified and measured. Data points related to mean ICP and amplitude of ICPW components, P1, P2 and P3, from before and after each maneuver were compared statistically by paired two-tailed Student t-test.

Results

The average mean baseline intracranial pressure for all patients was 8.2 ± 1.7 mm Hg (SE). Each patient presented a highly individual wave configuration. Head elevation by 15° significantly lowered the mean ICP by 6.74 ± 0.99 mm Hg

Table 1. Mean and standard deviation of mean intracranial pressure (ICP) and amplitude of ICPW components P1, P2 and P3 before and after hemodynamic maneuvers

Hemodynamic maneuvers	Δ ICP mm Hg, $\bar{x} \pm$ SEM	% Δ amplitude % ICPW components		
		P 1	P 2	P 3
Jugular compression	↑ 4.97±0.8 ***	↑	↑ 36 **	↑ 51 ***
Head up 15°	↓ 6.74±0.55 ***	↓ 3	↑ 22 *	↑ 30 *
Jugular compression at 15°	↑ 6.50±0.85 ***	↑ 15	↑ 24 **	↑ 19 *

* $p<0.02$; ** $p<0.01$; *** $p<0.001$.

($p<0.0001$). It also caused paradoxical increase of amplitude of P2 by 22% ± 3.2 ($p<0.02$) and P3 by 30% ± 4.1 ($p<0.02$), while P1 remained unchanged (Table 1).

Manual bilateral jugular compression in the horizontal position caused significant elevation of the mean ICP by 4.97 ± 0.8 mm Hg ($p<0.001$). It also produced a significant increase of the amplitude of components P_2 and P_3 by 36 ± 4.8% and 51 ± 3.9% respectively. Again the amplitude of P1 remained unchanged (Table 1). At 15° head elevation, jugular compression caused a greater increase of the mean ICP of 6.5 ± 0.85 ($p<0.001$) and also lead to significant increases of amplitude of P2 by 24 ± 3.1% ($p<0.01$) and P3 by 19 ± 2.8% ($p<0.02$), without altering P1.

Discussion

The findings of ICPW analysis during head maneuvers in hydrocephalic patients provided useful clues for the interpretation of hydrodynamic changes of the intracranial compartment. On 15° head elevation there was an increase in amplitude of P2 and P3, despite a fall in mean ICP. This suggests that 15° head elevation of hydrocephalic patients may facilitate retrograde transmission of venous pressure into the CSF, as the ICPW components P2 and P3 may in part originate from venous pulsations (Berring 1955, Dardenne et al. 1969). Head elevation in hydrocephalic patients causes lesser fall of the mean ICP as compared to the cerebral venous pressure, thus decreasing the pressure gradient across the venous CSF interface (Norcel et al. 1969, Shulman and Ransohoff 1965). According to the ICPW mathematical modeling of Klassen et al. narrowing of the pressure gradient increases the transmission of pulse pressure (Klassen et al., ICP VII Program). Furthermore, the shift of CSF volume into the spinal canal with head elevation is likely compensated by dilatation of the cerebral veins, which in turn increase their pulsatile surface. We, therefore, postulate that head elevation may magnify the retrograde transmission of venous pulsations into the head as a result of equalization of pressure gradients across the venous wall, as well as increasing venous pooling. As a result the amplitude of P2 and P3 increased at 15°.

Head elevation may facilitate the magnification of components P2 and P3 following jugular compression because both maneuvers dilate cerebral veins.

The ICPW findings described in this study give support to experimental results suggesting that the initial portion of the ICPW is formed mainly from pulsation originated in larger intracranial arteries, while the later portions are related to venous pulsations (Bering 1955, Dardenne et al. 1969). Thus, the increases of P2 and P3 observed with head elevation and jugular compression suggest that an increased effectiveness of transmission of venous pressure to the CSF takes place.

Acknowledgement. We wish to express our gratitude to the James A. and Muriel Richardson Trust Fund through the Winnipeg Foundation for funding of this project.

References

Bering EA Jr (1955) Choroid plexus and arterial pulsation of cerebrospinal fluid. Demonstration of the choroid plexuses as a cerebrospinal fluid pump. Arch Neurol Psychiat 73:165–172

Cardoso ER, Rowan JO, Galbraith S (1983) Analysis of the cerebrospinal fluid pulse wave in intracranial pressure. J Neurosurg 59:817–821

Dardenne G, Dereymaeker A, Lacheron JM (1969) Cerebrospinal fluid pressure and pulsatility. Eur Neurol 2:193–216

Norrel H, Wilson C, Wowieson J et al. (1969) Venous factors in infantile hydrocephalus. J Neurosurg 31:561–569

Shulman K, Ransohoff J (1965) Sagittal sinus venous pressure in hydrocephalus.

Intracranial and Venous Pressures
Part II: Extracranial Source of B-Waves

B. Unger and E.R. Cardoso

Cerebral Hydrodynamics Laboratory, Department of Surgery, University of Manitoba, Winnipeg, Manitoba R3A 1R9 (Canada)

Introduction

B-waves were first described by Lundberg as periodic elevations of intracranial pressure (ICP) of variable amplitude and lasting between 30 to 120 sec (Lundberg 1960). They were interpreted as manifestations of impaired intracranial compliance and were attributed to reflex changes in cerebral arterial resistance. It was also observed that cyclic alterations in breathing occur simultaneously with B waves but since Lundberg's original description, the mechanisms responsible for B-waves have received little attention.

We postulate that B-waves result from a primary respiratory dysrhythmia that leads to cyclic changes in venous pressure, which are then transmitted in a retrograde fashion into the intracranial compartment.

Materials and Methods

From a group of patients undergoing ICP monitoring for diagnosis of hydrocephalus, four subjects were selected on the basis of the presence of persistent B-waves on overnight monitoring. ICP was monitored by indwelling intraventricular catheter. The peripheral venous pressure was monitored simultaneously from the subclavian vein. Respiratory impedance plethysmography was also carried out on all four patients. The following hydrodynamic maneuvers were performed:

1. 15° elevation of the head of the bed.
2. Return to the horizontal position.
3. Drainage of enough cerebral spinal fluid (CSF) to produce a mean ICP comparable to that achieved by head elevation.

Results

Changes in respiratory excursion synchronous with B-waves, were observed in all patients. Peripheral venous pressure also showed cyclic variations similar in appearance, timing, and duration to the intracranial B-waves.

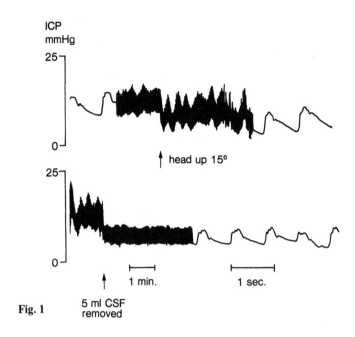

ICP
mmHg

↑ head up 15°

↑ 1 min.   1 sec.

Fig. 1   5 ml CSF
removed

The patients studied had a mean baseline ICP of 6.75 ± 2.6 mmHg. CSF drainage caused a mean ICP fall of 4.75 ± 1.9 mmHg while B-wave amplitude significantly declined by 3.66 ± 0.2 mmHg ($p < 0.001$). Head elevation reduced the mean ICP by 3.6 ± 1.3 mmHg but also resulted in a paradoxical increase in B-wave amplitude of 0.97 ± 0.2 mmHg ($p < 0.002$) (Fig. 1). No change in mean peripheral venous pressure or in venous wave amplitude was detected with head elevation or following CSF drainage.

Discussion

B-waves have long been thought to result from reduced intracranial compliance, implying that any maneuver designed to lower the mean ICP should bring about a reduction in B-wave amplitude. This was not confirmed in our study. Our results suggest that B-waves are more related to cyclic venous pulsations than to intracranial compliance. In Part I of our study it was shown that head elevation in hydrocephalic patients may facilitate the retrograde transmission of venous pressures into the intracranial compartment. This might also explain the increase in B-wave amplitude caused by elevation of the head. Thus, we suggest that B-waves may result from retrograde transmission of venous pulsations across cerebral venous walls.

Mean ICP is slightly greater than sagittal sinus venous pressure (SSVP) creating a small pressure gradient from ICP to SSVP. Head elevation in hydrocephalic patients causes a greater fall in the ICP than the SSVP, thus decreasing the ICP-SSVP gradient (Sainte-Rose et al. 1984). Since pulsatile transmission across cerebral venous walls is inversely proportional to the pressure gradient between blood and CSF, transmission of cerebral venous pulsations should increase with head elevation (Klassen et al. 1988). CSF drainage reduces the ICP, but not the SSVP. A fall in ICP to levels below the jugular venous pressure may result in an increase of the ICP-SSVP gradient, diminishing transmission of pulsations and causing a reduction in B-wave amplitude.

We suggest that intracranial B-waves are due to retrograde transmission of extracranial venous pulsations. These are likely due to cyclic respiratory changes caused by a primary defect in central respiratory control. Our results suggest that the IVP-SSVP gradient is more important than the state of intracranial compliance in the genesis of B-waves.

Acknowledgement. We are thankful to the Health Sciences Centre Research Foundation for funding this project.

References

Klassen PA et al. (1988) Mathematical modelling of the contribution of arterial diameter pulse to the configuration of the intracranial pulse wave (ICP III)

Lundberg W (1960) Continuous recording and control of ventricular fluid pressure in neurosurgical practice. Acta Psychiatr Scand [Suppl 14a] 36:1–193

Sainte-Rose C et al. (1984) Intracranial venous hypertension: Cause or consequence of hydrocephalus in infants? J Neurosurg 60:727–736

B-Waves in Healthy Persons

D. Mautner[1], U. Dirnagl[1], R. Haberl[1], P. Schmiedek[2], C. Garner[1],
A. Villringer[1], and K.M. Einhäupl[1]

[1] Departments of Neurology, and [2] Neurosurgery, University of Munich,
D-8000 München 70 (FRG)

Introduction

The etiology of $0.5-2$/minute oscillations of the ICP (B-waves, Lundberg, 1960) is controversial: some authors assume a correlation of B-waves to respiration, esp. to periodic breathing, by cerebral vasodilatation and constriction as a result of a periodic rise and fall in CO_2 (Kjaellquist et al. 1964, Børgesen and Espersen 1986). Others postulate an oscillator in the brainstem (Hayashi et al. 1986, Maeda et al. 1986). Another possibility for the origin of B-waves might be a myogenic rhythm of the intracranial vessels (Auer 1981). Their clinical significance is controversial, too. They are supposed to be a hint on a disturbed cerebrospinal fluid outflow and, therefore, a predictor for the success of shunting in normal pressure hydrocephalus (Brock 1977). In contrast they were also reported to signify a bad clinical condition (Hase et al. 1978) or to be of no significance at all (Hamer and Kühner 1967, Voldby and Enevoldsen 1982). It is also unclear whether these oscillations appear in healthy persons. Einhäupl and coworkers (1986) found oscillations in ICP simultaneous with cardiovascular as well as respiratory parameters and, therefore, postulated a CNS-rhythm as responsible for these oscillations. They suspected that B-waves might be a physiological phenomenon. In the following study, we wanted to test this hypothesis.

Methods

During B-wave activity, 20 patients were monitored for oscillations of the blood flow velocity in the middle cerebral artery by means of Transcranial Doppler Sonography (TCD) using the EME tc 2-64. Extracranial parameters such as systemic arterial pressure (SAP), heart rate, respiration and cutaneous circulation were also monitored. In addition, we investigated 20 healthy persons. In this group the same parameters except for the ICP and the SAP were monitored over a two hour time period. All parameters of both groups including the TCD-signal and the ICP were recorded on a multichannel paper strip. For the analysis of periodic fluctuations, the ICP and the TCD-signal were analog/digital converted and a spectral analysis (FFT) was performed in order to obtain the amplitudes and duration of the oscillatory activity.

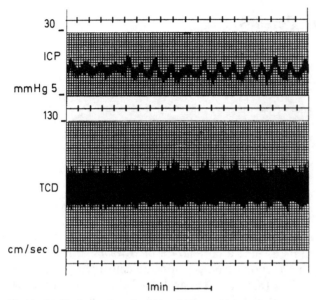

Fig. 1. Oscillations of cerebral blood flow velocity (TCD) simultaneously with B-waves in ICP

Results

All patients showed phases of oscillations in the cerebral blood flow velocity during B-wave activity in the ICP (Fig. 1) regardless whether the patient was artificially ventilated or breathing periodically. Oscillations with the same frequency were also seen in the extracranial parameters. 16 of 20 healthy persons showed 0.5–2/min blood flow velocity oscillations with a mean amplitude of 5.4 cm/sec. The mean flow velocity of the 20 subjects was 58.6 cm/sec. In two subjects we found amplitudes up to 13 cm/sec and 14 cm/sec that is 21% and 19% of their mean flow velocity, respectively. Only four subjects showed oscillations from the beginning of the recording, in the remaining 12 subjects oscillations started with a mean delay of 5 min. Oscillations appeared simultaneously in heart rate, cutaneous circulation, respiration and finger pulse (Fig. 2).

Discussion

During B-wave activity in the ICP, we were able to find 0.5–2/min oscillations in cerebral blood flow velocity measured by TCD. ICP and TCD were always oscillating together; there were no periods of TCD oscillations without ICP oscillations and vice versa. In healthy persons 0.5–2/minute-oscillations in blood flow velocity coincided with 0.5–2/min oscillations in the systemic parameters. The pattern of the oscillations in the noninvasive extracranial parameters were

210

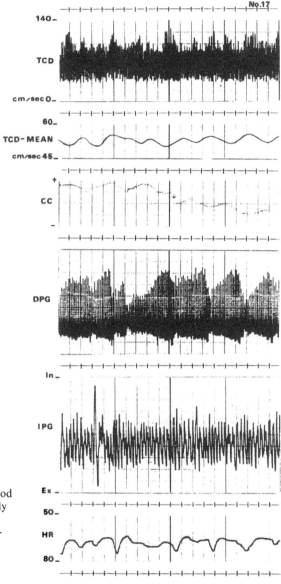

Fig. 2. Oscillations of cerebral blood flow velocity (TCD) simultaneously with 0.5–2/minute-oscillations in extracranial parameters (*CC*, cutaneous circulation; *DPG*, digital plethysmogram; IPG *respiration;* *HR*, heart rate)

identical in both groups. Therefore, we conclude that the finding oscillations in flow velocity in normals is an indirect proof for the concept that B-waves are a physiological phenomenon. They reflect oscillations in cerebral blood volume leading to intracranial pressure oscillation, even though they might be small in amplitude in normals because of good volume compensation capacity.

211

References

Auer LM (1981) Rhythmic patterns of pial vessels to neurogenic and metabolic stimuli and blood pressure changes. In: Cervos-Navarro J, Frischka E (eds) Cerebral Microcirculation and Metabolism. Raven Press, New York, pp 271–277

Børgesen SE, Espersen JO (1986) The correlation between A- and B-waves and arterial CO_2 tension. In: Miller JD, Teasdale GM, Rowan JO, Galbraith S, Mendelow D (eds) Intracranial Pressure VI. Springer, Berlin Heidelberg New York Tokyo, pp 298–304

Brock M (1977) Klinik und Therapie des normotensiven Hydrocephalus. Radiologe 17:460–465

Einhäupl KM, Garner C, Dirnagl U, Schmieder G, Schmiedek P, Kufner G, Rieder J (1986) Oscillations of ICP related to cardiovascular parameters. In: Miller JD, Teasdale GM, Rowan JO, Galbraith S, Mendelow D (eds) Intracranial Pressure VI. Springer, Berlin Heidelberg New York Tokyo, pp 290–297

Hamer J, Kühner A (1976) Mean intracranial resting pressure, episodic fluctuations, and intracranial volume/pressure response in patients with subarachnoid hemorrhage. In: Beks JWF, Bosch DA, Brock M (eds) Intracranial Pressure III. Springer, Berlin Heidelberg New York, pp 157–161

Hase U, Reulen H-J, Fenske A, Schuermann K (1987) Intracranial pressure and pressure volume relation in patients with subarachnoid hemorrhage. Acta Neurochir (Wien) 44:69–80

Hayashi M, Handa Y, Kobayashi H, Kawano H, Ishii H, Tsuji T (1986) Intracranial pressure and cerebral blood flow in patients with communicating hydrocephalus following intracranial aneurysm rupture. In: Miller JD, Teasdale GM, Rowan JO, Galbraith SL, Mendelow AD (eds) Intracranial Pressure VI. Springer, Berlin Heidelberg New York Tokyo, pp 476–480

Kjaellquist A, Lundberg N, Ponten U (1964) Respiratory and cardiovascular changes during rapid spontaneous variations of ventricular fluid pressure in patients with intracranial hypertension. Acta Neurol Scand 40:291–317

Lundberg N (1960) Continuous recording and control of ventricular fluid pressure in neurosurgical practice. Acta Psychiatr Scand [Suppl] 149/36: 1–193

Maeda M, Takahashi K, Miyazaki M, Ishii S (1986) The role of the central monoamine system and the cholinoceptive pontine area on the oscillation of ICP "pressure waves". In: Miller JD, Teasdale GM, Rowan JO, Galbraith SL, Mendelo AD (eds) Intracranial Pressure VI. Springer, Berlin Heidelberg New York Tokyo, pp 151–155

Voldby B, Enevoldsen EM (1982) Intracranial pressure changes following aneurysm rupture, part 1: Clinical and angiographic correlations. J Neurosurg 56:186–196

Correlation Between B-Waves
and Intracranial Pressure – Volume Relationships

U. Dirnagl[1], C. Garner[1], R. Haberl[1], D. Mautner[1], P. Schmiedek[2], and K.M. Einhäupl[1]

[1] Departments of Neurology, and [2] Neurosurgery, University of Munich, D-8000 München 70 (FRG)

Introduction

Intracranial pressure (ICP) in patients (Einhäupl et al. 1986) as well as in normal subjects (Gaab 1980, Dirnagel et al. 1988) often shows rhythmic fluctuations with a frequency of 0.5–2 per min, the so called B-waves (Lundberg 1960).

Due to the nonspecific occurrence of B-waves, the clinical significance of this phenomenon has been questioned (Hamer and Kühner 1976). Several authors (Børgesen et al. 1979, Venes 1979, Gaab 1980, Sorensen et al. 1980, Gjerris et al. 1986) suggested that intense B-wave activity is an indicator for a disturbance of the intracranial pressure/volume relationship (compliance). However, other authors (Miller and Pickard 1973, Wilkinson et al. 1979, Castel et al. 1980) proposed that there is no correlation between B-wave activity and intracranial compliance.

None of the studies quoted above discriminated between B-wave amplitudes and the duration of B-wave activity. In order to clarify the relationship of B-waves and intracranial pressure/volume relationships, it was the aim of this study to correlate the amplitudes of B-waves and the duration of B-wave activities separately with intracranial compliance.

Patients and Methods

The intraventricular ICP of 25 consecutive patients of our neurological intensive care unit was monitored continuously for 24 hr. Fifteen patients had intracranial hemorrhage for various reasons, 3 had inflammatory disease of the CNS (meningitis, encephalitis), 2 had intracranial tumors, 2 had trauma and 2 hypoxic encephalopathy. The ICP data were evaluated by means of computer assisted fast-Fourier analysis. B-wave activity for each patient was expressed as mean amplitude of B-waves (mm Hg) and percent B-wave-activity in the 24 hr observation period.

In each patient, the pressure volume index (PVI) as an indicator of intracranial compliance was determined according to the method of Marmarou (Maset et al. 1987). Three determinations of PVI (with 8 hr time intervals between each measurement) were performed in the 24 hr-ICP-analysis period. PVI was expressed as the mean of the three measurements.

B-wave amplitudes and B-wave duration respectively were correlated with PVI using Pearsons correlation coefficient. All results are expressed as mean ± standard error of the mean.

Results

All patients showed B-wave activity. The mean amplitude of B-waves in the 25 patients was 8.4 ± 0.9 mm Hg, B-waves were present in $34.4 \pm 4\%$ of the 24 hr observation period (mean duration).

There was a significant correlation between PVI and B-wave duration ($r = -0,75$, $p = 0.001$) between PVI and B-wave amplitudes (Fig. 1), whereas there was no correlation between PVI and B-wave duration ($r = 0.21$) (Fig. 2).

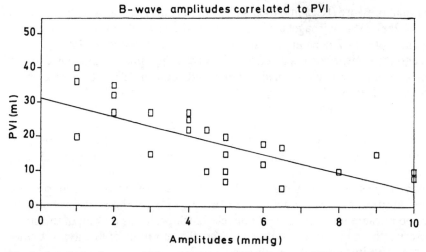

Fig. 1. Correlation between PVI and B-wave amplitudes ($r = -0.75$, $p = 0.001$)

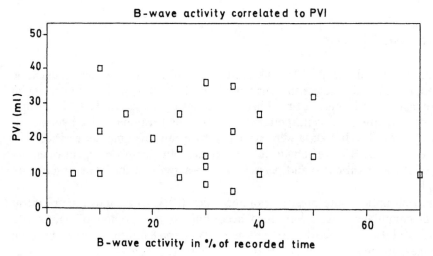

Fig. 2. Correlation between PVI and B-wave duration ($r = 0.21$)

Discussion

Knowledge on the relationship of B-wave activity and intracranial pressure volume relationships is essential for understanding the etiology of the B-wave as well as for determination of the clinical significance of this phenomenon. Our data support the theory that B-waves are caused by an oscillating cerebral vasomotor tone leading to an oscillating cerebral blood volume (Sayama and Aver 1983).

Small variations in volume lead to great changes in pressure when intracranial compliance is low, whereas states of normal compliance are associated with greater intracranial volume compensation capacity. This could account for the correlation of B-wave amplitudes and PVI. On the other hand, compliance seems not to be an etiologic factor in the generation of B-waves, since B-wave duration was not correlated with PVI. This finding fits well with the concept of B-waves as a physiological phenomenon (Gaab 1980, Einhäupl et al. 1986) which is amplified under pathological conditions. These conditions could now be identified as states of low compliance.

Many authors demonstrated intense B-wave activity as a valuable indicator for shunting in normal pressure hydrocephalus (Børgesen et al. 1979, Pickard et al. 1980, Nakamura et al. 1983). A disturbance of CSF outflow and, therefore, critical pressure volume relationships are believed to be one of the main mechanisms of NPH (Brock 1977). Our findings confirm this concept by documenting the association between compliance and B-wave amplitudes.

If B-waves with high amplitudes are indicative of low compliance, is there a further clinical significance in monitoring B-waves other than for shunting in NPH? Since PVI has been demonstrated as a valuable clinical parameter in the management of patients at risk for intracranial pressure/volume decompensation (Miller and Pickard 1973, Shapiro and Fried 1986, Maset et al. 1987), several methods have been developed for assessing PVI in the clinical situation. Pressure/volume studies proved to be safe and reliable (Shapiro et al. 1980). Where possible, this technique has to be preferred since it gives a direct measure of PVI. However, where this is not possible (esp. with the new epidural and intraparenchymal ICP-monitoring systems) B-wave amplitudes can be an indicator for intracranial pressure/volume relationships.

In summary, by discriminating between B-wave amplitudes and B-wave duration we found a correlation between B-wave amplitudes and PVI, whereas there was no correlation of B-wave duration and PVI. This lends support to the theory that B-waves are a physiological phenomenon which is amplified in states of low compliance. B-waves with high amplitudes, therefore, are indicative of a decompensation of the normal intracranial volume compensation capacity.

References

Børgesen SE, Gjerris F, Sørensen SC (1979) Cerebrospinal fluid conductance and compliance of the craniospinal space in normal-pressure hydrocephalus. J Neurosurg 51:521–525

Brock M (1977) Klinik und Therapie des intermittierend normotensiven Hydrocephalus. Radiologe 17:460–465

Castel JP, Dartigues JF, Vandendriesche M (1980) Pathological intracranial pressure waves in Arnold Chiari malformations. In: Shulman K, Marmarou A, Miller JD, Becker DB, Hochwald GM, Brock M (eds) Intracranial Pressure IV. Springer, Berlin Heidelberg New York, pp 569–574

Dirnagl U, Mautner D, Einhäupl KM, Bergmann M, Sigel K (1988) 0.5–2/minute oscillations of cerebral blood flow velocity in normals. In: Advances in transcranial doppler sonography. Springer, Berlin Heidelberg New York Tokyo (in press)

Einhäupl KM, Garner C, Dirnagl U, Schmiedek P, Kufner G, Rieder J (1986) Oscillations of ICP related to cardiovascular parameters. In: Miller JD, Teasdale GM, Rowan JO, Galbraith S, Mendelow AD (eds) Intracranial Pressure VI. Springer, Berlin Heidelberg New York Tokyo, pp 290–297

Gaab MR (1980) Die Registrierung des intrakraniellen Druckes. Habilitationsschrift, Würzburg

Gjerris F, Børgesen SE, Schmidt K, Sørensen PS, Gyring J (1986) Measurement of conductance to CSF outflow by the steady-state perfusion method in patients with normal or increased intracranial pressure. In: Miller JD, Teasdale GM, Rowan JO, Galbraith SL, Mendelow AD (eds) Intracranial Pressure VI. Springer, Berlin Heidelberg New York Tokyo, pp 411–416

Hamer J, Kühner A (1976) Mean intracranial resting pressure, episodic fluctuations, and intracranial volume/pressure response in patients with subarachnoid hemorrhage. In: Beks JWF, Bosch DA, Brock M (eds) Intracranial Pressure III. Springer, Berlin Heidelberg New York, pp 157–161

Hayashi M, Kobayashi H, Kawano H, Handa Y, Yamamoto S, Kitano T (1985) ICP patterns and isotope cisternography in patients with communicating hydrocephalus following rupture of intracranial aneurysm. J Neurosurg 62:220–226

Lundberg N (1960) Continuous recording and control of ventricular fluid pressure in neurosurgical practice. Acta Psychiatr Scand [Suppl] 149

Maset AL, Marmarou A, Ward JD, Choi S, Lutz HA, Brooks D, Moulton RJ, DeSalles A, Muizelaar JP, Turner H, Young HF (1987) Pressure-volume index in head injury. J Neurosurg 67:832–840

Miller JD, Pickard JD (1973) Intracranial volume/pressure studies in patients with head injury. Injury 52:265–268

Nakamura T, Yamaura A, Yamakami I, Nishiyama H, Isobe K, Ise H, Makino H (1983) Prognostic value of continuous ICP monitoring, computerized EEG topography, and regional CBF in communicating hydrocephalus. In: Ishii S, Nagai H, Brock M (eds) Intracranial Pressure V. Springer, Berlin Heidelberg New York Tokyo, pp 686–690

Pickard JD, Teasdale GM, Matheson M, Lindsay K, Galbraith S, Wyper D, Macpherson P (1980) Intraventricular pressure waves – the best predictive test for shunting in normal pressure hydrocephalus. In: Shulman K, Marmarou A, Miller JD, Becker DB, Hochwald GM, Brock M (eds) Intracranial Pressure IV. Springer, Berlin Heidelberg New York Tokyo, pp 488–491

Sayama I, Auer LM (1983) Oscillating cerebral blood volume: The origin of B-waves. In: Ishii S, Nagai H, Brock M (eds) Intracranial Pressure V. Springer, Berlin Heidelberg New York Tokyo, pp 307–311

Shapiro K, Marmarou A, Shulman K (1980) Characterization of clinical CSF dynamics and neural axis compliance using the pressure volume index: I. The normal pressure volume index. Ann Neurol 7:508–514

Shapiro K, Fried A (1986) Pressure – volume relationships in shunt-dependent childhood hydrocephalus. J Neurosurg 64:390–396

Sørensen SC, Gjerris F, Børgensen SE (1980) Etiology of B-waves. In: Shulman K, Marmarou A, Miller JD, Becker DB, Hochwald GM, Brock M (eds) Intracranial Pressure IV. Springer, Berlin Heidelberg New York Tokyo, pp 123–125

Venes JL (1979) B-Waves – A reflection of cardiorespiratory or cerebral nervous systems rhythm? Childs Brain 5:352–360

Wilkinson H, Schuman N, Ruggiero J (1979) Nonvolumetric methods of detecting impaired intracranial compliance or reactivity. J Neurosurg 50:758–767

Respiratory and Cardiovascular Oscillations During B-Waves

M. Hashimoto, S. Higashi, Y. Kogure, H. Fujii, K. Tokuda, H. Ito,
and S. Yamamoto

Department of Neurosurgery, School of Medicine, University of Kanazawa, Takaramachi 13-1,
Kanazawa City 920 (Japan)

Introduction

Lundberg defined B-waves as rhythmic oscillations of ICP with a frequency
of 0.5–2/min. These waves are found to occur simultaneously with periodic
breathing and cardiovascular oscillations. It was postulated that an autonomic
brain stem rhythm was the pacemaker of the ICP variations (Kjällquist et al.
1964). Hayashi et al. (1984) investigated the relationship between B-waves and
cardiovascular parameters, revealing that systemic blood pressure (SBP) and
heart rate (HR) oscillations accompanied by B waves connected with Cheyne
Stokes respiration (CSR). The main purpose of the present study is to elucidate
the phase relationships between B-waves and cardiovascular parameters and
deduce the genesis of this wave.

Materials and Methods

The series consist of 20 patients (SAH, 13; brain tumor, 4; head injury, 3) with
B-waves in continuous ICP recording. ICP was recorded with an indwelling
ventricular catheter connected to a pressure transducer (P-50, Nihon Kohden).
SBP, respiration (Impedance pneumography) and HR were studied polygraphi-
cally.

Results

B-waves with a frequency of 0.5–2/min and an amplitude of 5–70 mm Hg were
observed. Fig. 1 A shows a phase difference in time among synchronous oscillations of SBP, ICP, HR and respiration during B-waves. Some typical relationships were observed as follows: 1) In the phase of apnea ICP began to increase
without SBP changes. 2) ICP continued to increase with respirations. 3) SBP
increased transiently a few seconds prior to the B-wave peak. The deepest respiration began abruptly and tachycardia started at the point of SBP increase. ICP
increased more rapidly than before. 4) The B-wave peak was prior to the SBP

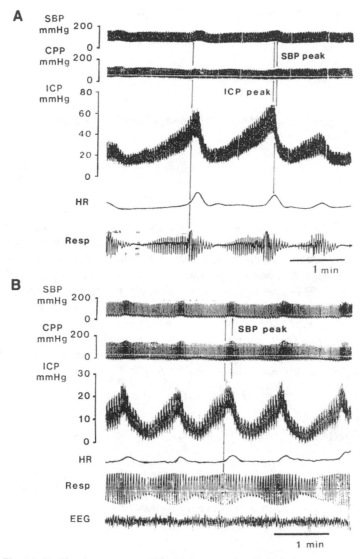

Fig. 1 A, B. Simultaneous recording of SBP, CPP, ICP, HR and respiration related to B-waves.
A Typical B-waves with apnea. **B** CSR variants respiration without apnea

peak and HR peak coincided roughly with the SBP peak. Similar relations were observed in B waves with CSR variant's respiratory pattern without apnea (Fig. 1B). These patterns were seen in 16 cases. In another 4 cases, HR peak coincided with ICP bottom.

Discussion

CSR is characterised by fluctuations of hemodynamic, respiratory, neurologic and acid base determinations (Dowell et al. 1971). Pupillary dilatation usually occurs during hyperpnea while constriction occurs in apnea (Werner 1951). Typical relationships of each parameter in our study suggest that the B-wave oscillation is triggered by a neurogenic factor which generates the transient SBP increase, tachycardia and the deepest respirations. B-waves occured in mechanically respired patients and were seen without CSR (Einhäupl et al. 1985). Auer et al. (1983) reported that B-waves originate from oscillations in the cerebral vascular resistance and the cerebral blood volume. In our study, the B-wave peak was prior to the SBP peak. These facts suggest that the active cerebral vasoconstriction occurs at the time of SBP increase. We speculate that the hyperpneic phase of B waves coincides with hyperactive state of sympathetic nervous system. Our results suggest that B-wave oscillations are derived from rhythmic cerebral vasoconstriction which is presumed to be caused by the intrinsic brain stem rhythm. Two types of HR oscillatory patterns suggest the instability of the brain stem.

References

Auer LM, Sayama I (1983) Intracranial pressure oscillations (B-waves) caused by oscillations in cerebrovascular volume. Acta Neurochir (Wien) 68:93–100

Dowell AR et al. (1971) Cheyne-Stokes respiration. A review of clinical manifestations and critique of physiological mechanisms. Arch Intern Med 127:712–723

Einhäupl KM et al. (1985) Oscillations of ICP related to cardiovascular parameters. In: Miller JD, Reasdale GM, Rowan JO, Galbraith SL, Mendelow AD (eds) Intracranial pressure VI. Springer, Berlin Heidelberg New York Tokyo, pp 290–297

Hayashi M et al. (1984) Blood pressure waves in intracranial hypertension In: Miyakawa K, Koepchen HP, Polosa C (eds) Mechanisms of blood pressure waves. Springer, Berlin Heidelberg New York Tokyo, pp 169–185

Kjällquist Å, Lundberg N, Pontén U (1964) Respiratory and cardiovascular changes during rapid spontaneous variations of ventricular fluid pressure in patients with intracranial hypertension. Arch Neurol Scand 40:291–317

Lundberg N (1960) Continuous recording and control of ventricular fluid pressure in neurosurgical practice. Acta Psychiatr Scand [Suppl] 149:1–193

Werner I (1951) Cheyne-Stokes respiration associated with rhythmic pupillary changes. Acta Psychiatr Neurol 26:213–217

The Role of Vasomotor Center and Adrenergic Pathway in B-Waves

S. Higashi, S. Yamamoto, M. Hashimoto, H. Fujii, H. Ito, Y. Kogure, and K. Tokuda

Department of Neurosurgery, School of Medicine, University of Kanazawa, Takaramachi 13-1, Kanazawa City 920 (Japan)

Introduction

Lundberg (1960) described rhythmic intracranial pressure (ICP) variations with a frequency of $2 \sim 0.5$/min at normal and increased ICP. These oscillations, called "B-waves", were found to occur with periodic breathing and cardiovascular oscillations. It was postulated that an intrinsic brain stem rhythm was the pacemaker of this ICP variation (Kjällquist et al. 1964). Although many papers have been published concerning the origins or mechanisms of B-waves, surprisingly few have analyzed the activities of the brain stem and phase difference between B-waves and other oscillations (Maeda et al. 1986, Yamamoto et al. 1983). Previous experiments in our laboratory (Yamamoto et al. 1983) showed that sympathetic nerve discharges (SND) exhibited oscillations of the same frequency as B-waves. Moreover, there was a phase difference between B-waves and other oscillations. The present paper is an extension of our previous experience, focusing on the origin of B-waves and the implications of the phase difference.

Materials and Methods

Experiments were performed in 18 cats with a body weight of $2.6 \sim 5.1$ kg. After induction of anesthesia with 10 mg/kg thiamylal sodium, the animals were intubated endotracheally, immobilized with 2 mg/kg pancronium bromide and ventilated with room air by a respirator. Supplemental doses of thiamylal sodium and muscle relaxant were given intermittently as required to keep the animals free from pain. One femoral artery and vein were cannulated for continuous recording of systemic blood pressure (SBP), sampling for blood gas checks, and drug administration. ICP was recorded by an epidural sensor (Königsberg Inst. P 3.5) placed in the left parietal epidural space. Efferent discharges of the sympathetic nerve (SND) (internal carotid nerve or renal nerve) and the phrenic nerve (PND) were recorded using bipolar silver wire electrodes from fine nerve strands. A plastic cannula was introduced into the subarachnoid space via the right parietal burr hole and connected to a syringe filled with mock CSF. ICP was increased stepwise using a Harvard infusion-pump for CSF infusion. The two burr holes were tightly sealed with dental cement. During the experiments the P_aCO_2 was

Eds.: J. T. Hoff and A. L. Betz
© Springer-Verlag Berlin Heidelberg 1989

kept constant by adjusting a respirator. Body temperature was kept around 38 °C by a heating pad.

In some animals thiamylal sodium (3 mg/kg) was administrated intravenously during ICP-oscillations.

The bilateral cervical sympathetic nerves were cut in three out of five animals which exhibited ICP-oscillations.

Results

In five of 18 animals B-wave-like ICP-oscillations, synchronous with SND-, PND- and SBP-oscillations, were provoked during increased ICP by CSF infusion. ICP-oscillations started at various levels of ICP, ranging from 47.5 to 115 mm Hg. The frequencies and amplitudes varied between 1 ~ 4/min, and

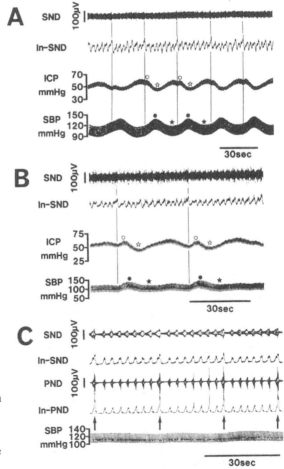

Fig. 1 A–C. B-waves associated with synchronous oscillations of SND, PND and SBP. Note the phase differences between SND and ICP-oscillations, and between ICP- and SBP-oscillations both during oscillations (**A**) and at the onset of oscillations (**B**) whereas oscillations of SND and PND are in phase (**C**)

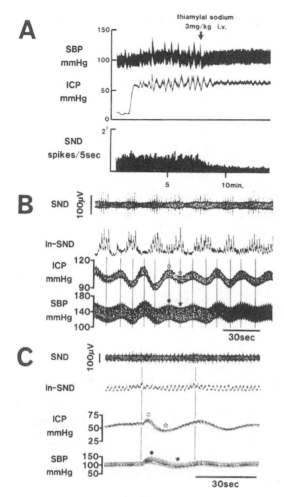

Fig. 2. A The effect of barbiturates on oscillations of SND, ICP and SBP. Note the disappearance of oscillations of SND, ICP and SBP immediately after injection of thiamylal sodium. **B** Disappearance of phase difference between ICP- and SBP-oscillations during cerebral vasomotor paralysis. **C** Oscillations of SND, ICP and SBP after bilateral cervical sympathectomy. The phase difference between ICP- and SBP-oscillations remains the same

4 ~ 22 mm Hg, respectively. The amplitude of the ICP-oscillations increased with a rising ICP baseline. A single example showing oscillations of SND, ICP and SBP is given in Fig. 1 A (during oscillations) and Fig. 1 B (at the onset). First the sympathetic nerve showed tonic burst discharges shortly before both ICP and SBP simultaneously began to rise and continued to increase. Then ICP began to fall and reached its trough earlier than SBP. In other words, there was a phase difference between ICP- and SBP-oscillations. SBP at its trough was similar to the original level, that is, monophasic variations. However ICP at its trough was lower than when it began to rise, and then it returned to the original level, that is, diphasic or triphasic variations. The second burst of the SND appeared immediately after the return of ICP and SBP to the original level. Then the second cycle of ICP- and SBP-oscillations started in the same manner described above. Thus, there were phase differences between ICP-oscillations and other oscillations. Whereas oscillations of SND and PND were in phase as shown in Fig. 1 C.

Immediately after the intravenous administration of thiamylal sodium (3 mg/kg) during these oscillations, the discharge frequencies of SND decreased to about half. In addition oscillations of ICP, SND and SBP disappeared (Fig. 2 A).

When ICP was increased to a level around SBP by CSF infusion, SND-, ICP- and SBP-oscillations grew to be more distinct (Fig. 2 B). However, there was no phase difference between ICP- and SBP-oscillations. After ICP was further increased by CSF infusion, ICP- and SBP-oscillations were replaced by monotonous variations, that is, cerebral vasomotor paralysis.

In order to investigate the role of the sympathoadrenergic pathway in the phase difference between ICP- and SBP-oscillations, bilateral cervical sympathectomy was performed. The phase difference remained the same after the sympathectomy.

Discussion

Lundberg (1960) noted that B-waves occurred in association with periodic breathing. In the majority of cases, B-waves disappeared once respirations were controlled, leading him to speculate that variations in P_aCO_2 would best explain the B-waves with periodic breathing. Further studies confirmed this (Brock et al. 1978). However Einhäupl et al. (1986) reported rhythmic oscillations in the cardiovascular parameters during B-wave activity even without Cheyne-Stoke respiration and therefore blood-gas variations. Moreover they found that respiration participates in this type of B-wave with small rhythmic changes in the tidal volume without a phase shift relative to the ICP. In the present study B-waves were provoked synchronously with oscillations of the sympathetic and phrenic nerve discharges in mechanically respired animals. Moreover B-waves were preceded by tonic burst discharges of the sympathetic nerve. Also barbiturates suppressed not only SND- and SBP-oscillations but also B-waves. These results indicate that B-waves originate from the intrinsic oscillatory rhythm of the brain stem, especially of the vasomotor center.

Shortly after a tonic burst of SND, ICP rose concomitantly with SBP. This can be explained by increased activity in the vasomotor center causing SBP to rise, blood inflow into the brain to increase, and ICP to rise. In spite of simultaneous rising of ICP and SBP, the subsequent variation of ICP was different from that of SBP. The present work emphasized different patterns of variations in a cycle of ICP- and SBP-oscillations (ICP: diphasic or triphasic, SBP: monophasic), which resulted in the phase difference between ICP- and SBP-osillations.

What does the phase difference imply? Auer and Sayama (1983) reported that B-waves could be provoked synchronously with oscillations of pial vascular diameter during stepwise increases in ICP. They speculated that B-waves originated from oscillations in the cerebral blood volume. On the other hand, Taneda et al. (1986) clearly showed that juglar compression increase ICP by distension of the cerebral vascular bed, and intracranial CSF shifted into the spinal subarachnoid space. They concluded that CSF played an important role in intracranial spatial compensation. Thus two possible mechanisms are proposed in the phase difference: 1) active vasoconstriction of cerebral vessels secondary to increased activities in the vasomotor center, 2) intracranial spatial compensation of CSF.

When ICP was increased to a level around SBP, in spite of distinct oscillations of SND, ICP and SBP, phase differences between ICP- and SBP-oscillations disappeared. This observation indicates that increased activities of the vasomotor center cannot provoke the active vasoconstriction of cerebral vessels during cerebral vasomotor paralysis.

In the active vasoconstriction, two possible neural pathways can be proposed: 1) sympathoadrenergic pathway via cervical sympathetic trunk, 2) central noradrenergic nervous system (Hartman et al. 1972). In the present study bilateral cervical sympathectomy did not affect the phase difference between ICP- and SBP-oscillations. Therefore, in this active vasoconstriction, the sympathoadrenergic pathway has little or no part in mediating the vasomotor center activities. It seems likely that the central noradrenergic nervous system plays this role.

References

Auer LM, Sayama I (1983) Intracranial pressure oscillations (B-waves) caused by oscillations in cerebrovascular volume. Acta Neurochir (Wien) 68:93–100

Brock M, Tamburus WM, Telles Ribeiro CR, Dietz H (1978) Circadian occurrence of pathologic cerebrospinal fluid pressure waves in patients with brain tumor. In: Frowein RA, Brock M, Klinger M (eds) Advances in Neurosurgery, Vol. 5. Springer, Berlin Heidelberg New York, pp 188–193

Einhäupl KM, Garner C, Dirnagl U, Schmieder G, Schmiedek P, Kufner G, Rieder J (1986) Oscillations of ICP related to cardiovascular parameters. In: Miller JD, Teasdale GM, Rowan JO, Galbraith SL, Mendelow AD (eds) Intracranial Pressure VI. Springer, Berlin Heidelberg New York, pp 290–297

Hartman BK, Zide D, Udenfriend S (1972) The use of dopamine β-hydroxylase as a marker for the central noradrenergic nervous system in rat brain. Proc Natl Acad Sci USA 69:2722–2726

Kjällquist Å, Lundberg N, Pontén U (1964) Respiratory and cardiovascular changes during rapid spontaneous variations of ventricular fluid pressure in patients with intracranial hypertension. Acta Neurol Scand 40:291–317

Lundberg N (1960) Continuous recording and control of ventricular fluid pressure in neurosurgical practice. Acta Psychiatr Scand [Suppl 149] 36

Maeda M, Takahashi K, Miyazaki M, Ishii S (1986) The role of central monoamine system and the cholinoceptive pontine area on the oscillation of ICP "pressure waves". In: Miller JD, Teasdale GM, Rowan JO, Galbraith SL, Mendelow AD (eds) Intracranial Pressure VI. Springer, Berlin Heidelberg New York, pp 151–155

Taneda M, Shimada N, Kinoshita Y, Taguchi J, Kuboyama K (1986) Radioisotopic observations on volume changes in cranial versus spinal CSF in response to intracranial pressure changes. A clinical study. In: Miller JD, Teasdale GM, Rowan JO, Galbraith SL, Mendelow AD (eds) Intracranial Pressure VI. Springer, Berlin Heidelberg New York, pp 128–131

Yamamoto S, Higashi S, Fujii H, Hayashi M, Ito H (1983) Vasomotor response in acute intracranial hypertension. In: Ishii S, Nagai H, Brock M (eds) Intracranial Pressure V. Springer, Berlin Heidelberg New York, pp 333–337

Intracranial Pressure Pulse Wave Form and Its dp/dt Analysis of Plateau Waves

M. Hashimoto, S. Higashi, Y. Kogure, H. Fujii, K. Tokuda, H. Ito,
and S. Yamamoto

Department of Neurosurgery, School of Medicine, University of Kanazawa, Takaramachi 13-1,
Kanazawa City 920 (Japan)

Introduction

It is generally accepted that plateau waves reflect vasodilatation with a subsequent increase in cerebral blood volume (CBV) (Lundberg et al. 1968). It has also been shown that the ICP-pulse wave form changes with intracranial compliance and vasotonicity (Avezaat et al. 1986). The configuration of the ICP-pulse wave represents three fairly consistent components (P1, P2 and P3) (Cardoso et al. 1983). The present study was performed to investigate how each component of the ICP-pulse wave changed during the up- and downward course of plateau waves.

Material and Methods

We studied 10 patients (brain tumor, 4; SAH, 3; Head injury, 2; intracerebral bleeding, 1) with plateau waves during continuous ICP monitoring. ICP was recorded with an indwelling ventricular catheter connected to a pressure transducer (P-50, Nihon Kohden). The differential (dp/dt) curve of ICP was calculated by a pressure processor (EQ-601G, Nihon Kohden). Systemic blood pressure, ECG and respiration (impedance pneumography) were monitored and simultaneously. Figure 1 shows the interrelationship of the ICP pulse wave and the dp/dt curve. Three positive peaks (U1, U2, U3) and three negative peaks (D1, D2, D3) were shown in the dp/dt curve corresponding to three ICP-pulse wave peaks. Each dp/dt peak represents the maximum rate of change of the ICP pulse pressure in one cardiac cycle.

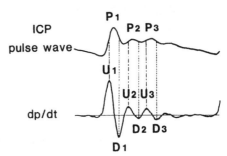

Fig. 1. Interrelationship of ICP pulse wave and dp/dt curve

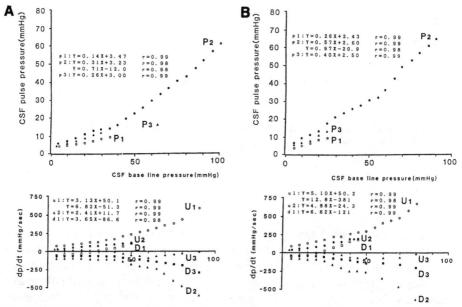

Fig. 2 A, B. ICP pulse pressure, dp/dt amplitude – ICP relationships in the typical plateau wave. A Upward course of plateau wave. **B** Downward course of plateau wave

Results

With an increase in ICP, the ICP-pulse wave form changed configuration continuously from a fundamental form to a monotonous one. Fig. 2 shows the ICP pulse pressure and dp/dt amplitude – ICP relationships in the typical plateau wave. During the upward course of plateau waves, P1–3, U1, U2 and D2 amplitudes are augmented linearly with intracranial hypertension. P2 and U1 were augmented more rapidly than the other components. P2 and U1 exhibited a notable breakpoint at about 50 mm Hg. On the other hand, U3 maintained the same value until 25–30 mm Hg and then decreased gradually to a negative value with intracranial hypertension. In the downward course of plateau waves, each pulse amplitude of P1–3, U1 and U3 exhibited higher values in contrast to the upward course. There were phase differences between U3 and U1, U2 during the respiratory cycle. At the beginning of expiration, U3 was elevated, but became depressed at the beginning of inspiration. On the other hand, U1 and U2 showed reverse relationships.

Discussion

The pressure volume response at a given level of ICP is determined by the elastance ($E = dp/dv$) of the intracranial system, i.e $dp/dt = E \cdot dv/dt$. Therefore, the

226

dp/dt value is determined by two factors. 1. E, the elastance coefficient. 2. The pulsatile changes in CBV (dv/ct). On the other hand, dv/dt reveals directly the pulsatile changes in CBV that result from the interaction between the pulsatile inflow and venous outflow of blood. In this study, P1, P2 and P3 rose linearly with intracranial hypertension. However, U3 decreased gradually and showed negative value over 25–30 mm Hg of ICP.

It has been suggested that respiratory changes of P3 result from the transmission of venous pressure changes from intrathoracic pressure variations with breathing (Harmer et al. 1977). This shows that P3 changes are under the influence of P2 augmentation and respiration. Moreover, the changes in U3 indicate that a disturbance of venous outflow begins at 25–30 mm Hg of ICP, and that the pulsatile flow pattern between diastole and systole changes with intracranial hypertension. Ludberg et al. (1968) found in patients that during plateau waves there was an increase in CBV due to vasodilatation. In our study, each pulse wave amplitude during the upward course was larger than that of the downward course. The result suggests that during plateau waves the ICP-pulse wave form reflects the state of the cerebral vasomotor tonicity and the venous outflow. The dp/dt analysis of ICP is useful for the investigation of the genesis of the ICP-pulse wave form and intracranial hemodynamics.

References

Avezaat CJ, van Eijndhoven JHM (1986) Clinical observations on the relationship between cerebrospinal fluid pulse pressure and intracranial pressure. Acta Neurochir (Wien) 79:13–29

Cardoso ER et al. (1983) Analysis of the cerebrospinal fluid pulse wave in intracranial pressure. J Neurosurg 59:817–821

Harmer J, Alberti E et al. (1977) Influence of systemic and cerebral factors on the cerebrospinal fluid pulse waves. J Neurosurg 46:36–45

Lundberg N, Cronqvist S, Kjällquist Å (1968) Clinical investigations on interrelations between intracranial pressure and intracranial hemodynamics. Prog Brain Res 30:69–75

The Roles of the Mutual Interaction Between the Locus Coeruleus Complex and the Chorioceptive Pontine Area in the Plateau Wave

M. Maeda, M. Miyazaki, and S. Ishii

Department of Neurosurgery and Casualty Center, Juntendo University School of Medicine, Izunagaoka, Shizuoka-Ken, 410-22 (Japan)

Introduction

Plateau waves are often observed in patients with intracranial hypertension from varying etiologies. Typical plateau waves are characterized by spontaneous and acute, rapid elevations in intracranial pressure (ICP).

Lundberg (1960) concluded that these spontaneous plateau waves or A-waves reflected vasodilatation with subsequent increases in cerebral blood volume (CBV). Human studies have shown plateau waves to be associated with increased CBV (Cooper and Hulme 1966), which tended to be greatest just before termination of the wave (Risberg et al. 1969), and these observations have been confirmed in animals (Löfgren and Zwetnow 1976).

Evidence now exists that there are at least two types of adrenergic innervation of cerebral vessels, one from the cervical sympathetic plexus innervating extracerebral arteries, but also reaching cerebral arterioles, and the other originating in the locus coeruleus and impinging directly on the walls of intramedullary arterioles (Katayama et al. 1984). The present experiments were designed to elucidate the roles of the locus coeruleus complex (LC) and the cholinoceptive pontine area (CPA) (Katayama et al. 1984) neurons in the plateau wave. The data suggests that the mutually inhibitory interactions between the LC and the CPA neurons may provide at least one endogenous neural basis for plateau waves.

Materials and Methods

The experiments were performed on 26 chloralose-anesthetized cats with or without Kaolin induced hydrocephalus. Continuous monitoring of intracranial pressure (ICP) by means of an epidural sensor, systemic arterial blood pressure (BP) and respiratory rate (Resp) were carried out. In the first series of experiments, single unit spikes were continuously recorded using tungsten-microelectrodes within the local coeruleus complex (LC) and the cholinoceptive pontine area (Katayama et al. 1984) (CPA, located ventromedially to the LC) during the occurrence of Lundberg's "A" waves. Successive discharge frequency was measured in each 100 to 500 msec. In the second series, after removal of the medial part of the cerebellum (anterior and posterior vermis), single unit spikes of the LC and

Eds.: J. T. Hoff and A. L. Betz

the CPA were recorded extracellularly using glass-micropipettes filled with Ringer solution. Stimulating electrodes were placed in the CPA, the LC, and the forelimb (or the hindlimb) nerves.

Results

Tonic discharges of the LC neuron were gradually suppressed at 15 to 30 sec prior to the onset of plateau waves (the rising phase), almost completely silenced during the plateau phase, and then began to recover at 10 to 30 sec prior to the falling phase (see also Maeda et al. 1985). Fig. 1 A shows the discharge pattern of fre-quencies were suppressed at 15 sec prior to the beginning of the rising phase.

Spike activities of the CPA neurons related to the plateau waves were shown in Fig. 1 B. The firing rate was increased in phase with the plateau waves. The spike frequency increased about 30 sec prior to the rising phase and decreased about 20 sec prior to the onset of the falling phase. During the plateau phase the unit spikes exhibited a high frequency-pattern. There were no remarkable changes in either BP or Resp during plateau waves.

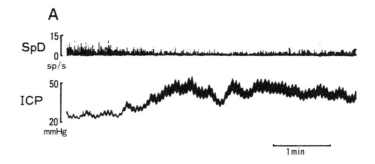

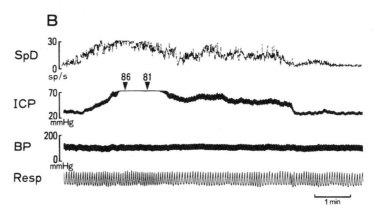

Fig. 1 Discharge pattern of a locus coeruleus complex-neuron (**A**) and a cholinoceptive pontine area-neuron (**B**) during plateau waves. Simultaneous recording of unit spike discharge (SpD), ICP, BP and Resp

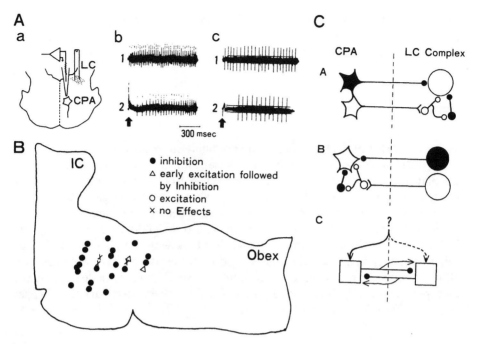

Fig. 2 Inhibitory effect of LC stimulation on the CPA neurons **A** *a*: experimental arrangement, *b, c*: Two individual CPA neurons. Spontaneous discharges (*upper traces, 1*) are inhibited by stimulation (*arrow*) of the LC (*lower traces, 2*). Upward reflection in each trace represents negativity. **B** Location and pattern of CPA-neurons studied by stimulation of LC. *IC:* inferior colliculus **C** Schematic drawings of mutually inhibitory connections between CPA and LC

The pattern of LC evoked effects in the CPA neurons was investigated by extracellular unit recording. Electrical stimulation of the ipsilateral LC evoked predominantly inhibition in the CPA neurons. Spontaneous spikes of the CPA neuron [Fig. 2 (Ab-1)] were inhibited following ipsilateral LC stimulation [Fig. 2 (Ab-2)]. Similar inhibition was observed in another CPA neuron as shown in Fig. 2 (Ac). Early excitation followed by inhibition was also observed.

Effects of ipsilateral (ipsi) or controlateral (contra) LC complex stimulation on CPA neurons are summarized as follows: inhibition (ipsi, 26/32; contra, 36/59), early excitation followed by inhibition (2/21, 12/59), excitation (0/32, 4/59) and no effects (4/32, 7/59). Location and pattern of the CPA neurons studied by stimulation of the LC are shown in Fig. 2 B. Stimulation of forelimb or hindlimb nerves also evoked early slight excitation followed by long lasting inhibition in the CPA neurons.

Discussion

Activation of the LC by means of microinjection of glutamate or carbachol produced a decrease in ICP (Maeda et al. 1985), while ICP increased (plateau

230

wave – like ICP – variations) following microinjection of carbachol into the CPA (Katayama et al. 1984, Maeda et al. 1985). In the present studies spontaneous activities of the LC-neurons were clearly suppressed during the plateau waves. On the other hand, the neurons which were recorded from the CPA fired in phase with the plateau waves. There was a mirror – image relation between the activities of the neurons in the LC and the CPA during the plateau waves. Some of the CPA-neurons send their axons to the LC neurons and inhibit them (Maeda et al. 1985). Similarly, spontaneous spikes of the CPA-neurons were predominantly inhibited following ipsi- or contra-lateral LC stimulation. Thus a mutually inhibitory mechanism exists in the midbrain and the pons at the level of the LC and the CPA neurons (Fig. 2c). An hypothesis has been presented that mutually inhibiting neural elements should produce alternating rhythmic activities (Wilson 1964). Taken together, these data suggest that the mutually inhibitory neural elements (the CPA and the LC) analyzed here may provide at least one endogenous neural basis for plateau waves seen during certain pathological conditions such as Kaolin induced hydrocephalus.

References

Lundberg N (1960) Continuous recording and control of ventricular fluid pressure in neurosurgical practice. Acta Psychiatr Scand [Suppl 149] 36:1–193

Cooper R, Hulme A (1966) Intracranial pressure and related phenomena during sleep. J Neurol Neurosurg Psychiatry 29:564–570

Risberg J, Lundberg N, Ingvar DH (1969) Regional cerebral blood volume during acute transient rises of the intracranial pressure (plateau waves). J Neurosurg 31:303–310

Löfgren J, Zwetnow NN (1976) Intracranial blood volume and its variation with changes in intracranial pressure. In Beks JWF, Bosch DA, Brock M (eds) Intracranial Pressure III. Springer, Berlin Heidelberg New York, pp 25–28

Hartmann BK, Zide D, Udenfriend S (1972) The use of dopamine hydroxylase as a marker for the central noradrenergic nervous system in a rat brain. Proc Natl Acad Sci USA 69:2722–2726

Katayama Y, Nakamura T, Becker DP, Hayes RL (1984) Intracranial pressure variations associated with activation of the cholinoceptive pontine inhibitory area in the unanesthetized drug-free cat. J Neurosurg 61:713–724

Maeda M, Takahashi M, Miyazaki M, Ishii S (1985) The role of the central Monoamine System and the Cholinoceptive Pontine Area on the Oscillation of ICP "Pressure Wave". In: Miller JD et al. (eds) Intracranial Pressure VI. Springer, Berlin Heidelberg New York, pp 151–155

Wilson DM (1964) Relative refractoriness and patterned discharge of locust flight motor neurons. J Exp Biol 41:191–205

Role of the Medulla Oblongata in Plateau Wave Development in Dogs

M. Hayashi, H. Ishii, Y. Handa, H. Kobayashi, and H. Kawano

Department of Neurosurgery, Fukui Medical School, Matsuoka-chou, Yoshida-gun, Fukui 910-11 (Japan)

Plateau waves, as described by Lundberg, are often observed in patients with increased intracranial pressure (ICP) due to brain tumors or benign intracranial hypertension. Two major causes have been proposed for the development of plateau waves; persistent intracranial hypertension and a cerebral vasomotor reaction. Plateau waves are often associated with changes in arterial blood pressure (ABP) and respiration, suggesting a role of the brain stem and a cerebral vasomotor reaction in the development of plateau waves. The object of this study was to identify the region of the brain stem that causes the cerebral vasomotor reaction responsible for the development of plateau waves.

Materials and Methods

Twenty mongrel dogs, weighing 7 to 10 g, were used in this study. They were anesthetized and tracheotomized and then fixed into the prone position in a stereotaxic frame. The experiments were carried out under spontaneous breathing. ICP was recorded through a needle inserted into the lateral ventricle. For monitoring ABP and periodic sampling of blood gases, a catheter was placed in the abdominal aorta via the femoral artery. The rate and pattern of respiration were recorded using a thermistor bridge. Cortical cerebral blood flow (CBF) was measured continuously with a temperature-controlled thermoelectric method using a tissue blood flow monitor. Stimulation was effected by a train of electrical pulses produced with a bipolar electrode inserted stereotaxically into the brain stem. The pulse duration and frequency were set at 1 m/sec and 50 Hz and the current intensity was increased from 0.1 to 1 mA. The duration of the stimulus was usually between 10 and 15 sec. The neck veins were occluded bilaterally with thread at the C-4 vertebral level so as to induce persistent intracranial venous hypertension. The mean ICP was 9 ± 2 mm Hg prior to the occlusion of the neck veins and 32 ± 6 mm Hg after occlusion. Autopsies were performed for confirmation of the sites of electrical stimulation in the brain stem.

Results

Stimulation of most areas of the brain-stem reticular formation in the medulla or pons always produced an increase in ICP associated with changes in ABP, ce-

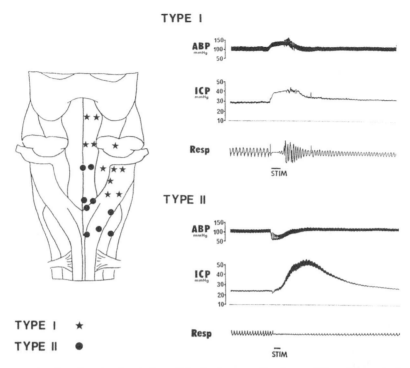

TYPE I

TYPE II

TYPE I ★
TYPE II ●

Fig. 1. Diagram showing the stimulated sites of the brain stem. Response of Type I is evoked by stimulation of the lateral reticular formation in the rostral medulla oblongata. Response of Type II, which is similar to the plateau waves in clinical practice, is evoked by stimulation of the medial reticular formation in the caudal medulla oblongata

rebral perfusion pressure (CPP), CBF, respiration and pulse rate. The changes were divided into two groups as follows (Fig. 1). One group (Type I) comprised those changes indicating an arterial pressor response, i.e. increases of CPP and CBF, hyperventilation, and bradycardia. The other group (Type II) included those changes showing an arterial depressor response, i.e. decreases of CPP and CBF, depressed ventilation, and bradycardia. Type I usually resulted from stimulation of a region of the lateral reticular formation in the rostral medulla and caudal pons and this area nearly corresponded to the pressor region of the vasomotor center. In contrast, Type II resulted from stimulation of the medial reticular formation in the caudal medulla. This region was close to the depressor area of the vasomotor center.

Discussion

Clinical observations suggest that a high pressure within the cranial cavity may elicit a secondary rise of ICP (plateau wave) in response to any change in intracranial dynamics, even if the increase is of only moderate magnitude. Lundberg et al. (1974) suggested that the plateau-wave phenomenon is related to a cerebral vasomotor response and it develops by dilatation of cerebral resistance vessels during a state of decreased compliance in the cranial cavity. Experimentally, it is observed that stimulation of the brain stem produces both dilatation of the cerebral vessels and a rise in ICP (Langfitt et al. 1968). Cerebral arteries are reportedly innervated by sympathetic nerves and intracerebral small arterioles or capillaries are also innervated by adrenergic nerves derived from the brain stem. These reports suggest that the tone or reactivity of cerebral arteries may be affected by the intrinsic activity of the brain stem and may elicit variations in ICP, ABP, and CBF. In this study, Type II was similar in many respects to the plateau waves observed in clinical practice. These similarities included a decline in ABP, CPP, and CBF, respiratory suppression, and bradycardia, as well as an increase in ICP. We suggest that the depressor area of the vasomotor center (Alexander 1946) may play a role in eliciting cerebral vasomotor reactions for the development of plateau waves in a state of intracranial hypertension.

References

Alexander RS (1946) Tonic and reflex functions of medullary sympathetic cardiovascular centers. J Neurophysiol 9:205–217
Langfitt TW, Kassel NF (1968) Cerebral vasodilatation produced by brain-stem stimulation: neurogenic control vs. autoregulation. Am J Physiol 215:90–97
Lundberg N, Kjallquist A, Kullberg G et al. (1974) Non-operative management of intracranial hypertension. In: Krayenbul H (ed) Advances and Technical Standards in Neurosurgery, Vol 1. Springer, Wien, pp 3–59

Electroencephalographic Changes During Plateau Waves – Plateau Waves Induced by Electrical Stimulation of the Brain Stem

Y. Kogure, H. Fujii, S. Higashi, M. Hashimoto, K. Tokuda, H. Ito, and S. Yamamoto

Department of Neurosurgery, School of Medicine, University of Kanazawa, Takaramachi 13-1, Kanazawa City 920 (Japan)

Introduction

It is known that activation of the cholinoceptive pontine area produces plateau wave-like ICP variations and EEG desynchronization. Our previous experiment showed that hippocampal regular θ activity during plateau waves suggested the possibility of an activated state of the brain stem reticular formation (Yamamoto et al. 1986). Plateau waves appear to be produced by some endogenous neural activity in the brain stem. The present study was designed to induce plateau waves by electrical stimulation of the brain stem reticular formation following experimental subarachnoid hemorrhage in dogs and to investigate changes in EEG during the plateau waves.

Materials and Methods

Ten adult mongrel dogs were lightly anesthetized, immobilized and artificially ventilated. EEG, intracranial pressure (ICP), systemic blood pressure (SBP) and cerebral perfusion pressure (CPP) were simultaneously recorded on electromagnetic tape before and after transorbital puncture of the internal carotid artery. EEG was recorded from cortical electrodes. Frequency analysis of the EEG was performed for 50 sec by a microcomputer (Nihon Kohden ATAC-450). Monopolar stimulating electrodes were oriented stereotaxically for an approach of the mesencephalic reticular formation (MRF). Stimulation parameters, i.e., intensity, duration and frequency, were 0.1 mA, 1 msec and 40–50 Hz, respectively. The total duration of each stimulation period was 5 sec. Electrode locations for each stimulation point were confirmed histologically.

Results

Spontaneous plateau waves occurred in two of ten dogs. Three points in the MRF were electrically stimulated at the ICP level of 30–50 mm Hg in one of the two dogs with spontaneous plateau waves.

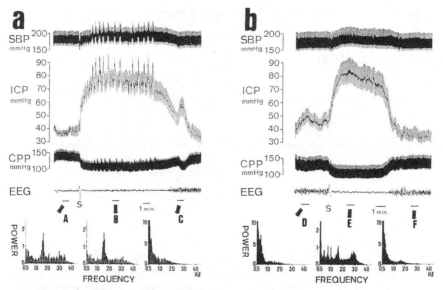

Fig. 1 a, b. Polygraphic recordings of SBP, ICP, CPP, and EEG with frequency analysis. Electrical stimulations (*dots*) were delivered during fast EEG activity (**a**) or slow EEG activity (**b**), S = electrical stimulation

Twenty-one electrical stimulations at two of the three points induced ten plateau waves, which occurred immediately after the electrical stimulation during fast or slow EEG activity. Eight plateau waves were induced during fast EEG activity (Fig. 1a). Before (*A*) and during the plateau wave (*B*), 15–16 c/s fast activity was dominant. After the plateau wave (*C*), slow activity under 5 c/s was dominant. During slow EEG activity electrical stimulation of the same points as Fig. 1a induced two plateau waves associated with EEG desynchronization (Fig. 1b). Before (*D*) and after the plateau wave (*F*), slow activity under 5 c/s was dominant. In contrast, EEG activity during the plateau wave (*E*) showed small spectrum power at frequency under 5 c/s and large spectrum power at frequency over 15 c/s.

Electrical stimulation at the other point induced only a small transient rise in ICP and no remarkable changes in EEG.

Discussion

The start of ICP increase coincided with EEG desynchronization in REM sleep-related plateau waves, which were associated with increased cerebral blood volume (CBV) (Cooper et al. 1966). They inferred that the plateau waves were caused by cerebral vasodilatation associated with an increased metabolic rate. In our study, electrical stimulation at certain points in the MRF during slow EEG activity induced plateau waves coincident with EEG desynchronization. During

236

fast EEG activity, however, plateau waves were induced in spite of no remarkable changes in the EEG. In addition, plateau waves occurred immediately after brief (5 sec) electrical stimulation. These findings suggest that the rapid onset of the plateau waves may not be accounted for by the increase in metabolism alone. For the reasons mentioned above, it seems that CBV increases during plateau waves are due to rapidly occurring neurogenic vasodilatation of cerebral vessels later augmented by increases in cerebral metabolism. Therefore, there appears to be some endogenous neural activity in the brain stem which influences CBV and metabolism.

References

Cooper R, Hulme A (1966) Intracranial pressure and related phenomena during sleep. J Neurol Neurosurg Psychiatry 29:564–570

Katayama Y, Nakamura T, Becker DP, Haters RL (1984) Intracranial pressure variations associated with activation of the cholinoceptive pontine inhibitory area in the unanesthetized drug-free cat. J Neurosurg 61:713–724

Yamamoto S, Uno E, Fujii H, Higashi S, Hashimoto M, Futami K, Kogure Y, Obinata C (1986) Electroencephalographic changes during pressure waves of ICP following experimental subarachnoid hemorrhage. In: Miller JD et al. (eds) Intracranial Pressure VI. Springer, Berlin Heidelberg New York, pp 345–350

Changes of Evoked Potentials During Pressure Waves

Y. Handa, M. Hayashi, S. Hirose, N. Shirasaki, H. Kobayashi, and H. Kawano

Department of Neurosurgery, Fukui Medical School, Fukui 910-11 (Japan)

In cases of intracranial hypertension, continuous recording of intracranial pressure (ICP) reveals marked fluctuation of ICP including plateau waves and B-waves (Lundberg 1960). The appearance of these fluctuations of ICP are thought to be affected by the state of the brain stem function. This study is designed to clarify the state of regional brain functions, especially the brain stem, during the appearance of either plateau waves or B-waves by evaluation of evoked potential.

Materials and Methods

The ICP and systemic blood pressure (SBP) were recorded continuously in eight patients with intracranial hypertension. In three patients with plateau waves, auditory brain stem evoked potential (BAEP) and somatosensory evoked potential (SEP) were measured when ICP was high during plateau waves and when it was low during the interval phase between two plateau waves. In five patients demonstrating B-waves, BAEP and SEP were measured during the time of increased ICP with marked appearance of B-waves, and during the time of low ICP without B-waves produced by cerebrospinal drainage or mannitol administration. Measurements of evoked potentials were performed more than five times at each phase in each case. The ABEP were obtained by averaging 1,000 responses at the vertex and the ear lobe to 85 dB clicks of 0.1 m/sec duration given through an earphone to one ear. Absolute latencies (I–III and V waves) and interwave latencies (I–III, III–V and I–V waves) were measured in each recording. The SEP were obtained from the average of 256 responses over the somatosensory scalp area contralateral to the stimulated median nerve at the wrist. Latencies of P15 and N20 and the interwave latency of P15 to N20 were calculated in each recording. The mean value of each latency was compared between two phases of each case using Student's t-test.

Results

The mean ICP during the interval phases of plateau waves ranged from 18 to 42 mm Hg and the cerebral perfusion pressure (CCP, difference between SBP and

Eds.: J. T. Hoff and A. L. Betz
© Springer-Verlag Berlin Heidelberg 1989

Table 1. Summary of the evaluations of latencies of evoked potentials in each case with plateau waves or B-waves

Case	ABEP						SEP		
	I	III	V	I–III	III–V	I–V	P_{15}	N_{20}	$P_{15}–N_{20}$
Plateau waves									
1	ns	ns	ns	ns	ns	ns	*	*	ns
2	ns	ns	ns	ns	ns	ns	ns	ns	ns
3	ns	ns	ns	ns	ns	ns	ns	ns	ns
B-waves									
4	ns	*	*	*	ns	*	*	ns	ns
5	ns	ns	*	*	ns	**	*	ns	ns
6	ns	ns	ns	ns	ns	ns	ns	ns	ns
7	ns	ns	*	ns	ns	ns	*	*	ns
8	ns	ns	*	ns	ns	*			

ns: $p > 0.05$; *: $p < 0.05$; **: $p < 0.01$.

ICP) from 62 to 90 mm Hg. During the plateau waves, the mean ICP increased to between 65 and 84 mm Hg, while the mean CPP decreased to between 30 to 43 mm Hg. Absolute and interwave latencies of ABR measured during the phase of the plateau waves showed no significant ($p > 0.05$) prolongation compared with the latencies measured during the interval phases of plateau waves in all three cases. In one of the three cases with plateau waves, latencies of P15 and N20 of SEP showed significant prolongation ($p < 0.05$) during the plateau waves.

In five cases with B-waves, the mean ICP during low ICP without B-waves ranged from 6 to 16 mm Hg and mean ICP during increased ICP level with B-waves ranged from 16 to 46 mm Hg, whereas the mean CPP showed no difference between those during the low ICP and increased ICP with B-waves. Four of five cases showed significant ($p < 0.05$) prolongation of absolute latencies of V wave of the ABEP with or without prolongation of III wave, and three cases showed significant prolongation of interwave latencies of I–III or I–V waves, measured during increased ICP level with B-waves, compared those measured during the low ICP without B-waves. Two of four cases showed significant prolongation of P15 of the SEP and one case showed significant ($p < 0.05$) prolongation of P15 and N20 of the SEP measured during increased ICP level with B-waves compared to those measured during the low ICP without B-waves.

Discussion

It has been demonstrated that a significant decrease in cerebral blood flow causes a prolongation of latency of evoked potentials as a result of an increase in central conduction time (Hargandle et al. 1980). Experimental studies revealed that a marked increase in ICP also produced a prolongation or disappearance of the waves of the evoked potential, which may be caused by a decrease in cerebral blood flow by a reduction of cerebral perfusion pressure (Sohmer et al. 1982). In this study, latencies of the ABEP showed no prolongation during the plateau waves despite a marked reduction of CPP. These results suggest that there was no significant reduction of cerebral blood flow or functional disturbance of the brain stem during the plateau waves, and may explain why there is no Cushing reflex and why patients are often alert during plateau waves. On the other hand, during the time of increased ICP level with B-waves, there were significant prolongations of latencies of the ABEP or the SEP indicating a delay of central conduction time in the brain stem, although there was no difference in CPP between low ICP without B-waves and increased ICP with B-waves. B-waves are usually accompanied with the fluctuation in SBP, rhythmic breathing and heart rate as observed in our cases. These results suggest that dysfunction or instability of the brain stem produced B-wave phenomenon.

References

Hargandie JR, Branston NM, Symon L (1980) Central conduction time in primate brain ischemia – a study in baboons. Stroke 11:637–664
Lundberg N (1960) Continuous recording and control of ventricular fluid pressure in neurosurgical practice. Acta Psychiat Neurol Scand [Suppl 149] 36:1–193
Sohmer H, Gafni M, Goittein K, Fainmesser P (1983) Auditory nerve-brainstem evoked potentials in cats during manipulation of the cerebral perfusion pressure. Electroencephalogr Clin Neurophysiol 55:198–202

Comparative Study with Experimental and Clinical Plateau Waves Relating to Sleep

K. Shima, H. Ueno[1], H. Chigasaki, and S. Ishii[1]

Department of Neurosurgery, National Defense Medical College, 3-2 Namiki, Tokorozawa, Saitama[1], and Juntendo University, Tokyo (Japan)

Introduction

Plateau waves or A-waves (Lundberg 1960) have been observed sometimes during sleep, more frequently during rapid eye movement (REM) sleep in patients with increased intracranial pressure (ICP). We reported previously that experimental plateau waves were successfully produced in hydrocephalic cats and monkeys during calcium-induced sleep (Shima et al. 1980, Ishii 1983). In order to clarify the relationship between plateau waves and sleep, we compared our experimental plateau waves with clinical ones.

Materials and Methods

Animal Experiments

Fourteen cats and 5 monkeys (*Macaca irus*) anesthetized with ketamine were used in this study. Hydrocephalus was induced by intracranial injection of sterile kaolin suspension. At the acute stage of hydrocephalus between 5 and 8 days after kaolin injection, sleep was induced according to the method described previously (Ishii 1983, Shima et al. 1980). Double-walled cannulae were stereotaxically inserted bilaterally into the dorsomedial hypothalamic area, and perfused with a modified Krebs-Ringer's solution with excess calcium, which has about 4 times higher calcium content than the extracellular fluid in the brain. Perfusion was carried out with a pump for 30–40 min at a rate of 50 μl/min. ICP from the lateral ventricle, systemic blood pressure (BP), respiration, EEG, ocular movements (EOG), EMG of the nuchal muscle, and cerebral blood flow (CBF) in the frontal cortex by the cross thermocoupled method were continuously monitored under spontaneous respiration.

Clinical Materials

Eleven patients, aged 10 to 65 years, with plateau waves were studied. ICP, BP, respiration, EEG, EOG, ECG and heart rate (HR) were continuously monitored. The ICP was measured either as ventricular fluid pressure or as epidural pressure.

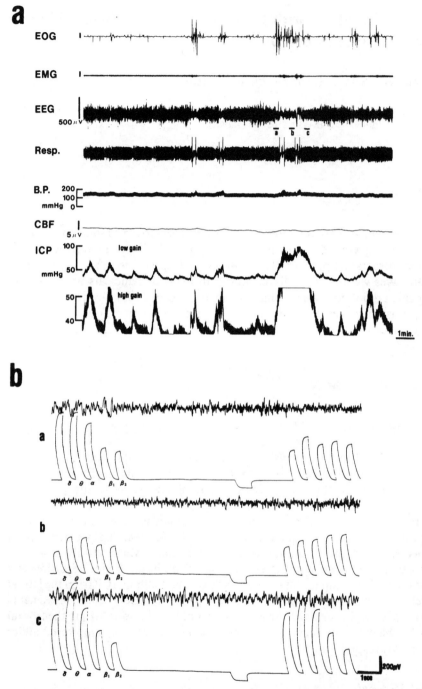

Fig. 1. a Polygraphic recording in the hydrocephalic monkey 2 h after perfusion. Note the plateau wave accompanied by rapid eye movements and irregular breathing pattern. Horizontal bars (*a–c*) in this figure correspond to EEG tracings indicated in **b**. **b** EEG recordings at faster paper speed. The records were taken (*a*) at the rapid rise phase of plateau wave, (*b*) during the plateau phase and (*c*) at the rapid fall phase

Results

Animal Experiments

In 7 of 14 cats and in 4 of 5 monkeys, behavioral and physiological signs such as sleep were evoked within 5–30 min following the start of perfusion and lasted as long as 3 to 5 hr. The perfused sites which caused sleep were limited to the posterior part of the hypothalamus, which were less than 1.0 mm in diameter around each cannula. Plateau waves were observed only in animals (3 cats and 4 monkeys) with induced sleep and a resting ICP higher than 15 mm Hg. The typical plateau wave developed within 1 min and lasted for 1 to 4 min as shown in Fig. 1 a. During the plateau wave, the ICP rose to between 50 and 120 mm Hg. Each plateau wave was accompanied by decreased high-amplitude slow waves on EEG, appearance of eye movements and irregular breathing patterns. A few seconds before the cessation of the plateau wave, there was the disappearance of desynchronization of the EEG (Fig. 1 b). In half of the plateau waves in monkeys, a decrease in the CBF was coincident with the plateau wave.

Clinical Materials

The clinical plateau wave was also observed most frequently during REM or light slow-wave sleep. In 5 of 11 patients, plateau waves occurred only during the REM stage of sleep. At the acute stage of increased ICP, no plateau wave was seen for several days until there was a good recovery from the suppressed sleep-waking cycle. Plateau waves during slow-wave sleep were also accompanied by a decrease in the amplitude of the EEG. The respiration showed a decrease in the rate and irregular patterns throughout the plateau wave. Changes in heart rate were usually minimal.

Discussion

It has been pointed out that the plateau wave is provoked by cerebral vasodilatation closely related to REM sleep (Risberg et al. 1969). Our experimental plateau waves occurred under sleep induced by the change of ions in the hypothalamus, and the physiological alterations throughout the waves were similar to those observed in patients. Ishii (1966) produced acute brain swelling in monkeys due to vasodilatation by lesions of the hypothalamus. This structural coincidence between sleep and vasomotor control mechanisms suggests that a functional change of the hypothalamus may play an important role in the occurrence of the plateau wave.

References

Ishii S (1966) Brain swelling; studies of structural, physiologic and biochemical alterations. In: Caveness WH, Walker AF (eds) Head Injury Conference Proceedings. Lippincott, Philadelphia Toronto, pp 275–299

Ishii S (1983) Oscillation of intracranial pressure and local cerebral metabolism. In: Ishii S, Nagai H, Brock M (eds). Springer, Berlin Heidelberg New York, pp 893–900

Lundberg N (1960) Continuous recording and control of ventricular fluid pressure in neurosurgical practice. Acta Psychiatr Neurol Scand [Suppl 149] 36:1–193

Risberg J, Lundberg N, Ingvar DH (1969) Regional cerebral blood volume during acute transient rises of the intracranial pressure (plateau waves). J Neurosurg 31:303–310

Shima K, Akiyama I, Ueno H, Ishii S (1980) Intracranial pressure changes during experimental sleep in cats and primates. Neurol Med Chir (Tokyo) 20:1215–1222

Failure in Aborting Plateau Waves by a Temporary Increase in Cerebral Perfusion Pressure

M. Matsuda and H. Handa

Department of Neurosurgery, Shiga University of Medical Science, Ohtsu, Shiga 520-21 (Japan)

Clinical Materials and Observations

A 36-year-old man with oligodendroglioma of the left frontal lobe showed typical plateau waves (PW) of up to 67 mm Hg (85 mm Hg systolic) lasting 15 to 25 min with an interval of 30 to 50 min (Fig. 1). During the PWs he complained of headache and became slightly drowsy. The values of the parameters recorded at each phase of the PWs are shown in Table 1. During the interval that the intra-

Table 1. Pressure changes at each phase of the plateau waves. Values are means ± SD, expressed as the mean pressure (a third of the difference between the systolic and diastolic pressures added to the diastolic pressure) in mm Hg. ($n=6$)

	before PW	PW peak	PW terminal	after PW
SABP	79.0±5.7	84.0±7.7	81.0±5.9	76.4±2.6
ICP	24.4±4.3	57.6±9.0	40.8±8.7	5.2±1.9
CPP	54.6±3.2	26.4±5.3	40.2±7.5	71.2±2.3

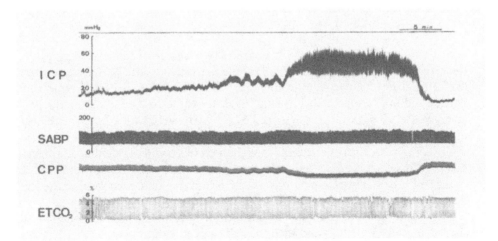

Fig. 1. Simultaneous recording of ICP, SABP, CPP and $ETCO_2$. No Cushing response was observed

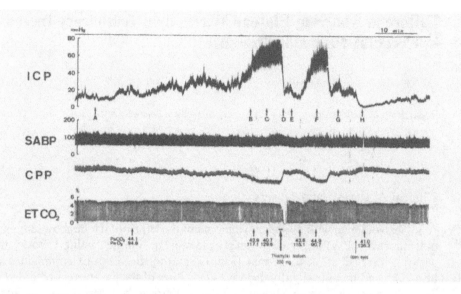

Fig. 2. The PW was interrupted, but not completely aborted, by thiamylal injection

Table 2. Pressure changes during the PW interrupted by thiamylal. Values are expressed as the mean pressure in mm Hg

	before PW'	Thiamylal 250 mg i.v.			before PW''	PW'' peak	PW'' terminal	after PW''
		PW' peak	↓	after PW'				
SABP	68	82		75	~ 67	80	78	70 ~ 73
ICP	23	63		17	~ 12	57	51	17 ~ 3
CPP	45	19		58	~ 55	23	27	53 ~ 70

cranial pressure (ICP) gradually increased there was a concomitant decrease in the cerebral perfusion pressure (CPP) while the systemic arterial blood pressure (SABP) did not change significantly. End-tidal (ET) CO_2 and the respiratory rhythm did not change, either. As the CPP decreased to 54.6 ± 3.2 mm Hg; PW emerged and its peak pressure reached 57.6 ± 9.0 mm Hg with a further decrease in CPP to 26.4 ± 5.3 mm Hg. Thereafter, the plateau gradually declined to 40.8 ± 8.7 mm Hg with a concomitant slight increase in CPP. A sudden disappearance of PW followed. No Cushing response was observed in the terminal phase of the PW. The ICP was, at its lowest, 5.2 ± 1.9 mm Hg immediately after the PW disappeared.

Thiamylal sodium, 250 mg, was intravenously administered over one min at the height of a PW (PW'), and then the PW' suddenly disappeared (Fig. 2, Table 2). The ICP went down from 63 to 17 mm Hg, the SABP changed slightly from 82 to 75 mm Hg and the CPP concomitantly increased from 19 to 58 mm Hg.

However, this CPP level was less than that (71.2 ± 2.3 mm Hg) recorded immediately after the other PWs ended in the natural course, and the next PW (PW″) emerged only 4 min later in contrast to an interval of more than 30 min in the naturally occurred PWs. Furthermore, this particular PW″ lasted for only 7 min compared with the naturally occurring PWs which lasted more than 15 min. Therefore, it is possible that this short-lived PW″ was a continuation of the preceding PW′ which had been temporarily interrupted by thiamylal. The PW was not completely aborted by an increase in CPP.

Discussion

The CPP changes observed in this case support the hypothesis that a decrease in CPP includes cerebral vasodilatation and the vasoconstricting effect of thiamylal fading away, the PW″ emerged probably by an autoregulatory mechanism. Thus, it appears that the emergence of PW is closely related to the level of CPP, not to the ICP itself, since an ICP of 12 mm Hg immediately before the short-lived PW″ emerged was much lower than before the natural PWs occurred.

There seems to be some other cooperating mechanism. Cerebral vasodilatation and the PW are correlated with some intrinsic neural mechanism in the brain stem during increased ICP (Hayashi et al. 1987, Maeda et al. 1986, Nagao et al. 1987). Although the dilated cerebral vessels reacted to thiamylal with vasoconstriction and PW′ disappeared, the neural discharge for vasodilatation continued and PW″ emerged shortly after the preceding PW′. At the end of this particular PW″ the CPP was 53 mm Hg, critical for induction of a PW. The ICP actually started to rise, but the PW did not emerge probably because the neural discharge for vasodilatation was already off.

The present study may indicate that the level of CPP and some intrinsic neural mechanism closely cooperate in the emergence of the PW during increased ICP with decreased intracranial compliance.

References

Hayashi M, Ishii H, Handa Y, Kobayashi H, Kawano H, Kabuto M (1987) Role of the medulla oblongata in plateau-wave development in dogs. J Neurosurg 67:97–101
Maeda M, Takahashi K, Miyazaki M, Ishii S (1986) The role of the central monoamine system and the cholinoceptive pontine area on the oscillation of ICP "Pressure waves". In: Miller JD, Teasdale GM, Rowan JO, Galbraith SL, Mendelow AD (eds) Intracranial pressure VI. Springer, Berlin Heidelberg New York Tokyo, pp 151–155
Nagao S, Nishiura T, Kuyama H, Suga M, Murota T (1987) Effect of stimulation of the medullary reticular formation on cerebral vasomotor tonus and intracranial pressure. J Neurosurg 66:548–554
Rosner MJ, Becker DP (1983) The etiology of plateau waves: A theoretical model and experimental observations. In: Ishii S, Nagai H, Brock M (eds) Intracranial pressure V. Springer, Berlin Heidelberg New York Tokyo, pp 301–306

The Plateau Wave is Not Solely an Intracranial Phenomenon

J. Vajda, I. Nyary, and E. Pasztor

National Institute of Neurosurgery, Budapest, 1426 Pf. 25 (Hungary)

Introduction

The final cause of the plateau waves of Lundberg appears to be an increase in cerebral blood volume (Avezaat and Eijndhoven 1986, Risberg et al. 1969). This increase may be due to a brain stem mediated arterial dilatation in response to a falling cerebral perfusion pressure (Furuse et al. 1982, Hayashi et al. 1987, Rosner and Becker 1984). Alternatively it may be caused by increased venous outflow resistance at the bridging vein-sagittal sinus junction (Laas and Arnold 1981, Nyary and Vajda 1986, Shapiro et al. 1966). Our recent findings support the latter view.

Materials and Methods

A 25-year-old male underwent right retrograde brachial angiography with his right forearm in a cast. With catheters in the brachial artery and vein, the forearm in its cast served as a model of the intracranial space. The brachial vein pressure in the forearm corresponded to cerebral venous pressure or ICP. Venous compression at the elbow led to periodic elevations of forearm venous pressure (ICP). A similar experiment was performed in the casted hindlegs of 5 dogs. Arterial and venous flow was controlled by perivascular cuffs on the proximal artery and vein. Alternate reductions of arterial and venous flows were performed with systemic arterial pressure held constant at 140/90 mm Hg.

Results

Similar pressure responses to changes in flow inflow and outflow were seen in all cases. After venous occlusion venous pressure rose to 50 mm Hg (Fig. 1). At high venous pressures the pulse profile was dominated by the arterial pressure wave rather than the respiratory intrathoracic pressure changes seen at resting levels. This pulse profile at high venous pressures resembles the profile seen in increased ICP. When the venous cuff was deflated even minimally the plateau wave resolved rapidly and completely.

Eds.: J. T. Hoff and A. L. Betz

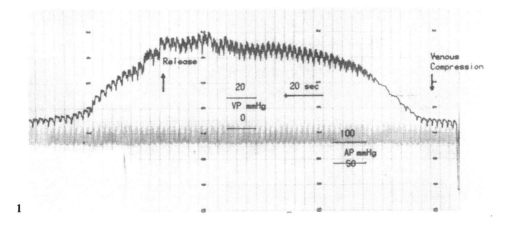

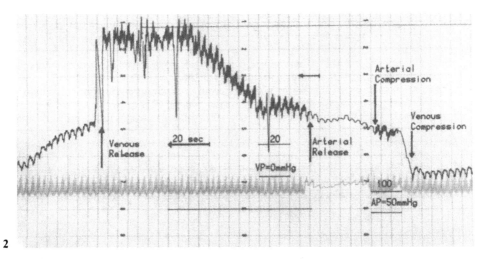

Fig. 1. Pressure recordings from the intravenous segment under the plaster in the forearm (*dark line*) and from the brachial artery at the elbow (*grey line*). Charts should be read from the right to the left. Venous compression invokes plateau-like waves

Fig. 2. Arterial compression during development of plateau wave halts rise in pressure and removes arterial pulse effect from venous pressure wave. Opening artery causes great increase in venous pressure

If venous compression was followed by arterial compression, the rising venous pressure levelled off and remained stable. Venous pressure then rose to a very high plateau after arterial compression was released (Fig. 2).

Discussion

These findings support the view that venous compression and increased venous outflow resistance is the cause of plateau waves in increased ICP. When arterial

249

pressure remained constant increased venous resistance evoked plateau-like rises of venous pressure and tissue pressure within the closed space. Plateau development could be prevented by occluding arterial inflow during increased venous outflow resistance. Even small decreases in venous resistance served to terminate the plateau. Brain stem reflex vasodilation cannot explain the development of plateau waves in this model and lack of linear pressure increase suffices to discount the presence of a purely mechanical response. The arterialized pulse profile of venous pressure or tissue pressure can be produced in any closed space, not only in the intracranial space.

References

Avezaat CJJ, Eijndhoven JHM (1986) Clinical observations on the relationship between CSF pulse pressure and ICP. Acta Neurochir 79:13–29

Furuse M, Kuchiwaki H, Hasuo M, Nakaya T, Toyama K, Asano Y, Teraoka M, Kageyama N, Ikeyama A (1982) The pathogenesis of pressure waves. Neurol Med Chir (Tokyo) 22:37–42

Hayashi M, Ishii H, Handa H, Kobayashi H, Kawano H, Kabuto M (1987) Role of the medulla oblongata in plateau-wave development in dogs. J Neurosurg 67:97–101

Laas R, Arnold H (1981) Compression of the outlets of the leptomeningeal veins – the cause of intracranial plateau waves. Acta Neurochir (Wien) 58:187–201

Nyary I, Vajda J (1986) Clinical evidence of compressed lacunar veins causing plateau waves. ICP VI., pp 142–145

Risberg J, Lundberg N, Ingvar DH (1969) Regional CBV during acute transient rises of the ICP (plateau). J Neurosurg 31:303–310

Rosner JM, Becker DP (1984) Origin and evolution of plateau waves. J Neurosurg 60:312–324

Shapiro HM, Langfitt TW, Weinstein JD (1966) Compression of cerebral vessels by intracranial hypertension. II: Morphological evidence for collapse of vessels. Acta Neurochir (Wien) 15:223–233

Slow Oscillation of Compliance and Pressure Rate in the Naturally Closed Cranio-Spinal System

K. Lewer Allen[1] and E.A. Bunt[2]

George Hospital[1], George and Rand Afrikaans University[2], Johannesburg (South Africa)

Experimental

Previously reported work on periodic movement of human brain and variations of density and ventricular shape revealed by rapid CT-scanning (Lewer Allen and Bunt 1985) has suggested that a periodic variation of brain compliance occurs. To test this, we examined 19 normal and off-normal case categories (involving 23 experiments) selected from a group many of whose brain property (pressure/volume but excluding time) diagrams had previously been investigated.

The infusion procedure – a set of controlled volume injections, each interrupted long enough to allow a system to stabilize at a pressure value close to the resting pressure in the natural response time of the system – was used as a 'meter' to take, in effect, point readings of the compliance and pressure recovery of the cranio-spinal system over a total period of up to about 2–300 sec. Compliance was measured by $C = \Delta V / \Delta p$, where V is the injection volume in ml (+ or −) and Δp ("pressure rate") is the resulting pressure change in mm Hg over the infusion interval.

Data Handling of Experimental Results

The initial assumption was that brain pressure and compliance variation could be described as periodic and thus be subject to Fourier analysis. Series of values of C and Δp at equal time intervals were established for analysis by linear interpolation of clinical data. The techniques employed to decompose the data into contributions associated with frequency were:

a) A Fast Fourier computer procedure (Statistical Graphics Corporation 1986), and
b) An analysis of non-harmonic functions (Worthing et al. 1959).

Procedure (b) was used to check the results obtained by Procedure (a) in the control case (Case 1, Near-normal) and Table 1 lists all resulting periodicities (in seconds) for both variables C and Δp for this case. The accuracy of periodicities is estimated to be within a range of 1–2%.

Table 1. The periodicities yielded for case 1 (near-normal) by procedure (*a*) are as shown:

Case	Compliance periods, sec.	Δp periods, sec.
1 (*a*) (diastolic)	186, 323[+], 613, 1996	311, 545, 1066, 2199
1 (*b*) (systolic)	175, 317[+], 619, 1922	211, 433, 1066, 2220

The corresponding periods given by procedure (*b*) are 305.75 sec. and 302.00 sec

Fourier analysis yielded a large number of Fourier components of longer period than those of the cardiac and respiratory waves. These are all outside the band studied by Bray (1986). It will be seen that Procedure (b) in Case 1 yielded for values of C dominant periods of 305.75 sec and 302 sec which closely corresponded to the Fast Fourier components of 323 and 317 sec. – an indication of the relative accuracy of the two procedures. However, the observed variation of wave patterns during induced stress cycles suggests that a physiological interpretation of periodic motions is necessary.

Periodic Response of System to Stress

Figure 1 shows (on an injection time base) upper curves of systolic and diastolic pressures for Case 1, as measured by telemetry. The lower curve shows (to the same time base) the derived compliance curves. Small pressure changes clearly correspond to large compliance values ("soft" property and vice versa). Also on the same time base are shown horizontal broken lines representing the duration of 'evident' wave trains over the spectral range shown (logarithmic scale).

The normal 'resting range' of an individual is considered to lie within the bandwidth 200–300 sec. (shorter periods than these characterize an unstable state of over-softness). This "toned" region is also characterized by the appearance of desirable waves in the 15–32 sec band ("3rd waves" – Lewer Allen et al. 1967) – possibly an auto-regulatory fine adjustment. As stress accumulates outside this region, waves of 305 sec. appear to be dominant within the 305–698 sec. band. This band is associated with a pressure rise which coincides with the summation of a great number of waves (including the 3rd wave), with pressure peaking even to 80 mm Hg (Fig. 1). Despite accumulating stress the pressure is then seen to drop away as the important intermediate band of 300–698 sec. falls out. The summation cycle then reappears. Indeed, a conspicuous prolonged absence of this intermediate range characterizes cases of N.I.H., B.I.H., post-traumatic dementia, and Alzheimer's disease, all of which developed signs and symptoms of deficient cerebral function associated with distortion of brain/ventricular shape indicative of longstanding dynamic imbalance. The physiological significance of the longest waves is obscure.

Fluid releases (Lewer Allen et al. 1978) (which occur at high intracranial pressure) leading to alternating 'softening' and 'hardening' are now believed to be a normally occurring periodic phenomenon (and not merely a 'safety valve' type

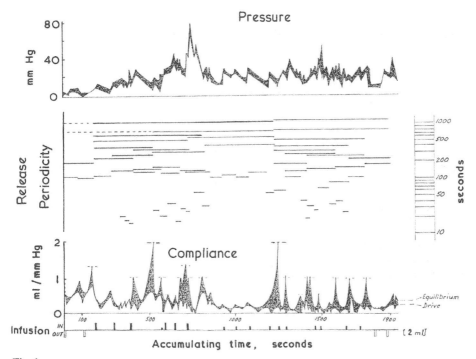

Fig. 1

of operation to relieve infusion-induced stress). Such releases occur in the 200–300 sec. band of operation. The normal operation through rest and through stress to major fluid release is seen to span a periodic spectrum from 275 to 698 sec.

A previous experiment based on a different technique led to the concept of a vascularly-energized traveling wave able to move circulatory fluid (Lewer Allen et al. 1978). The combined evidence of this and the present experiment points to the existence of an important mechanism of the compression wave being preceded and followed by a softening of the brain to facilitate circulatory penetration as well as to prevent harmful pressure peak accumulation.

Conclusions

i) Periodicity of brain C and Δp (independent of the irregular infusion rate) has been demonstrated, although phase differences could not be studied. Certain (intermediate) bands in the periodic spectrum can be shown to have physiological purpose; if these are suppressed over long period, pathological effects can develop.

ii) Major fluid releases activated by pressure changes are now believed to be a normally occurring periodic phenomenon. Such releases maintain compliance at a dynamically satisfactory level.

253

iii) The observed C and Δp periodic variations correlate well with those of brain movement registered by the use of a different method (Lewer Allen and Bunt 1985).

References

Bray R (1986) Fast Fourier transform of ICP waveform. In: Miller et al. (eds) Intracranial Pressure VI. Springer, Berlin Heidelberg New York Tokyo, p 260–264

Lewer Allen K, Bunt EA (1978) Dysfunctioning of the fluid mechanical craniospinal system as revealed by stress/strain diagrams. South African Mechanical Engineer, 28:159–166

Lewer Allen K, Bunt EA (1985) Rhythmic brain movement and density variations shown by rapid sequential CT scanning in the human subject. In: Miller JD et al. (eds) Intracranial Pressure VI. Springer, Berlin Heidelberg New York Tokyo, p 437–440

Lewer Allen K, Goldman HI (1967) Phasic pressure characteristics of the cerebrospinal fluid system. South African J Surg 5:151–158

Statistical Graphics Corporation, Inc. Statgraphics program, 1986.

Worthing AC, Geffner J (1959) Treatment of experimental data. J Wiley, New York

Remarks on Amplitude–Pressure Characteristic Phenomenon

M. Czosnyka [1], P. Wollk-Laniewski [2], L. Batorski [3], W. Zaworski [1], and C. Nita [1]

Institute of Electronics Fundamentals, Warsaw University of Technology [1],
Department of Anesthesiology and Intensive Care, Child's Health [2], Clinic of Neurosurgery,
Child's Health Centre [3], Warsaw (Poland)

A pulse wave is the most characteristic component of the intracranial pressure (ICP) signal. Many authors have devoted their work to questions concerning its mechanisms and clinical validation, however, most of these questions remain still open. It should also be emphasized, that almost all the theoretical works dealing with the cerebrospinal space model except a few (Hoffmann 1985, Sorak 1986) do not discuss the phenomenon of pulsatile changes of cerebral blood volume (CBV). The model introduced by Marmarou (1976) describes only the cerebrospinal fluid (CSF) circulation and phenomena concerning the CSF container such as infusion or bolus tests, but cerebral blood flow (CBF) is not included in the model. Therefore, the amplitude-pressure (AMP-P) characteristic cannot be explained in the same way as a linear relationship between the cerebrospinal elastance and the pressure level.

From the point of view of the pressure–volume relationship, the amplitude of the pulse wave (AMP) is a pressure rise in response to the maximal increase of CBV during one heart cycle. This increase can be expressed (Avezaat and Eijndhoven 1984) as the maximum value of the integral of the differences between the arterial inflow and venous outflow rates (for one heart beat). Both rates are time dependent and both are affected by complex factors including features of the autoregulation loop, non-linear compliances of the vessel bed, and pressure dependent resistance of the bridging veins. Even if the pressure–volume characteristic (where volume is meant as the volume of CSF) has the monoexponential character, the AMP-P is affected by so many phenomena, especially in continuous ICP monitoring that its shape and slope cannot provide information on the cerebrospinal compensation ability alone, but rather on CBF regulation mechanisms.

The purpose of this work was to collect all the observations supporting this thesis made during five years of clinical work on ICP signal analysis and interpretation.

Material and Method

Over 150 children with ICP monitored continuously or for short periods form the clinical basis for our considerations. The group consists of patients who had tumors of posterior fossa removed (67), Reye's syndrome and encephalitis (6), head injuries (4), craniostenosis (9), and hydrocephalus (74). ICP was measured intraventricularly (69), epidurally (15) or using a lumbar catheter (74).

The pressure was monitored using HP 1200 or S and W 9000 bedside monitors. It was analyzed using a computerized system for neurosurgical intensive care and diagnostics of our own design (Czosnyka et al. 1986). Various types of signal processing were applied, according to clinical needs. The following points summarize the most important results concerning the pulse wave analysis.

I) Measurement of the Pulse Wave Amplitude

Many questions arose from the problem of precise and efficient measurement of the pulse wave amplitude for the purpose of AMP-P relationship analysis. Three methods were compared in a group of 18 constant rate infusion tests. Amplitude was calculated as: – peak to peak value from one pulse (AMPpp), – amplitude of the first harmonic component using the short time spectral analysis (AMPh), and the root mean square of energy of one pulse evolution (AMPa).

The correlation coefficient between AMPh and ICP during the test was the highest, however, it did not differ significantly from the remaining coefficients (mean: 0.965 for AMPh, 0.912 for AMPa and 0.907 for AMPpp).

It was also observed that the coefficient of harmonic distortion did not change significantly during the test. All these support the thesis that the spectral analysis can be regarded as the best method of measuring pulse wave amplitude for the purpose of AMP-P evaluation.

This method additionally allows for neglecting the influences of the remaining components and on-line calculations of the heart rate and respiratory amplitude.

II) The "Floating AMP-P" Relationship

In 22 selected patients, monitored continuously in postoperative care operations for tumors of the posterior fossa, data were analyzed using the method of "floating AMP-P characteristic". In the method, the statistical relationship between AMP and ICP is calculated in short period (about 10 min). The characteristic is considered to be homogeneous as long as the correlation coefficient between AMP and ICP (RAP) remains significantly higher than 0.6.

This characteristic can be treated as stable if RAP is satisfactorily high within a period longer than 20 min.

The AMP-P line in this group of patients was highly variable with time. It was registered in 40% of the total monitoring time. The average period was about 42 min. Its average slope was 0.18 with a standard deviation of 0.11.

Some characteristic fluctuations of the ICP signal parameters were noticed to follow the changes of the stable AMMP-P characteristic: 1) changes of the heart rate (52%); 2) changes of the respiratory wave (43%); and 3) rapid changes of the mean ICP level (27%).

III) AMP-P Characteristic in Infusion Tests

The AMP-P linear relationship was observed during 96% of 74 infusion tests. But its slope was significantly higher than in continuous monitoring: mean 0.391 with a standard deviation 0.132. The slope of the AMP-P was not correlated with the cerebrospinal elasticity calculated during the test.

It was best correlated with the opening level of the pulse wave amplitude. The baseline pressure, P_0, calculated as the pressure of the intercept of the AMP-P line and the pressure axis was, in 17 cases (over 30%), out of the range which can be regarded as a physiological range for the sagittal sinus pressure (lower than -8 mm Hg).

IV) Non-Linear Character of the AMP-P

In many cases the characteristic is strongly non-linear. The lower breakpoint, below which the slope is equal to zero, can be observed only in a few infusion tests, after the withdrawal of a portion of CSF.

Frequently the amplitude increases more than proportionally to the rise of the mean ICP. A linear relationship between the slope of a short-term AMP-P characteristic was found in the monitoring of craniostenosis (6 out of 9 cases). A similar phenomenon can be observed in infusion tests when the induced rise of ICP produces (as a central reflex) a decrease in the heart rate.

In continuous monitoring, especially when developing brain edema is suspected, the upper breakpoint, above which the slope becomes negative is commonly observed (Fig. 1 b).

V) Interpretation of the RP – Short Term Correlation Coefficient Between the Amplitude and the Mean ICP

This coefficient, expressing the character of the short-term AMP-P relationship, found its application in neurosurgical intensive care.

In the steady state RAP is close to 0, pointing out the lack of a significant amplitude–pressure relationship. If an uncompensated volume process is introduced (either internally or externally – as infusion tests) RAP increases to values significantly close to 1. Such a process usually forces an increase of ICP level, but not necessarily. Further increase of ICP usually causes a decrease of RAP to negative values and a decrease of the AMP (Fig. 1 a). This can be interpreted as an exhaustion of the autoregulatory reserve.

Conclusions

The summary made in the above five points suggests that the amplitude of the pulse wave and its relationship with the mean ICP level reflect in most situations, especially in continuous monitoring, the state of CBF regulation.

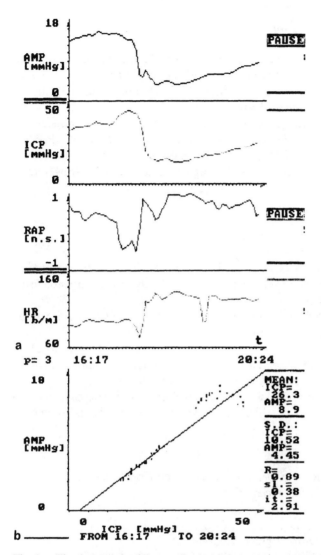

Fig. 1. a The time trends of the amplitude (*AMP*), the mean pressure level (*ICP*), the correlation coefficient between the mean pressure and the amplitude (*RAP*), and the heart rate (*HR*) registered in head injured child with clinical symptoms of brain edema (confirmed in CT). During the slow increase of ICP above the level of 37 mm Hg, RAP became negative and AMP was decreasing. After mannitol administration, ICP decreased, AMP decreased, HR increased, and RAP became positive (common *abscissa* = time in hr and min sampling period, 5 min). **b** The amplitude/pressure characteristic, registered during the same period as the time trends. Above the pressure level or about 37 mm Hg, an upper breakpoint was observed (*ordinate* = amplitude, *abscissa* = pressure)

The positive slope of AMP-P can be theoretically modelled by the dependence between the perfusion pressure and vascular bed resistance (when autoregulation holds) and by the ICP-dependent resistance of bridging veins. The upper breakpoint of the AMP-P line can be interpreted as a cut-off point of the autoregulation range (with respect to CPP decrease).

258

These considerations also allow us to propose the term of "uncompensated volume process", the processes producing changes in cerebrospinal space and affecting the CBF control parameters, which produce, in most cases, changes of the pulse wave amplitude correlated to mean ICP.

References

Avezaat CJ, van Eijndhoven JHM (1984) Cerebrospinal fluid pulse pressure and craniospinal system. Doctor's Thesis. Erasmus University, Jongbloed en Zoon Publishers, The Hague

Czosnyka M, Laniewski P (1986) Intracranial pressure analysis for intensive care purposes. Proc. of IV Mediterranean Conference on Medical and Biological Engineering, Sevilla, pp 76–79

Hoffmann O (1985) Ein mathematisches Modell zur Simulation und Analyse der intrakraniellen Liquor- und Hämodynamik. Eine medizinisch-theoretische Studie. Hab. thesis, Justus-Liebig Universität Gießen

Marmarou A (1976) A theoretical and experimental evaluation of the cerebrospinal fluid system. PhD Thesis. Drexel Univ., Philadelphia

Sorek S et al. (1985) Models of cerebrospinal system mechanics. Scientific Report. Technion-Israel Institute of Technology, Haifa

Non-Provocative Assessment
of Intracranial Volume – Pressure Relationships

A.P. Rosiello, E.L. McCleary, and P.R. Cooper

Department of Neurosurgery, Boston University, 720 Harrison Ave., Suite 710, Boston 02118 (USA)

Although intracranial volume–pressure relationships can be directly determined, volume–pressure testing is an invasive and potentially dangerous maneuver requiring a ventricular or lumbar catheter. Therefore, we examined three non-provocative mathematical techniques for estimating the volume–pressure relationship by analyzing the shape and character of the ICP waveform.

Using Marmarou's fundamental pressure–volume relationship (Marmarou et al. 1975, 1978), Avezaat and van Eijndhoven (1979) derived a linear relationship between CSF pulse amplitude and ICP. If the volume bolus due to the cardiac impulse remains constant, CSF pulse amplitude becomes a linear function of ICP. The slope of this line is defined as the pulse amplitude index (PAI) and can be used to estimate the shape of the pressure–volume curve.

Many investigators have shown that this linear relationship persists through ranges of pressure that are within clinical interest. Brawanski, Gaab, and Heissler (1983) noted that changes in the slope of this relationship parallel changes in the shape of the pressure–volume curve as described by the elastance.

Szewczykowski et al. (1976) have also suggested a linear relationship between the standard deviation of ICP and ICP. Measuring ICP instability in this manner is analagous to the pulse amplitude relationship, but includes respiratory and sub-respiratory variations of ICP. The slope of this line may be defined as the standard deviation index (SDI).

Fast Fourier transformation of the ICP waveform identifies its fundamental and harmonic frequencies which occur in three frequency ranges. The respiratory and heart rates with their respective harmonics form the respiratory and vascular components. Frequencies below the respiratory component, with a rate of 1.2 cycles per minute (cpm), are referred to as the subrespiratory component. Auer and Gallhofer (1981) studied cat pial vessels in vivo, and described slow variations of arteriolar tone with a frequency in the ½ to 2 cpm range. Lundberg B-waves also occur with a frequency of ½ to 2 cpm. If Lundberg B-waves are related to alterations in intracranial vascular volume, the magnitude of the sub-respiratory component may reflect the volume–pressure relationship.

Fourteen patients underwent continuous ICP monitoring with a dedicated real-time microprocessor system for periods of 8 to 120 h. Monitoring was per-

---

Fig. 1. a Distribution of the pulse amplitude index (PAI). b Distribution of the standard deviation index (SDI). c Distribution of the sub-respiratory component (SRC). Note – normal curve is superimposed on all distributions

Eds.: J. T. Hoff and A. L. Betz
© Springer-Verlag Berlin Heidelberg 1989

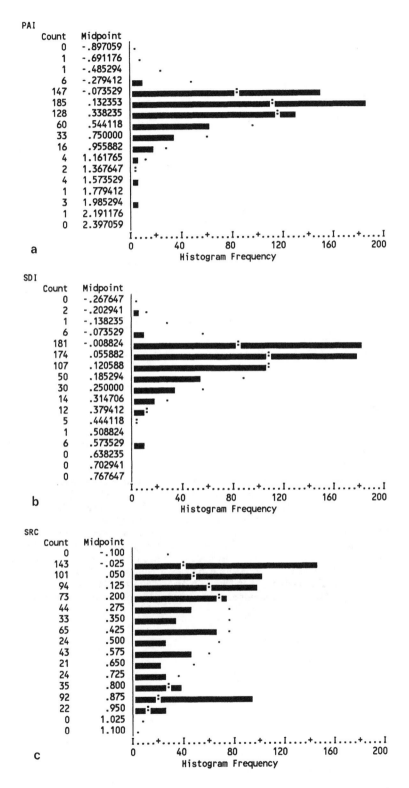

formed in 10 patients due to head trauma (1 patient fully recovered, 2 recovered with mild disability, 2 with moderate disability, 2 with severe disability, and 3 died), in 3 patients due to complicated hydrocephalus, and in 1 patient due to complicated pseudotumor. ICP was recorded with volume-coupled, fiber-optic, and electrical strain gauge techniques. The magnitude of the sub-respiratory component (as a percentage of total power) was determined in all 14 patients, while the pulse amplitude index (PAI) and standard deviation index (SDI) were determined in 11 patients.

Data from all patients were then pooled to discern the mean, standard deviation, and distribution of each parameter. The means and standard deviations are summarized below:

parameter	cases	mean	standard deviation
PAI	594	0.265	0.406
SDI	593	0.091	0.136
SRC	814	0.344	0.318

Figure 1 displays the distribution of each parameter compared to a normal curve with the same mean and standard deviation. Distribution of the PAI and SDI is similar to a normal curve, which is the expected distribution of a physiologic parameter. Failure of the SRC to distribute normally is probably due to inadequate resolution of sub-respiratory frequencies.

References

Auer LM, Gallhofer B (1981) Rhythmic activity of cat pial vessels in vivo. Eur Neurol 20:448–468
Avezaat CJJ, van Eijndhoven JHM, Wyper DJ (1979) Cerebrospinal fluid pulse pressure and intracranial volume–pressure relationships. J Neurol Neurosurg Psychiatry 42:687–700
Brawanski A, Gaab MR, Heisler HE (1983) Computer-analysis of ICP-modulations: Clinical significance and prediction of ICP-dynamics. In: Ishii S, Nagai H, Brock M (eds) Intracranial Pressure V. Springer, Berlin Heidelberg New York, pp 186–190
Marmarou A, Shulman K, LaMorgese J (1975) Compartmental analysis of compliance and outflow resistance of the cerebrospinal fluid system. J Neurosurg 43:523–534
Marmarou A, Shulman K, Rosende RM (1978) A nonlinear analysis of the cerebrospinal fluid system and intracranial pressure dynamics. J Neurosurg 48:332–344
Szewczykowski J, Dytko P, Kunicki A, Korsak-Sliwka J, Sliwka S, Dziduszko J et al. (1976) A method of estimating intracranial decompensation in man. J Neurosurg 45:155–158

The Viscoelasticity of Normal and Hydrocephalic Brain Tissue

C.M. Zee and K. Shapiro

Humana Advanced Surgical Institutes, Humana Hospital Medical City Dallas,
7777 Forest Lane, Dallas, Texas 75320 (USA)

Introduction

Many studies have investigated the role of brain compliance and the pressure
volume index (PVI) in the hydrocephalic process (Shulman and Marmarou 1971,
Guinane 1974, Shapiro et al. 1985, Shapiro and Fried 1986). However, very little
is known about the changes in the brain tissue characteristics which take place
during hydrocephalus. These properties are of interest because, although the PVI
has been shown to increase with hydrocephalus and does describe changes in
brain compliance, it does not explain what occurs during the disease process to
account for these changes. In hydrocephalus, the brain tissue can be severely
deformed. Therefore, it is probable that the mechanical properties of the brain
tissue are compromised and weakened. This may be a cause for the increased
brain compliance associated with hydrocephalus and may facilitate ventricular
enlargement. Knowledge of brain tissue properties is essential in the understanding of ICP dynamics and pathologies. Yet, despite their importance, few
studies have been performed to look at these properties (Keonman 1966;
Ommaya 1968; Fallenstein et al. 1969; Metz et al. 1970, Marmarou et al. 1980).
This is because there are many problems associated with studying brain tissue due
to its highly compliant nature. We have developed a system using a gas bearing
electrodynamometer, GBE, which addresses many of these problems and allows
the direct determination of the viscoelastic properties of brain tissue. In this study
the viscoelastic properties of normal and hydrocephalic brain tissue were evaluated in vivo using the GBE.

Methods

Six normal and seven cats rendered hydrocephalic through an intracisternal kaolin injection were used in this study. All hydrocephalic animals were tested three
weeks after kaolin injection. The animals were anesthetized with pentobarbital
and intubated. All animals were ventilated using a Bear jet ventilator, in order to
reduce brain pulsations, and fixed in a stereotactic frame. Arterial blood pressure,
ICP, and blood gases were monitored.

The GBE is an instrument that measures the force acting on and the resulting
displacement of a moving gas suspended armature. The GBE armature oscillates

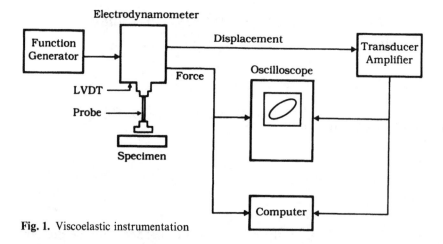

Fig. 1. Viscoelastic instrumentation

in response to a changing magnetic field in the surrounding coil. The coil is activated by a function generator operating in the sinusoidal mode. The function generator controls the frequency and amplitude of the armature force since the force is directly related to the electrical current applied to the coil. The resulting displacement is measured by a linear variable displacement transformer (LVDT) which is mounted coaxially with the force coil in the GBE. The output of the coil, force, and the LVDT, displacement are displayed on the x and y axes of an oscilloscope resulting in a hysteresis loop (Fig. 1). The data were sampled using a DEC PDP11-23 computer at 200 Hz and the following parameters were measured on line: 1) The dynamic spring rate (DSR) in gm/mm is the slope of the major axis of the loop and an indicator of the stiffness of the material. 2) The loop opening in mm which results from energy being lost in the specimen and indicates the viscous response of the tissue. 3) The loss angle in degrees which is the phase lag between the applied force and the resulting deformation. 4) The loss rate and the elastic spring rate in gm/mm which are the x and y components of the dynamic spring rate and indicators of stiffness.

The dura was exposed and opened through a 10 mm burr hole located 10 mm posterior to the coronal suture extending medially to within 4 mm of the sagittal suture on the right side of the skull. The GBE probe was applied normal to the brain surface and a (0.5–2.0 gm) 10 Hz sinusoidal force was applied. The applied force and the resulting deformation were sampled on line for 15 min.

Results

Significant differences in the viscoelastic properties of brain tissue were observed between intact and hydrocephalic animals (Table 1). The dynamic spring rate of normal brain tissue was determined to be 4.468 gm/mm ± 0.494 (SE). In hydrocephalus, the DSR decreased significantly ($p < 0.0001$) to 2.77 gm/mm ± 0.518 (SE), indicating that the brain became less stiff with hydrocephalus. The loop

264

Table 1. The viscoelastic values of normal and hydrocephalic brain tissue

	Dynamic spring rate (gm/mm)	Loop opening (mm)	Loss angle (degrees)	Loss rate (gm/mm)	Elastic spring rate (gm/mm)
Normal brain tissue	4.468	0.91	13.948	0.989	4.347
Hydrocephalic brain tissue	2.770	0.157	20.982	0.978	2.583
Percent difference[a]	−38	+72.5	+50.4	−1	−40.6

[a] Alpha < 0.05.

opening for normal tissue was found to be 0.091 mm $\pm$ 0.011 (SE) and increased significantly ($p < 0.0001$) to 0.157 mm $\pm$ 0.013 (SE) showing that the tissue became more viscous with hydrocephalus. This decrease in stiffness and increase in viscosity are also indicated by the increase in loss angle and the decrease in the loss rate and elastic spring rate.

Discussion

The gas bearing electrodynamometer has proven to be an advantageous means of studying the viscoelasticity of brain tissue in vivo. The GBE addresses many of the problems associated with the study of very soft biological tissue and yields highly reproducible results. These studies show that hydrocephalic brain tissue appears less stiff and more viscous than normal brain tissue as evidenced by a decrease in the DSR and an increase of the loop opening. These changes in the mechanical properties of the hydrocephalic tissue indicate tissue weakening which may facilitate ventricular enlargement. The weakening of the tissue may also account for the increase in brain compliance associated with hydrocephalus. Although these studies show significant tissue changes with hydrocephalus the time course of these changes has not been addressed. Future studies will be performed to analyze the time course and recovery characteristics of these changes in brain tissue properties seen in hydrocephalus.

References

Fallenstein GT, Hulce VD, Melvin JW (1969) Dynamic mechanical properties of human brain tissue. J Biomech 2:217–236
Guinane JE (1974) Cerebrospinal fluid resistance and compliance in subacutely hydrocephalic cats. Neurology 24:138–142
Koenman JB (1970) Viscoelastic properties of brain tissue. Masters Thesis, Case Institute of Technology
Marmarou A, Takagi H, Hargens CW, Shulman K (1980) Effects of cerebral edema upon viscoelastic properties of brain tissue. In: Shulman K, Marmarou A, Miller JD, Becker DP, Hochwald GM, Brock M (eds) Intracranial Pressure IV. Springer, Berlin Heidelberg New York

Metz H, McElhanry J, Ommaya AK (1970) A comparison of the elasticity of live, dead, and fixed brain tissue. J Biomech 3:453–458

Shapiro K, Fried A, Marmarou A (1985) A biomechanical and hydrodynamic characterization of the hydrocephalic infant. J Neurosurg 66:69–75

Shapiro K, Fried A (1986) Pressure volume relationships in shunt department childhood hydrocephalus. J Neurosurg 64:390–396

Shulman K, Marmarou A (1971) Pressure volume considerations in infantile hydrocephalus. Dev Med Child Neurol 13 [Suppl 25]:90–95

Intracranial Elastance:
Spline Interpolation vs Exponential Function

M.R. Gaab and H.E. Heissler

Neurosurgical Department, Hanover Medical School, Konstanty-Gutschow-Str. 8,
D-3000 Hannover 61 (FRG)

Introduction

The main pathophysiological effects of increased ICP are explained by the
pressure/volume-function of the intracranial space. Pressure waves, fluctuation
of ICP pulse amplitudes and the sudden decompensation of space occupying
lesions are caused by the nonlinear relationship between ICP and intracranial
volume. The evaluation of the patient's actual volume/pressure function ("elastance") is, therefore, an important supplement to ICP monitoring in acute brain
damage (Avezaat et al. 1980, Gaab and Heissler 1984) as well as in diagnostics,
e.g. for CSF disorders (Avezaat et al. 1980, Gaab et al. 1982).

For objective mathematical evaluation of intracranial elastance, progress has
been achieved by Marmarou's exponential P/V model (Marmarou 1976). However, the criteria for this model may not be given by the biological substrate (Hopp
and Berninger 1987, Sprent 1969) and large deviations are usually found with the
bolus tests based on Marmarou's equations (Gaab et al. 1982). In adding a
"constant term", we could improve the accuracy of the P/V diagram using bolus
injection (Gaab et al. 1982). However, the exponential function per se as well as
any model presuming a definite mathematical correlation may fail in describing
the biological conditions. We therefore investigated the spline interpolation as a
model-free method for evaluating intracranial elastance and the pressure/volume
diagram.

Rationale and Methods

Rationale

The functional relation between two biological values (here: ICP/bolus volume)
can mathematically be described by "calibration curves" (here: the "P/V diagram"). In order to find these curves, two different mathematical methods are
available: Interpolation and approximation. The exponential function gives a
model-based "least square error" approximation; the estimated P/V diagram
(Fig. 1 b, d) does, more or less, fit the actual data (with "r" as a parameter for the
"goodness of fit").

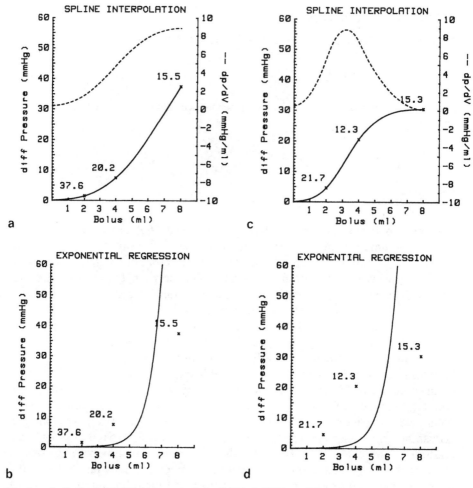

Fig. 1. a, b Patient with "high pressure defect" (65 y.): "Bilinear" P/V diagram with a threshold volume response and linear pressure increase in spline interpolation (**a**). Inaccuracy of exponential function (**b**). **c, d** Patient with hydrocephalus (43 y.): Sigmoidal shape of the interpolation function due to (?) increasing CSF outflow at high ICP (**c**). New equilibrium not shown by the inaccurate exponential model (**d**)

The natural (cubic) spline interpolation is a polynomial interpolation procedure with minimal curvature. This interpolation function is characterized by 3rd order polynomials between the measured values. The coefficients are determined with respect to the initial conditions and monotonicity. Hence, a generally model free evaluation of exogenously induced ICP transients will be accomplished. Therefore, the results are directly related to the measured values and not to a predetermined mathematical model.

Practical Method

In 53 patients with ventricular dilatation (differential diagnosis: active hydrocephalus), a bolus injection test was performed: In all patients, the epidural ICP (GAELTEC ICT/b transducer, left frontal position [Gaab and Heissler 1984]) was recorded for 48–72 hr. In the lateral recumbent position and with continued epidural ("intracranial") pressure recording, a lumbar puncture was performed with two 20 g cannulas at neighboring levels. One needle was used for the spinal pressure record (MEDEX X800-50 transducer), the other for the bolus injection: Mock CSF was rapidly injected, beginning with a 1 ml bolus. With respect to a maximal ICP peak pressure after bolus injection of 40 mm Hg, the bolus volume was increased in geometrical order (2, 4, 8 ml). The subsequent injection was started when the ICP was again within the range of the resting pressure. Using the difference between Po before the bolus and the peak pressure Pp after injection, the P/V diagram was calculated by exponential function (Fig. 1 b, d) and by spline interpolation (Fig. 1 a, c) for the spinal and for the intracranial pressure record. Additionally, the pressure-volume index PVI according to Marmarou (1973) was calculated for comparison. To distinguish the different parts of the spline interpolated P/V-diagram trace, the first derivative dP/dV was calculated and plotted in the diagram. In both the interpolation and the approximation procedure, the origin of the diagram was included in the data set to improve the fit.

Results

According to the mathematical concept, the exponential function (Fig. 1 b) results in a monotonously rising P.V. characteristic in all patients. The only individual difference is given by the steepness of the curve which is defined by the exponent ("k-slope"). In some patients, however, (Fig. 1 c, d), the mono-exponential model clearly fails and does not approximate the biologic conditions. The unsatisfying fit of this method is shown by the poor correlation coefficient. The mean r in 52 patients was found to be 0.69 ranging from 0.59 up to a poor maximum of 0.72.

According to the individual fit of each segment, the spline interpolated P/V diagrams (Fig. 1 a, c) are more sensitive to the actual values. The curve characteristics can be divided into quasi-linear, quasi-exponential (Fig. 1 a), bilinear and sigmoid (Fig. 1 c) shapes. The slope does vary considerably between the curve segments. Although definite pathophysiological parameters cannot yet be derived from these P/V characteristics, the potential for new information on craniospinal biomechanics is suggested. In one patient (Fig. 1 a, b), almost no CSF outflow was found (no plateau with constant rate infusion test), whereas another (Fig. 1 c, d) had a normal CSF outflow conductance.

Conclusions

The interpretation of the results should be done with respect to the obviously different and often not at all "exponential" behavior of the cerebrospinal system with volume load. There are patients with normal or altered CSF outflow and patients with virtually no CSF conductance. In addition to CSF dynamics, the cerebral blood volume, the cerebrovascular resistance and the mechanical characteristics of brain tissue and of the dura influence the pressure–volume relation.

As in most biological systems, the exponential model may only be valid in a limited range (Hopp and Berninger 1987, Sprent 1969). The complex behavior of the cerebrospinal space at different levels of resting ICP, with different "loading volumes" and with different dV/dt obviously exceeds the limits of an exponential relation. Here the spline interpolation method provides an accurate and more differentiated determination of the actual pressure–volume relationship. The spline interpolated P/V diagrams offer a good qualitative description. The pathophysiological significance of the different types of P/V curves obtained should be investigated further.

References

Avezaat CJJ, Eijndhoven JHM, Wyper DP (1980) Cerebrospinal fluid pressure and intracranial volume–pressure relationship. J Neurol Neurosurg Psychiatry 42:687–700

Gaab MR, Haubitz I et al. (1982) Pressure/volume test and pulse wave analysis of ICP. In: Driesen W, Brock M, Klinger M (eds) Advances in Neurosurgery, vol 10. Springer, Berlin Heidelberg New York, pp 367–377

Gaab MR, Heissler HE (1984) ICP monitoring. CRC Crit Rev Biomed Engin 11:189–250

Hopp V, Berninger G (1987) Mathematical functions for describing processes in nature and technology. GIT Fachz Lab 8:682–691

Jordan-Engeln G, Reutter F (1978) Mathematik für Ingenieure. 2. Aufl. Bibliographisches Institut, Mannheim Wien Zürich

Marmarou A (1973) A theoretical model and experimental evaluation of the cerebrospinal fluid system. Ph. D. Thesis, Drexel University, Philadelphia

Ohmayer G, Gränzer W (1987) Mathematical methods for the determination of calibration-curves in the biological analysis. GIT Labor-Medizin 9:397–404

Sprent P (1969) Models in regression and related topics. Methuen, London

Brain Tissue Elasticity and CSF Elastance

E.K. Walsh and A. Schettini

College of Engineering, University of Florida, Gainesville, Florida 32611 (USA)

Introduction

A common parameter reported in studies of intracranial volumetric buffering capacity is the CSF or brain elastance, designated as Ecsf. Ecsf is determined as dP/dV, the slope of the pressure-volume response. Since the pressure-volume response is nonlinear, Ecsf is pressure-dependent. CSF elastance is considered a measure of the volume storage capacity determined by the elastic properties of the system and as such is affected by the compressibility of the vascular volume as well as the subpial brain tissue. A question arises as to the correlation between CSF elastance and the actual elastic properties of the subpial brain tissue.

In our work we use an experimental configuration which more directly measures the response of the subpial tissue as a result of compression of the tissue by a pressure-sensing transducer. As the transducer is inserted through the subarachnoid space and against the dura, it causes a compression of the subpial tissue resulting in a force which is directly related to the depth of insertion of the base. The resulting nonlinear force/deformation response is analogous to the pressure-volume response caused by a bolus injection of fluid into the subarachnoid space, but in this case, isolates the subpial tissue response. The resulting response is a measure of brain tissue elasticity.

Clearly, it would be useful if changes in this parameter could be correlated with controlled changes in the intracranial environment, such as an intracranial mass lesion, and, if so, the question arises as to how such changes might compare with changes in CSF elastance under the same test conditions. We have investigated this during incremental inflation of an epidural balloon. The results show clear differences between the behavior of the system elastance, E_{csf}, and brain tissue elasticity as indicated by G_0. Further, additional measurements made following circulatory arrest showed a significant decrease in E_{csf} while G_0 increased, demonstrating a situation where brain tissue elasticity is indeed sensitive to controlled changes in the intracranial environment.

Materials and Methods

Ten dogs were included in the study. During the incremental inflation (0.5 ml) of an extradural balloon, simultaneous measurements of brain elastic response

(BER) parameters and CSF dynamics were carried out. In five additional dogs these measurements were combined with the monitoring of brain cortical impedance following circulatory arrest. The details of animal preparation and measurement of the various parameters have been described in an earlier report (Walsh et al. 1986). Here we limit the discussion to the parameters of interest, i.e., BER, Ecsf, and the measurement of cortical impedance.

Although brain tissue exhibits viscoelastic response, for observation times short compared to the characteristic relaxation time of the material, the response can be considered to be elastic (Schettini and Walsh 1973). In this case, brain elastic response (BER) can be measured extradurally with a coplanar pressure-displacement transducer (Walsh and Schettini 1984). The resulting nonlinear pressure-insertion depth response (BER curve) is reminiscent of the pressure-volume response of the ICP resulting from a bolus injection into the lateral ventricle, and is closely approximated as an exponential response. The initial point on the BER curve is (P_s, δ_s), where δ_s is the point (insertion-depth) beyond which any additional insertion causes a compression of the underlying subpial tissue and P_s is the corresponding pressure. The tangent to the BER curve at this point represents the initial linear elastic parameter, designated as G_0. This is the parameter to be reported here. Note that this is analogous to the determination of Ecsf as dP/dV, the slope of the pressure-volume curve, if that value was determined at the initial point of fluid volume insertion.

Ecsf was calculated from the equation (Sullivan et al. 1977)

$$Ecsf = \frac{P_0 (\ln (P_p/P_0))}{\Delta V} , \tag{1}$$

where P_0 is the baseline pressure and P_p is the peak pressure resulting from a bolus injection of normal saline (0.5 ml at 0.1 ml/s) into the ventricle.

To measure the specific cortical impedance, we used Ranck's method of four platinum iridium microelectrodes in a tetrapolar array and a two-phase lock-in amplifier (Ranck 1963). The electrode system was calibrated in vitro against known concentrations of a salt solution, in order to obtain the transfer factor and convert the experimental data (voltage) into specific impedance.

Results

The principle results are given in Fig. 1 which shows the ventricular pressure, Pvcsf (P_0 in eqn.1), Ecsf, and G_0, during incremental balloon expansion in 10 dogs. Clearly, while Pvcsf and Ecsf show a continual increase from the onset of balloon inflation, G_0 remains essentially unchanged.

The second significant result is that following circulatory arrest E_{csf} decreased while G_0 and the specific cortical impedance both increased over a 30 min period. The rise in impedance after circulatory arrest is related to an approximate 50% reduction in brain extracellular space due to glial swelling without any change in tissue water content (Van Harreveld and Ochs 1956). This intracellular water and

272

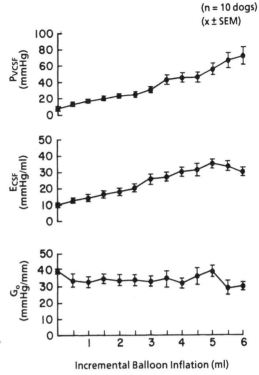

Fig. 1. Ventricular CSF pressure, Pvcsf, CSF elastance, Ecsf, and brain elasticity, G_0, during incremental expansion of an epidural balloon in 10 dogs

ion shift will increase cellular tension and may account for the increase in tissue elasticity, G_0. The fall in CSF elastance is likely related to the lack of flow in cerebral circulation.

Changes in G_0 also occur during Nipride, Arphonad, and graded bleeding induced hypotension (Walsh and Schettini 1984).

Discussion

The present hypothesis that brain elastance, as indicated by Ecsf, does not represent brain tissue elasticity has been suggested before. Chopp et al. (1983) proposed a hydraulic model for the cerebrovascular bed to explain the volume-pressure test from which the PVI and the Ecsf were determined. They concluded that the volume-pressure test was not a measure of the elasticity of the cerebral tissue. Here we have direct evidence that CSF elastance bears no relation to brain tissue elasticity (G_0).

References

Chopp M, Portnoy HD, Branch C (1983) Hydraulic model of the cerebrovascular bed: An aid to understanding the volume-pressure test. Neurosurgery 13:5–11

Ranck JB (1963) Specific impedance of rabbit cerebral cortex. Exp Neurol 7:144–152

Schettini A, Walsh EK (1973) Pressure relaxation of the intracranial system in vivo. Am J Physiol 225:513–517

Sullivan HG, Miller JD, Becker DP, Flora RE, Allen GA (1977) The physiological basis of intracranial pressure change with progressive epidural brain compression. J Neurosurg 47:532–550

Van Harreveld A, Ochs S (1956) Cerebral impedance changes after circulatory arrest. Am J Physiol 187:180–192

Walsh EK, Schettini A (1984) Calculation of brain elastic parameters in vivo. Am J Physiol 247:R693–R700

Walsh EK, Schettini A, Beck J, Salton RA (1986) Brain elastic behavior and CSF dynamics during progressive epidural balloon expansion. In: Miller JD, Teasdale GM, Rowan JO, Galbraith SL, Mendelow AD (eds) Intracranial pressure VI. Springer, Berlin Heidelberg New York

High Frequency Ventilation vs Conventional Mechanical Ventilation: Their Influence on Cerebral Elastance

R. García-Sola, J.J. Rubio, F. Gilsanz, P. Mateos, M.A. González, and C. Hernández

Department of Neurosurgery, Hospital de la Princesa; Department of Experimental Surgery, Clínica Puerta de Hierro, Autonomous University, Madrid (Spain)

High-frequency ventilation (HFV) has lesser hemodynamic repercussions and lower risk of barotrauma production, although it does not seem to affect the mean intracranial pressure (ICP) (Babinski et al. 1984). This fact, however, does not preclude a beneficial effect of HFV on the intracranial dynamic state.

The purpose of this study was to observe the effects of HFV on the mean ICP in situations of progressive intracranial hypertension (ICHT), as well as on cerebral elastance (CE).

Material and Methods

After anesthetic induction with thiopental sodium, 12 healthy dogs were maintained under general anesthesia with fentanyl and pancuronium bromide. The endotracheal tube was equipped with a lateral cannula for high-frequency jet ventilation (HFJV) using a prototype designed by one of the authors (Rubio et al. 1984).

The following parameters were monitored: blood pressure (BP), heart rate (HR), blood gases, mean and peak inspiratory airway pressures (Paw and PIP, respectively) and epidural ICP. This last parameter was registered and sampled in a monitoring unit designed by the authors (García Sola et al. 1981) which afforded: a) ICP/time relationship; and b) cerebral pulse wave amplitude/ICP relationship (Amp/ICP).

Two groups of 6 experiments each were performed:

a) *IPPV*. After 30 min in stable condition with conventional mechanical ventilation using intermittent positive pressure (IPPV), a situation of progressive ICHT was provoked by inflation of an epidural latex balloon at a rate of 4.5 cc/hr. Given the type of continuous infusion into the epidural balloon, the ICP/time relationship was equal to the pressure/volume (P/V) curve. The experiment was finalized once hemodynamic alterations were observed as a consequence of the high level of ICHT reached.

b) *HFJV*. After 30 min in basal conditions with IPPV, the switch was made to HPJV without producing changes in blood gases. After the animal was maintained in a basal condition for an additional 30 min with HFJV, inflation of the epidural balloon was begun at the same rate as in the IPPV control group.

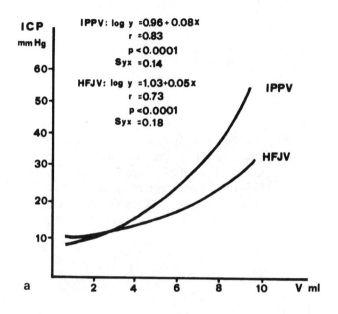

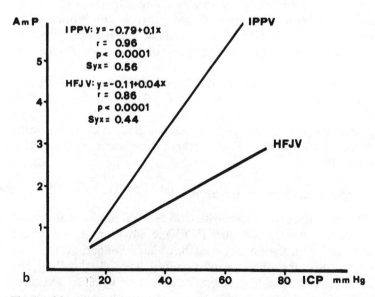

Fig. 1. a Mean pressure/volume curve with IPPV and HFJV. **b** Mean AmP/ICP relationships of both goups

Results and Discussion

Basal Situation. The change from IPPV to HFJV provoked a significant decrease in Paw and PIP ($p < 0.05$). No significant changes were observed in the mean BP, HR, $PaCO_2$, PaO_2, pH or mean ICP. Nevertheless, the Amp was significantly lower ($p < 0.001$), attributable to the almost complete disappearance of the respiratory component of the cerebral pulse wave.

Intracranial Hypertension. In the absence of changes in mean BP, HR, PaO_2, $PaCO_2$ or pH throughout all of the experiments, the following observations were made:

a) The P/V ratio is an exponential curve with a correlation coefficient greater than 0.9 in every case. With HFJV, the mean P/V curve presents a lesser slope than in the IPPV group (Fig. 1 a). This indicates that global CE is lower with HFJV.
b) The Amp/ICP relationship is a straight line with a correlation coefficient greater than 0.95 in all the experiments. The mean Amp/ICP curve of the HFJV group had a lesser slope than with IPPV, this difference being statistically very significant ($p < 0.001$) (Fig. 1 b).

Given that the Amp/ICP relationship may be assimilable to the CE/ICP relationship when there are no hemodynamic variations (Gilsanz et al. 1986), these results show that with HFJV, the more severe the ICHT situation, the slower the increase in CE when compared with IPPV.

This intracranial hemodynamic behavior, clearly more favorable in HFJV when compared to that resulting with IPPV, may be attributed, among other things, to the existence of lower PIP and Paw which favor a better cerebral venous return (Babinski et al. 1984).

However, the positive influence of reduced fluctuation of the cerebral parenchyma is also very suggestive, given the disappearance of the respiratory component of the BP pulse wave and of that of the ICP. This situation of greater barostability achieved by HFV could increase the capacity of resistance of the cerebral parenchyma in situations of adverse dynamic circumstances.

Acknowledgements. This work was financed by the FIS and the CAICYT.

References

Babinski MF, Smith RB, Albin MS (1984) High frequency ventilation. A review. Contemp Neurosurg 6:1

García Sola R, Bravo G, Linacero G, Hernández C (1981) On line analysis of the ICP evolution with a microcomputerized monitoring unit. In: Dietz H et al. (eds) Neurological Surgery. Thieme, Stuttgart, p 299

Gilsanz F, García Sola R, Lora Tamayo JI et al. (1986) Effects of etomidate, sodium penthotal and lidocaine on cerebral elastance. In: Miller JD et al. (eds) Intracranial pressure VI. Springer, Berlin Heidelberg New York, pp 736–739

Rubio JJ, Villota ED, Galdos P et al. (1984) Ventilación a alta frecuencia con sistema jet (HFJV). Desarrollo de un prototipo y estudio de su comportamiento físico. Medicina Intensiva 8:253–259

Brain Elasticity Changes in a Canine Model of Pseudotumor Cerebri

J.S. Nichols and F.H. Sklar

Division of Neurological Surgery, University of Colorado, Health Sciences Center,
P.O. Box C-307, 4200 East Ninth Avenue, Denver, Colorado 80262 (USA)

Introduction

Pseudotumor cerebri is characterized by intracranial hypertension unassociated with a space occupying lesion. The pathophysiology of pseudotumor remains controversial. Evidence of primary involvement of the cerebrovascular bed, the brain parenchyma and the cerebrospinal fluid compartment have been postulated.

In a previous study, using a constant rate lumbar infusion, we have shown a CSF absorptive defect in 7 of 9 patients with pseudotumor which is indistinguishable from patients with hydrocephalus (Sklar et al. 1980). Yet, in pseudotumor the ventricles fail to enlarge. In addition, pseudotumor patients have lower elasticity slopes (elasticity slope is defined as the slope equivalent to linear relationship between the exponential pressure-volume function of elastance (dP/dV) and ICP) when compared to patients with hydrocephalus.

To explore the possibility that it is the difference in the pressure-volume function that may result in some patients with CSF absorptive defects and intracranial hypertension developing ventriculomegaly and hydrocephalus while others develop pseudotumor, a canine model of pseudotumor was investigated in which ICP, CSF absorptive capacity and elasticity slope were measured.

Methods

Patients undergoing bilateral radical neck dissections can develop intracranial hypertension. Likely this relates to increased cerebral venous outflow resistance caused by ligating both jugular veins. These patients show a pseudotumor picture and do not develop hydrocephalus. To reproduce this phenomenon, we inflated a blood pressure cuff around the neck of 6 anesthetized dogs in order to increase the cerebral venous outflow resistance in a graded step-wise fashion.

Animals were anesthetized with sodium pentobarbital, intubated, mechanically ventilated and positioned prone in a stereotactic frame. A femoral arterial catheter was used to monitor blood pressure and obtain arterial blood gases. Blood pressure, blood gases and body temperature were maintained within normal physiological ranges. The lateral ventricle was cannulated with an 18 gauge

Eds.: J.T. Hoff and A.L. Betz

spinal needle connected via high pressure tubing to a Statham pressure transducer and Sanborn polygraph. ICP was controlled using a 14 gauge Touhy needle placed percutaneously in the cisterna magna. A servo-controlled infusion pump with reciprocal syringe arrangement controlled continuous infusion or withdrawal of normal saline. A PDP 11/34 dual drive computer (Digital Equipment Corporation) activated the solenoid valve switching device allowing constant artifact free infusion or withdrawal of fluid. Measuring the rate of pump infusion or withdrawal provides the arithmetic difference between CSF formation and absorption. The slope of the curve of pump rate vs ICP represented the absorptive capacity in ml/min/mm Hg. The x-intercept represented the resting pressure or that point where absorption equaled formation.

In addition to controlling ICP, the PDP 11/34 computer collected mean ICP at one second intervals and recorded data points at 10 msec intervals. For each level of neck compression, CSF absorptive capacity and resting pressure were determined from a minimum of 8 different constant pressure plateaus. At least 10 rapid rate infusions were done at each level of neck compression.

Results

Increasing venous outflow resistance by graded neck compression from 0 to 100 mm Hg increased the resting intracranial pressure from a mean of 8 mm Hg at 0 mm Hg neck compression to a maximum of 27 mm Hg at 80 mm Hg ($n=27$, $p=0.03$). At neck compression pressures greater than mean arterial pressure there was a decrease in the resting intracranial pressure, likely a result of reduction of pulsatile arterial flow.

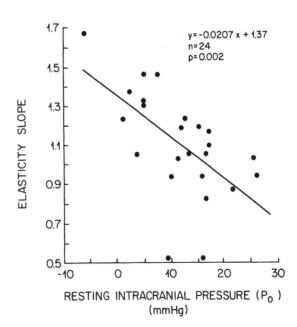

$$y = -0.0207\,x + 1.37$$
$$n = 24$$
$$p = 0.002$$

Fig. 1. Pooled data of elasticity slope versus resting intracranial pressure using a graded neck compression model of pseudotumor cerebri

RESTING INTRACRANIAL PRESSURE (P_0) (mmHg)

279

Conversely, a variable response in the development of a CSF absorptive defect was observed with graded neck compression. In 4 animals there was a 50% decrease in the absorptive capacity between 0 and 80 mm Hg neck compression, while 2 dogs had less than a 20% decrease in neck compression.

When elasticity slopes from individual dogs were compared to venous outflow resistance there was a decrease in the elasticity slope with increasing neck compression, followed by an increase in the elasticity slope for neck compression values as a function of resting intracranial pressure resulted in a linear relationship with correlation coefficient of 0.002 (Fig. 1). This suggests that as resting intracranial pressure increases there is a decrease in the elasticity slope in this model. This parallels previous clinical studies where lower elasticity slopes were noted in patients with pseudotumor.

Conclusion

Neck compression appears to be one model of pseudotumor cerebri and the physiological data parallels the clinical studies. The animals develop intracranial hypertension with a variable response in the CSF absorptive capacity. With graded venous occlusion by neck compression, the resulting intracranial hypertension is associated with a decrease in the elasticity slope rather than an increase as is seen in hydrocephalus. Perhaps an augmentation of the cerebrovascular bed results from increased venous outflow resistance and this directly affects the pressure–volume relationship. These pressure-volume changes may protect against the development of ventriculomegaly.

Reference

Sklar FH, Diehl JT, Beyer CW, Clark WK (1980) Brain elasticity changes with ventriculomegaly. J Neurosurg 53:173–179

Cerebral Elasticity and Ventricular Size
Part I: Normalization of Ventricles Following Shunting

M.R. Del Bigio and E.R. Cardoso

Cerebral Hydrodynamics Laboratory, Section of Neurosurgery, University of Manitoba,
Health Sciences Centre, Winnipeg, Manitoba R3A 1R9 (Canada)

Introduction

The anatomical and developmental literature indicate that the human brain un-
dergoes numerous age-related changes, including a decrease in water content and
an increase in myelin and glial cell composition in the post-natal period. The
mature composition of brain is achieved by the age of approximately 2–3 years.
Furthermore, the human brain often shows evidence of atrophy by the sixth
decade of life.

We hypothesize that these developmental changes in the cellular composition
of human brain may contribute to changes in its elastic properties. We investigated this hypothesis indirectly by measuring the change in the size of the cerebral
ventricles following cerebrospinal fluid shunting of hydrocephalic patients.

Methods

Thirty-one hydrocephalic patients ranging in age from 1 week to 82 years were
studied prospectively. A variety of etiologies were included (10 occult communicating hydrocephalus, 4 post-traumatic, 9 congenital, 4 tumoral, 4 posthemorrhagic). All patients underwent CT scanning prior to shunting. Seven days
following insertion of a low pressure valve ventriculo-peritoneal shunt with anti-
siphon device, the CT scan was repeated. Using computerized planimetry, the
area of the lateral ventricles and cerebrum was determined on four consecutive
CT slices beginning at the level of the caudate nucleus. The proportion of cerebrum occupied by ventricle was determined in the pre- and post-shunted brain.
The percent change in ventricular size following shunting was then calculated.

Results

The thirty-one patients underwent a total of thirty-two shunting procedures.
Under the age of two years ($n = 5$) the reduction in size of ventricles following
shunting was relatively small ($8.5 \pm 6.3\%$) (mean $\pm$ SEM). Between the ages of

Intracranial Pressure VII
Eds.: J.T. Hoff and A.L. Betz
© Springer-Verlag Berlin Heidelberg 1989

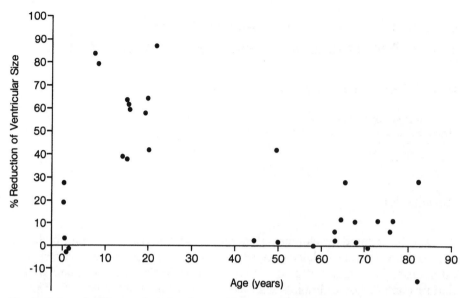

Fig. 1. Scatter plot diagram depicting the percentage reduction of the area of cerebrum occupied by ventricle seven days following CSF shunting as a function of age. The 32 patients fall roughly into three clusters which include infants, older children and young adults, and older adults

eight and 22 years ($n=10$) the ventricles were much smaller after shunting ($61.2 \pm 5.2\%$). In the older age group aged 44 to 82 years ($n=16$) the ventricles were reduced to a small degree ($9.7 \pm 3.5\%$). Although a distinct pattern was evident as demonstrated in Fig. 1, there was no linear relationship between age and the degree to which the ventricles were reduced in size after shunting. Nor was there a good correlation between ventricle size reduction and initial ventricle size ($r = -.05$) or duration of symptoms ($r = -.35$).

Discussion

Retrospective studies have failed to demonstrate a relationship between clinical improvement and ventricle size reduction after shunting (Shenkin et al. 1975, Tans and Poortvliet 1988). The immature brain may be less elastic due to its higher water content and lower glial cell and myelin density. Between the age of two and four years the brain attains a mature cellular structure and presumably mature elastic properties. The elderly brain, in contrast may lose its elasticity due to atrophy (Cardoso et al. 1988). The rate of reduction of ventricle size in the hydrocephalic brain following shunting supports the hypothesis that the brain is less elastic before age two and after the fifth decade. Obviously other factors such as unfused skull sutures in the neonatal period may play a role. It is worthwhile to note that many of older patients had small ventricles on CT scans obtained several months after shunting. This suggests that atrophy was not the sole reason for slow reduction in the size of the ventricles.

In summary, despite the use of the same shunt system, ventricles of hydrocephalic patients reduce initially at a rate that appears to be age-related. The structural and cellular changes in the brain due to development and aging may influence the elasticity of the brain and thus the rate at which hydrocephalic ventricles return to normal.

References

Cardoso ER, Del Bigio MR, Schroeder G (1988) Cerebral elasticity and ventricular size. Part II. Age-related development of extracerebral fluid collections. Intracranial Pressure VII

Samorajski T, Rolsten C (1973) Age and regional differences in the chemical composition of brains of mice, monkeys, and humans. In: Ford DH (ed) Neurobiological aspects of maturation and aging. Prog Brain Res 40:253–265

Shenkin HA, Greenberg JD, Grossman CB (1975) Ventricular size after shunting for idiopathic normal pressure hydrocephalus. J Neurol Neurosurg Psychiatry 38:833–837

Tans JTJ, Poortvliet DCJ (1988) Reduction of ventricle size after shunting for normal pressure hydrocephalus is related to CSF dynamics before shunting. J Neurol Neurosurg Psychiatry 51:521–525

Cerebral Elasticity and Ventricular Size
Part II: Age-Related Development of Extracerebral
Fluid Collections

E.R. Cardoso, M.R. Del Bigio, and G. Schroeder

Cerebral Hydrodynamics Laboratory, Health Sciences Centre, Department of Surgery,
University of Manitoba, Winnipeg, Manitoba R3A 1R9 (Canada)

Introduction

Communicating hydrocephalus (CH), pseudotumor cerebri (PC) and slit-ventricle syndrome (SVS) share the common pathophysiological features of impaired CSF absorption, and reduced cerebral compliance (Collman et al. 1980, Martins 1980, Sklar et al. 1980). Ventriculomegaly, however, develops in CH, but not in PC or SVS. This suggests that other variables, besides decreased CSF absorption, are responsible for the development of ventriculomegaly in CH. Furthermore the development of chronic subdural hematomas (CSH) is much more likely to occur in neonates and the elderly despite a much greater incidence of head trauma in young adults.

We compared the age distribution of these four diseases in order to search for a possible age-related distribution. We postulated that the size of cerebral ventricles in communicating hydrocephalus (CH) and the other cerebro-spinal fluid (CSF) disorders might be related to volume and elastic properties of the brain, besides the decrease in CSF absorption. Furthermore, we also postulated that cerebral volume and elastic properties may also contribute to the age distribution of chronic subdural hematomas (CSH).

Materials and Methods

The medical literature was searched for reports containing explicit information regarding age of patients with CH, PC, SVS and CSH. Data were entered if ages of individuals were specified or if patient age was divided in groups of five or fewer years. Ages were then re-grouped in decades and further subdivided for the first ten years.

Fig. 1. A The age distribution of communicating hydrocephalus (*CH*) is closely related to chronic subdural hematomas (*CSH*). B The age distribution of slit-ventricle syndrome (*SVS*) approximates that for pseudo-tumor cerebri (*PC*)

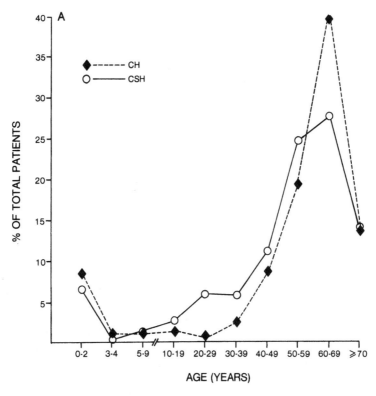

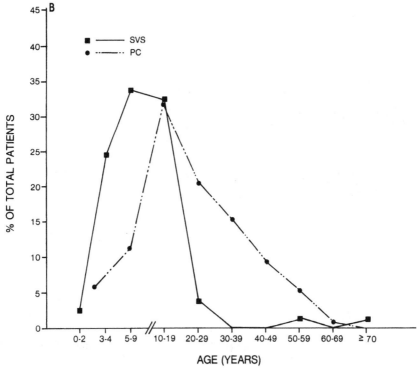

285

Results

A total of 66 studies involving 1306 patients included 349 cases of CH, 569 cases of CSH, 289 cases of PC, and 77 cases of SVS (references available on request). An age-related incidence was found: CH and CSH predominated in neonates less than 18 months old and adults older than 55 years, while PC and SVS occurred mainly in older children and young adults (Fig. 1). The latter patient groups seem to show a greater resistance to ventricular dilatation in the presence of decreased CSF absorption. This may be related to the larger volume and the state of maturity of the cerebrum in this age group. On the other hand, neonates and the elderly more readily develop subdural collections or, in association with impairment of CSF absorption, enlarged ventricles.

Discussion

There is experimental and clinical evidence that ventricular enlargement depends upon the amount of resistance to centrifugal cerebral displacement offered by the overlying dura and skull. Removal of skull and dura over the convexity in hydrocephalic cats causes much greater ventriculomegaly (Hochwald et al. 1972). In the clinical setting, subtemporal craniectomy leads to ipsilateral ventricular expansion in patients with impaired CSF absorption (Linder et al. 1983).

For ventriculomegaly to develop, gradients of pressure within the cerebral tissue must exist in order to displace the parenchyma outward. The centrifugal displacement of cerebral tissue is probably facilitated by two conditions: 1) decreased resistance to expansion by structures surrounding the brain and 2) diminished resistance of cerebral tissue to deformity. Both conditions might also facilitate the accumulation of blood in the subdural space. They are present during neonatal and senile life and may therefore explain the predisposition to development of ventriculomegaly and CSH in those age groups. Our results suggest that the age-related incidence of the four diseases investigated might depend upon cerebral and extracerebral developmental factors, such as open cranial sutures, cerebral atrophy, cerebral water and myelin contents. Similarly, the development of ventriculomegaly may depend upon cerebral elastic properties besides the primary disturbance of CSF dynamics.

Acknowledgment. We are indebt to the Health Sciences Centre Research Foundation for its support to the Cerebral Hydrodynamics Laboratory.

References

Collman H, Mauersberger W, Mohr G (1980) Clinical observations and CSF absorption studies in the slit ventricle syndrome. Adv Neurosurg 8:183–186

Hochwald GM, Epstein F, Malhan C, Ransohoff J (1972) The role of skull and dura in experimental feline hydrocephalus. Dev Med Child Neurol [suppl 27] 14:65–69

Linder M, Diehl J, Sklar FH (1983) Subtemporal decompression for shunt-dependent ventricles: Mechanism of action. Surg Neurol 19:520–523

Martins AN (1973) Resistance to drainage of cerebrospinal fluid: Clinical measurement and significance. J Neurol Neurosurg Psychiatry 36:313–318

Sklar FH, Beyer CW, Clark WK (1980) Physiological features of the pressure-volume function of brain elasticity in man. J Neurosurg 53:166–172

Intracranial Pressure Changes from a Temporal Lobe Mass in Cats

J.D. Miller, H.R. Holaday, and D.F. Peeler

Department of Neurosurgery, University of Mississippi Medical Center, 2500 North State Street, Jackson, Mississippi 39216-4505 (USA)

Temporal lobe mass lesions may result in neurologic deterioration in the absence of elevated intracranial pressure. One possible mechanism is direct compression of the midbrain by the enlarged temporal lobe. We have attempted to study such a mechanism in an animal model by creating an expanding left temporal lobe mass while measuring pressures within the left temporal lobe, midbrain, and either the right frontal lobe or right lateral ventricle.

Materials and Methods

All procedures were approved by the Animal Care Committee of the University Medical Center.

Twelve cats of either sex were anesthetized using ketamine (22 mg/kg) and acepromazine (0.2 mg/kg) intraperitoneally. Following insertion of femoral venous and arterial lines, the animals were placed in a stereotactic headholder in the sphinx position. The scalp was incised in the midline and retracted bilaterally. Cranial holes were drilled in the right frontal area, anterior and posterior left temporal region, and 3 mm left of midline in the parietal area. Pressure monitoring flaccid cuff balloons were inserted into the anterior left temporal lobe and stereotactically into the midbrain at the level of the superior colliculus in all animals. Six animals had placement of a flaccid cuff pressure monitoring balloon in the right frontal lobe, while the remaining six had insertion of right lateral ventricular cannulae. All had placement of an inflatable mass balloon into the posterior left temporal region. Cranial holes were sealed with dental acrylic.

Pressures in the right frontal region (right frontal intraparenchymal or right lateral ventricular pressure), left temporal lobe, and midbrain were monitored before and during inflation of the mass balloon by an infusion pump. Inflation at a rate of 0.072 cc/min was continued until either the left temporal or midbrain pressure reached 40 mm Hg. Pressures were then monitored for at least 1 hr.

Each animal had an intravenous Evan's blue 2% (1 ml/kg) injection, and following sacrifice, the brain was placed in 10% formalin. The brains were later sectioned in the coronal plane and examined grossly to demonstrate evidence of intracerebral hemorrhage and proper placement of the pressure monitoring and mass balloons.

Results

Ten animals, five with right frontal lobe pressure monitor and five with intraventricular cannulae, were used for data analysis. Two were excluded; one developed a leak from the mass balloon and the other a leak in the left temporal lobe pressure monitor. The average volume injected into the mass balloon was 1.2 cc (range 0.5–2.0 cc). At a constant infusion rate of 0.072 cc/min, the time required for inflation was 7 to 28 min (average of 16.6 min).

In each animal, the midbrain pressure rose much higher than the generalized ICP reflected by a right frontal lobe or right ventricular pressure monitor (see Fig. 1). In only 3 of the 10 animals did the generalized pressure reach 10 mm Hg. The mean pressure change over time showed close correlation between left temporal and midbrain pressures, while the right frontal pressure changed minimally (Fig. 2A). Pressures were averaged at every minute over the 45 min session. Portions of the curves reflecting increasing pressure were compared with respect to slope. The curves were statistically different from one another ($p < 0.01$).

Pressure values were averaged for each group at the time either left temporal or midbrain pressure reached 40 mm Hg. The maximum pressure change averaged 32.4 mm Hg and 25.2 mm Hg in the left temporal lobe and midbrain, respectively (Fig. 2B). The maximum mean pressure change in the right frontal region was 6.8 mm Hg (6.2 mm Hg in the right frontal lobe and 7.4 mm Hg in the right lateral ventricle). The data from the three groups was compared using analysis of variance and paired t-tests for differences between individual means. The groups are significantly different ($F = 8.89$, $p < 0.005$). The maximum left temporal and midbrain mean differential pressures were both significantly greater than right frontal pressure ($p < 0.025$).

Pathological evaluation revealed one animal with a 1 mm diameter extravasation of Evan's blue over the right frontal lobe surface and another with less than 1 mm extravasation on the left parietal surface from either drilling or placement of the pressure monitoring balloons. One cat had a 5 mm diameter hemorrhage in the temporal lobe in the cavity of the mass balloon and another had slight

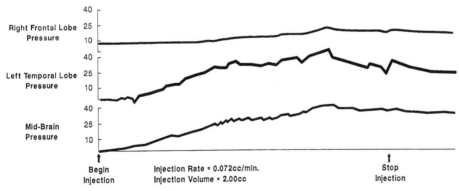

Fig. 1. Example of pressure changes from expanding left temporal mass. In this animal the left temporal lobe pressure reached 40 mm Hg while midbrain pressure concomitantly rose to 35 mm Hg. Right frontal lobe pressure increased slightly to 14 mm Hg

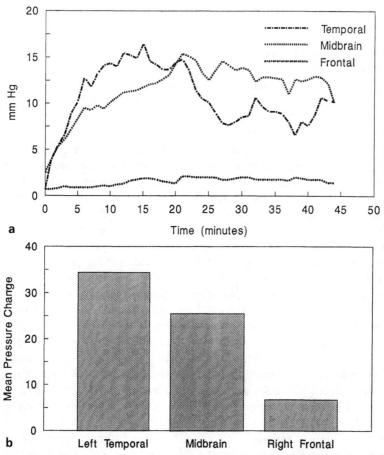

Fig. 2 a, b. Intracranial pressures. **a** Mean pressure changes over time showing minimal elevation of the right frontal pressure (right frontal lobe and right lateral ventricle) as compared to
sharp rise of left temporal and midbrain pressure. Pressures were averaged at every minute over
the session. **b** Maximum differential mean pressure changes in three intracranial regions consequent to an expanding left temporal lobe mass. Pressure values were averaged at the time either
the left temporal or midbrain pressure reached 40 mm Hg

layering of blood in the left temporal mass balloon cavity. Other animals had no
evidence of Evan's blue extravasation or intracerebral hemorrhage.

Discussion

We have previously reported a method of recording intracerebral pressure in
animals via a flaccid cuff balloon catheter (Miller et al. 1985). These silicone
catheters are easily inserted into various intracranial regions to record local
pressure. With such pressure monitors in the right and left hemispheres, we have

recorded differential pressures during inflation of subdural and epidural mass balloons (Miller et al. 1987). Similarly, Iannotti et al. (1985) found 8 mm Hg pressure differences between the hemispheres following middle cerebral artery occlusion in cats. Differential pressures may be of pathophysiologic importance during evolving intracranial masses.

Patients with temporal lobe mass lesions may experience sudden neurologic deterioration in the presence of low intracranial pressure (Klauber et al. 1984, Marshall et al. 1986). Possible mechanisms include axonal distortion, axonal or vessel shearing, and ischemia which may result from brainstem displacement or direct compression. Clinical and experimental data reveal evidence of brain shift associated with decreased consciousness and alterations of cerebral blood flow and ICP (Misu et al. 1986, Ropper 1986). Recently, Thompson and Salcman (1988) demonstrated brainstem hemorrhages following brainstem distortion with arterial tethering and suggested a spectrum of lesions from ischemia to macro-hemorrhages.

In the current study, we have attempted to show midbrain compression as evidenced by an elevated pressure within the midbrain during expansion of a temporal lobe mass. Concomitant recording from the right frontal lobe or lateral ventricle failed to reveal significant pressure changes in these regions at the time of elevated left temporal lobe or midbrain pressures. Once the midbrain or left temporal lobe pressure rose to the predetermined level of 40 mm Hg, inflation was terminated, and the pressures began to descend toward baseline. Such changes would be compatible with neurologic changes in patients with temporal lobe contusions or other masses in the presence of normal ICP. Of course, this does not exclude other simultaneous mechanisms which might impair cerebral functions.

References

Iannotti F, Hoff JT, Schielke GP (1985) Brain tissue pressure in focal cerebral ischemia. J Neurosurg 62:83–89

Klauber MR, Toutant SM, Marshall LF (1984) A model for predicting delayed intracranial hypertension following severe head injury. J Neurosurg 61:695–699

Marshall LF, Cotten JM, Bowers-Marshall S, Seelig JM (1986) Pupillary abnormalities, elevated intracranial pressure and mass lesion location. In: Miller JD, Teasdale GM, Rowan JO, Galbraith SL, Mendelow AD (eds) Intracranial Pressure VI. Springer, Berlin Heidelberg New York Tokyo, pp 656–660

Miller JD, Pattisapu J, Peeler DF, Parent AD (1985) Intracranial pressure monitoring by flaccid cuff catheter in an animal model. J Neurosurg 63:242–245

Miller JD, Peeler DF, Pattisapu J, Parent AD (1987) Supratentorial pressures. Part 1: Differential intracranial pressures. Neurol Res 9:193–197

Misu N, Kuchiwaki H, Hirai N, Ishiguri H, Takada S, Kageyama N (1986) Local shift of the brain and its relation to the tentorial edge. Miller JD, Teasdale GM, Rowan JO, Galbraith SL, Mendelow AD (eds) Intracranial Pressure VI. Springer, Berlin Heidelberg New York Tokyo, pp 318–324

Ropper AH (1986) Lateral displacement of the brain and level of consciousness in patients with an acute hemispheral mass. NEJM 314:953–958

Thompson RK, Salcman M (1988) Dynamic axial brainstem distortion as a mechanism in the production of brainstem hemorrhages: role of the carotid arteries. Neurosurgery 22:629–632

Increase in ICP Produced by Electrical Stimulation of the Brain Stem Reticular Formation in Cats with Spinalization and Vagotomy

M. Maeda and S. Matsuura

Department of Physiology, Osaka City University Medical School, 1-4-54, Asahi-machi, Abeno-ku, Osaka 545 (Japan)

Introduction

The effects of focal electrical stimulation on intracranial pressure (ICP) and arterial blood pressure (ABP) have been extensively examined by applying the stimulus to the brain stem (Maeda et al. 1985, Maeda et al. 1986, Matsuura et al. 1986, Maeda et al. 1988 a), cerebral cortex and hypothalamus (Maeda et al. 1986, Maeda et al. 1988 b) in cats. The early change in ICP produced by the electrical stimulation was explained by the change in cerebral blood volume (CBV) due to neurogenic cerebral vasodilatation or constriction and by the change in the driving pressure associated with the stimulus-induced alteration of ABP and respiratory movement (Maeda et al. 1988 a). The ABP and respiration can be maintained at normal levels during electrical stimulation in spinalized and vagotomized cats. Therefore, the present study was undertaken to explore the changes in ICP in response to brain stem activation by focal electrical stimulation in spinalized and vagotomized cats in order to deduce the locations in the brain stem reticular formation which are related to cerebral vasodilatation.

Materials and Methods

Experiments were performed on cats anesthetized with urethane and chloralose. The ABP, ICP, cerebral blood flow (CBF) by heat clearance method, cerebral blood volume (CBV) by photoelectric method, heart rate (HR), end-tidal CO_2, and central venous pressure (CVP) were continuously recorded on a multipurpose polygraph recorder. Electrical stimulation (duration, 0.4 ms; frequency, 40 Hz; intensity, 200 µA), was applied at the same brain stem sites before and after spinalization and vagotomy. The stimulated sites were histologically identified.

Results

The sites investigated were classified into three groups according to the control patterns of ABP response: arterial pressor sites, arterial depressor sites, and no response sites of which stimulation produced no change in ABP.

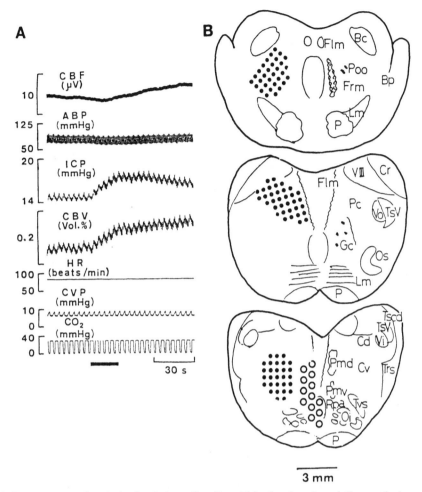

Fig. 1. A Responses to electrical stimulation of a site within the dorsal medullary reticular formation in spinalized and vagotomized cat. The period of stimulation is indicated by the horizontal bar. Rises in ICP, CBV, and CBF were produced with no apparent changes in ABP, HR, CVP, and respiration. **B** Schematic drawing of the regions in which electrical stimulation produced an increase in ICP in cats with spinalization and vagotomy. This is presented in coronal sections (45° to the horizontal plane) of the cat brain stem. Filled circles and open circles indicate the regions which yielded an increase in ICP following spinalization and vagotomy, in arterial pressor and depressor area, respectively. Abbreviations (*n.* = nucleus): *Cv*, n. medullae oblongatae centralis subnucleus ventralis; *Frm*, formatio reticularis mesencephali; *Gc*, n. gigantocellularis; *Pc*, n. parvocellularis; *Pm*, n. paramedium reticularis; *Pmd*, n. paramedium reticularis subnucleus dorsalis; *Pmv*, n. paramedium reticularis subnucleus ventralis; *Poo*, n. pontis centralis oralis; *Rpa*, n. raphe pallidus

In the arterial pressor sites, electrical stimulation following spinalization and vagotomy produced a rise in ICP with no change in ABP and respiration in 41% (Fig. 1 A), a fall in ICP in 1%, and no change in ICP in the other 58%. There were three principal regions which yielded an increase in ICP in the arterial pressor area of the brain stem reticular formation: the central part of the pontine reticular formation, the dorsal medullary reticular formation, and the central part of the medullary reticular formation (Fig. 1 B). The central part of the pontine reticular formation constitutes the area extending from the nucleus pontis centralis oralis to the nucleus pontis centralis caudalis. The dorsal medullary reticular formation corresponds mainly to the nucleus parvocellularis and the dorsal part of the nucleus gigantocellularis. The central part of the medullary reticular formation corresponds mainly to the nucleus medullae oblongatae centralis subnucleus ventralis.

In the arterial depressor sites, electrical stimulation following spinalization and vagotomy produced an increase in ICP in 52% and no change in ICP in the other 48%. The region that yielded an increase in ICP was the paramedial and ventral medial region of the medullary reticular formation. This region corresponds mainly to the nucleus paramedium reticularis and the nucleus raphe pallidus.

Discussion

There are three principal regions that yield an increase in ICP after spinalization and vagotomy in the arterial pressor area of the cat brain stem reticular formation and one principal region in the arterial depressor area. The ABP and respiration were sustained at steady levels during electrical stimulation in spinalized and vagotomized cats. This suggests that excitation of cell bodies or fibres within these regions produces cerebral vasodilatation.

References

Maeda M, Matsuura S, Tanaka K, Nishimura S (1985) Plateau waves and cerebral autoregulation. J Cereb Blood Flow Metab [Suppl 1] 5:S65–S66
Maeda M, Tanaka K, Nishimura S, Matsuura S (1986) Pressure wave-like changes in ICP produced by electric stimulation of the brainstem, hypothalamus and cerebral cortex in cats. In: Miller JD, Teasdale GM, Rowan JO, Galbraith SL, Mendelow AD (eds) Intracranial Pressure VI. Springer, Berlin Heidelberg New York Tokyo, pp 156–160
Maeda M, Matsuura S, Tanaka K, Katsuyama J, Nakamura T, Sakamoto H, Nishimura S (1988a) Effects of electrical stimulation on intracranial pressure and systemic arterial blood pressure in cats. Part 1: Stimulation of brain stem. Neurol Res 10: in press
Maeda M, Matsuura S, Tanaka K, Katsuyama J, Nishimura S (1988b) Effects of electrical stimulation on intracranial pressure and systemic arterial blood pressure in cats. Part II: Stimulation of cerebral cortex and hypothalamus. Neurol Res 10: in press
Matsuura S, Kuno M, Yasunami T, Maeda M (1986) Changes in intracranial pressure and arterial blood pressure following electric stimulation to restricted regions in the cat brainstem. Jpn J Physiol 36:857–869

Computer Simulation of Intracranial Pressure Using Electrical R-C Circuit

M. Kimura, N. Tamaki, S. Kose, T. Takamori[1], and S. Matsumoto

Department of Neurosurgery, [1] Faculty of Engineering, Kobe University School of Medicine, Kobe (Japan)

Introduction

Physical and mathematical analysis of the intracranial cavity was started by Hakim et al. (1986) and Marmarou et al. (1975). However, in these studies, the intracranial cavity is regarded as only one component. In 1988, Rekate et al. (1988) reported a 6 compartment analysis of the intracranial cavity.

The purpose of this study was to apply a physical and mathematical model which can explain many clinical experiences and estimate the pressure of the components that can not be monitored in patients.

Method

Arterial pressure shows a biphasic pattern. Jugular venous pressure reveals a triphasic pattern (Marmarou et al. 1975). The venous wave form is more affected by respiration than the arterial wave form.

The compliance of each cavity is regarded as an electrical capacitance C and the flow resistance of each canal is regarded as an electrical resistance R.

Cerebrovascular System Model

The cerebrovascular model is composed of 3 condensers connected in parallel and 4 electrical resistances (Fig. 1 a).

Modeling of the cerebrovascular system is based on the next 4 assumptions.
(1) The total value of the 4 vascular resistances is regarded as a constant. In equation form,

$$R_{ic\text{-}ca} + R_{ca\text{-}cc} + R_{cc\text{-}cv} + R_{cv\text{-}jv} = \text{constant.}$$

(2) When ICP is increasing, outflow blood volume is less than the inflow blood volume. The values of $R_{cc\text{-}cv}$ and $R_{cv\text{-}jv}$ are considered to be relatively high. When ICP is decreasing, outflow blood volume is greater than the inflow blood volume.

The value of R_{cc-cv} and R_{cv-jv} are considered to be relatively low. They are given by

$$R_{ic-ca}+R_{cv-jv}=\text{constant}, \quad R_{ca-cc}+R_{cc-cv}=\text{constant}.$$

(3) The compliance of the arterial blood bed is regarded as constant. In equation form,

$$C_a=\text{constant}$$

(4) As the wall of the vein and capillary is thin and soft, it is affected by ICP.

Ventricular System Model

The ventricular system model is composed of 5 condensers connected in parallel, 4 electrical resistances and several electrical diodes (Fig. 1 b).

Modeling of the ventricular system is based on 3 assumptions.
(1) A negative correlation exists between pressure and compliance. The compliance of each ventricle is variable due to ICP. Compliance is regarded as proportional to the ratio of each volume. In equation form,

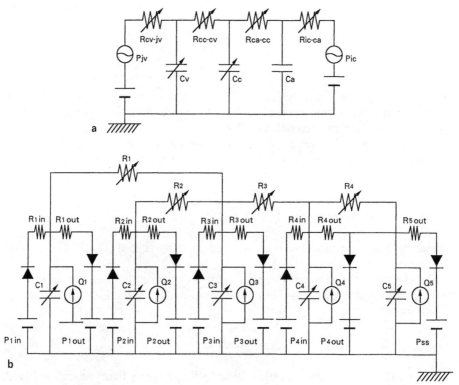

Fig. 1 a, b. Cerebrospinal system models using the electrical R-C circuit. **a** Cerebrovascular systems. **b** Ventricular systems

296

$$C_1 = 10/(K \times P_{c1}), \quad C_2 = 10/(K \times P_{c2}), \quad C_3 = 0.4/(K \times P_{c3}),$$
$$C_4 = 1/(K \times P_{c4}), \quad C_5 = 60/(K \times P_{c5}).$$

(2) The wall of each space is oscillated by the periventricular blood volume changes. Periventricular blood volume changes are regarded as proportional to the ratio of each surface space. They are given by

$$Q1 = 10 \times KQ \times Q, \ Q2 = 10 \times KQ \times Q, \ Q3 = 1 \times KQ \times Q, \ Q4 = 1.5 \times KQ \times Q,$$
$$Q5 = 60 \times KQ \times Q.$$

(3) The flow resistance of the canal is proportional to its length (l) and is inversely proportional to its surface area (s). It is given by

$$R = Kr \times l/s.$$

All Systems of the Model

In the cerebrovascular model, the total value of $l_{ic\text{-}ca}$ in the period of one heart beat is equal to that of $l_{cv\text{-}jv}$ at the stable state. Though in the short period, $l_{ic\text{-}ca} - l_{cv\text{-}jv}$ means the change of cerebral blood volume. In equation form,

$$Q = l_{ic\text{-}ca} - I_{cv\text{-}jv}.$$

The periventricular blood pressure is equal to that of the capillary vascular bed. The sagittal sinus pressure is equal to that of the venous vascular bed. The calculation is performed by the Runge-Kutta method using a 16-bit personal computer.

Result

The gradient of the pulse amplitude markedly decreased and fluctuation occurred due to respiration. The calculated result is similar to the clinical record obtained from the patient.

When mean pressure is high, the ICP wave form reveals biphasic waves which resemble the arterial wave with little influence of respiration. The more the mean ICP value decreases, the more its amplitude also decreases. A triphasic wave form (P_1, P_2, P_3) is gradually identified and it is slightly affected by respiration. Eventually it is affected by respiration. When the mean ICP value is about 5 mm Hg, P_1, P_2 and P_3 are identified and much affected by respiration.

A very slight pressure gradient between the 3rd and 4th ventricles is identified. The pressure gradient between one side of the aqueduct and the other side is the power source of the to-and-fro CSF movement in the aqueduct.

Discussion

The CSF pulsations become more venous in character as ICP pulsation increases and more arterial in character as ICP pulsation decreases. Therefore, P_1 may be considered to have originated from the venous pressure.

References

Hakim S, Venegas JB, Burton JD (1976) The physics of the cranial cavity, hydrocephalus and normal pressure hydrocephalus: mechanical interpretation and mathematical model. Surg Neurol 5:187–210

Hurst JW, Schlant RC (1974) Examination of the arterial pulse. In: Hurst JW, Logue RB, Schlant RC et al. (eds): The Heart, Arteries, and Veins, ed 3. New York. McGraw Hill, pp 170–189

Marmarou A, Shulman K, LaMorgese J (1975) Compartmental analysis of compliance and outflow resistance of the cerebrospinal fluid system. J Neurosurg 43:523–534

Rekate HL et al. (1988) The application of mathematical modeling to hydrocephalus research. Concepts Pediat Neurosurg 8:1–14

Session III: CSF Dynamics and Hydrocephalus

Chairmen: M. Pollay, F. Gjerris, C.J.J. Avezaat, and T. Tsubokawa

Changes of CSF Migration, Energy Metabolism and High Molecular Protein
of the Neuron in Hydrostatic Intracranial Hypertension
N. Hayashi, T. Tsubokawa, T. Tamura, Y. Makiyama, and H. Kumakawa

Increased Brain Water Self Diffusion Measured by Magnetic Resonance
Scanning in Patients with Pseudotumor Cerebri
P. Soelberg-Sørensen, C. Thomsen, F. Gjerris, J.F. Schmidt, and O. Henriksen

Neuropsychological Testing in Normal Pressure Hydrocephalus
N.R. Graff-Radford, J.C. Godersky, D. Tranel, P.J. Eslinger, and M.P. Jones

^{123}I-IMP-SPECT and Lumbar Subarachnoid Pressure in Adult Hydrocephalus
O. Hirai, M. Nishikawa, M. Munaka, S. Watanabe, T. Kaneko, A. Fukuma,
and H. Handa

Concentrations of Neurotransmitters in Ventricular and Lumbar Cerebrospinal
Fluid in Patients with Normal Pressure Hydrocephalus
A. Gjerris, P. Soelberg-Sørensen, and F. Gjerris

CSF Oxygen Tension and ICP
A.I.R. Maas, D.A. de Jong, and W.A. Fleckenstein

Possible Physiological Role of the Cushing Response During Parturition
R.C. Koehler, A.P. Harris, M.D. Jones Jr., and R.J. Traystman

Electrocardiographic Changes are Associated with Elevated Blood Pressure
Rather Than a Direct Effect of Raised Intracranial Pressure
C.P. McGraw, P.R. Palakurthy, and C. Maldonado

Exchange vs Cotransport of Na and Cl Across the Barriers Interfacing Cerebrospinal Fluid and Brain with Blood

C.E. Johanson, V.A. Murphy, D. Bairamian, and M.H. Epstein

Department of Clinical Neurosciences, Program in Neurosurgery, Brown University and Rhode Island Hospital, 593 Eddy Street, Providence, Rhode Island 02902 (USA)

Introduction

The flow of water from the capillaries into various compartments in the CNS is in large part dependent on the net transport of ions across barrier systems. Disruption of the normal flow of fluid into the brain can lead to altered ICP. Therefore, it is not surprising that carrier protein molecules in the cells of the barrier systems should regulate the translocation of ions from blood to CSF and brain tissue.

The initial step for entry of Na and Cl into CNS occurs at the basolateral membrane of choroid plexus (CP) and the luminal membrane of the cerebral endothelium (Johanson 1988b). It has been postulated that secondary active transport systems, i.e., Na-H exchange and/or NaCl cotransport, move Na from plasma into the barrier cell (choroid epithelial and brain endothelial) down the electrochemical gradient for Na as established by the extrusion arm of the Na-K pump at the opposite pole of the cell (see Fig. 1).

The concerns of this paper are to present evidence in support of Na-H exchange in both the blood-CSF and blood-brain barriers; to summarize information that $Cl-HCO_3$ occurs as a parallel operator with Na-H exchange; and to discuss the possibility that NaCl cotransport also exists in the barrier cells. With enhanced knowledge about the transporters, it should be feasible to devise more effective strategies for pharmacologically treating fluid imbalances in the CNS.

Procedures

In vitro and in vivo methodologies were used to quantify rates of permeation of tracer ^{22}Na and ^{36}Cl into the choroid plexus (CP), CSF and brain. Adult Sprague-Dawley rats, 150 to 275 g, were sacrificed under ketamine anesthesia (100–120 mg/kg). The diminutive-sized samples of CP were removed and handled by analytical microtechniques as comprehensively described in a recent review on methodologies (Johanson 1988b). NEN supplied the radioisotopes.

Intracranial Pressure VII
Eds.: J.T. Hoff and A.L. Betz
© Springer-Verlag Berlin Heidelberg 1989

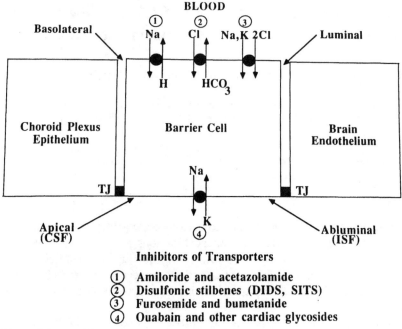

Fig. 1. Schema of ion transport systems in the blood-CSF (choroid plexus) and blood-brain barriers. Polarity of barrier cells is portrayed as the blood-facing membrane and that abutting the extracellular fluid of the CNS, i.e., the CSF or ISF (interstitial fluid). TJ = tight junctions between choroid epithelial or brain endothelial cells. In this working model, Na is transported from blood into barrier cell by secondary active transporters, i.e., either Na-H exchange (anti-port) or Na-K-2Cl cotransport. Na is subsequently extruded into the CNS extracellular fluid by the primary active Na-K pump. Transporters # *1, 2* and *3* are non-electrogenic but the Na-K pump is electrogenic. Filled circles represent carrier proteins presumably actively involved in conformational changes resulting in vectorial transport as indicated. The relative and absolute concentrations of ions on either side of the external limiting membrane of the cell determine transport rate. Inhibitors of the respective transporters are summarized below the diagram

The In Vitro CP-CSF System

Just after extirpation, each lateral ventricle plexus tissue as immersed in synthetic CSF for incubation with test substance(s). The advantages of the isolated CP include capabilities for finely regulating CSF ions, pCO_2, temperature and agent concentration; also, alterations associated with blood flow, neural tone, drug metabolism and extracellular protein binding are not complicating variables. Typically, each CP was preincubated for 15 min in CSF containing the drug, and then transferred rapidly to incubation medium having tracer in addition to test agent. The exact conditions are described further in the figure legends.

The In Vivo CP-CSF-Brain System

By analyzing the kinetics of distribution of tracer Na and Cl from blood to CP, CSF and brain, one can define functional relationships between the blood-CSF and blood-brain barriers to ions. If a particular drug reduces tracer uptake by *both* plexus and CSF, then the inhibitory effect can be putatively ascribed to interference with basolateal transporters. For blood-brain barrier analysis, the fronto-parietal cortex was selected because it is far enough from ventricular CSF so that the latter does not contribute to tracer uptake by cortical tissue (Smith and Rapoport 1986). The two-compartment model assumes that tracer entry into brain across the cerebral endothelium is proportional to plasma concentrations and that backflux is negligible in the short experiment (Cserr et al. 1987).

The general approach was to: i) stabilize the plasma concentration of isotope by 12 min, ii) quantitate the volume of distribution (V_d) of tracer at 12, 18 and 24 min after administration, iii) determine the apparent time of isotope circulation (Gjedde 1981), and iv) calculate the transfer rate (K_{in}) as $V_d \div$ apparent time. K_{in} (ml/g/hr) is comparable to permeability-surface area product because K_{in} for Na (and Cl) is $\ll$ blood flow to CP or brain.

Results and Discussion

Evidence for Na-H Exchange

The existence of Na-H exchange (Aronson 1983) can be demonstrated in several ways: by testing for inhibition by amiloride on the in vitro and in vivo transport of ^{22}Na into CP, CSF and brain; by determining if amiloride can deplete the steady-state level of stable Na in the CP epithelium; and by ascertaining if reduction of the H ion gradient across the barrier cell slows exchange for Na.

The in vitro CP took up ^{22}Na rapidly from the 37°C CSF medium, attaining a V_d of 50% by 1 min (Fig. 2). When the temperature was lowered to 27°C, the rate fell by more than one half (Q_{10} of 2.1). Both the rapidity of uptake and temperature sensitivity are consistent with carrier-mediated Na transport. Amiloride (1 mM) depressed ^{22}Na transport rate by 52% (compare slopes in Fig. 2). Hypothermia (27°C) plus amiloride caused greater inhibition, with the ^{22}Na uptake being suppressed by 83%. The amiloride-induced inhibition is characteristic of drug interference directly with Na-H exchange.

There were similar findings for the CP in the intact animal. Thus, amiloride administered i.p. at 100 mg/kg (to give a plasma [amiloride] of about 1 mM) decreased the K_{in} for ^{22}Na in CP from 0.19 to 0.10 ml/g/hr; see Fig. 2. As a consequence of less uptake of tracer by the plexus, the rate of penetration of ^{22}Na into CSF was lowered by 27% (Fig. 2). With respect to transport across the blood-brain barrier, amiloride brought about a 29% decrease on average in the K_{in} for ^{22}Na in parietal cortex. Overall, amiloride treatment for 1 hr resulted in substantial attenuation in the ability of Na to penetrate the in vivo CNS barrier systems.

Disruptions in rate of exchange of H for Na, as by amiloride or acidosis, lead to depletion of cell Na. The CP is a structurally-appropriate tissue readily excisable and analyzable for intracellular Na by compartmentation analysis (Johanson 1988 b). The steady-state level of stable Na was reduced in choroidal tissues

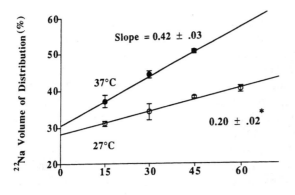

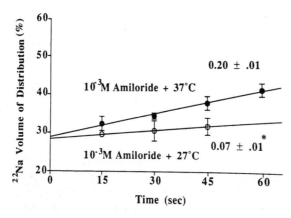

Fig. 2. Time course of uptake of ^{22}Na by the adult rat lateral ventricle CP incubated in artificial CSF at 37°C or 27°C, with and without 1 mM amiloride. Uptake is expressed as % volume of distribution ($100 \times$ dpm/g CP $\div$ dpm/ml CSF). Rate of uptake, i.e., the slope of the least-squares regression, has units of volume/ tissue wt./time (i.e., ml/g/sec) and is thus similar to the K_{in} data presented for the in vivo system (Fig. 3). *$P < 0.05$, by analysis of covariance. Each filled and unfilled circle is the mean $\pm$ SEM for $n = 3$ or 4 tissues

exposed to amiloride. In vitro as well as in vivo analyses demonstrated depleted levels of stable Na following treatment with amiloride. Cellular Na was reduced by 5 mM, from a baseline of 45 mM, in intact animals treated with amiloride. Even greater reductions in [Na]$_i$ were elicited in vitro by this Na-H inhibitor (Murphy and Johanson 1988 b).

Metabolic acidosis is a useful model for testing Na-H in vivo. Because of the relatively impermeable external limiting membranes of barrier cells (Fig. 1), there is a significantly diminished H ion gradient across the blood-facing membrane during acute metabolic acidosis (Murphy and Johanson 1988 c). The presence of Na-H exchange on the vascular side of the barrier should manifest itself in acidosis as slower permeation of tracer Na across the barrier, because of the less favorable H ion gradient to pull Na into the choroid epithelial (or cerebral endothelial) cell. Indeed we have found less rapid penetration of ^{22}Na into plexus and cortex (Murphy and Johanson 1988 a). For example, after 1 hr of HCl acidosis, the K_{in} for ^{22}Na (ml/g/hr) decreased by 48% in CP (0.19 to 0.099), by 20% in cisternal CSF (1.32 to 1.06), and by 29% in fronto-parietal cortex (from 0.132 to 0.094); all the decreases were significant at the 0.05 level (Fig. 3). Such apparent coupling of Na transport to the transmembrane H ion distribution constitutes further evidence for Na-H exchange in the blood-CSF and blood-brain barriers.

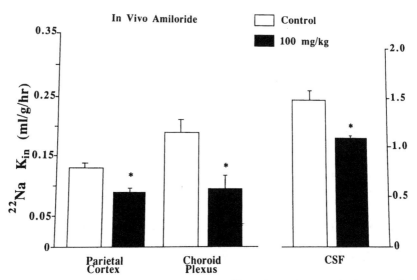

Fig. 3. Influx coefficients, K_{in}, are rates of transfer of ^{22}Na from blood to brain (cortex), choroid plexus and CSF (sampled from cisterna magna) 12 min after tracer administration. K_{in} = volume of distribution (V_d) of ^{22}Na apparent time of circulation. V_d = dpm/g tissue (or CSF) dpm/g plasma H_2O. Apparent time was calculated as

$$\int_0^T Cp^* \, dt \div Cp^* \text{ at } T,$$

where T = 12 min and $Cp^* = [^{22}Na]$ in plasma at 12 min. Amiloride (or vehicle control) was injected I.P. 1 hr before the end of experiment. Means ± SEM for $n = 8$ for CSF and 15–20 rats for the tissue data. *$P < 0.05$, amiloride vs vehicle control by Student's t test. K_{in} values for cortex at 12, 18 and 24 min were not significantly different and so were pooled

With an Ussing-type chamber preparation, Wright (1977) elevated the [HCO_3] on the blood side and furnished ^{22}Na kinetic evidence for basolateral Na-H in the bullfrog CP. In a series of experiments with carbonic anhydrase inhibitors and acidoses, Johanson (1984) used the DMO method to establish that acetazolamide alkalinizes choroid cell pH thereby enabling the hypothesis that elevated pH$_i$ decreases basolateral Na-H exchange. Blood-brain barrier studies with amiloride have been few. However, Betz (1983a) employed a modified intracarotid bolus injection method to demonstrate 0.1 μM amiloride- but not pH-sensitive uptake of ^{22}Na; overall, on the basis of the in vivo bolus approach and in vitro isolated capillaries, he concluded that Na-H exchange was on the anti-luminal membrane of the cerebral endothelium.

Does Na-H Exchange Operate in Parallel with Cl-HCO$_3$ Exchange?

In other epithelia such as kidney and small intestine, the parallel operation of cation and anion antiporters (Fig. 1) has been described. There is substantial evidence for Cl-HCO$_3$ exchange in CP, based on analyses of in vitro steady-state

307

[HCO$_3$]$_i$ (Johanson et al. 1985), and on in vitro and in vivo kinetics of ^{36}Cl uptake by the CP and CSF system (Deng 1986). CSF formation is reduced appreciably by amiloride and by DIDS (Deng 1986), likely by drug interference with the operation of Na-H and Cl-HCO$_3$ exchangers. With functional coupling of baso-lateral cation and anion exchangers, one expects that the disulfonic stilbene, DIDS (inhibitor of anion exchange), would interfere with Na transport (indirect-ly) as well as Cl transport (directly) from blood into the CP-CSF system; in fact, this has been observed (Deng 1986). Conversely, as another reflection of parallel Na-H and Cl-HCO$_3$ exchange, it is predicted that amiloride would indirectly curtail Cl transport into CSF concurrently with its inhibition of Na transport (Murphy and Johanson 1988 a; 1988 b).

The Possibility of Two Different Transporters for Moving Na into Barrier Cells

In addition to Cl-HCO$_3$ exchange, many epithelia have a cotransporter moving Na "downhill" concurrently with K and Cl "uphill" into the cell. The cotransport nature of Na and Cl in the CP was initially hypothesized by Smith et al. (1982). Furosemide's ability to inhibit CSF flow under some conditions has also led investigators to propose Na and Cl cotransport in the plexus. However, the inability to exclude volume depletion (from marked diuresis) or intense vasocon-striction of vessels ($\downarrow\downarrow$ CP blood flow) as explanations for inhibiting CSF secre-tion has made the case for cotransport equivocal. Vogh and Langham (1981) as well as Miller et al. (1986) reported negligible alteration of CSF flow after treat-ment with loop diuretics. Johnson et al. (1987) found that bumetanide decreased transport of tracer Cl across the blood-CSF barrier. However, because bumeta-nide may also affect Cl-HCO$_3$ exchange, one has to be cautious about inter-preting loop diuretic experiments. Substantially reduced plasma [Na] decreased ^{36}Cl transport across the blood-CSF barrier (Smith and Rapoport 1984), suggest-ing NaCl cotransport. By microelectrode analysis of Cl activity, Saito and Wright (1987) concluded that NaCl cotransport exists in amphibian CP. Using the iso-lated rat CP, we also find evidence for cotransport (Johanson et al. 1988) as bumetanide and furosemide (0.1 mM) reduce by 30–40% the uptake of ^{22}Cl and ^{86}Rb (or K) (Fig. 4).

Surprisingly, the effects of loop diuretics on ion transport across the blood-brain barrier have not been widely investigated. The carotid bolus injection tech-nique was used by Betz (1983 a) to show that 1 mM furosemide reduced Na extraction, relative to that of L-glucose, across the cerebral capillary wall; how-ever, ^{86}Rb extraction was not altered by furosemide. With isolated capillaries (where principally the abluminal membrane is exposed), Betz (1983 b) reported no effect of 1 mM furosemide on ^{22}Na uptake by isolated microvessels. Alter-natively, the ion substitution approach (e.g., depletion of plasma [Na] to very low levels) provides a way to identify the tightly-coupled NaK$_2$Cl cotransport; thus, very low extracellular [Na] reduces the obligatory inward transport of Cl or K. Along this line Smith and Rapoport (1984) did not find NaCl cotransport in the BBB, because their reduced plasma [Na] did not alter ^{36}Cl transport across the BBB.

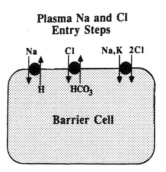

**Plasma Na and Cl
Entry Steps**

Evidence For Transporters in CNS Barriers

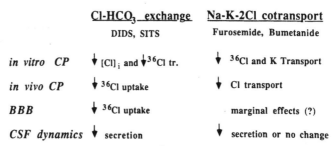

	Cl-HCO₃ exchange DIDS, SITS	Na-K-2Cl cotransport Furosemide, Bumetanide
in vitro CP	↓ [Cl]ᵢ and ↓³⁶Cl tr.	↓ ³⁶Cl and K Transport
in vivo CP	↓ ³⁶Cl uptake	↓ Cl transport
BBB	↓ ³⁶Cl uptake	marginal effects (?)
CSF dynamics	↓ secretion	↓ secretion or no change

Fig. 4. Schematic diagram and summary of information for carrier transport of Na and Cl across the blood-CSF and blood-brain barriers. Exchange and cotransport systems for translocating Na and Cl into the CNS are drawn for the basolateral and luminal membranes, respectively for CP and BBB endothelium. Sufficient information has been obtained to permit the working hypothetical scheme as depicted. Evidence for Cl-HCO₃ exchange has been obtained mainly by Deng (1986) and by Johanson et al. (1985). Indirect pharmacological evidence for Na-Cl cotransport in the CP-CSF system has been found by Johanson et al. (1988); Melby et al. (1982); Johnson et al. (1987). Lack of support for furosemide- and bumetanide-sensitive cotransport in the CSF system has been noted by Miller et al. (1986); Vogh and Langham (1981)

Ion Transport, Fluid Secretion and Intracranial Pressure

The inhibitory effects of amiloride and acidosis on Na transport into CP, CSF and brain are consistent with the presence of basolateral Na-H exchange in the CNS barrier systems. There is substantial evidence that Na-H exchange operates in parallel with Cl-HCO₃ in the CP, and likely in the BBB. The larger capacities (V_{max}) of antiporters in the blood-CSF barrier make the choroidal tissue the most suitable site for altering fluid movement into CNS. On the other hand, NaCl transport across the BBB is probably involved with a relatively slow rate of fluid formation and with maintenance of the interstitial fluid of brain with a stable composition.

Most likely the substantial fluid production by the plexus stems from the generative action of the Na and Cl exchange systems, with water following osmotically. The abundance of carbonic anhydrase in the CP assures an extensively catalyzed supply of H and HCO₃ for exchange with basolateral Na and Cl.

Acetazolamide is an effective inhibitor of the anhydrase, but its undesirable side effects have encouraged the search for new drugs to arrest fluid production and control ICP. It would be pharmacotherapeutically significant if there is more than one carrier system for translocating vascular Na (or Cl) into the CNS. The existence of several carriers in the barrier cell would seemingly present multiple pharmacological opportunities for regulating ion fluxes (1988a). NaCl cotransport could actually be involved with functions other than fluid secretion, e.g., cell volume regulation. Therefore it is essential to identify functional characteristics of the transporters once their presence has been established.

A fruitful area for future research is to ascertain mechanisms by which hormones and neurotransmitters modulate CSF formation. There is a paucity of information about biochemical control of CSF secretion, especially as to how the carriers are linked to hormone-2nd messenger effector systems. The CP is apparently more vulnerable than the BBB to the effects of ischemia, and so more information is needed to determine how such susceptibility may be related to failure of the primary and secondary active transport systems underlying the CSF secretory process.

References

Aronson P (1983) Mechanisms of active H^+ secretion in the proximal tubule. Am J Physiol 245 (Renal Fluid Elec 14):F647–F659

Betz AL (1983a) Sodium transport from blood-brain: inhibition by furosemide and amiloride. J Neurochem 41:1158–1164

Betz AL (1983b) Sodium transport in capillaries isolated from rat brain. J Neurochem 41:1150–1157

Cserr HF, DePasquale M, Patlak CS (1987) Volume regulatory influx of electrolytes from plasma to brain during acute hyperosmolality. Am J Physiol 253 (Renal Fluid Elec 22):F530–F537

Deng QS (1986) Drug modification of chloride transport in the choroid plexus-cerebrospinal fluid system of the rat. Ph. D. Thesis, University of Utah

Gjedde A (1981) High and low affinity transport of D-glucose from blood to brain. J Neurochem 36:1463–1471

Johanson CE (1984) Differential effects of acetazolamide, benzolamide and systemic acidosis on hydrogen and bicarbonate gradients across the apical and basolateral membranes of the choroid plexus. J Pharmacol Exp Ther 231:502–511

Johanson CE, Parandoosh Z, Smith QR (1985) Cl-HCO$_3$ exchange in choroid plexus: Analysis by the DMO method for cell pH. Am J Physiol (Renal Fluid Elec) 249:F478–F484

Johanson CE, Bairamian D, Parmelee J, Sweeney S, Epstein M (1988) Use of bumetanide and furosemide to test for NaK$_2$Cl cotransport in the isolated rat choroid plexus. Soc Neurosci Abs vol 14

Johanson CE (1988a) Potential for pharmacological manipulation of the blood-cerebrospinal fluid barrier. In: Neuwelt E (ed) Implications of the blood-brain barrier and its manipulation, vol. 1, Basic Science Aspects. Plenum, New York, in press

Johanson CE (1988b) The choroid plexus-arachnoid-cerebrospinal fluid system. In: Boulton A, Baker G, Walz W (eds) Neuromethods: The neuronal microenvironment, vol 9. Humana Press, Clifton, NJ, pp 33–104

Johnson DC, Singer S, Hoop B, Kazemi H (1987) Chloride flux from blood to CSF: inhibition by furosemide and bumetanide. J Appl Physiol 63:1591–1600

Melby JM, Miner LC, Reed DJ (1982) Effect of acetazolamide and furosemide on the production and composition of cerebrospinal fluid from the cat choroid plexus. Can J Physiol Pharmacol 60:405–409

Miller TB, Wilkinson HA, Rosenfield SA, Furuta T (1986) Intracranial hypertension and cerebrospinal fluid production in dogs: Effects of furosemide. Exp Neurol 94:66–80

Murphy VA, Johanson CE (1988a) Acidosis, acetazolamide and amiloride: effects on ^{22}Na transfer across the blood-brain and blood-CSF barriers. Submitted to J Neurochem

Murphy VA, Johanson CE (1988b) Alteration of sodium transport by the choroid plexus with amiloride. Submitted to Biochim Biophys Acta

Murphy VA, Johanson CE (1988c) Altered Na-H antiport in the choroid epithelial-CSF system during acute metabolic acidosis or alkalosis. Submitted to Am J Physiol (Renal Fluid Elec)

Saito Y, Wright EM (1987) Regulation of intracellular chloride in bullfrog choroid plexus. Brain Res 417:267–272

Smith QR, Johanson CE (1980) Effect of ouabain and potassium on ion concentrations in the choroidal epithelium. Am J Physiol (Renal Fluid Elec) 238:F399–F406

Smith QR, Woodbury DM, Johanson CE (1982) Kinetic analysis of [^{36}Cl], [^{22}Na] and [^{3}H]mannitol uptake into the in vivo choroid plexus-cerebrospinal fluid system: Ontogeny of the blood-brain and blood-CSF barriers. Dev Brain Res 3:181–198

Smith QR, Rapoport SI (1984) Carrier-mediated transport of chloride across the blood-brain barrier. J Neurochem 42:754–763

Smith QR, Rapoport SI (1986) Cerebrovascular permeability coefficients to sodium, potassium and chloride. J Neurochem 46:1732–1742

Vogh BP, Langham MR (1981) The effect of furosemide and bumetanide on cerebrospinal fluid formation. Brain Res 221:171–183

Wright EM (1977) Effect of bicarbonate and other buffers on choroid plexus Na$^+$/K$^+$ pump. Biochim Biophys Acta 468:486–489

Omeprazole, an Inhibitor of H^+-K^+-ATPase, Markedly Reduces CSF Formation in the Rabbit

C. Owman, M. Lindvall-Axelsson, and B. Winbladh

Department of Medical Cell Research, University of Lund, Biskopsgatan 5, S-223 62 Lund (Sweden)

CSF formation can be inhibited by ouabain, suggesting an involvement of transport systems dependent on sodium-potassium activated adenosine triphosphatase (Na^+-K^+-ATPase) (Cserr 1975). Recently, it has been found that the gastric mucosa of pig, dog and guinea-pig contains another specific ATPase, which is H^+-K^+ dependent (Saccomani et al. 1979). Inhibition of this enzyme with omeprazole, a substituted benzimidazole, markedly and selectively reduces histamine- and db-cAMP-stimulated gastric acid secretion (Wallmark et al. 1983). In view of similarities between the secretory responses in the gastric mucosa and choroid plexus epithelia to drugs affecting the autonomic nervous sytem, and since the choroid plexus seems to play a role in the regulation of the pH in the CSF, it was considered of interest to determine whether H^+-K^+-ATPase-like activity is present in the choroid plexus by measuring the effect of the selective inhibitor, omeprazole, on choroid plexus ATPase activity, transport function, and rate of CSF formation.

The experiments were performed on 56 randomly pigmented rabbits of either sex, weighing 2.5–3.5 kg. A modification of the spectrophotometric method of Bonting et al. (1961) was used for determination of ATPase. The plexus was homogenized in ice-cold distilled water using a Potter-Elvehjem homogenizer. Before analysis, each homogenate was resuspended in 100 μl/mg imidazole buffer solution (imidazoale 25 mM; EDTA, 1 mM). After vigorous shaking, 50 μl of the homogenate was mixed with 0.2 ml of three different solutions, all having the same basic composition (in mM): ATP, 2; $MgCl_2$, 3.75; KCl, 25; NaCl, 163; EDTA, 0.2; TRIS, 41.3; and histidine, 5 mg/ml. Two of the solutions, in addition, contained either 1 mM of an inhibitor of Na^+K^+-ATPase (ouabain, Sigma) and/or 1 mM of an inhibitor of H^+-K^+-ATPase (H 168/68, 5-Methoxy-2-[[4-methoxy-3,5-dimethyl-2-pyridinyl]-methyl]sulfinyl-1H-benzimidazole); omeprazole, Hässle, Sweden. The specific ATPase activities were calculated from the difference in phosphate concentration between the solution containing no inhibitors and that containing ouabain, omeprazole, and NaSCN, respectively.

For uptake studies, plexus tissues were pre-incubated for 10 min in a Krebs-Henseleit buffer (pH 7.4) under continuous gassing with 95% O_2 and 5% CO_2 at 37°C in a shaking bath. Thereafter, ^{14}C-choline (methyl-^{14}C-choline chloride; Radiochemical Centre, Amersham) or ^{14}C-benzylpenicillin (benzyl-^{14}C-penicillin potassium; Radiochemical Centre, Amersham) was added (final concentration 10^{-5} M) and the incubation was continued for 20 min. The tissues were removed, rinsed in cold Krebs-Henseleit buffer, gently blotted on filter

Eds.: J. T. Hoff and A. L. Betz

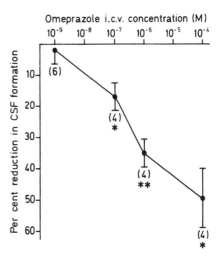

Fig. 1. Changes in the rate of cerebrospinal fluid (*CSF*) production during intracerebroventricular (*i.c.v.*) perfusion of the selective H^+-K^+-ATPase inhibitor, omeprazole, at various concentrations in the CSF infusate. The values are related to the control values of CSF production obtained in each animal prior to administration of omeprazole and are shown as mean per cent changes $\pm$ SE; number of animals indicated within parentheses. Significant differences from the control values were determined according to the paired t-test (based on the absolute values for the CSF formation): *$0.01 < p < 0.05$, **$0.001 < p < 0.01$

paper, wrapped in plastic film to avoid drying, weighed on a microbalance, and dissolved in Soluene 350 (Packard). Radioactivity was measured by liquid scintillation counting using conventional methods. Tissue/medium ratios were calculated as the quotient between the tissue (wet weight) and the incubation medium.

A modification of Pappenheimer's intraventricular ^{14}C-inulin method was used during ventriculocisternal perfusion for measurement of CSF formation (Lindvall et al. 1979). Omeprazole was given in varying concentrations in the perfusate from 10^{-4} to 10^{-9} M, corresponding to 0.2×10^{-1} to 0.2×10^{-6} mg $\times kg^{-1}$. In another set of experiments the drug was given as an i.v. injection of 2×10^{-1} to 2×10^{-3} mg/kg.

The mean rate of CSF formation during the 2-hr steady state period before administration of enzyme inhibitor was 9.9 ± 0.5 (SEM) µl/min. Various concentrations of omeprazole were added to the inulin-containing perfusion solution in 18 animals during a subsequent 2 hr experimental period. There was a dose-related pronounced reduction in CSF formation (Fig. 1), being about 50% at the highest concentration of the inhibitor tested (10^{-4} M), while it was not significantly altered at the concentration of 10^{-9} M. Intravenous injection of omeprazole significantly decreased CSF production (but to a smaller extent than the highest concentrations used intraventricularly; Fig. 2), by around 25% at the highest doses of 2×10^{-2} mg/kg and 2×10^{-1} mg/kg (Fig. 2). Higher doses were not tested.

The activity of ouabain-sensitive Na^+-K^+-ATPase comprised, omeprazole in low concentrations, 2×10^{-5} and 2×10^{-6} M, did not affect total or Na^+-K^+-activated ATPase activity. At the 2×10^{-4} M concentration, a variable influence was seen. At the 2×10^{-3} M omeprazole concentration, a considerable decrease (46%) in total ATPase activity occurred. Addition of ouabain further decreased the activity, but less than ouabain alone, showing that both H^+-K^+-ATPase and Na^+-K^+-independent ATPase activities were affected (Table 1). Pretreatment of omeprazole with acid significantly increased its inhibitory activity at a concentration of 2×10^{-3} M but not at lower concentrations. Acidi-

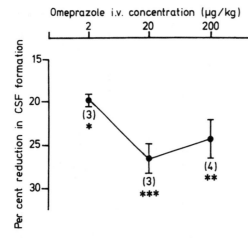

Fig. 2. Changes in the rate of CSF formation after i.v. injection of various omeprazole concentrations. The values were obtained as in Fig. 1 and show mean percent values $\pm$ SE; number of animals indicated within parentheses. Significant differences from the control value before omeprazole injection according to the paired t-test (based on the absolute values for the CSF formation): $*p < 0.05$; $**0.001 < p < 0.01$; $***p < 0.001$

Table 1. Inhibition of ATPase activity by different concentrations of ouabain, omeprazole, ouabain and omeprazole, or omeprazole pretreated with acid

Inhibitor concentration (M)	Percent inhibition			
	Ouabain	Omeprazole	Omeprazole + Ouabain	Omeprazole pretreated with acid
2×10^{-3}	32 ± 2 (19)	46 ± 2 (18)	67 ± 2 (3)	62 ± 2 (16)
2×10^{-4}	32 ± 2 (4)	11 ± 3 (4)	39 ± 4 (3)	11 ± 1 (16)
2×10^{-5}	25 ± 2 (3)	7 ± 7 (2)	25 ± 2 (3)	2 ± 1 (13)
2×10^{-6}	11 ± 5 (2)	0 ± 0 (3)	7 ± 1 (3)	–

Mean $\pm$ S.E.; number of determinations indicated within parentheses

fication of the incubation medium to pH 6.5 and 4, respectively, during the preincubation gave a small decrease in total ATPase activity with decreasing pH. However, the pattern and magnitude of inhibition by omeprazole was the same as at pH 7.5. Addition of $NaHCO_3$ (40 mM) to the ouabain-inhibited incubate increased ATPase activity significantly, $28 \pm 9\%$ (SD; $n=8$), suggesting the presence of bicarbonate-activated ATPase (HCO_3-ATPase). Consequently, this increase in activity was partly inhibited by NaSCN 10^{-2} M, a known HCO_3-ATPase inhibitor. However, omeprazole 2×10^{-4} M did not influence the increase in ATPase activity caused by $NaHCO_3$, $34 \pm 8\%$ (SD; $n=4$).

The choroid plexus uptake of choline (organic base; 10^{-5} M) or benzylpenicillin (organic acid; 10^{-5} M) in vitro was significantly reduced by 58 and 65%, respectively, with acid-pretreated omeprazole (2×10^{-3} M) in the incubation medium. On the other hand, the plexus uptake of choline was not influenced by omeprazole at 2×10^{-5} M and pretreatment of the inhibitor with acid did not change the results.

Omeprazole thus decreased CSF production significantly even at low concentrations when infused intraventricularly or when given intravenously. The highest dose given i.v. was about the same as that recommended for clinical use in man. An influence on CSF production via the ATPase system could be possible if the choroid plexuses accumulated omeprazole to a high concentratation. However, at 2×10^{-5} M omeprazole, no reduction in choline uptake was obtained in choroid plexuses in vitro. Omeprazole needs transformation in acid milieu to obtain specific H^+-K^+-ATPase inhibiting properties. No such compartment is known to exist in the choroid plexus.

An intact sodium pump seems to be necessary for at least part of the CSF production by the choroid plexus. High concentrations of ouabain do not completely inhibit CSF production when the latter is determined by cerebroventricular perfusions (Pollay et al. 1985). It has been suggested that up to half of the total CSF might be derived from extrachoroidal sources in the brain. Hypothetically, omeprazole might interfere with these less well known mechanisms. The maximal inhibition of CSF production obtained with omeprazole was around 50%, which is less than the maximal effect obtained with ouabain (Pollay et al. 1985). This further supports the theory that CSF is produced by several different mechanisms.

Other possible mechanisms could be an influence of the drug on choroid plexus blood flow or a more general toxic metabolic influence. However, no influence on the general circulation or general toxic effects were seen in the intact animals even at the highest i.v. dose or highest intraventricular infusion rate of omeprazole. This is in sharp contrast to the profound general effects seen in animals receiving high concentrations of ouabain by ventriculocisternal perfusion (Cserr 1975) with comparable influence on CSF production rates.

References

Bonting SL, Simon KA, Hawkins NM (1961) Studies on sodium-potassium-activated adenosine triphosphatase. Arch Biochem Biophys 95:416–423

Cserr HF (1975 Physiology of the choroid plexus. In: Netsky MG, Shuangshoti S (eds) The Choroid Plexus in Health and Disease. Wright, Bristol, pp 175–195

Cserr HF, Ostrach LH (1974) Bulk flow of interstitial fluid after intracranial injection of blue dextran 2000. Exp Neurol 45:50–60

Lindvall M, Edvinsson L, Owman C (1979) Effect of sympathomimetic drugs and corresponding receptor antagonists on the rate of cerebrospinal fluid production. Exp Neurol 64:132–145

Pollay M, Hisey B, Reynolds E, Tomkins P, Stevens FA, Smith R (1985) Choroid plexus Na^+/K^+-activated adenosine triphosphatase and cerebrospinal fluid formation. Neurosurgery 17:768–772

Saccomani G, Helander HF, Crago S, Chang HH, Dailey DW, Sachs G (1979) Characterization of gastric mucosal membranes. J Cell Biol 83:271–283

Wallmark B, Jaresten B-M, LOarsson H, Ryberg B, Brändström, Fellenius E (1983) Differentiation among inhibitory actions of omeprazole, cimetidine, and SCN^- on gastric acid secretion. Am J Physiol 245:G64–G71

Glucocorticoid Effects on Choroid Plexus Function

M. Lindvall-Axelsson, P. Hedner, and C. Owman

Department of Medical Cell Research, University of Lund, Biskopsgatan 5, S-223 62 Lund
(Sweden)

It was shown more than four decades ago that adrenocortical extracts counteract the development of brain edema upon exposure of the cerebral cortex through a craniotomy (Prados et al. 1945). Glucocorticoids have since been widely applied in clinical neurosurgery to cope with intracranial hypertension. However, the mechanism of action on intracranial pressure and also their effects on the choroid plexus and the production of cerebrospinal fluid (CSF) are still poorly understood.

In a series of experiments on rabbits, we have shown that the production rate of CSF is markedly enhanced by sympathetic denervation (Lindvall et al. 1978), which is associated with an increased transport capacity of the choroid plexus as measured by choline uptake (Lindvall et al. 1981) and sodium-potassium ATPase activity (Lindvall et al. 1982). The present study was carried out to explore the possibility that betamethasone is able to counteract these three aspects of choroid plexus function as an important part of the glucocorticoid effect on intracranial pressure dynamics.

Methods

The study was performed on 22 male Sprague-Dawley rats and 56 rabbits of either sex.

Eleven of the rats were pretreated for 5 days with betamethasone phosphate (Betapred; Glaxo, England) 0.3–0.4 mg/kg body weight per day administered in the drinking water. Thirty-one of the rabbits were pretreated for the same time with betamethasone phosphate 2 mg/kg body weight per day with addition of subcutaneous betamethasone-21-phosphate in a dose of 0.5 mg/kg twice a day during the last two days of treatment.

Tissue uptake of the organic base, choline, was studied by incubation in the presence of the ^{14}C-labelled compound (Winbladh 1974) and expressed as tissue-medium ratios (T/M). ATPase activity was measured by a modification of the spectrophotometric method (Bonting et al. 1961). The rate of bulk CSF production was determined in rabbits by intraventricular dilution of ^{14}C-inulin during ventriculo-cisternal perfusion according to Pappenheimer (Lindvall et al. 1979). Before sacrifice of the animals, 1–2 ml of blood was collected from the left ventricle of the heart under light anesthesia. In the perfusion experiments on rabbits, blood samples were taken from the femoral artery throughout. Plasma concentrations of corticosterone (rat) were determined fluorometrically according to Hedner (1961) and plasma concentrations of cortisol (rabbit) with a radioimmunoassay kit obtained from New England Nuclear (North Billerica, MA 01862). Blood glucose levels were estimated by Dextrostix (Ames, Elkhart, Indiana, USA) in a reflectometer (Hedner et al. 1974). Concentrations of Na^+ and K^+ in serum were analyzed by flame photometry.

Results

The corticosterone concentration in rat serum was reduced by 62% after pretreatment with betamethasone; in rabbit the reduction in serum cortisol was 69%.

The activity of Na^+-K^+-ATPase in the rat's choroid plexuses was significantly reduced by 24% after daily treatment of the animals for 5 days with oral betamethasone (Fig. 1). Total ATPase showed only a slight (13%), but nevertheless significant, decrease in activity. The mean T/M ratio for choline in the rat choroid plexus showed a slight reduction of 16% though not statistically significant.

In rabbit, there was a highly significant decrease of 31% in Na^+-K^+-ATPase activity in the lateral choroid plexuses after combined oral and subcutaneous treatment with betamethasone (Fig. 1). A significant reduction in Na^+-K^+-ATPase activity was also found in the third ventricle plexus while that of the

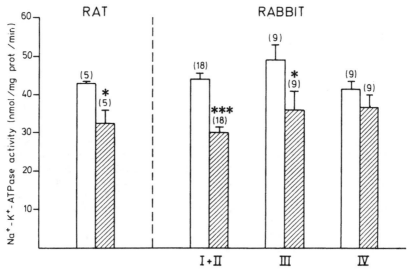

Fig. 1. Na^+-K^+-ATPase activity in choroid plexus of rat (tissue from all ventricles) and rabbit (tissue from lateral (*I+II*), third (*III*) or fourth (*IV*) ventricle) after treatment for 5 days with betamethasone-phosphate (*dashed bars*) in comparison with choroid plexus tissue from control animals (*open bars*). Differences between mean values according to Student's *t*-test: * $p < 0.05$; *** $p < 0.001$. Number of determinations (plexuses) within parenthesis

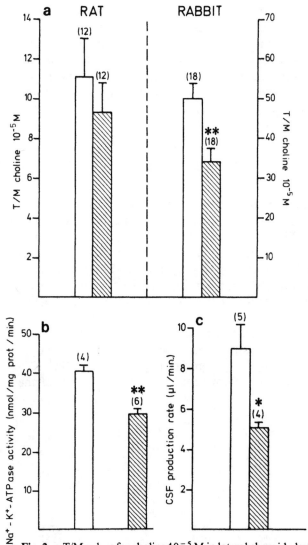

Fig. 2. a T/M values for choline 10^{-5} M in lateral choroid plexuses after treatment of the animals for 5 days with betamethasone-phosphate (*dashed bars*) in comparison with lateral plexuses from control animals (*open bars*). Differences between mean values using Student's t-test: ** $0.001 < p < 0.01$. Number of determinations (plexuses) within parenthesis. **b** Na$^+$-K$^+$-ATPase activity in sympathectomized, lateral choroid plexus of rabbit after 5 days of treatment with betamethasone-phosphate (*dashed bar*) in comparison with denervated, control plexus (*open bar*). Differences between mean values using Student's t-test: ** $0.001 < p < 0.01$. Number of determinations (plexuses) within parenthesis. **c** Rate of CSF production in a group of rabbits pretreated for 5 days with betamethasone-phosphate p.o. and s.c. (*dashed bar*) and in a control group of animals (*open bar*) Significant difference between mean values according to Student's t-test: * $p < 0.05$. Number of animals within parenthesis

fourth ventricle showed only a slight, non-significant, decrease of 13% (Fig. 1). No parallel change in total ATPase activity could be demonstrated. The mean T/M for choline (10^{-5} M) in the lateral choroid plexuses was reduced by 31% after 5 days of steroid treatment (Fig. 2a), similar to the alteration in Na^+-K^+-ATPase activity. The effect of sympathetic denervation, which increases ATPase activity and choline uptake in the rabbit choroid plexus, was counteracted by cortisone treatment. This was particularly evident for the ATPase activity (Fig. 2b).

There was a significant decrement by 43% in the rate of CSF formation in vivo, from 9.0 ± 1.2 µl/min to 5.1 ± 0.3 µl/min, in the group of steroid-treated animals compared to the control group (Fig. 2c).

Concentrations of Na^+ and K^+ in serum were only slightly influenced by the steroid treatment: mean serum Na^+ increased significantly, while serum K^+ decreased, though not significantly. The blood glucose levels were significantly enhanced in the same groups of rabbits.

The increase in body weight of rabbits was significantly higher after 5 days of glucocorticoid treatment (7%) as compared to matched control animals (3%). There was no significant difference in plexus wet weight.

Discussion

Daily treatment of rabbits with betamethasone for 5 days clearly reduced CSF formation measured with Pappenheimer's radioactive inulin dilution technique during ventriculo-cisternal perfusion. The dose used was high enough to markedly diminish the endogenous cortisol production. It can be assumed that an extended period of treatment is required, even though labelled cortisol accumulates in the choroid plexus within minutes after injection (Schwartz et al. 1972). Although cortisone rapidly affects membrane permeability (Eisenberg et al. 1970), it seems likely that the influence on CSF formation involves more complex intracellular receptor mechanisms and associated secretory processes.

The reduction in CSF formation was parallelled by a lower ATPase activity in the choroid plexus and a reduced uptake of choline. The effects were significant in the rabbit and showed the same tendency (though not statistically significant for choline uptake) in the rat.

It has been suggested by Johanson et al. (1974) that the effect of corticosterone on Na^+-K^+-ATPase and CSF formation may be secondary to a lowering of K^+ in the CSF during hypokalemia. In their experiments on chronically deoxycorticosterone-treated rats (2 weeks) K^+ decreased in CSF by only a few per cent in spite of a significant and pronounced hypokalemia. The authors hypothesize that the reduction in K^+ concentration might have approached a critical level causing a "turning off" of the Na^+-K^+ pump in the apical membrane of the epithelium. In our study, we did not measure cellular, tissue or CSF cationic concentrations. On the other hand, we noted only a slight and non-significant reduction in serum K^+ concentration after 5 days of treatment with betamethasone probably because of its weaker mineralocorticoid effect compared to deoxycorticosterone. Thus, it is probable that the demonstrated effects on CSF formation, choline transport, and Na^+-K^+-ATPase activity are, for the most part, dependent on the glucocorticoid component of the steroids.

The presently observed in vivo reduction by betamethasone in Na^+-K^+-ATPase activity agrees with the marked inhibition seen in vitro in both cat and rabbit choroid plexus with dexamethasone in the incubation medium (Mayman 1972), though a direct blocking effect of dexamethasone when given in vitro cannot be excluded. The in vitro reduction in ATPase activity may also have been mediated by an interference with membrane phospholipids and cholesterol necessary for its activity (Fien and Seiler 1977).

In conclusion, there is strong reason to believe that glucocorticoids can indeed reduce transport functions in the choroid plexus, including Na^+-K^+-ATPase activity, which is directly related to the formation of CSF, and that this action could represent one important component in its well-known effect on intracranial hypertension.

References

Bonting SL, Simon KA, Hawkins NM (1961) Studies on sodium-potassium activated adenosine triphosphatase. Arch Biochem Biophys 95:416–423

Eisenberg HM, Barlow CF, Lorenzo AV (1970) The effect of dexamethasone on altered brain vascular permeability. Arch Neurol 23:18–22

Fiehn W, Seiler D (1977) (Na^+,K^+)-ATPase activity and sterol composition of membranes. Naunyn-Schmiedebergs Arch Pharmacol 297:S21

Hedner P (1961 Experiences with a fluorometric method for determining corticosteroids in man and rat. Acta Pharmacol 18:65–74

Hedner P, Scherstén B, Thulin T (1974) Dextrostix Reflectance Meter as an aid in diagnostic hypoglycemia. Acta Med Scand 195:29–31

Johanson CE, Reed DJ, Woodbury DM (1974) Active transport of sodium and potassium by the choroid plexus of the rat. J Physiol (Lond) 241:359–372

Lindvall M, Edvinsson L, Owman C (1978) Sympathetic nervous control of cerebrospinal fluid production from the choroid plexus. Science 201:176–178

Lindvall M, Edvinsson L, Owman C (1979) Effect of sympathomimetic drugs and corresponding receptor antagonists on the rate of cerebrospinal fluid production. Exp Neurol 64:132–145

Lindvall M, Owman C, Winbladh B (1981) Sympathetic influence on transport functions in the choroid plexus of rabbit and rat. Brain Res 223:160–164

Lindvall M, Owman C, Winbladh B (1982) Sympathetic influence on sodium-potassium activated adenosine triphosphatase activity of rabbit and rat choroid plexus. Brain Res Bull 9:761–763

Mayman CI (1972) Inhibitory effect of dexamethasone on sodium-potassium activated adenosine triphosphatase of choroid plexus in cat and rabbit. Fed Proc 31:691

Prados M, Strowger B, Feindel W (1945) Studies on cerebral edema, reaction of the brain on exposure to air: Physiological changes. Arch Neurol Psychiat (Chicago) 54:290–300

Schwartz ML, Tator CH, Hoffman HJ (1972) The uptake of hydrocortisone in mouse brain and ependymoblastoma. J Neurosurg 36:178–183

Winbladh B (1974) Choroid plexus uptake of acetylcholine. Acta Physiol Scand 92:156–164

Sex Steroids and Transport Functions in the Rabbit Choroid Plexus

C. Owman and M. Lindvall-Axelsson

Department of Medical Cell Research, University of Lund, Biskopsgatan 5, S-223 62 Lund (Sweden)

Fluctuations in intracranial pressure have been suggested to occur during the menstrual cycle, in pregnancy, during use of oral contraceptives, and in obese young women (Greene 1975). Studies were, therefore, performed on isolated choroid plexus tissue from rabbits to elucidate the effects of estrogen and progesterone on the uptake and accumulation of the organic base, choline, and on the activities of various types of ATPase.

Tissue uptake of choline was studied by incubation in the presence of the ^{14}C-labelled compound (Winbladh 1974) and expressed as tissue/medium ratios (T/M). ATPase activity was measured by a modification of the spectrophotometric method of Bonting et al. (1961). The rate of bulk CSF production was determined in rabbits by intraventricular dilution of ^{14}C-inulin during ventriculocisternal perfusion according to Pappenheimer (Lindvall et al. 1979).

The results are summarized in Fig. 1. The mean T/M for choline at a concentration of 10^{-5} M in the incubation medium was 114.7 ± 9.9 in the lateral ventri-

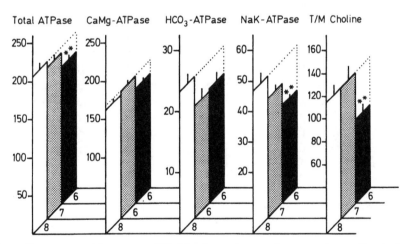

Fig. 1. Effects of treatment with estrogen (*filled bars*) or estrogen plus progesterone (*hatched bars*) on the various parameters measured in rabbit choroid plexus from the lateral ventricles compared with tissue from control animals (*open bars*) receiving vehicle only. The activities of the various types of ATPase were expressed in nmoles/mg protein/min; the choline accumulation as tissue/medium ratio (T/M) comparing radioactivity per mg protein in the plexus with the radioactivity per µl medium. Values are means ± SEM, number of animals indicated at *bottom of bars*. Student's *t*-test: ** $0.001 < p < 0.01$

cle plexuses of the control group. Two weeks of daily estrogen treatment (0.5 µg/kg s.c.) did not change the mean T/M (115.3 ± 14.8) significantly, while addition of progesterone (2 mg/kg s.c.) during the last week markedly reduced the T/M for choline by 35% to 74.6 ± 5.6.

The activity of the transport enzyme, Na^+-K^+-ATPase, was determined in the same lateral plexuses. Following estrogen, the Na^+-K^+-ATPase activity showed a slight, but non-significant, decrease by 17% while addition of progesterone significantly reduced the activity by a further 14% to a total of 31%, compared to animals receiving no hormone treatment. There was also a small, but non-significant, reduction in HCO_3^--activated ATPase activity after estrogen treatment, but no further change after addition of progesterone. Ca^{++}-Mg-ATPase was unchanged in the treated animals.

The choroid plexuses of the third and fourth ventricle presented similar changes in activities and are not illustrated.

Progesterone treatment of estrogen-primed rabbits thus significantly lowers the ATPase activity and the uptake and accumulation of radiolabelled choline in the rabbit choroid plexus, whereas estrogen alone has no substantial effect. This was not related to weight changes in the plexus tissue. In attempts to distinguish various functional classes of ATPase activities it was evident that the reduction was particularly associated with the Na^+-K^+-activated ATPase. This enzyme is localized in the plasma membrane of the plexus epithelium (Milhorat et al. 1975) and is directly correlated with the rate of fluid secretion by the choroid plexus (Wright 1978).

The effect of progesterone in combination with estrogen may thus be related to hose fluctuations in intracranial pressure proposed to occur during the above-mentioned conditions, including for unknown – presumably hormonal – reasons obese young women (Greene 1975). There may be several kinds of cellular mechanisms involved in the action of progesterone on the choroid plexus function. One could be an interaction with aldosterone in terms of competition between progesterone and aldosterone at cellular receptors (Landau and Lugibihl 1958, Laidlaw et al. 1962). Another mechanism might be related to the increase in β-adrenoceptor activity seen under the influence of progesterone (Helm et al. 1982) in view of the fact that activation of the β-receptors in rabbit choroid plexus inhibits the rate of CSF production (Lindvall et al. 1979). Progesterone may also have effects on the functional turnover of noradrenalin in the sympathetic nervous system supplying the choroid plexus with fibres which inhibit the rate of CSF formation (Lindvall et al. 1978).

References

Bonting SL, Simon KA, Hawkins NM (1961) Studies on sodium-potassium activated adenosine triphosphatase. Arch Biochem Biophys 95:416–423

Greene R (1975) The endocrinology of headache. In: Pearce J (ed) Modern topics in migraine, chapter 7. Heinemann, London, pp 64–71

Helm G, Owman C, Sjöberg N-O, Walles B (1982) Quantitative pharmacological character-ization of β-receptors and two types of α-receptors mediating sympathomimetic smooth muscle response in the human Fallopian tube at various cyclic stages. Acta Physiol Scand 114:425–432

Laidlaw JC, Ruse JL, Gornall AG (1962) The influence of estrogen and progesterone on aldosterone excretion. J Clin Endocrinol 22:161–171

Landau RL, Lugibihl K (1958) Inhibition of the sodium-retaining influence of aldosterone by progesterone. J Clin Endocrinol 18:1237–1245

Lindvall M, Edvinsson L, Owman Ch (1978) Sympathetic nervous control of cerebrospinal fluid production from the choroid plexus. Science 201:176–178

Lindvall M, Edvinsson L, Owman C (1979) Effect of sympathomimetic drugs and corresponding receptor antagonists on the rate of cerebrospinal fluid production. Exp Neurol 64:132–145

Milhorat TH, Davis DA, Hammock MK (1975) Localization of ouabain-sensitive Na-K-ATPase in frog, rabbit and rat choroid plexus. Brain Res 99:170–174

Windbladh B (1974) Choroid plexus uptake of acetylcholine. Acta Physiol Scand 92:156–164

Wright EM (1978) Transport processes in the formation of the cerebrospinal fluid. Rev Physiol Biochem Pharmacol 83:1–34

Axonal Coexistence of Certain Transmitter Peptides in the Choroid Plexus

C. Nilsson, R. Ekman, M. Lindvall-Axelsson, and C. Owman

Department of Medical Cell Research, University of Lund, Biskopsgatan 5, S-223 62 Lund (Sweden)

Both adrenergic and cholinergic nerves have been described in the choroid plexus (Lindvall and Owman 1981) and a few studies have reported the presence of nerves immunoreactive to vasoactive intestinal polypeptide (VIP), neuropeptide Y (NPY) and substance P (SP) (Lindvall et al. 1978, Edvinsson et al. 1983, 1987). The aim of the present study was to investigate the peptidergic nerve supply of the choroid plexus using immunocytochemistry and radioimmunoassay. The origin and possible coexistence of the neuropeptides in this secretory tissue were studied as a basis for future functional investigations in vivo and in vitro.

Choroid plexus tissue from rats, guinea pigs, rabbits, and adult pigs was used. The pig plexuses were obtained from a local slaughterhouse. Following anesthesia the laboratory animals were perfused with 0.9% saline, followed by Stefanini's fixation solution for immunohistochemistry. The plexuses from all ventricles were dissected out and immersion fixed in the same fixative for a further 2 hr. The brain was taken from the skull of the pigs 30–40 min after killing, and the choroid plexuses from the lateral and fourth ventricles were removed and immersed in ice-cold Stefanini's solution for 24 hr. The plexuses were then rinsed. Sections of the choroid plexus or the whole brain of the rats were cut in a cryostat and placed on chromalyn-gelatin coated glass slides. After rinsing in phosphate buffered saline with 0.25% Triton-X, 100 sections were incubated with the antisera in a moist chamber for 20 hr at 4°C followed by 2 hr at room temperature. Thereafter the procedure followed the indirect immunofluorescence method of Coons et al. (1955). As secondary antibodies, we used swine anti-rabbit antibodies (1:20, DAKO, Denmark) conjugated with either fluorescein isothiocyanate (FITC) or tetramethylrhodamine isothiocyanate (TRITC). In order to visualize the antibody towards NPY raised in sheep a donkey anti-sheep antibody conjugated with FITC (1:80, SIGMA) was used.

The possible coexistence of NPY, VIP, PHI and DBH (dopamine-β-hydroxylase, a specific marker enzyme for adrenergic nerves) in nerve fibers was investigated by sequential staining with elution of the primary antibody by a 30 sec treatment of the sections with potassium permanganate as described by Tramu et al. (1980). Further double staining was performed by applying sheep antisera towards NPY, visualized with donkey anti-sheep antibodies conjugated with FITC, followed by staining with antibodies towards either VIP, PHI or DBH which were visualized with swine anti-rabbit antibodies conjugated with TRITC.

For radioimmunoassay (RIA), the laboratory animals were anesthetized but perfused only with 0.9% saline at 4°C to wash out the blood. The tissue from

Eds.: J. T. Hoff and A. L. Betz
© Springer-Verlag Berlin Heidelberg 1989

these animals and from the pigs was boiled in 0.9% saline for 10 min, followed by homogenization. The homogenates were centrifuged at 4°C, $1000 \times g$ for 30 min and the supernatants were collected. The pellets were dissolved in 0.5 M acetic acid and the peptide extracted. The supernatants were mixed and lyophilized. For the NPY assay, a rabbit antiserum raised against synthetic porcine NPY (gift from Dr. P.C. Emson, Cambridge, U.K.) conjugated to bovine serum albumin with carboxyimide was used at a final dilution of 1:40000. Immunoreactive VIP was quantitated using antiserum (no. 7852, Milab, Malmö, Sweden) at a final dilution of 1:72000. In the case of CGRP, we used a rabbit antiserum (code no. A 13, Milab, Malmö, Sweden) raised against albumin-conjugated synthetic rat CGRP. The antiserum was used at a final dilution of 1:30000. Immunoreactive SP was determined using a rabbit antiserum raised against synthetic SP (code no. SP-2, a kind gift from Dr. E. Brodin, Stockholm, Sweden).

Nerve fibers immunoreactive to NPY and VIP were found in all species studied. It was not possible to investigate the VIP-immunoreactivity in the rabbit, since a suitable antibody was lacking for this species. A moderately dense innervation of both neuropeptides was found in the choroid plexus of the lateral and third ventricles in pig as well as for NPY in rabbit, while only a few nerve fibers were found in the fourth ventricle choroid plexus of these species, as well as in all plexuses from rat and guinea-pig. In choroid plexus from pig, PHI showed approximately the same distribution as NPY and VIP but with a lower density of nerve fibers. There was no specific immunoreactivity with the antisera towards SP and CGRP.

Nerve fibers immunoreactive to NPY and VIP showed a markedly similar distribution. Dense nerve plexuses could be found around larger and medium-sized arteries, while smaller arteries and veins were more sparsely innervated. A varying density of single fibers could also be found in the plexus stroma and in close approximation to microvessels and epithelium.

Analysis by RIA (Table 1) revealed quite constant levels of NPY in the choroid plexus of all species studied, with an average content of 11 and 18 pmol-equivalents (pmoleqv)/g in the pig and rabbit, respectively. In spite of the paucity of nerve fibers shown by immunohistochemistry, results with RIA showed a concentration for NPY of 49 pmoleqv/g for rat and 38 pmoleqv/g in the

Table 1. Preliminary data on the concentration of immunoreactive neuropeptides in choroid plexus tissue from four animal species. Values (p mol eqv/g) are means $\pm$ SEM, $n = 3-6$

Animal	Plexus	NPY	VIP	CRGP	SP
Rabbit	all	13.9 ± 2.8	0.57 ± 0.03	5.5 ± 1.6	1.8
	lateral	8.0 ± 0.3			
	third	33.2 ± 5.4	5.5		
	fourth	11.1 ± 2.2			
Rat	all	49.4 ± 7.9	0.37	0	0
Guinea-pig	all	37.5	0.40	1.7	3.0
Pig	lateral	11.2 ± 4.3	1.8 ± 0.5	0.3 ± 0.08	0.1
	fourth	18.2 ± 8.3	2.4 ± 1.2	0.3	0.08

guinea-pig. Regional differences in concentration of NPY could also be seen between choroid plexus from the different ventricles of the brain. In the rabbit, concentrations were highest in choroid plexus tissue from the third ventricle, while the concentration was approximately three times lower in choroid plexus from the lateral and fourth ventricles. Measurable concentrations of VIP were found in choroid plexus from all species except rat, the highest levels being found in pig (1.8–2.4 pmoleqv/g). CGRP and substance P were found only in some of the analyzed samples with low and rather varying concentrations (Table 1).

Studies in the pig with both the sequential and double staining methods revealed a very similar distribution for NPY and VIP immunoreactivity, with a great majority of the nerve fibers and varicosities containing both NPY and VIP. A few nerve fibers could be found to contain both NPY and DBH, while VIP and DBH were never present in the same nerve fiber. Also in the guinea-pig, NPY and VIP were found to coexist. PHI immunoreactivity always coexisted with NPY or VIP.

Excision of the superior cervical ganglion in 5 rabbits completely abolished the NPY-immunoreactive nerve fibers in the ipsilateral choroid plexus of the lateral ventricle. These results stand in contrast to the RIA analysis, which showed only a moderate (31%) decrease in NPY concentration in the ipsilateral choroid plexus, while the NPY concentration in the corresponding iris was 88% lower after sympathectomy compared to control.

NPY is a well known co-transmitter to noradrenalin in both peripheral and cerebral vessels (Edvinsson et al. 1987). We therefore expected to find NPY- and DBH-immunoreactivity in the same nerve fibers. However, in the pig, NPY and DBH only coexisted in a few of the nerves. Instead there was an extensive co-localization of NPY- and VIP-immunoreactivity in nerves of the choroid plexus from pig. PHI derives from the same precursor molecule as VIP and is thus often localized in the same nerve fibers as VIP (Itoh et al. 1983). In the present study, PHI was also found to coexist with NPY, which further confirms the co-localization of NPY and VIP. It should be noted that although matching varicosities are considered as evidence for coexistence, definite proof can only be provided by electronmicroscopic immunohistochemistry. Different nerve fibers may run in parallel with the respective varicosities lying adjacent to each other.

Coexistence of NPY, VIP and PHI has previously been described in intra-mural neurons of the small intestine (Ekblad et al. 1984), and recently Leblanc et al. (1987) described coexistence of NPY and VIP in cranial parasympathetic neurons, notably those in the sphenopalatine ganglion which is known to inner-vate cerebral vessels (Hara et al. 1985). The mammalian choroid plexus harbors an extensive cholinergic innervation, as shown by the acetylcholinesterase tech-nique, maybe indicating that the largest input of NPY-immunoreactive nerves to the choroid plexus is with a cholinergic parasympathetic innervation. There is also reason to suspect species variation in the proportion of NPY-immu-noreactive nerves arriving via the sympathetic and parasympathetic innervation. This is indicated by the denervation studies in rabbit where all of the NPY immonoreactivity disappeared after sympathectomy. However, RIA showed only a decrease of 31% of NPY immunoreactivity in the chroid plexus after sympa-thetic denervation. In contrast, the NPY concentration in iris fell by 88%. Both the choroid plexus of the lateral ventricles and the iris receive essentially an ipsilateral sympathetic innervation originating entirely in the superior cervical ganglion. However, the present results indicate a significant difference between the two tissues in the proportion of NPY-containing nerve fibers with a sympathetic origin. It is possible that the parasympathetic NPY nerves have a low concentration of NPY in rabbit, not detectable with the antisera used for immunohistochemistry. Alternatively, the NPY-like material in the sympathetic and parasympathetic innervation may consist of different fragments of the NPY precursor molecule, the fragments not being detectable by the antisera. At present, little is known about the degradation of NPY, although it has been reported to be stable in human postmortem brain tissue (Dawbarn et al. 1984). It seems unlikely that NPY was degraded during the extraction procedures used, as judged from recovery data (more than 80%). In any event the presence of several NPY-like immunoreactive peptides should be considered when performing routine RIAs on tissue extracts. Variations in the concentrations of these NPY-like fragments relative to NPY could provide conflicting results.

Concerning the possible functions of the above described neuropeptides in the choroid plexus, VIP has been shown to stimulate production of cyclic AMP in whole choroid plexus (Lindvall et al. 1985) and in cultured bovine plexus epithelial cells (Crook and Pruisner 1986). Furthermore, VIP is a powerful vasodilator in cerebral arteries (Suzuki et al. 1984) including the choroidal artery (Lindvall et al. 1978). NPY has been found in a large number of peripheral and central vessels, located in the noradrenergic, sympathetic nerves. Both a direct contractile effect and a modulation of the sympathetic contractile effect on blood vessels has been described (Edvinsson et al. 1987). In the gut, NPY has been found to modulate epithelial ion transport (Friel et al. 1986). Thus, VIP and NPY may be involved in both flow regulation and epithelial function in the choroid plexus.

References

Coons AH, Leduc EG, Connolloy JM (1955) Studies on antibody production. I. A method for histochemical demonstration of specific antibody and its application to a study of hyperimmune rabbit. J Exp Med 102:49–60

Crook RB, Pruisner SB (1986) Vasoactive intestinal peptide stimulates cyclic AMP metabolism in choroid plexus epithelial cells. Brain Res 384:138–144

Dawbarn D, Hunt SP, Emson PC (1984) Neuropeptide Y – regional distribution, chromatographic characterization and immunohistochemical demonstration in post-mortem after chronic sympathectomy. Exp Eye Res 37:213–215

Ekblad E, Håkanson R, Sundler F (1984) VIP and PHI coexist with an NPY-like peptide in intramural neurones of the small intestine. Regul Pept 10:47–55

Edvinsson L, Rosendahl-Helgesen S, Uddman R (1983) Substance P localization, concentration and release in cerebral arteries, choroid plexus and dura mater. Cell Tissue Res 234:1–7

Edvinsson L, Copeland JR, Emson PC, McCulloch J, Uddman R (1987) Nerve fibers containing neuropeptide Y in the cerebrovascular bed: immunocytochemistry, radioimmunoassay, and vasomotor effects. J Cereb Blood Flow Metabol 7:45–57

Friel DD, Miller RJ, Walker MW (1986) Neuropeptide Y: a powerful modulator of epithelial ion transport. Br J Pharmacol 88:425–431

Hara JH, Hamill GS, Jacobowitz DM (1985) Origin of cholinergic nerves to the rat major cerebral arteries: coexistence with vasoactive intestinal polypeptide. Brain Res Bull 14:179–188

Itoh N, Obata K, Yanaihara N, Okamoto H (1983) Human preprovasoactive intestinal polypeptide contains a novel PH1-27-like peptide, PHM-27. Nature 304:547–549

Leblanc GG, Trimmer BA, Landis SC (1987) Neuropeptide Y-like immunoreactivity in rat cranial parasympathetic neurons: coexistence with vasoactive intestinal peptide and choline acetyltransferase. Proc Natl Acad Sci USA 84:3511–3515

Lindvall M, Alumets J, Edvinsson L, Fahrenkrug J, Håkanson R, Hanko J, Owman C, Schaffalitzky de Muckadell OB, Sundler F (1978) Peptidergic (VIP) nerves in the mammalian choroid plexus. Neurosci Lett 9:77–82

Lindvall M, Owman C (1981) Autonomic nerves in the mammalian choroid plexus and their influence on the formation of cerebrospinal fluid. J Cereb Blood Flow Metab 1:245–266

Lindvall M, Gustafsson Å, Hedner P, Owman C (1985) Stimulation of cyclic adenosine 3′, 5′-monophosphate formation in rabbit choroid plexus by beta-receptor agonists and vasoactive intestinal peptide. Neurosci Lett 54:153–157

Suzuki Y, McMaster D, Lederis K, Rorstad OP (1984) Characterization of the relaxant effects of vasoactive intestinal peptide (VIP) and PHI on isolated brain arteries. Brain Res 322:9–16

Tramu G, Pillez A, Leonardelli J (1980) An efficient method for the successive or simultaneous location of two antigens by immunocytochemistry. J Histochem Cytochem 26:322–324

Effect of Sympathetic Denervation on the Cerebral Fluid Formation Rate in Increased Intracranial Pressure

H. Sakamoto and S. Nishimura

Department of Neurosurgery, Osaka City University Medical School, 1-5-7 Asahi-machi, Abeno-ku, Osaka (Japan)

Introduction

The effect of increased intracranial pressure (ICP) on the formation rate (Vf) of cerebrospinal fluid (CSF) has not been firmly established. This is because there are several influential factors on Vf in addition to ICP and also ventriculocisternal perfusion, the most reliable method for estimating Vf, has the drawback of possibly reducing Vf in prolonged perfusion with ICP kept constant (Martins et al. 1977). Cervical sympathetic nerve activity has an influence on the neurogenic control for CSF formation by the choroid plexus (Lindvall et al. 1978), and this nerve activity changes in increased ICP (Sakamoto et al. 1986b). We have shown that Vf decreases with a moderate increase in ICP (Sakamoto et al. 1986a). In the present study, using the perfusion method we measured the changes of Vf in animals with cervical sympathetic denervation in order to investigate whether or not the reduction of Vf in raised ICP was mediated primarily by sympathetic nerves.

Method

The experiments were performed on adult cats of either sex weighing 2.7 to 4.5 kg. In the control group, 6 animals were paralyzed with pancuronium bromide after tracheostomy and mechanically ventilated with a mixture of oxygen and nitrous oxide. A 25 gauge needle, which was connected to a strain gauge transducer for measurement of CSF pressure and also to a motorized syringe for the perfusion of the CSF space, was inserted into each lateral ventricle. With ICP maintained at the opening pressure, ventriculocisternal perfusion was continued at a perfusion rate of 0.107 ml/min for 6 hr while the steady state was documented. Relative concentrations of blue dextran in the outflow sample were determined by a spectrophotometer and Vf (μl/min) was calculated by Pappenheimer's method (Heisey et al. 1962). The relation between perfusion time and VF was estimated in the control group.

In the experimental group, 11 animals were sympathectomized by bilateral removal of the superior cervical ganglion. Sham operations were done in 9 animals (sham group). On the 8th postoperative day the perfusion was prepared in a procedure similar to that of the control group. Vf was determined at the ICP of the opening pressure, and was then measured at the increased ICP of 14 mm Hg and 24 mm Hg by stepwise increases in the height of the cisternal outflow cannulae. The reference point of ICP was the external auditory meatus.

Result

The control group showed a significant decrease in Vf ($p < 0.001$) at a rate of 4.20% per hr for 6 hr of perfusion, although ICP, blood pressure, arterial pH and pCO_2 and blood osmotic pressure were kept constant. The raw value of Vf was experimentally obtained and the calculated value of Vf was estimated from the raw Vf at the opening pressure would have diminished at a rate of 4.20% per hour if perfusion had been continued at the opening pressure, as was observed in the control group (Table 1). The raw value of the Vf was significantly lower than the corresponding calculated value of Vf at an ICP of 24 mm Hg in both the sympathectomized and sham groups, but at each level of ICP there were no significant differences in the raw Vf between these two groups (Table 1). Vf was found to be a function of cerebral perfusion pressure (CPP; mm Hg). A regression line for the experimental group was Vf $= -1.1 + 0.0194 \times$ CPP; $r = 0.58$, and that for the sham group was Vf $= -0.2 + 0.0116 \times$ CPP, $r = 0.51$. The slope of each line was significantly different from 0 (experimental group; $p < 0.001$, sham group; $p < 0.025$), but there was no significant difference between these two slopes. There was no significant difference in blood pressure, arterial pCO_2 and pH or blood osmolarity between these two groups.

Table 1. Effect of increased intracranial pressure on CSF formation rate

Group	Intracranial pressure (mm Hg)	Cerebral perfusion pressure (mm Hg)	CSF formation rate (µl/min)	
			raw	calculated
Sham	opening pressure (5.9±1.7)	141±23	17.1±2.9	–
	14	137±17	12.8±1.9	14.5±2.3
	24	124±16	10.1±3.4*	13.7±2.5
Experimental	opening pressure (6.0±1.7)	136±14	18.4±5.0	–
	14	125±15	11.4±4.6*	16.3±6.1
	24	111±16	8.4±3.7*	15.0±4.2

Values are means ±SD. * Significantly different from calculated value of CSF formation rate, $p < 0.05$, paired-t test

Summary

Eliminating the possible error of a reduced CSF formation rate using the perfusion method, we demonstrated that the CSF formation rate decreased significantly with increased ICP up to 24 mm Hg. Neither the CSF formation rate nor the slope of the regression line between cerebral perfusion pressure and formation rate showed a significant difference between the animals with and without sympathetic innervation to the choroid plexus. The results suggest that sympathetic nerves have a minor effect on bulk formation of CSF and a decrease in cerebral perfusion pressure is the major cause for diminished formation rate with increased ICP up to 24 mm Hg.

References

Heisey SR, Held D, Pappenheimer JR (1962) Bulk flow and diffusion in the cerebrospinal fluid system of the goat. Am J Physiol 203:775–781

Lindvall M, Edvinsson L, Owman C (1978) Sympathetic nervous control of cerebrospinal fluid production from the choroid plexus. Science 201:176–178

Martins AN, Newby N, Doyle TF (1977) Sources of error in measuring cerebrospinal fluid formation by ventriculocisternal perfusion. J Neurol Neurosurg Psychiatry 40:645–650

Sakamoto H, Nakamura T, Marmarou A, Becker DP (1986a) Comparison of CSF formation and outflow resistance measured by ventriculo-cisternal perfusion and volume manipulation techniques. In: Miller JD, Teasdale GM, Rowan JO, Galbraith SL, Mendelow AD (eds) Intracranial Pressure VI. Springer, Berlin Heidelberg New York Tokyo, p 108–110

Sakamoto H, Tanaka K, Nakamura T, Nishimura S, Matsuura S (1986b) Direct observation of autonomic nerve activity in experimental acute brain swelling. In: Miller JD, Teasdale GM, Rowan JO, Galbraith SL, Mendelow AD (eds) Intracranial Pressure VI. Springer, Berlin Heidelberg New York Tokyo, p 166–173

CSF Production in Patients with Increased Intracranial Pressure

S.E. Børgesen and F. Gjerris

University Clinic of Neurosurgery, Rigshopitalet, DK-2100 Copenhagen (Denmark)

The relationship between intracranial pressure (ICP), resistance to CSF outflow (R_{out}), CSF formation rate (RF), and the pressure in the sagittal sinus (P_{ss}) is generally accepted to be linear (Børgesen 1984, Ekstedt 1978, Kosteljanetz 1985).

The function may be expressed as:

$$ICP = FR * R_{out} + P_{ss} \qquad (1)$$

The regression is given by the FR. The linearity of the function shows that the formation rate is constant even as the intracranial pressure goes up. However, this is in contradiction with the often observed decline in CSF production in patients drained following subarachnoid hemorrhage, where often less than 100 ml CSF drainage is adequate for keeping the intracranial pressure at acceptable levels.

Børgesen and Gjerris (1987) found, in a series of 230 patients, a mean CSF production rate of 0.30 ml/min. It was shown that the production rate tended to decline in patients with increased intracranial pressure.

This series has now been extended to 333 patients.

The results of ICP monitoring and measurement of R_{out} are presented here.

Methods

In all 333 patients, the mean intracranial pressure (MICP) was monitored for more than 24 hr via an intraventricular catheter connected to a pressure transducer. Following the pressure recording, the resistance to CSF outflow was measured by a lumboventricular perfusion (Børgesen 1984, Kosteljanetz 1985).

Material

The investigations were carried out in patients with normal pressure hydrocephalus ($n=240$) or with increased intracranial pressure in conjunction with acute hydrocephalus ($n=29$), acute subarachnoid hemorrhage ($n=21$), and benign intracranial hypertension ($n=43$).

Intracranial Pressure VII
Eds.: J.T. Hoff and A.L. Betz
© Springer-Verlag Berlin Heidelberg 1989

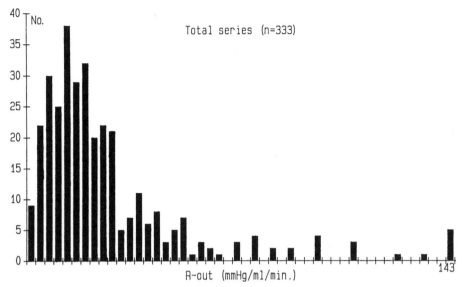

Fig. 1. Distribution of R_{out} in the total series of 333 patients, divided into two groups with either normal (< 12 mm Hg) or increased (> 12 mm Hg) MICP

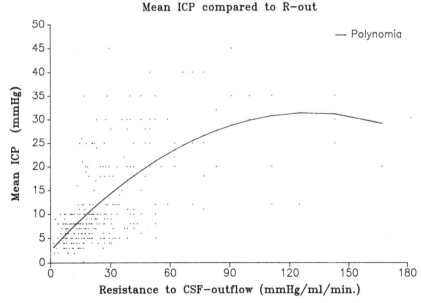

Fig. 2. Scatterplot of MICP by R_{out}. The best curvefit is given by: $MICP = 2.53 + 0.44 * R_{out} - 0.002 * R_{out}^2$ ($r_{xy} = 0.67$, $p < 0.001$)

Results

In Fig. 1, the distribution of resistance to outflow in the total material is shown.

R_{out} varied between 1 and 143 mm Hg/ml/min, mean 28.36, standard deviation (SD) 25.96. The mean R_{out} in patients with increased intracranial pressure was 49.71 (SD = 34.65). The mean R_{out} in patients with normal pressure hydrocephalus was 20.04 (SD = 15.00). This difference is statistically significant (T-test, $P < 0.001$).

In Fig. 2, the MICP is compared to R_{out}. The linear regression correlating MICP to R_{out} is described by:

$$ICP = 0.23 * R_{out} + 5.9 \tag{2}$$

The correlation coefficient of this function is 0.61 ($P < 0.001$). However, better fit is obtained with the polynomial:

$$ICP = 2.53 + 0.44 * R_{out} - 0.002 * (R_{out})^2 \tag{3}$$

The correlation coefficient of this function is 0.67 ($P < 0.001$).

If the regression line is computed for patients with intracranial pressure above 12 mm Hg, the slope of the regression line is 0.11. The correlation coefficient of this function is 0.42.

Discussion

The relationship between intracranial pressure, resistance to outflow, formation rate, and the pressure in the sagittal sinus may be expressed by the formula given above (formula 1). This correlation shows a stale formation rate, expressed as the regression of the linear correlation between ICP and R_{out}. The function has been tested in the present series on data collected from 333 patients where ICP and R_{out} were measured. From formula 2, the regression of the linear correlation shows a mean CSF production rate of 0.23 ml/min. The correlation coefficient of this function to the whole material was 0.61. However, a better curvefit was obtained by using a second order polynomial, as given in formula 3. The curve expressed by this function is shown in Fig. 2 and clearly indicates that the production rate of CSF decreases with increasing intracranial pressure.

It may thus be concluded that while a linear relationship exists between ICP and R_{out}, indicating resistance to outflow to be a major factor responsible for increases in ICP, it is shown that in a series of patients with different causes of increased intracranial pressure and also different length of histories, the production of CSF tends to decrease with increasing intracranial pressure.

In patients with increased intracranial pressure this decrease in production may amount to more than 50% of the base line formation rate.

The mechanism behind the reduction in CSF production may be explained to some extent by a pressure dependent reduction of the fraction of CSF that

334

originates from the ventricular walls and the brain surface. The filtration process in the choroid plexus may also be influenced by the pressure increase. While the production of CSF continues in high pressure hydrocephalus, it is also partly reduced by the resulting pressure increase. A balance exists between the R_{out}, ICP and FR, where the R_{out} is determined by the causal disorder and the ICP is modified by the FR.

Summary

In 333 patients the resistance to outflow of CSF (R_{out}) was compared to the mean intracranial pressure (MICP). The correlation between R_{out} and MICP is normally accepted to be linear, indicating a constant CSF formation rate (FR). In the present study, the best correlation between MICP and R_{out} is given by a second degree polynomia. The result may be interpreted as an indication of decreasing FR with increasing intracranial pressure.

Acknowledgement. The study has received financial support from ESKOFOT A/S, Denmark.

References

Børgesen SE (1984) Conductance to outflow of CSF in normal pressure hydrocephalus. Acta Neurochir (Wien) 71:1–45

Børgesen SE, Gjerris F (1987) Relationships between intracranial pressure, ventricular size, and resistance to CSF outflow. J Neurosurg 67:535–539

Ekstedt J (1978) CSF hydrodynamic studies in man. 2. Normal hydrodynamic variables related to CSF pressure and flow. J Neurol Neurosurg Psychiatry 41:345–353

Gjerris F, Børgesen SE, Hoppe E et al. (1982) The conductance to outflow of CSF in adults with high-pressure hydrocephalus. Acta Neurochir (Wien) 64:59–67

Kosteljanetz M (1985) Pressure – volume conditions in patients with subarachnoid and/or intraventricular hemorrhage. J Neurosurg 63:398–403

Changes in Intracranial CSF Volume After LP

R. Grant[1], B. Condon, I. Hart, and G.M. Teasdale

Institute of Neurological Sciences, Southern General Hospital, Glasgow (UK)
[1] Present address: Department of Clinical Neurosciences, Western General Hospital, University of Edinburgh (UK)

Introduction

Post-LP headache has always been considered to be due to "low intracranial pressure" secondary to a reduction in total craniospinal CSF volume. Previously, it has not been possible to quantitate the volume of cranial CSF lost after LP and, therefore, it has not been possible to calculate how much total intracranial CSF volume is lost 24 hr after LP [$\Delta tCSF_{(v)}$] or to say if this is related to the development of post LP headache.

The aim of this study was to quantitate the volume of intracranial CSF lost 24 h after LP [$\Delta CSF_{(v)}$] by a Magnetic Resonance Imaging (MRI) technique and to investigate the relationship with headache.

Subjects and Methods

Twenty patients with neurological disorders were studied. There were eight males aged from 25–71 years (mean 41.5 years) and 12 females aged from 14–64 years (mean 38.5 years). Each patient had intracranial CSF volume measured by MRI before lumbar puncture and within 24 hr afterwards. Spinal puncture was performed in the lumbar region with an 18 gauge needle. 10 ml of CSF was removed and the patient was kept in bed for at least 14 hr.

At the time of the second scan the presence of headache was noted.

Magnetic Resonance Imaging

Total cranial CSF volume [$tCSF_{(v)}$], ventricular CSF volume [$vCSF_{(v)}$], cortical sulcal CSF volume [$csCSF_{(v)}$] and posterior fossa CSF volume [$pfCSF_{(v)}$] measurements were performed using MRI as previously described (Condon et al. 1986).

Results

The tCSF$_{(v)}$ decreased in 19 of the 20 patients (range 1.8–158.6 ml) (Fig. 1). Most CSF was lost from the cortical sulcal spaces (Table 1). The ΔtCSF$_{(v)}$ was not related to the patient's age or to the initial resting volume. The patient with an increase in tCSF$_{(v)}$ (8.8 ml) after LP did not develop headache and the two patients who lost > 50 ml had the most severe and prolonged headache. There was a significant overlap between the remaining patients.

Table 1. Mean intracranial CSF volume measurements before and after LP

	tCSF$_{(v)}$ ml mean (±SEM)	csCSF$_{(v)}$ ml mean (±SEM)	vCSF$_{(v)}$ ml mean (±SEM)	pfCSF$_{(v)}$ ml mean (±SEM)
Pre LP	179.8 (17.0)	147.6 (14.3)	17.0 (2.3)	15.2 (1.5)
Post LP	151.6 (16.6)	122.1 (14.1)	15.8 (2.2)	14.0 (1.2)

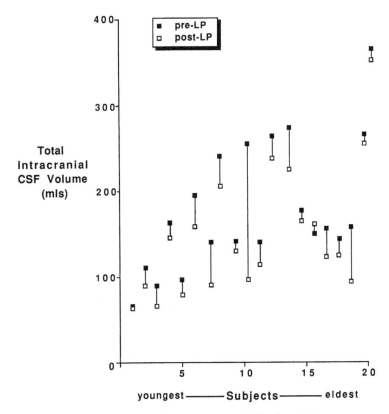

Fig. 1. Change in total intracranial CSF volume following LP (individual results)

337

Conclusions

This study demonstrates, for the first time, the extent of reduction in intracranial CSF volume following LP and the relationship with post LP headache. Most of the CSF is lost from the cortical sulci (especially from the convexity). The results of this study support the role of reduced intracranial CSF volume in the pathogenesis of post-lumbar puncture headache.

Reference

Condon B et al. (1986) Intracranial CSF volumes determined using Magnetic Resonance Imaging. Lancet I:1355–1358

Changes in Intracranial CSF Volume During Hypercapnia and Hypocapnia

R. Grant[1], B. Condon, J. Patterson, J. Rowan, and G.M. Teasdale

University Department of Neurosurgery, Institute of Neurological Sciences, Glasgow (UK)
[1] Present address: Department of Clinical Neurosciences, Western General Hospital, University of Edinburgh (UK)

Introduction

To what extent does a change in cerebral blood volume affect intracranial CSF volume? A Magnetic Resonance Imaging (MRI) method was used to assess changes in total intracranial CSF volume during 7% CO_2 inhalation and during hyperventilation with 60% O_2.

The aim of the study was to measure the direction and magnitude of change of intracranial CSF volume in response to hypercapnia and hypocapnia.

Methods and Subjects

Total intracranial CSF volume was measured using the IRCP 300/400/5000 pulse sequence with the 240 mm thick slice select and imaging in the sagittal plane (Condon et al. 1986). This MR sequence produces an image of cranial CSF only. Intracranial CSF volume was calculated from the signal intensity from within the head.

a) CSF Volume and CO_2 Inhalation

Twelve healthy subjects were studied (9 males and 3 females). A rubber mouthpiece was placed in the subject's mouth and then connected to a two-way valve. Tubing extended from the inspiratory limb of the two-way valve to outside the MRI radiofrequency shield. During the assessment of "resting" intracranial CSF volume, the inspiratory limb of the tubing was left open so that the subject was able to breath fresh air. A repeat scan was taken during inhalation of 7% CO_2 from a Douglas bag attached to the inspiratory limb of tubing. End-tidal pCO_2 was measured by capnograph recorder.

b) CSF Volume and Hyperventilation During High Flow Oxygen

Twelve healthy subjects were studied before and during hyperventilation with 60% O_2. The method used was similar to that of CO_2 inhalation, but O_2 was

Intracranial Pressure VII
Eds.: J.T. Hoff and A.L. Betz
© Springer-Verlag Berlin Heidelberg 1989

delivered via the inspiratory limb. The degree of reduction in $PaCO_2$ was measured by "arterialised" venous blood sampling before and during hyperventilation with 60% O_2.

Results

A reduction in total CSF volume was recorded in all subjects following inhalation of 7% CO_2. This ranged from -0.7 ml to -23.7 ml (mean -9.3 ml, SD 7.67) and represented a percentage reduction in total intracranial CSF volume of -0.9 to -19.4% (mean -8.8%). End-expiratory CO_2 increased in all cases (mean 13.25 mm Hg, SD 4.18). There was no correlation between an individual subject's change in end-expiratory CO_2 and the reduction in CSF volume.

During hyperventilation total intracranial CSF volume increased in all subjects. This ranged from $+0.7$ ml to $+26.7$ ml (mean $+12.7$ ml, SD 6.84). As a percentage of the total CSF volume this was $+0.3$ to $+13.6\%$ (mean $+7.6\%$). The estimated change in pCO_2 was 10.2 mm Hg (SD 1.2).

Conclusions

This study provides direct confirmation of the modified Monro-Kellie doctrine and a measure of the extent of the reciprocal interactions between CSF volume and cerebral blood volume (CBV) in human subjects. The mean change in intracranial CSF volume is similar to that found in CBV under similar circumstances. Greenberg demonstrated a change in CBV of 0.0495 ml/100 g brain/torr pCO_2 (Greenberg et al. 1978). Hypercapnia induces an increase in CBV and an increase in intracranial pressure. The degree of alteration in CBV in individuals will depend on differences in brain size, vascular compliance, intracranial pressure and vascular responsiveness to changes in arterial CO_2 tension. These factors may account for the observed variability of change of the CSF volume in this study.

References

Condon B et al. (1986) Use of Magnetic Resonance Imaging to measure intracranial CSF volume. Lancet I:1355–1357
Greenberg J et al. (1978) Local cerebral blood volume response to carbon dioxide in man. Circ Res 43(2):324–331

Intracranial CSF Volume Distribution in Normal Pressure Hydrocephalus

R. Grant[1], B. Condon, D.M. Hadley, and G.M. Teasdale

University Department of Neurosurgery, Institute of Neurological Sciences, Glasgow (UK)
[1] Present address: Department of Clinical Neurosciences, Western General Hospital, University of Edinburgh (UK)

Introduction

The diagnosis of Normal Pressure Hydrocephalus (NPH) is supported by CT scanning which demonstrates enlarged ventricles out of proportion to the degree of cortical atrophy, however, quantitation of the degree of atrophy or hydrocephalus by CT is difficult and often inaccurate. Intracranial CSF volumes can now be accurately and reproducibly measured using MRI (Condon et al. 1986, Grant et al. 1987).

Intracranial CSF volume measurements were performed on patients with NPH to determine whether it is possible to distinguish NPH from changes found in normal aging or in dementia of other causes.

Subjects and Methods

Fourteen patients with clinical and radiological features suggesting NPH were studied (10 females, 4 males). Ages ranged from 59 to 78 years (mean 68.9 years). Pressure monitoring was carried out in eight patients and in the remainder the diagnosis was not in doubt. Twelve patients with dementia of other causes were scanned (8 females, 4 males). Ages ranged from 54–89 years (mean 71.7 years). There was a wide range of severity of dementia. Twenty-five healthy subjects were also scanned (15 females, 10 males). Ages ranged from 50–91 years (mean 64.4 years).

Using a specially designed MRI pulse sequence (IRCP 300/400/5000) images of intracranial CSF only were obtained. Total intracranial CSF volume [$tCSF_{(v)}$], cortical sulcal CSF volume [$csCSF_{(v)}$] and ventricular CSF volume [$vCSF_{(v)}$] were measured and the ventricular:cortical sulcal ratio (v:cs ratio) calculated as previously described (Grant et al. 1987).

Results

Patients with NPH frequently had a 'smooth concave' cut-off of CSF at the foramen magnum in contrast to the acute 'V-shaped' cut-off found in normals

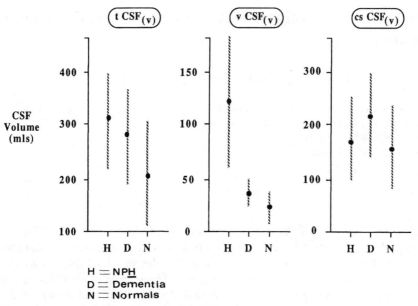

Fig. 1. Mean and xl SD of intracranial CSF volume measurements in NPH, dementia and normal subjects

Table 1. Mean intracranial CSF volume measurements in patients with NPH, dementia and normal subjects

	tCSF$_{(v)}$ mean ($\pm$SEM)	csCSF$_{(v)}$ mean ($\pm$SEM)	vCSF$_{(v)}$ mean ($\pm$SEM)	v:cs ratio
NPH	318.4 (21.4)	172.2 (19.4)	121.9 (13.3)	0.98 (0.24)
Dementia	280.7 (25.2)	218.8 (22.2)	40.6 (2.7)	0.20 (0.02)
Normals	206.2 (19.3)	165.5 (16.2)	24.6 (2.8)	0.15 (0.01)

and in patients with dementia. There was a significant overlap in tCSF$_{(v)}$ and csCSF (v) in all groups (Fig. 1 and Table 1). vCSF$_{(v)}$ ranged from 46.1–202.7 ml in patients with NPH compared with 27.8–61 ml and 9.7–67.6 ml in patients with dementia and healthy subjects respectively. vCSF$_{(v)}$ was age dependent in the latter two groups only. The v:cs ratio was always >0.34 in patients with NPH (range 0.34–3.19), <0.31 in patients with dementia (range 0.15–0.31) and <0.25 in healthy subjects (range 0.06–0.25).

Conclusions

This study demonstrates that while vCSF$_{(v)}$ is a good indicator of hydrocephalus, the v:cs ratio better differentiates patients with NPH from asymptomatic subjects with hydrocephalus ex vacuo or with dementia of other causes. The v:cs ratio may also be a useful indicator of progression of the NPH when serial scans are performed.

References

Condon B et al. (1986) Intracranial CSF volumes determined by Magnetic Resonance Imaging. Lancet I:1355–1358

Grant R et al. (1987) Human cranial CSF volumes measured by MRI: sex and age influences. Magn Reson Imaging 5:465–468

Benign Intracranial Hypertension: Brain Swelling and Cranial CSF Volume

R. Grant[1], B. Condon, J. Rowan, and G.M. Teasdale

University Department of Neurosurgery, Institute of Neurological Sciences, Glasgow (UK)
[1] Present address: Department of Clinical Neurosciences, Western General Hospital, University of Edinburgh (UK)

Introduction

Changes to the intracranial CSF volume in benign intracranial hypertension (BIH) are important to concepts of the disease, but evidence is controversial. Is total intracranial CSF volume increased (Davidoff 1956) or is the cerebral ventricular volume decreased (Reid et al. 1980)? Intracranial CSF volume can now be measured using an MRI method (Condon et al. 1986).

The aim of this study was to measure total, cortical sulcal and ventricular CSF volumes in patients with BIH and compare them with those of healthy subjects.

Subjects and Methods

Fourteen female patients aged from 14–46 years (mean 27 years) were studied. Seven of these patients had "definite" BIH (headaches of raised intracranial pressure with intracranial pressures of >18 cm CSF, papilledema and a normal CT and MRI scan) and seven had "probable" BIH (all the above except papilledema). Thirty age-related females acted as control subjects. MRI intracranial CSF volumes were measured prior to lumbar puncture/pressure monitoring. Total intracranial CSF volume [$tCSF_{(v)}$], cortical sulcal CSF volume [$csCSF_{(v)}$] and ventricular CSF volume [$vCSF_{(v)}$] were calculated from the MR image.

Results

The mean $tCSF_{(v)}$ and $csCSF_{(v)}$ were smaller in patients with BIH than in the healthy subjects, however, this was not statistically significant ($p=0.059$ and $p=0.11$ respectively). $vCSF_{(v)}$ was significantly smaller in patients with BIH ($p<0.0001$: Mann-Whitney Test) (Table 1).

The mean intracranial CSF volumes were less in patients with probable BIH (i.e. without papilledema), however, the mean age was also less and thus it was difficult to compare results satisfactorily.

There was no evidence of a localised or generalised increase in brain water content on the T_2 weighted structural scans.

Eds.: J.T. Hoff and A.L. Betz
© Springer-Verlag Berlin Heidelberg 1989

Table 1. Mean intracranial CSF volume measurements in patients with BIH and in normal subjects

	$tCSF_{(v)}$ mean ($\pm$SEM)	$csCSF_{(v)}$ mean ($\pm$SEM)	$vCSF_{(v)}$ mean ($\pm$SEM)
BIH	87.7 mls (30.7)	71.2 mls (7.2)	6.0 mls (0.7)
Normal	107.5 mls (26.5)	85.2 mls (4.2)	11.9 mls (0.7)

Conclusions

Ventricular CSF volume is significantly decreased in many but not all patients with BIH. This study provides evidence against an increase in intracranial CSF volume with distended cortical sulcal spaces (Davidoff 1956) and supports the theory that the brain is swollen. Whether the brain is swollen or congested cannot be detected directly, however, there was no evidence of increased intracellular or extracellular water in the brain on T_2 weighted images. The relationship of changes in CSF volume, total cranial cavity size, and severity of disease still requires investigation.

References

Condon B et al. (1986) Intracranial CSF volumes determined by Magnetic Resonance Imaging. Lancet I: 1355–1358

Davidoff LM (1956) Pseudotumour cerebri. Benign intracranial hypertension. Neurology 6:605–615

Reid AC et al. (1980) Volume of the ventricles in benign intracranial hypertension. Lancet II:7–8

CSF Distribution in Acute and Chronic Obstructive Hydrocephalus and the Response to Shunting

R. Grant[1], B. Condon, D.M. Hadley, and G.M. Teasdale

University Department of Neurosurgery, Institute of Neurological Sciences, Glasgow (UK)
[1] Present address: Department of Clinical Neurosciences, Western General Hospital, University of Edinburgh (UK)

Introduction

Re-distribution of intracranial CSF volumes is the fundamental change in obstructive hydrocephalus. Until recently it was not possible to measure CSF volumes and, therefore, not possible to compare acute and chronic hydrocephalus and the response to treatment. Using a Magnetic Resonance Imaging (MRI) technique (Condon et al. 1986), we have measured the total intracranial CSF volume [$tCSF_{(v)}$], the ventricular CSF volume [$vCSF_{(v)}$], the cortical sulcal CSF volume [$csCSF_{(v)}$] and the ventricular:cortical sulcal CSF ratio [v:cs ratio].

The aim of the study was to measure intracranial CSF volume distribution in five patients with acute, four patients with chronic, and one patient with acute on chronic obstructive hydrocephalus and to determine the effects of ventriculoperitoneal shunting.

Subjects and Methods

In five patients, hydrocephalus was known to be over six months duration (chronic) and in five patients less than three months (acute). One of the patients with chronic hydrocephalus developed acute decompensation. Four patients had aqueduct stenosis (chronic), one bilateral acoustic neuromas (acute on chronic), and five acute hydrocephalus (two brain stem gliomas, one pineal region tumour, one cerebellar secondary and one cerebellar hematoma).

Four of those presenting 'acutely' had papilledema. Seven patients had intracranial CSF volume measurements repeated 4–10 days (mean 7 days) after operation.

Two sagittal CSF volume sequences (IRCP 300/400/5000) were performed. The first had a slice select of 240 mm, thus giving an image of the total cranial CSF volume. The second scan had a slice select set to a diameter that would include the ventricles and exclude overlying and underlying cortical sulci. The CSF volumes were calculated as described by Condon et al. 1986.

Intracranial Pressure VII
Eds.: J.T. Hoff and A.L. Betz
© Springer-Verlag Berlin Heidelberg 1989

Results

The results of the tCSF$_{(v)}$ and csCSF$_{(v)}$ are shown in Figures 1 and 2. The characteristic features in patients with acute hydrocephalus were a normal tCSF$_{(v)}$, an increased vCSF$_{(v)}$ in all cases (range 44.9–89.7 ml) and a csCSF$_{(v)}$ >1 SD below the mean for the patient's age. The v:cs ratio was increased in all cases (normal <0.30) and in the most severe case was >1.0. In the two acute cases studied after shunting, CSF volume measurements returned to the normal range in all parameters.

In patients with chronic aqueduct stenosis, tCSF$_{(v)}$ was always increased (348.0–927.3 ml) as was vCSF$_{(v)}$ (range 168.5–748.3 ml) and the csCSF$_{(v)}$ was characteristically >1 SD above the mean for the patient's age. The v:cs ratio in the patients with aqueduct stenosis was >0.9. Following V-P shunting the tCSF$_{(v)}$ remained elevated, the vCSF$_{(v)}$ and the v:cs ratio fell significantly but did not always return to within the normal range.

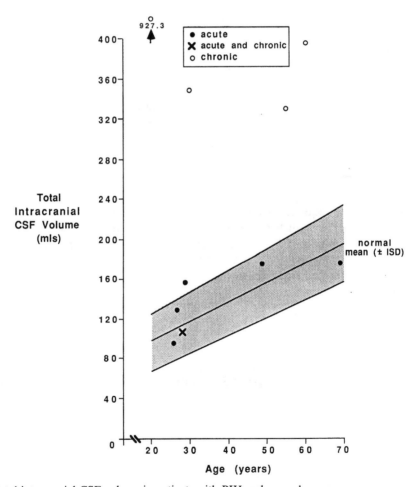

Fig. 1. Total intracranial CSF volume in patients with BIH and normal range

347

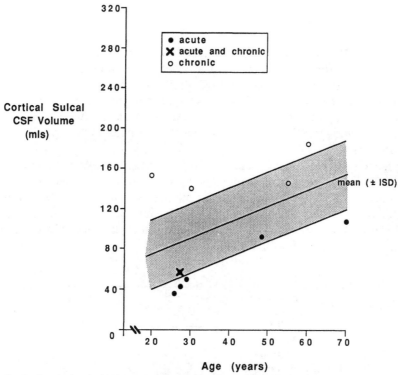

Fig. 2. Cortical sulcal CSF volume in patients with BIH and normal range

Conclusions

CSF volume sequences using MRI can reliably demonstrate hydrocephalus and may help to distinguish 'acute' obstructive hydrocephalus from 'chronic' obstructive hydrocephalus. CSF volume measurement has a valuable role in the assessment of hydrocephalus for diagnostic, management, and research purposes and can be performed to establish the success of post-operative ventricular decompression.

Reference

Condon B et al. (1986) Intracranial CSF volumes determined using Magnetic Resonance Imaging. Lancet I:1355-1358

Reproducibility and Reliability of Measurement of Resistance to CSF Outflow by Subarachnoid Perfusion

F. Gjerris, S.E. Børgesen, J.F. Schmidt, O. Fedders, and M.J. Albeck

University Clinic of Neurosurgery, Rigshospitalet, DK-2100 Copenhagen (Denmark)

It is generally agreed that the main site of CSF absorption is the arachnoid villi. The CSF resorptive capacity can be evaluated by several methods which, during the last decade, have been evaluated especially in patients with hydrocephalus (for review: see Børgesen 1984, Kosteljanetz 1987). Measurement of conductance to CSF outflow, or the reciprocal value resistance to CSF outflow (R_{out}), is a parameter which especially has shown its use as a predictive value of clinical results after shunting in patients suffering from normal pressure hydrocephalus (Børgesen and Gjerris 1982), and also in the treatment of patients with pseudotumor cerebri (Sørensen et al. 1989). However, as stressed by Børgesen (1984) the measurements must be reliable and reproducible. In a previous study we found an acceptable concordance of repeated investigations of R_{out} in 28 patients (Gjerris et al. 1986).

The purpose of the present study was to present the data from our repeated measurements of R_{out} and, in a prospective study, to compare the lumbo-ventricular with the ventriculo-ventricular method.

Methods

A) The material of repeated measurements comprises 80 patients with normal pressure hydrocephalus (NPH), 34 patients with high pressure hydrocephalus (HPH), and 16 patients with pseudotumor cerebri (benign intracranial hypertension (BIH). Most of the patients with NPH or HPH had R_{out} measured by the lumboventricular (LV) perfusion test (Børgesen et al. 1978, 1989). While in the BIH group the lumbo-lumbar infusion (LL) test was used (Gjerris et al. 1985, Sørensen et al. 1989).

B) The prospective study comprises 16 patients with NPH. ICP was measured via a cannula in the right frontal horn of the ventricular system through a precoronal burr hole. ICP was measured by a disposable pressure monitoring system (Bentley Lab., Uden, Holland) and the amplifying system was from DANICA (Medical Division, Denmark).

After monitoring of ICP for 6 hr, R_{out} was measured by a ventriculo-ventricular perfusion test with the patients in the supine position (Gjerris et al. 1981). After a known steady state ICP was obtained, an infusion of Ringer lactate (V_{in}) was started at a rate of 1.82 ml per min. The outflow volume (V_{in}) was sampled from the outflow tube in periods of 3 min and measured at 6–7 different pressures, obtained by elevating the outlet of the outflow tube. With the assumption of a constant CSF formation of 0.4 ml per min, the absorbed CSF-volume per min (V_{abs}) could be calculated from the formula: $V_{abs} = V_{in} + 0.4 - V_{out}$. Thereafter, V_{abs} was related to the different steady-state levels of ICP and the slope of the best fitted line through the 6–7 pairs of values expresses the conductance to CSF. The resistance to outflow is calculated from the formula: $C_{out} * R_{out} = 1$.

The test was performed twice, each run separated by a resting interval of 15 min (VV_1 and VV_2). These early runs were only performed in the first 10 of the 16 patients.

On the next day, 2 further ventriculo-ventricular perfusion tests were performed (VV_3 and VV_4). In addition, measurement of R_{out} was performed by a lumbo-ventricular perfusion test with the patient in a lateral recumbent position (LV_1 and LV_2), again separated by a resting period of 15 min.

The statistics were computed on the SPSS/PC+ (SPSS Inc., Chicago, Illinois, USA).

Results

A) In the 80 NPH-patients a comparison of the repeated VV values after 24 hr ICP monitoring showed a good correlation (correlation coefficient = 0.74). The mean R_{out} was $20 \, \text{mm Hg} \times \text{ml}^{-1} \times \text{min}$ in the first LV test and $20 \, \text{mm Hg} \times \text{ml}^{-1} \times \text{min}$ in the second LV test.

In the 34 HPH-patients the correlation coefficient of the repeated investigations was 0.89. The mean R_{out} was $39 \, \text{mm Hg} \times \text{ml}^{-1} \times \text{min}$ in the first run and $28 \, \text{mm Hg} \times \text{ml}^{-1} \times \text{min}$ in the second.

In the 16 BIH-patients a comparison of repeated R_{out} measurements showed a very good correlation (correlation coefficient = 0.79). The mean R_{out} of LL_1 was $33 \, \text{mm Hg} \times \text{ml}^{-1} \times \text{min}$ and of LL_2, $31 \, \text{mm Hg} \times \text{ml}^{-1} \times \text{min}$.

B) R_{out} in both VV_1 and VV_2 were lower than R_{out} in all the investigations performed later, independently of whether they were performed as LV- or as VV-perfusion tests. No differences between LV_1, LV_2 and VV_3, VV_4 were found in the 16 patients.

Discussion

The calculation of R_{out} implies a constant rate of CSF production, irrespective of the increases in ICP during the study. We have, in a previous study, shown a decreasing formation rate in patients with raised ICP (Børgesen and Gjerris 1987), but we never found a decreased formation rate in the patients under the relatively short increase of ICP during a perfusion test. The CSF- and cerebral blood volumes are also presumed to be constant and, with the open system we use

350

for the perfusion test of R_{out}, these vascular reactions seem to be avoidable. Børgesen (1984) found in 8 patients with NPH that C_{out} did not vary more than 5% when it was measured twice. Nearly the same was found in 28 patients with repeated R_{out} measurements performed with only a short interval between the two runs (Gjerris et al. 1986).

The present study confirms the concordant findings of repeated measurements in BIH patients by Sklar et al. (1979), who found in 5 patients that C_{out} was unchanged despite several months between the 2 runs. However, the patients with HPH had significantly lower R_{out} in the second examination. This might be explained by opening of new resorptive channels in the arachnoid villi induced by elevations of ICP during the first examination of R_{out}.

The differences in the R_{out} values in the 16 consecutively investigated patients with a lower R_{out} value after 6 hr than after 24 hr of ICP monitoring might be explained by leakage of CSF after the newly made burr hole. This will lead to a too high estimation of absorption and, thereby, falsely low values of R_{out}. The problem of CSF-leakage is very important during the lumbo-ventricular perfusion test and has especially been underlined by Børgesen (1984) regarding the lumbar cannula.

The identical R_{out} values obtained using the ventriculo-ventricular or the lumbo-ventricular perfusion tests 24 hr after the application of the burr hole show that only one perfusion test is necessary in the investigation of hydrocephalic patients. The advantage of having the patients in the supine position is obvious. The lumbar perfusion test must, however, be saved for patients with BIH and can be performed as a lumbo-lumbar test which in the present study was found very reproducible. The presumption is that the conductance of the infusion cannula is sufficiently high (Børgesen 1984). In the present study the lumbo-lumbar test of R_{out} was reproducible but the test has not been compared with either the ventriculo-ventricular or the lumbo-ventricular tests.

In conclusion we have demonstrated that, after the insertion of the ventricular catheter, more than 6 hr must elapse before measurement of R_{out} should be performed by a ventriculo-ventricular perfusion test. However, after 24 hr we found lumbo-ventricular and ventriculo-ventricular perfusion tests reproducible and comparable in NPH-patients. In HPH-patients the second measurement had a significantly lower R_{out} value. In BIH-patients the lumbo-lumbar test of R_{out} was very reliable and repeated tests were concordant.

These findings suggest that one measurement of R_{out} is sufficient. One value gives reliable information in patients with NPH and BIH and nothing more could be gained by repetitive measurements.

Acknowledgement. The study has received financial support from the Research Foundation of Lundbeck and ESKOFOT A/S.

References

Børgesen SE (1984) Conductance to outflow of CSF in normal pressure hydrocephalus. Acta Neurochir (Wien) 71:1–41

Børgesen SE, Gjerris F (1982) The predictive value of conductance to outflow of CSF in normal hydrocephalus. Brain 105:65–86

Børgesen SE, Gjerris F (1987) The relationships between intracranial pressure, ventricular size and resistance to CSF outflow. J Neurosurg 67:535–539

Børgesen SE, Gjerris F, Schmidt JF (1989) Measurement of resistance to CSF outflow by subarachnoid perfusion. In: Gjerris F, Børgesen SE, Sørensen PS (eds) Outflow of the cerebrospinal fluid. Copenhagen, Munksgaard, in press

Børgesen SE, Gjerris F, Sørensen SC (1978) The resistance to cerebrospinal fluid absorption in humans. Acta Neurol Scand 57:88–96

Gjerris F, Børgesen SE, Hoppe E, Boesen F, Nordenbo AM (1982) The conductance to outflow of CSF in adults with high-pressure hydrocephalus. Acta Neurochir (Wien) 64:59–67

Gjerris F, Børgesen SE, Schmidt K, Sørensen PS, Gyring J (1986) Measurement of conductance to cerebrospinal fluid outflow by the steady-state perfusion method in patients with normal or increased intracranial pressure. In: Miller JD, Teasdale GM, Rowan JØ, Galbraith SL, Mendelow AD (eds) Intracranial Pressure VI. Springer, Berlin Heidelberg New York Tokyo, pp 411–416

Gjerris F, Sørensen PS, Vorstrup, S, Paulson OB (1985) Conductance to CSF-outflow, intracranial pressure and cerebral blood flow in patients with benign intracranial hypertension. Ann Neurol 17:158–162

Kosteljanetz M (1987) Intracranial pressure: cerebrospinal fluid dynamics and pressure–volume relations (Thesis). Acta Neurol Scand [Suppl] 75

Sklar FH, Beyer CW, Ramanathan M, Cooper PR, Clark WK (1979) Cerebrospinal fluid dynamics in patients with pseudotumor cerebri. Neurosurgery 5:208–216

Sørensen PS, Gjerris F, Schmidt JF (1989) Resistance to CSF outflow in benign intracranial hypertension. In: Gjerris F, Børgesen SE, Sørensen PS (eds) Outflow of the cerebrospinal fluid. Copenhagen, Munksgaard, in press

Measurement of Resistance to CSF Outflow – Clinical Experiences in 333 Patients

S.E. Børgesen, F. Gjerris, O. Fedders, J.F. Schmidt, M.J. Albeck, and P. Soelberg-Sørensen

University Clinic of Neurosurgery, Rigshospitalet, DK-2100 Copenhagen (Denmark)

Increasing interest in pathological conditions due to possible impairment of CSF reabsorption has prompted a demand for a clinically usable, low risk and not too time-consuming method for measurement of resistance to CSF outflow (R_{out}).

The steady pressure – steady perfusion test (Børgesen et al. 1988) for measurement of R_{out} has been performed in 333 patients. The clinical experiences, the complications, the distribution of R_{out}, and the relation between R_{out} and the clinical effect of shunting is presented here.

Material

From Table 1 the clinical data on etiology divided into two intracranial pressure groups are listed. The material comprises several different types of possible etiologies for impaired CSF-reabsorption.

Table 1. Clinical data on the etiology to possible CSF resorption deficit divided into two groups of mean intracranial pressure (MICP). BIH: benign intracranial hypertension. HPH: high pressure hydrocephalus. SAH: subarachnoid hemorrhage. TUM: intracranial tumor. TUMSP: spinal tumor. Known: suspected etiology to normal pressure hydrocephalus, Unknown: no etiology to normal pressure hydrocephalus. Trauma: head trauma

	MICP > 12	MICP ≤ 12	Total
BIH	44	0	44
HPH	16		16
MEN	4	4	8
SAH	21	37	58
TUM	5	1	6
TUMSP	3		3
Known		36	36
Trauma		15	15
Unknown		147	147
Total	93	240	333

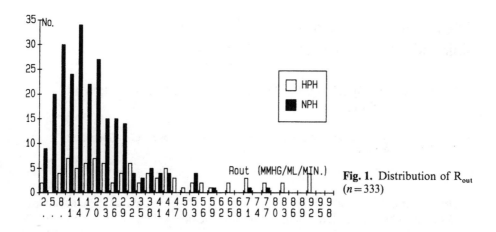

Fig. 1. Distribution of R_{out} ($n = 333$)

Results

The distribution of R_{out} can be seen in Fig. 1. R_{out} was higher in patients with intracranial pressure above 12 mm Hg (t-test, $p < 0.001$). The lowest value of R_{out} where clinical effect following shunting therapy may be expected is 12 mm Hg/ml/min. Below this value no benefit from shunting was observed. The limit is well defined and may be considered as the upper normal level for R_{out}.

Complications

No fatal complications were observed. In 4 patients a clinical, meningeal reaction was found. In one of these cases, staphylococcus aureus infection was disclosed and successfully treated. In the remaining patients the symptoms subsided within a few days.

In 2 patients the insertion of an intraventricular catheter resulted in an intracerebral hematoma. In 1 case the hematoma had to be surgically evacuated.

In 4 patients the lumbo-ventricular perfusion had to be re-done as the plot of absorbed volume versus intracranial pressure did not show a straight line. In these cases the perfusion test was re-done after at least 1 week.

Discussion

The present series represents 333 consecutively investigated patients. The material constitutes several different clinical conditions, from normal pressure hydrocephalus and benign intracranial hypertension to patients in bad condition following subarachnoid hemorrhage. In this material, R_{out} showed considerable variation. When plotted against mean intracranial pressure a non-linear correla-

354

tion was demonstrated. The correlation indicates decreasing formation rate of CSF as the intracranial pressure increases.

The result of shunting compared to R_{out} shows that the upper normal value of R_{out} is about 12 mm Hg/ml/min, as no patients with values below this level benefitted from shunting.

The steady pressure – steady perfusion test for measurement of resistance to CSF outflow has proven to be a safe, relatively quick, and easy procedure. It can be performed with a minimal risk of infection. As the diagnostic sensitivity and specifity has proven to be very good (Børgesen 1984) the test is of great clinical value.

Acknowledgement. The study has received financial support from ESKOFOT A/S, Denmark.

References

Børgesen SE (1984) Conductance to outflow of CSF in normal pressure hydrocephalus. Acta Neurochir (Wien) 71:1–45
Børgesen SE, Gjerris F, Sørensen SC (1978) The resistance to outflow of cerebrospinal fluid absorption in normal pressure hydrocephalus. Acta Neurol Scand 57:88–96

Further Analysis of the Bolus Injection Technique for Resistance Measurements

M. Kosteljanetz

Department of Neurosurgery, Aalborg Sygehus, DK-9100 Aalborg (Denmark)

An analysis of intracranial pressure (ICP) and cerebrospinal fluid (CSF) dynamics is essential in order to understand the events that lead to changes in ICP and pathological conditions in the CSF compartment (Kosteljanetz 1987). The bolus injection or pressure-volume index (PVI) technique (Marmarou et al. 1978) is a safe and fast method to determine resistance to outflow of CSF (R_{out}) and has previously been employed by the author in various clinical conditions (Kosteljanetz 1987).

R_{out} is determined by injecting a bolus of fluid intraventricularly and observing the pressure decrement that follows the sudden rise in ICP brought about by the bolus. According to the model equations (Marmarou et al. 1978), R_{out} can be calculated based on any ICP value that follows after peak pressure. In the equation, P_t designates the ICP at time t. The practical consequence of this is that P_t can be extracted from the ICP tracing at a point where the trajectory is without movement artefacts or transient ICP changes, be they spontaneous or induced by the volume loading. The present study was undertaken in order to test this statement.

Material and Method

The tracings analyzed in the present study were selected from a larger sample of PVI tests undertaken as part of a normal-pressure hydrocephalus study reported elsewhere in this volume (Kosteljanetz et al. 1988). The tracings were selected because they were without irregularities except for the transient ICP rise sometimes seen immediately after the peak pressure P_p. As a general rule P_t was extracted at times $t = 1$, $t = 2$ and $t = 3$ min after the peak. The corresponding R_{out} values are disignated R_1, R_2, etc. In some instances the ICP was followed for up to nine min.

The studies were conducted under general anesthesia. A total of 19 tracings in 9 patients were selected. Since the studies were performed under anesthesia the tracings were as a rule more regular than normally seen in awake subjects.

The opening ICP (P_0) varied from 0.5 to 11.0 mm Hg. The peak pressure (P_p) brought about by the volume loading varied from 6.0 to 22.5 mm Hg. The pressure increase ($P_p - P_0$) was 4.5–13.5 mm Hg (all ICP values diastolic).

      Eds.: J. T. Hoff and A. L. Betz
      © Springer-Verlag Berlin Heidelberg 1989

Table 1. Resistance to outflow of CSF (mm Hg/ml/min) based on different P_T values extracted at varying times, T after peak pressure (Bolus method)

Patient	R_1	R_2	R_3	R_4	R_5	R_6	R_7	R_8	R_9
A	10.1		9.8						
	14.3	11.4	8.4			8.2			
	17.3	14.1	10.9						
B	5.5	5.4	5.9						6.6
	11.1	9.6	8.3						
C	4.9	2.7	2.6						
	3.5	2.5			2.5				
	4.0	3.1	2.2						
D		4.5	2.9						
		11.9	5.4	4.0					
E	3.3	4.6	5.2				5.7		
	4.0	3.5	3.8						
F		46.1	38.0				15.5		
G		131.0	71.1					52.2	
H	15.3	17.7	14.6		10.1				
	34.1	18.3	18.0		17.3				
J	48.3	29.5	24.2		25.9	21.4			
				30.9	17.7				
		29.1		35.6					

$R_{1, 2, 3...}$ indicates R_{out} values based on P_T values extracted at times $T = 1, 2, 3 ...$ minutes after peak pressure P_P

Results

The results are presented in Table 1. It appears that there were sometimes considerable differences between R_1 and later values, especially when R_{out} was high. Only when R_{out} was below 10 mm Hg/ml/min were the differences minor. Although the general trend was a decrease in R_{out} with time, the opposite was also observed.

Discussion

A comprehensive analysis of the bolus model has been undertaken by Avezaat and van Eijndhoven (1984) and is beyond the scope of the present paper. In the following I shall only briefly summarize possible causes for the time dependent R_{out} variation: 1) the ICP decay after peak ICP is caused by factors other than CSF absorption (e.g., pressure relaxation, compliance, vasoconstriction), 2) the model equations do not apply in the present clinical setting (e.g., general anesthesia), 3) constant compliance and resistance as presumed in the model may not be true and 4) CSF leaks may account for erroneous ICP values, especially in the first minutes.

357

References

Avezaat CJJ, van Eijndhoven JHM (1984) Cerebrospinal fluid pulse pressure and craniospinal dynamics. A theoretical, clinical and experimental study. A Jongbloed en Zoon Publ, The Hague, The Netherlands, pp 1–339

Kosteljanetz M (1987) Intracranial pressure: Cerebrospinal fluid dynamics and pressure-volume relations. Acta Neurol Scand [Suppl 111] 75:1–23

Kosteljanetz M, Westergaard L, Kaalund J, Nehen AM (1988) The significance of outflow resistance measurements in the prediction of outcome after CSF-shunting in patients with NPH. Intracranial pressure VII

Marmarou A, Shulman K, Rosende RM (1975) A nonlinear analysis of the cerebrospinal fluid system and intracranial pressure dynamics. J Neurosurg 48:332–344

Comparison of Resistance to Outflow (R_{out}) Measured by Ventricular and Lumbar Perfusion

O. Fedders, J.F. Schmidt, M.J. Albeck, and F. Gjerris

University Clinic of Neurosurgery, Rigshospitalet, DK-2100 Copenhagen (Denmark)

Introduction

Several methods are available when studying the resorptive capacity of cerebrospinal fluid. In clinical practice, measurement of the resistance to CSF outflow (R_{out}) has been shown to be useful (Børgesen and Gjerris 1982). This prospective study was performed to verify the reproducibility and reliability of the method.

Material and Method

10 patients with normal pressure hydrocephalus (NPH) participated. A ventricular cannula was placed through a precoronal rightsided burrhole. The intracranial pressure (ICP) was measured for 6 hr and subsequently 2 runs of ventriculo-ventricular perfusion tests (VV_1 and VV_2) (Gjerris et al. 1982) were performed in the following way:

With the patient in the supine position and with a known and stable ICP, an infusion of Ringers lactate (V_{in}) was started at a rate of 1.82 ml/min. The outflow volume (V_{out}) was sampled in periods of 3 min and measured at 6–7 different intracranial pressures obtained by elevating the outflow tube.

On the assumption that the CSF formation rate is constant (0.4 ml/min) the absorbed CSF volume (V_{abs}) can be calculated from the formula:

$$V_{abs} = V_{in} + 0.4 - V_{out} .$$

V_{abs} was then related to ICP and the slope of the best fitted line through the 6–7 points expresses the conductance to CSF outflow (C_{out}) (Fig. 1).

R_{out} is calculated from $C_{out} * R_{out} = 1$.

After the first 2 perfusion tests, monitoring of the ICP was continued and, on the next day, 2 further ventriculo-ventricular perfusion tests were performed (VV_3 and VV_4).

In addition, 2 examinations of R_{out} were performed by a lumbo-ventricular perfusion test with the patient in a lateral recumbent position (LV_1 and LV_2) (Børgesen et al. 1978).

All perfusion tests were separated by a resting period of 15 min.

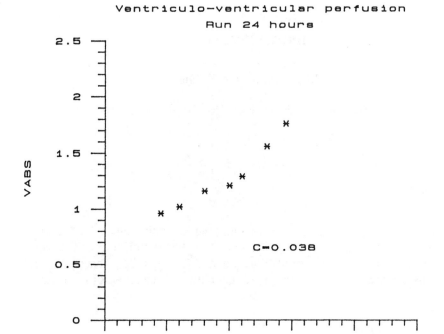

Fig. 1. An example of the relation between V_{abs} and ICP. The slope of the best fitted line through the points expresses the conductance to CSF outflow

Results

R_{out} in VV_1 and VV_2 was lower than R_{out} in all the later performed tests (VV_3, VV_4, LV_1, LV_2).

No differences between LV_1, LV_2, VV_3 and VV_4 were found ($p=0.38$).

Discussion

The calculation of R_{out} demands a constant rate of CSF production, irrespective of the increased ICP during the study. Two other factors have to be constant, i.e. the CSF volume and the cerebral blood volume. Børgesen (1984), found in 8 patients with NPH that C_{out} did not vary more than 5%. The difference in R_{out}-values after 6 and 24 hr with the lower value after 6 hr can be explained by leakage of CSF due to the newly placed ventricular cannula. This will lead to an overestimation of CSF absorption, and produce a falsely low value in the calculation of R_{out}. The identical values obtained using the ventriculo-ventricular and the lumbo-ventricular perfusion test 24 hr after the application of the ventricular cannula makes the use of the lumbar puncture obsolete in NPH patients. The advantage of having the patients in the supine position are obvious. The lumbar approach can be saved for lumbo-lumbar perfusion tests in patients with benign intracranial hypertension.

Conclusion

1. More than 6 hr have to elapse after the insertion of a ventricular cannula before a reliable ventriculo-ventricular perfusion test is performed.
2. After 24 hr, the ventriculo-ventricular perfusion test is reliable and comparable to the lumbo-ventricular test.
3. In patients with NPH, we recommend one ventriculo-ventricular perfusion test after 24 hr of ICP monitoring.

References

Børgesen SE, Gjerris F, Sørensen SC (1978) The resistance to cerebrospinal fluid absorption in humans. Acta Neurol Scand 57:88–96

Børgesen SE, Gjerris F (1982) The predictive value of conductance to outflow of CSF in normal pressure hydrocephalus. Brain 105:65–86

Børgesen SE (1984) Conductance to outflow of CSF in normal pressure hydrocephalus. Acta Neurochir (Wien) 71:1–41

Gjerris F, Børgesen SE, Hoppe E, Boesen F, Nordenbo A (1982) The conductance to outflow of CSF in adults with high-pressure hydrocephalus. Acta Neurochir (Wien) 64:59–67

CSF Dynamics and Ventricular Size in Experimental Sagittal Sinus Occlusion Models

N. Kojima, K. Fujita, N. Tamaki, and S. Matsumoto

Department of Neurosurgery, Kobe University, School of Medicine, Chuoku, Kusunokicho, 7-5-1 Kobe (Japan)

Introduction

The relationship of increased cerebral venous pressure to ventricular enlargement and the role of a distensible skull have remained controversial (Bering and Salibi 1959, Guthrie et al. 1970). Clinically, it is well known that increased intracranial venous pressure may lead to hydrocephalus in younger infants and to benign intracranial hypertension in older patients (Rosman et al. 1978). However, there have been very few reports on changes in CSF dynamics and ventricular size after sagittal sinus occlusion because a good experimental model of sagittal sinus occlusion has not been available. The aim of this study is to evaluate the changes in CSF dynamics and ventricular size and to define the role of craniectomy in a new model of sagittal sinus occlusion.

Methods

Adult mongrel dogs weighing 6–10 kg were intubated under pentobarbital anesthesia and maintained on controlled ventilation using pancronium bromide for paralysis. A small burr hole was made in the anterior one-third of the superior sagittal sinus. A polyethylene catheter was inserted into the superior sagittal sinus and placed 1 cm posterior to the coronal suture. α-cyano-acrylate monomer (0.3–0.7 ml for partial occlusion and 0.8–1.0 ml for complete occlusion) was injected through the catheter. The burr hole was sealed with dental cement. This was carried out as an embolization technique to produce sagittal sinus occlusion (Fujita et al. 1985). Dogs were divided into the following four groups: A) controls (30 dogs), B) acute models of sinus occlusion (22 dogs), C) chronic models of sinus occlusion without craniectomy (6 dogs), D) chronic models sinus occlusion with craniectomy (8 dogs). In group D, a large frontoparietal craniectomy was added before sinus occlusion as a model of the distensible skull. Changes in the cisterna magna pressure, superior sagittal sinus pressure, and CSF dynamics according to Marmarou's method (Marmarou et al. 1978) were evaluated with a Statham transducer before and after these procedures. In chronic models, similar pressure measurements and examinations of CSF dynamics were also performed 10 and 30 days after sinus occlusion. Ventricular size was confirmed at autopsy. Evans blue dye was injected into the cisterna magna one hour prior to killing.

Eds.: J. T. Hoff and A. L. Betz
© Springer-Verlag Berlin Heidelberg 1989

Results

A) Controls

The general relationship between cisterna magna and superior sagittal sinus pressures was similar in all animals examined. The mean resting pressure in the cisterna magna was 9.1 ± 2.1 mm Hg and that in the superior sagittal sinus was 4.7 ± 2.2 mm Hg. Cisterna magna pressure was always higher than superior sagittal sinus pressure. The pressure-volume index (PVI) averaged 1.3 ± 0.4 ml and the CSF outflow resistance (R_b) averaged 105 ± 38 mm Hg/ml/min.

B) Acute Model of Sinus Occlusion

Occlusion of the dural sinus(es) produced intracranial hypertension. In the partial occlusion models (sagittal sinus $\pm$ transverse sinus occlusion) the mean cisterna magna pressure immediately after occlusion was 31 ± 12 mm Hg and it was 21 ± 2.2 mm Hg. In the complete occlusion models (sagittal sinus + transverse sinus + cortical vein occlusion) the mean pre-occlusion cisterna magna pressure was 10 ± 2.8 mm Hg and the post-occlusion pressure was elevated remarkably with a mean value of 57 ± 14 mm Hg. Usually complete occlusion dogs died several hours after occlusion.

In the partial occlusion models, the superior sagittal sinus pressure before occlusion was 4.6 ± 1.9 mm Hg and the immediate post-occlusion value was 39 ± 7.5 mm Hg. It was 27.8 ± 5.6 mm Hg in the stable state. There were significant rises in these pressures with sinus occlusion ($p < 0.001$). The normal pressure gradient from the cisterna magna to the superior sagittal sinus became reversed after sinus occlusion.

In the partial occlusion models the mean PVI and R_b increased significantly after sinus occlusion ($p < 0.05$, $p < 0.01$), while there were no statistically significant changes in the complete occlusion dogs (Table 1).

Table 1. Changes of the pressure-volume index and CSF outflow resistance in the sinus occlusion dogs

	PVI[a] (ml)		R_b[b] (mm Hg/ml/min)	
	pre occlusion	post occlusion	pre occlusion	post occlusion
Partial occlusion	$n = 16$		$n = 18$	
	1.29 ± 0.23	1.52 ± 0.37[c]	94.8 ± 26.6	200 ± 157[d]
Complete occlusion	$n = 4$		$n = 4$	
	1.47 ± 0.34	1.51 ± 0.66	101 ± 28	531 ± 539

[a] PVI: pressure-volume index; [b] RB: CSF outflow resistance; [c] Significant difference ($P < 0.05$); [d] Significant difference ($P < 0.01$).

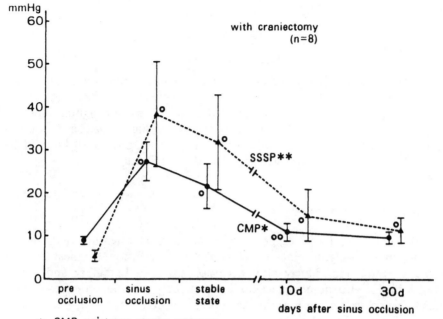

* CMP : cisterna magna pressure
** SSSP : superior sagittal sinus pressure o : significant difference (P<0.001)
                                           oo : significant difference (P<0.05)

a

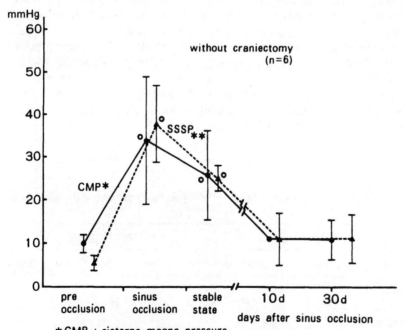

*CMP : cisterna magna pressure
**SSSP : superior sagittal sinus pressure
o : significant difference (P<0.005)

b

364

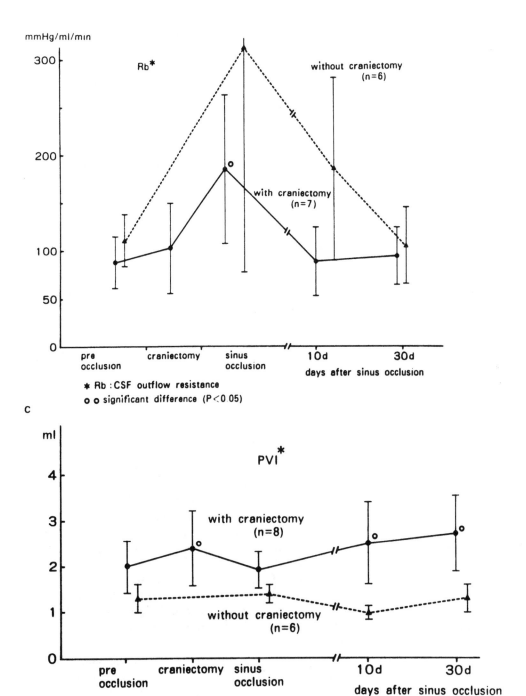

c

d

Fig. 1 a–d. Chronological changes of the cisterna magna pressure, superior sagittal sinus pressure, CSF outflow resistance, and pressure-volume index in sinus occlusion dogs with and without craniectomy

365

Sinus occlusion produced elevation of pressures in the cisterna magna and superior sagittal sinus for as long as 30 days. Serial determination of pressures showed a general downward trend. Increased sagittal sinus pressure and the reverse gradient of pressure from the CSF to the superior sagittal sinus remained in the sinus occlusion dogs with craniectomy (Fig. 1 a, b).

Craniectomy resulted in a significant increase in the PVI ($p < 0.05$). Prior to craniectomy, the mean PVI was 2.0 ± 0.6 ml and it was 2.4 ± 0.8 ml in the postcraniectomy preparation. The increased PVI was noted 10 and 30 days after sinus occlusion. The sinus occlusion dogs without craniectomy did not show significant changes in the PVI throughout the experiment (Fig. 1 d).

Craniectomy had no significant effect on the R_b. Although the R_b increased with sinus occlusion, this increase was not maintained 10 or 30 days after sinus occlusion in either model (Fig. 1 c).

Postmortem examinations of the brains showed a variety of ventricular sizes, however, there was no distinct ventricular enlargement in the chronic models of sinus occlusion regardless of whether they had craniectomy or not.

Evans blue dye was not seen in the subarachnoid space of the cerebral hemispheres but was present on the basal surface of the brain in the sinus occlusion dogs. In contrast, the dye distributed widely throughout the subarachnoid space in the control dogs.

Discussion

According to previous studies CSF pressure is slightly higher than sagittal sinus pressure in the normal state (Bering and Salibi 1959, Bedford 1934, Guthrie et al. 1970, Shulman et al. 1964). This pressure gradient between the CSF and dural sinuses is considered to be the driving force responsible for outflow of CSF from the intracranial subarachnoid space to the dural venous sinuses (Davson et al. 1970). Theoretically, reversal of this relationship or reduction of the normal pressure gradient by elevating pressure in the cranial venous sinuses would be expected to lead to a disturbance of CSF absorption and subsequent ventriculomegaly. However, most attempts to produce hydrocephalus by venous blockade have been unsuccessful and have provided little information as to the changes of CSF dynamics or the causes of the failure to produce hydrocephalus (Beck and Russell 1946).

In the present study, the resting values of CSF pressure and sagittal sinus pressure agree with previous published values. These pressures increased and a reversal of the pressure gradient occurred following sinus occlusion in association with increased CSF outflow resistance. Determination of CSF outflow resistance has been used by many investigators as an index of an absorptive defect. The CSF pressure and the superior sagittal sinus pressure fell with time although normal levels were not reached in our experiment in agreement with other authors (Bering and Salibi 1959, Guthrie et al. 1970). The general downward trend to these pressures and CSF outflow resistance may be due to the development of collateral circulation of the CSF on the basal surface of the brain as supported by the distribution of the Evans blue dye. Distinct ventricular enlargement did not appear in our sagittal sinus occlusion dogs. It has been recognized that, in the dog, there are important paths of CSF absorption in the perineural channels of the optic nerves and olfactory nerves leading to the nasal mucosa and cervical lymph nodes (Schurr et al. 1953).

In conclusion, sinus occlusion in the dog may be a model of benign intracranial hypertension rather than hydrocephalus. Craniectomy by itself may be insufficient to produce ventricular enlargement in this experimental model.

References

Beck DJK, Russell DS (1946) Experiments on thrombosis of the superior longitudinal sinus. J Neurosurg 3:337–347

Bedford THB (1934) The great vein of Galen and the syndrome of increased intracranial pressure. Brain 57:1–24

Bering EA, Salibi B (1959) Production of hydrocephalus by increased cephalic-venous pressure. Arch Neurol 81:693–698

Davson H, Hollingsworth G, Segal MD (1970) The mechanism and drainage of cerebrospinal fluid. Brain 93:665–678

Fujita K, Kojima N, Tamaki N, Matsumoto S (1985) Brain edema in intracranial venous hypertension. In: Inaba Y, Klatzo I, Spatz M (eds) Brain edema. Springer, Berlin Heidelberg New York Tokyo, pp 228–234

Guthrie TC, Dunbar HS, Karpell B (1970) Ventricular size and chronic increased intracranial venous pressure in the dog. J Neurosurg 33:407–414

Marmarou A, Shulman K, Rosende RM (1978) A nonlinear analysis of the cerebrospinal fluid system and intracranial pressure dynamics. J Neurosurg 48:332–344

Rosman NP, Kathryn N, Shands N (1978) Hydrocephalus caused by increased intracranial venous pressure: a clinicopathological study. Ann Neurol 3:445–450

Schurr PH, McLaurin RL, Ingraham FD (1953) Experimental studies on the circulation of the cerebrospinal fluid. J Neurosurg 10:515–525

Shulman K, Yarnell P, Ransohoff (1964) Dural sinus pressure in normal and hydrocephalic dogs. Arch Neurol 10:575–580

The Importance of Outflow Resistance of the Shunt System for Elimination of B-Waves

K. Tanaka and S. Nishimura

Department of Neurosurgery, Osaka City University Medical School, 1-5-7 Asahi-machi, Abeno-ku, Osaka 545 (Japan)

Introduction

There are several papers which report the effectiveness of shunt surgery especially in patients who show B-Waves in ICP recording (Chawla et al. 1974, Lamas and Lobato 1979, Børgesen and Gjerris 1982). Nevertheless, the fate of B-Waves after shunting has seldom been reported (Symon and Dorsch 1975). In another part of this volume, we reported the effects of the shunt system on CSF hydrodynamics (Tanaka et al. 1989), that is, the installation of a shunt decreases not only mean ICP but also outflow resistance (R_{out}), and increases the pressure-volume index (PVI). After the shunt system is installed, a new R_{out} for the patient, $R_{out\,(gross)}$, will be established, governed by the following equation:

$$1/R_{out\,(gross)} = 1/R_{out\,(h)} + 1/R_{out\,(shunt)}, \tag{1}$$

where $R_{out(h)}$ is the R_{out} of the patient before shunt and $R_{out\,(shunt)}$ is the R_{out} of the shunt system itself. In this paper, CSF fluctuation is more thoroughly analyzed, focusing on the changes in B-Waves after a shunt. The importance of R_{out}, not only of the patient, but also of the shunt system itself, will be emphasized.

Material and Methods

Fifteen hydrocephalic patients of various causes (3 high pressure, 12 NPH) underwent shunt surgery using Heyer-Schulte's on-off flushing reservoir with antisiphon, and low pressure Pudenz peritoneal catheter. A ventricular catheter was inserted into the lateral ventricle, opposite to the shunted side, for monitoring ICP and CSF manipulation. ICP was continuously monitored for 24 hr, both before and after opening the on-off valve. The highest and the lowest values of the ICP fluctuation, except for the pressure waves, were sampled every 30 min throughout the period of ICP monitoring. The mean ICP ($mICP_{24}$) was arbitrarily defined as the mean pressure of all these pressure readings. Two prominent B-Waves were sampled every 30 min and the peak pressure (BPp) and the trough pressure (BPo) of the B-Waves were measured (Fig. 1 A). By definition, a B-Wave is the pressure wave occurring at a frequency of one half to two per minute. As it is unlikely that the volume of brain parenchyma of CSF changes within such

Intracranial Pressure VII
Eds.: J. T. Hoff and A. L. Betz
© Springer-Verlag Berlin Heidelberg 1989

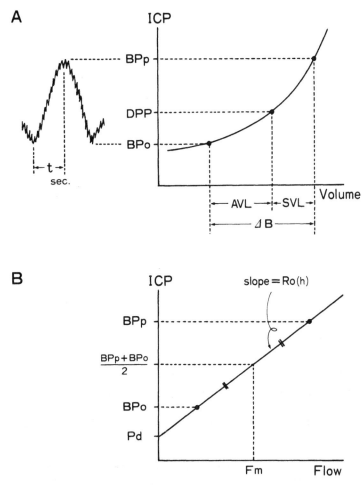

Fig. 1. A The B-Wave was projected onto the pressure-volume curve. The ΔB, the volume which elicits a B-Wave, can be divided into two portions, *AVL* (acceptable volume limit) and *SVL* (shunt volume load). *DPP:* desired peak pressure. **B** During the rising phase of a B-Wave, when the ICP goes up from trough pressure (BPo) to peak pressure (BPp), the mean flow at which CSF will be expelled from the intracranial cavity through the system which has an outflow resistance of $R_{out(h)}$ will be given by the equation: $Fm=((BPp+BPo)/2-Pd)/R_{out(h)}$, where Pd is the dural sinus pressure

a short period of time ($15\sim60$ sec), the volume which elicited a B-Wave (ΔB) is thought to be the volume of intracranial blood. If the volume which will be expelled (V_{exp}) during the time t in sec, the rising phase of the B-Wave, can be calculated, it is feasible to use Marmarou's PVI equation (Marmarou et al. 1975) to compute ΔB by changing its form to:

$$\Delta B = PVI \times \log_{10} (BPp/BPo). \tag{2}$$

Before the shunt system is installed, the mean flow (Fm ml/min) at which CSF will be expelled from the intracranial cavity during the rising phase of the B-Wave, through the system which has an outflow resistance of $R_{out\,(h)}$, will be calculated as shown in Fig. 1 B. Then the V_{exp} will be:

$$V_{exp} = (lf + Fm)/60] \times t, \tag{3}$$

where lt is the rate of fluid formation, 0.35 ml/min (Cutler et al. 1968). On the pressure-volume curve as shown in Fig. 1 A, ΔB can be divided into two portions, the acceptable volume limit (AVL) which will not raise ICP above normal or desired peak pressure (DPP), and the volume which should be shunted, the shunt volume load (SVL). Because V_{exp} has been expelled, the total CSF volume which should be expelled from the intracranial cavity during the time t, TVE (total volume egress), is:

$$TVE = SVL + V_{exp}, \tag{4}$$

We computed the $R_{out\,(gross)}$, with which TVE can be expelled without raising ICP above DPP. Then the $R_{out\,(shunt)}$ can also be calculated by changing the equation (1) as:

$$R_{out\,(shunt)} = [R_{out\,(gross)} \times R_{out\,(h)}]/[R_{out\,(h)} - R_{out\,(gross)}], \tag{5}$$

Results

In these 15 patients, shunt surgery was performed 16 times. All of these patients showed B-Waves in ICP recording. After shunt surgery, all of them satisfied our criteria of shunt effectiveness, i.e., $mICP_{24}$ decreased, PVI increased and R_{out} decreased. The $mICP_{24}$ of pre- and post-opening of the on-off valve were

Table 1. Post-operative changes in outflow resistance and B-Waves

	Ro (h)	Actual Ro (gross)	Calculated Ro (gross)	% reduction of B-Wave (%)	% difference of Ro (%)
	(mm Hg/ml/min)				
1	6.7042	1.1085	0.9341	−100.0	18.67
2	8.0502	1.5207	1.9121	−100.0	−20.47
3	22.6166	5.0684	1.9066	0.0	165.83
4	4.6499	1.0680	0.6035	−100.0	76.97
5	3.6669	1.3847	0.7491	−78.5	84.85
6	1.1475	1.0329	0.4858	0.0	112.62
7	7.2919	2.7302	1.0519	−40.0	159.55
8	4.1372	2.2743	0.8264	−81.8	175.21
9	5.1363	1.7949	0.8796	−75.5	104.06
10	21.0475	3.8172	4.0553	−100.0	−5.87
11	5.7881	0.5732	1.5208	−77.8	−62.31
12	3.7613	2.2895	2.1786	−100.0	5.09
13	4.3517	1.2660	0.7164	−81.2	76.72
14	6.6536	1.4158	1.3983	−89.7	1.25
15	20.4740	2.3091	1.5360	−100.0	50.33

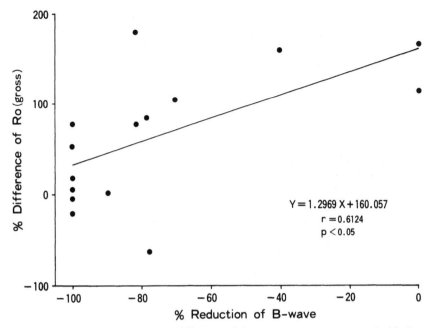

Fig. 2. The correlation between the percent difference of the actual $R_{out\,(gross)}$ compared with the calculated $R_{out\,(gross)}$, Y-axis, and the percent reduction in the number of B-Waves which exceeded DPP, X-axis, was significant ($p < 0.05$, $r = 0.6124$)

157.0 ± 51.5 (mean $\pm$ SD) and 80.7 ± 32.90 mm H_2O, respectively, and the mean reduction of $mICP_{24}$ compared to the pre-opening value was $46.4 \pm 19.4\%$. This post-operative $mICP_{24}$ did not correlate at all with the closing pressure of the shunt system which was measured in the operating room. Even after the valve was opened, B-Waves never disappeared in 24 hr of ICP recording in all patients. The peak pressure of B-Waves decreased except for one case, from 24.96 ± 9.40 to 12.98 ± 4.24 mm Hg post-operatively and the reduction was $42.7 \pm 24.7\%$. The magnitude of the B-Waves (BPp – BPo) also decreased except for two cases, from 5.91 ± 3.31 to 2.60 ± 1.12 mm Hg and the reduction was $48.7 \pm 31.4\%$. The PVI increased except for one case, from 26.58 ± 12.59 to 45.24 ± 24.08 ml post-operatively; the increment was $75.97 \pm 58.75\%$. The R_{out} decreased in all cases from 8.365 ± 6.958 to 1.977 ± 1.185 mm Hg/ml/min, a $67.6 \pm 21.7\%$ reduction.

The R_{out} was more thoroughly analyzed in terms of $R_{out\,(h)}$, the pre-opening value of the patient; actual $R_{out\,(gross)}$, the value measured after the on-off valve was opened; and the calculated $R_{out\,(gross)}$ which is the mean of the $R_{out\,(gross)}$ calculated for all B-Waves sampled throughout the recording period (Table 1). Out of all B-Waves, consisting of about 40 to 60 observations in each period of pre- and post-opening of the valve, the percentage of the number of B-Waves which required a shunt to keep the ICP below the DPP was calculated. Before valve-opening, $89.3 \pm 13.6\%$ of B-Waves sampled needed CSF diversion to keep the ICP below DPP; 200 mm H_2O. After the valve was opened, 7 patients showed no B-Waves which exceeded DPP and in another 5 patients, less than 20% of B-Waves sampled needed CSF diversion. The correlation between the percent reduction in the number of B-Waves which exceed DPP and the percent difference of the actual $R_{out\,(gross)}$ compared to the calculated $R_{out\,(gross)}$ was studied. As shown in Fig. 2, there was a significant correlation between these two parameters ($p < 0.05$, $r = 0.6124$).

Discussion

The $mICP_{24}$ after shunting did not correlate at all with the closing pressure of the shunt system, but the percent reduction of $mICP_{24}$ did significantly correlate with the percent reduction of R_{out}. This seems to imply that the dynamic aspect of post-operative mean ICP has nothing to do with the closing pressure of the shunt system but with the percent reduction of R_{out}. Besides this, the R_{out} seems to have an important meaning for the elimination of the B-Wave. The actual $R_{out\,(gross)}$ was compared with the calculated $R_{out\,(gross)}$ which is the ideal value obtained by calculation to keep the peak pressure of the B-Waves below the DPP. The correlation between the percent reduction in the number of B-Waves, the peak pressure of which exceeded DPP, and the percent difference of the actual $R_{out\,(gross)}$ compared with the calculated $R_{out\,(gross)}$ was highly significant. This means that the closer the actual $R_{out\,(gross)}$ is to the ideal calculated $R_{out\,(gross)}$, the greater is the rate of elimination of B-Waves. By changing DPP in the equations, not only the peak pressure of the B-Waves but also the upper limit of ICP fluctuation can be controlled.

Although there are many papers which report abnormal R_{out} in the hydrocephalic patients, to the best of our knowledge, there have been few papers which elucidated the importance of $R_{out\,(shunt)}$. The $R_{out\,(h)}$ and the calculated $R_{out\,(gross)}$ can be obtained from continuous ICP monitoring for at least 24 hr. Because the $R_{out\,(shunt)}$ can be calculated from these two figures, it is now possible to select the shunt system which has the most suitable $R_{out\,(shunt)}$ for each particular patient. The $R_{out\,(shunt)}$ seems to depend primarily upon the caliber of the shunt tube according to Poiseuille's law. The shunt tube which is now commercially available has been designed to keep ICP within normal limits with a rate of CSF formation up to twice the normal value. The mean volume of the TVE in this study was 5.71 ± 3.64 ml, and this volume should be expelled within the time t, 35.3 ± 12.1 sec. A part of the TVE will be absorbed via a physiological route which has an outflow resistance of $R_{out\,(h)}$, and the rest will be expelled via a shunt tube. The flow of CSF in the shunt tube during the rising phase of B-Wave reached 9.7 ± 5.0 ml/min. This is as much as 28 times the normal rate of CSF formation and about 12 times the flow predicted by shunt manufacturers. We are not yet sure whether or not complete elimination of B-Waves is mandatory for the treatment of hydrocephalus, but if this is the case, surgeons should be aware of R_{out} not only of the patient but also of the shunt system itself. The supply of shunt systems of various calibers, i.e., of various $R_{out\,(shunt)}$ not of various closing pressures should be considered.

References

Børgesen SE, Gjerris F (1982) The predictive value of conductance to outflow of cerebrospinal fluid in normal pressure hydrocephalus. Brain 105:65–86

Chawla JC, Hulme A, Cooper R (1974) Intracranial pressure in patients with dementia and communicating hydrocephalus. J Neurosurg 40:376–380

Lamas E, Lobato RD (1979) Intraventricular pressure and CSF dynamics in chronic adult hydrocephalus. Surg Neurol 12:287–295

Marmarou A, Shulman K, LaMorgese J (1975) Compartmental analysis of compliance and outflow resistance of the cerebrospinal fluid system. J Neurosurg 43:523–534

Symon L, Dorsch NWC (1975) Use of long-term intracranial pressure measurement to assess hydrocephalic patients prior to shunt surgery. J Neurosurg 42:258–273

Tanaka K, Hayashi H, Ohata K, Sakamoto H, Nishimura S (1989) Intracranial pressure on pre- and post-shunt surgery in patients with normal pressure hydrocephalus (NPH). This volume, pp 399–401

Benign Intracranial Hypertension:
CSF Dynamics and CSF Pulse Wave Morphology

C. Anile, G. Maira, A. Mangiola, and G.F. Rossi

Institute of Neurosurgery, Catholic University, Largo Gemelli 8, 00168 Rome (Italy)

Introduction

Benign intracranial hypertension (BIH), otherwise called "pseudotumour cerebri", is a pathological condition characterized by the presence of chronic or intermittent signs of raised intracranial pressure (ICP), such as headache, papilledema, and spontaneous cerebrospinal fluid (CSF) leakage, without any evidence of an intracranial space occupying mass lesion or CSF protein concentration increase. This condition is frequently observed in female patients suffering from endocrine disorders (obesity, hypertrichosis, irregular menses, and sometimes galactorrhea) and is often associated with a typical radiological feature depicting an intrasellar arachnoidal herniation (the so-called "empty sella") (Anile and Maira 1986). Some authors have suggested that an impairment in CSF absorptive capacity due, probably, to an increase in the venous outflow resistance resulting from an obstacle at postcerebral level in the dural sinuses, could be the most important pathogenetical factor in BIH (Junck 1986). In spite of this assumption, however, patients diagnosed as affected by this syndrome show, at neuroradiological examinations, normal, or even small ventricles (Hansen et al. 1987).

Methods and Materials

To investigate this apparent discrepancy already noted by others, we compared ICP dynamics in a series of 54 patients with BIH to those in a series of 30 patients affected by normal pressure hydrocephalus (NPH). In particular we analyzed the following data:

1) *CSF absorptive reserve* by infusing mock CSF at a constant rate into the spinal subarachnoidal space to get a plateau pressure and then calculating the ratio of the difference between the plateau and resting pressure and the rate of infusion;
2) *Intracranial elastance* by measuring the slope of the linear regression between CSF diastolic and pulse pressure values (recorded by intraventricular or spinal catheter) in resting conditions and during spontaneous (REM phase of sleep)

Eds.: J. T. Hoff and A. L. Betz

or artificially induced (jugular compression [Q] and/or intraventricular infusion [IVI]) ICP increases;

3) *CSF pulse wave (CSFPW) morphology* by means of Fourier's spectral analysis in resting and dynamic conditions as described above.

All patients with BIH had normal or small sized ventricles as estimated by the ventricular index of Sklar et al. (1980) (normal values: <0.5) and CSF protein concentration in the normal range for our laboratory standards. Twenty patients because of the severity of the signs of intracranial hypertension (mainly papilledema and CSF rhinoliquorrhea), were operated on for placement of lumbo- or ventriculo-peritoneal or ventriculo-atrial shunts utilizing, in all cases, high pressure devices. The signs of raised ICP were immediately relieved by CSF shunting although in some cases, disturbances due to orthostatic hypotension could be seen. For this reason in recent years we more often utilize ventriculo-atrial shunts which, theoretically, should be unaffected by the spatial position of the body.

In patients with NPH the diagnosis was suspected on the basis of clinico-radiological signs (Hakim-Adam's triad and ventricular enlargement) and confirmed by a significant improvement in the clinical status after a CSF shunting procedure.

Results

All the patients with BIH had diastolic ICP values in resting conditions >15 mm Hg. None of the patients with NPH reached this level.

CSF Absorptive Reserve

An impairment in the CSF absorptive reserve (normal values in our laboratory >0.11 ml/min/mm Hg) was found in all the patients with BIH and in about 50% of those with NPH.

Intracranial Elastance

Patients with BIH and NPH showed similar values of intracranial elastance during both the REM phase of sleep and intraventricular testing. In contrast, a significant difference was observed between the two groups of patients after compressing the jugular veins in the neck; during this manoeuvre, in fact, the slope of the linear regression between pulsatile and diastolic ICP pressure is higher in patients with BIH as compared to those with NPH. Nevertheless, in all the three dynamic conditions, the diastolic ICP values were higher in patients with BIH. This indicates a relative reduction of the intracranial "pulsatility" in BIH compared to that observed in patients with NPH.

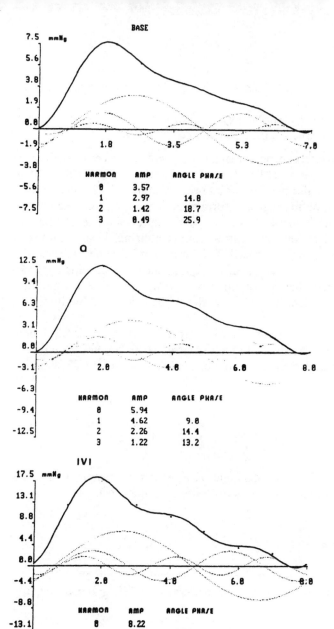

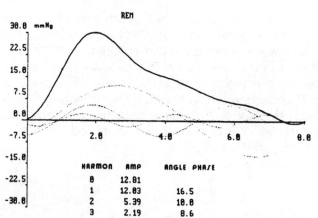

Fig. 1. Example of CSFPW morphological changes in a patient with BIH from resting (*BASE*) to dynamic conditions. *Continuous line:* CSFPW original shape. *Dotted lines:* 1st, 2nd and 3rd harmonic of the CSFPW spectrum

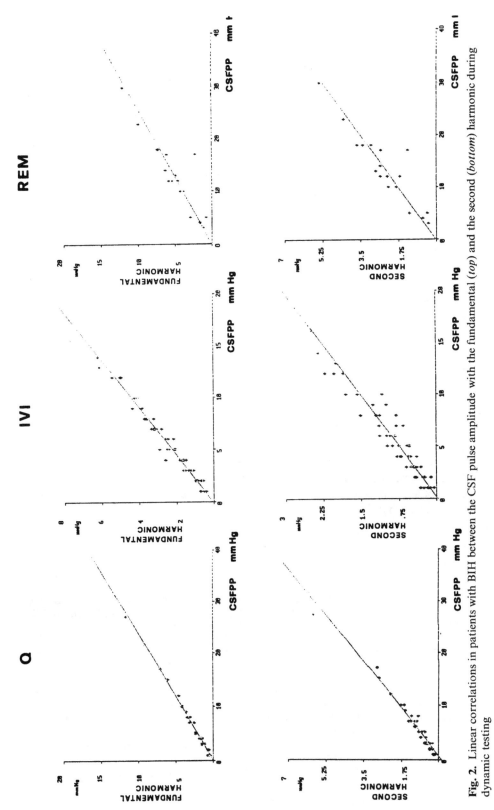

Fig. 2. Linear correlations in patients with BIH between the CSF pulse amplitude with the fundamental (*top*) and the second (*bottom*) harmonic during dynamic testing

377

A typical bi- or tri-phasic CSFPW was observed in all patients with BIH in resting conditions. Unlike the results obtained in patients with NPH (see this book) in which the contour of the wave becomes rounded during ICP increases, in patients with BIH, the CSFPW shape remains constant in all three different examined dynamic conditions (Fig. 1). Moreover, the ratio between the first and the second harmonic does not change during dynamic testing as demonstrated by the linear correlations found in all the patients between each of these two frequencies and the CSF pulse pressure amplitude, both in basal and at maximum ICP level (Fig. 2).

Discussion

Our results confirm that an impairment in the CSF absorptive reserve is not always associated with an increase in ventricular size (Rossi et al. 1987). On the contrary, they suggest that ventricular enlargement is probably due to an alteration in the CSFPW impedance transmission through the intracranial system. In fact, in patients with BIH we can observe both a reduction of intracranial "pulsatility" and a stability of the CSFPW morphology during dynamic testing. This association is also observed in patients with NPH (see this book) during jugular compression. We can speculate along with Portnoy et al. (1982), that this particular situation is determined by the increase in the dural sinus pressure (downstream to the so-called Starling resistor at the lacunae laterales level) thereby affecting the venous outflow impedance. A chronic condition, therefore, of increased dural sinus pressure, as hypothesized in patients with BIH, could explain the peculiar feature of a disturbance in CSF absorptive reserve and increased ICP levels with normal, or even small cerebral ventricles.

References

Anile C, Maira G (1986) "Empty sella" and benign intracranial hypertension: endocrine and CSF dynamic study. In: Miller JD, Teasdale GM, Rowan JO, Galbraith SL, Mendelow AD (eds) Intracranial pressure VI. Springer, Berlin Heidelberg New York Tokyo, pp 486–490

Hansen K, Gjerris F, Sørensen PS (1987) Absence of hydrocephalus in spite of impaired cerebrospinal fluid absorption and severe intracranial hypertension. Acta Neurochir (Wien) 86:93–97

Junck L (1986) Benign intracranial hypertension and normal pressure hydrocephalus: theoretical considerations. In: Miller JD, Teasdale GM, Rowan JO, Galbraith SL, Mendelow AD (eds) Intracranial pressure VI. Springer, Berlin Heidelberg New York Tokyo, pp 447–450

Portnoy HD, Chopp M, Branch C, Shannon M (1982) Cerebrospinal fluid pulse waveform as an indicator of cerebral autoregulation. J Neurosurg 56:666–678

Rossi GF, Maira G, Anile C (1987) Intracranial pressure behaviour and its relation to the outcome of surgical CSF shunting in normotensive hydrocephalus. Neurol Res 9:183–187

Sklar FH, Diehl JT, Beyer CW, Clark WK (1980) Brain elasticity changes with ventriculomegaly. J Neurosurg 53:173–179

CSF Dynamics in Patients with Suspected Normal Pressure Hydrocephalus

E.J. Delwel, D.A. de Jong, C.J.J. Avezaat, J.H.M. van Eijndhoven, and A. Korbee

Department of Neurosurgery, University Hospital Rotterdam, Rotterdam (The Netherlands)

Introduction

Although both the pathophysiology and diagnosis of the so-called normal pressure hydrocephalus (NPH) syndrome remain the subject of much controversy, most authors agree that disturbed CSF dynamics, particularly impaired CSF absorption, play a central role. Determination of CSF outflow resistance (R_{out}) ranks high on the list of tests designed for the selection of patients who might benefit from a CSF shunting procedure (Børgesen and Gjerris 1981). Another important parameter of CSF dynamics is the elastance coefficient (E_1, inverse PVI) which determines the slope of the craniospinal volume-pressure curve (Avezaat and van Eijndhoven 1984). Finally, the CSF pulse pressure, reflecting craniospinal elastance, has been found to be increased in patients with NPH (Belloni et al. 1976).

Aim

The aim of the present study was to examine the significance of R_{out}, E_1 and the slope of CSF pulse pressure versus ICP with regard to the selection of patients with suspected NPH for a CSF shunt.

Material and Methods

Sixty-seven patients with CT-verified hydrocephalus and clinical symptoms of NPH (gait disturbance, urinary incontinence and dementia) were subjected to a constant rate lumbar infusion test. Infusion rates were either 1.46 ml/min or 2.05 ml/min. The parameters of CSF dynamics were computed, by curve-fitting, from the time-pressure data stored in a parallel-lined computer using the following model equations:

$$R_{out} = \frac{P_\infty - P_b}{F_{in}} \text{ mm Hg/ml} \cdot \text{min}$$

$$P(t) = \frac{[F_{in} + C(P_b - P_o)][P_b - P_o]}{C(P_b - P_o) + F_{in}\, e^{-E_1[F_{in} + C][P_b - P_o]t}} + P_o \text{ mm Hg}$$

Intracranial Pressure VII
Eds.: J.T. Hoff and A.L. Betz

P(t) = pressure at time (t) P_∞ = steady state pressure
P_o = constant term P_b = baseline pressure
C   = $1/R_{out}$ F_{in} = infusion rate

Fifty patients were selected for CSF shunting using the following criteria:

R_{out} < 8 mm Hg/ml · min ----- no shunt
R_{out} ≥ 12 mm Hg/ml · min ----- shunt

Else: continuous pressure monitoring: > 5% B-waves – shunt
                                      ≤ 5% B-waves – no shunt

However, in five patients with strong clinical evidence for NPH, a CSF shunt was inserted in spite of these criteria.

Results

Thirty patients (60%) clinically improved as a result of shunting. Figure 1 shows the distribution of R_{out} in the 50 patients operated upon. No correlation was found between R_{out} and the effect of shunting.

Similarly, according to Fig. 2, the effect of a shunting procedure could not be predicted on the basis of E_1.

Figure 3 shows the distribution of the slope of the CSF pulse pressure versus ICP relationship in both improved and not-improved patients. The difference in slope was not statistically significant.

OPERATED PATIENTS

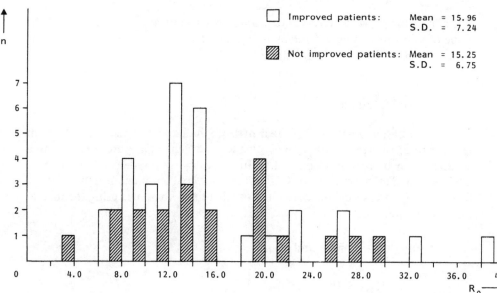

Improved patients: Mean = 15.96
                          S.D. = 7.24

Not improved patients: Mean = 15.25
                          S.D. = 6.75

Fig. 1. Distribution of R_{out} in the 50 patients who were selected for operation

[mmHg/ml·min]

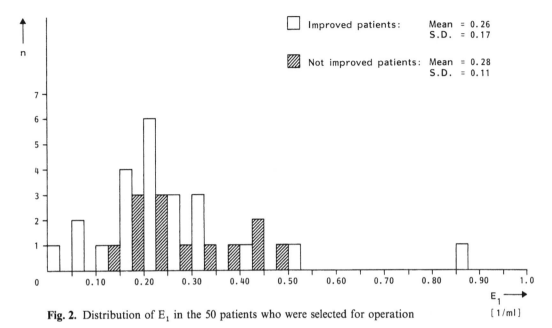

Fig. 2. Distribution of E_1 in the 50 patients who were selected for operation

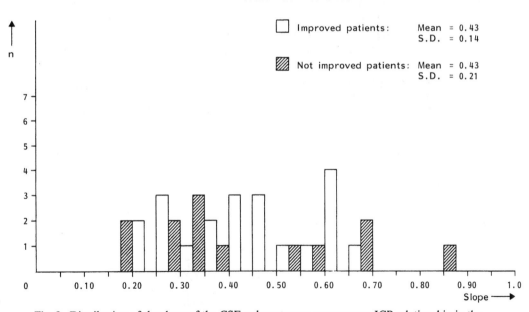

Fig. 3. Distribution of the slope of the CSF pulse pressure versus mean ICP relationship in the 50 patients who were selected for operation

	Improved	Not improved
Dilatation of temporal horns on CT	20	11
No dilatation of temporal horns on CT	6	6
	26	17

Sensitivity	$\dfrac{20}{20+6} \times 100\% = 77{,}0\%$
Specificity	$\dfrac{6}{10+6} \times 100\% = 35{,}3\%$

Fig. 4. Presence of dilated temporal horns on CT in improved and not-improved patients

In the present study, only dilation of the temporal horns on CT proved to be a consistent finding in NPH patients improving after shunting (Fig. 4) which is in accordance with the observation of Tans (1977). The specificity of this finding was, however, low.

Conclusions

From the present study it appears that neither a single parameter of CSF dynamics, nor a combination of parameters, has a predictive value with regard to the effect of a shunting procedure in patients with NPH.

The role of R_{out} as determined by the constant rate lumbar infusion method, in both diagnosis and prognosis of NPH can also be questioned on the basis of the finding that improvement after shunting occurred in patients with R_{out} values lower than 12 mm Hg/ml · min.

Looking for dilatation of the temporal horns on CT-scan in patients suspected of NPH would seem to be worthwhile.

References

Avezaat CJJ, van Eijndhoven JHM (1984) Thesis. A. Jongbloed and Zoon Publishers, The Hague, The Netherlands

Børgesen SE, Gjerris F (1982) The predictive value of conductance to outflow of CSF in normal pressure hydrocephalus. Brain 105:65–86

Belloni G, DiRocco C, Focacci C, Galli G, Maira G, Rossi GF (1976) Surgical indications in normotensive hydrocephalus. A retrospective analysis of the relations of some diagnostic findings to the results of surgical treatment. Acta Neurochir (Wien) 33:1–21

Tans JTJ (1979) Differentiation of normal pressure hydrocephalus and cerebral atrophy by computed tomography and spinal infusion tests. J Neurol 222:109–118

The Significance of Outflow Resistance Measurements in the Prediction of Outcome After CSF-Shunting in Patients with Normal Pressure Hydrocephalus

M. Kosteljanetz, L. Westergaard, J. Kaalund, and A.M. Nehen

Departments of Neurosurgery, Neuroanesthesia and Neuroradiology, Aalborg Sygehus, DK-9100 Aalborg (Denmark)

Selection of patients with normal-pressure hydrocephalus (NPH) for CSF shunting still remains a problem. Only few authors have been able to demonstrate a clear correlation between the presence of low conductance (or the reciprocal, increased resistance to CSF outflow ($= R_{out}$)) and the success rate after surgery (Børgesen and Gjerris 1982).

The author has previously demonstrated a linear relationship between R_{out} and intracranial pressure (ICP) in patients with NPH (Kosteljanetz 1986) and it is the contention of the author that the ICP *de facto* is (mildly) increased in patients with NPH who will benefit from shunting. This is in concert with the findings of other authors (e.g. Chawla et al. 1974). It therefore seems logical that there should exist a relationship between increased R_{out} and surgical success.

In order to test this hypothesis the authors undertook a controlled clinical study where the control group consisted of patients with NPH symptoms and signs, who underwent shunt surgery in spite of normal R_{out}.

Material and Method

The study group comprises eleven patients (selected from a larger NPH study where some patients did not undergo surgery) (Table 1) who fulfilled the following criteria: 1) clinical symptoms compatible with NPH (deteriorating mental faculties + various combinations and degrees of urinary problems and gait disturbances), 2) ventriculomegaly on CT and 3) small (less than 3 mm wide) or absent cortical sulci on CT (Kosteljanetz and Ingstrup 1985, Børgesen et al. 1980).

All eleven patients who fulfilled these criteria underwent ventriculo-peritoneal shunting under general anesthesia. Before the shunt was inserted an intraventricular cannula was placed and connected to an ICP monitoring system. The bolus injection technique (Marmarou et al. 1978, Kosteljanetz 1986) was employed to determine R_{out}. Three boluses were injected leading to three R_{out} values and the mean of these values constitutes the R_{out} value presented herein. During anesthesia, end-tidal pCO_2 was monitored and kept at a fairly constant level close to the patient's pCO_2 level prior to surgery. After the tests were performed the shunt was inserted.

After surgery all patients were followed for at least three months and underwent follow-up CT in order to confirm proper shunt function. (The study was approved by the Committee of Scientific Ethics in our county.)

Table 1. Some clinical data, results of outflow resistance measurements (R_{out}) and shunt surgery in eleven patients with normal-pressure hydrocephalus

Patient number	Sex	Age	Etiology	R_{out} mm Hg/ml/ min	Pre/post-operative grade	Outcome
1	F	64	Unknown	9.7	3/2	Improved
2	F	54	Unknown	7.2	3/3	No change
3	M	53	SAH	2.4	4/2	Improved
4	F	56	SAH	Infin.	2/2	Question.
5	F	47	SAH	4.2	3/3	Question.
6	F	45	Meningitis	4.5	2/2	Question.
7	F	40	SAH	12.2	4/2	Improved
8	M	71	Unknown	infin.	3/n. a.	Death
9	M	80	Unknown	34.9	4/n. a.	Death
10	M	72	Unknown	> 20.0	3/n.a.	Complic.
11	M	63	Unknown	17.0	4/2	Improved

Grade according to Stein and Langfitt 1974 (see text).
SAH: Subarachnoid hemorrhage; Infin.: Infinite (see text); n.a.: Not accessible

Results

The results of R_{out} measurements and that of surgery appear in the Table. "Infin." means that there was no decay in ICP after bolus injection for several minutes so that R_{out} could not be calculated. The measure for outcome was an improvement of grade (according to Stein and Langfitt 1974). Three patients escaped postoperative grading due to complications or death. Three patients (Nos. 4, 5, 6) and their relatives reported improvement but that was not reflected in any change of the rating (= questionable).

Discussion

The study did not confirm the expected correlation between the result of R_{out} measurement and outcome after surgery, nor did it confirm the previously documented correlation between CT finding and R_{out} measurement with respect to the size of the cortical sulci. There are several possible explanations: R_{out} measured under the study conditions only reflects a moment of the "true". ICP and R_{out} may be influenced by anesthesia. Undiscovered CSF leaks may account for falsely low ICP values and thus erroneous R_{out} values. The model equations do not apply in the present setting (see also Kosteljanetz: "Further analysis ..." elsewhere in this volume).

References

Børgesen SE, Gjerris F (1982) The predictive value of conductance to outflow of CSF in normal pressure hydrocephalus. Brain 105:65–86

Børgesen SE, Gyldensted C, Gjerris F, Lester J (1980) Computed tomography and pneumoencephalography compared to outflow of CSF in normal pressure hydrocephalus. J Neuroradiol 20:17–22

Chawla JC, Hulme A, Cooper R (1974) Intracranial pressure in patients with dementia and communicating hydrocephalus. J Neurosurg 40:376–380

Kosteljanetz M (1986) CSF dynamics and pressure–volume relationships in communicating hydrocephalus. J Neurosurg 64:45–52

Kosteljanetz M, Ingstrup HM (1985) Normal pressure hydrocephalus: Correlation between CT and measurements of cerebrospinal fluid dynamics. Acta Neurochir (Wien) 77:8–13

Marmarou A, Shulman K, Rosende RM (1978) A nonlinear analysis of the cerebrospinal fluid system and intracranial pressure dynamics. J Neurosurg 48:332–344

Stein SC, Langfitt TW (1974) Normal-pressure hydrocephalus. Predicting the results of cerebrospinal fluid shunting. J Neurosurg 41:463–470

Does Compliance Predict Ventricular Reduction After Shunting for Normal Pressure Hydrocephalus

J.T.J. Tans and D.C.J. Poortvliet

Department of Neurology and TNO Research Unit for Clinical Neurophysiology, Westeinde Hospital, 32 Lijnbaan, NL-2512 VA The Hague (The Netherlands)

Introduction

Ventricular size before, as well as after, shunting for normal pressure hydrocephalus (NPH) correlates poorly with clinical improvement and resistance to outflow of cerebrospinal fluid (Rcsf) (Børgesen 1984, Shenkin et al. 1975). Most authors agree that compliance, which can be expressed as the pressure-volume index (PVI), is also not related to ventricular size (Kosteljanetz 1986, Shapiro et al. 1985, Tans and Poortvliet 1983), but its relationship with ventricular reduction after shunting has not been investigated. One might hypothesize that reduction will be greater in patients with a tight brain and that dilated ventricles surrounded by a compliant brain are less likely to diminish in size.

Previous investigators studied the magnitude of ventricular reduction, but did not consider its time course, which may be quite variable. The aim of this study, therefore, was to collect data on both the magnitude and the rate of reduction of ventricular size and relate these to PVI and Rcsf.

Patients and Methods

We selected 35 adult patients with NPH who met the following criteria:
1. Performance of constant flow infusion yielding an Rcsf > 13 mm Hg/ml/min.
2. Administration of multiple bolus infusions from which one PVI was calculated (Tans and Poortvliet 1985).
3. Insertion of a medium pressure ventriculoatrial shunt.
4. No complications during follow-up.
5. Availability of at least three CT scans with a mean of four; five linear measurements on CT were combined in one ventricular index; the maximum reduction ratio (RRm) was obtained from dividing the pre by the smallest postoperative ventricular index.

Fig. 1 A–C. Ventricular index before (*on y-axis*) and at variable intervals after shunting. *Group A, n*=11, rapide and marked reduction of ventricular size. *Group B, n*=16, slow and moderate to marked reduction. *Group C, n*=8, minimal to mild reduction

Eds.: J. T. Hoff and A. L. Betz
© Springer-Verlag Berlin Heidelberg 1989

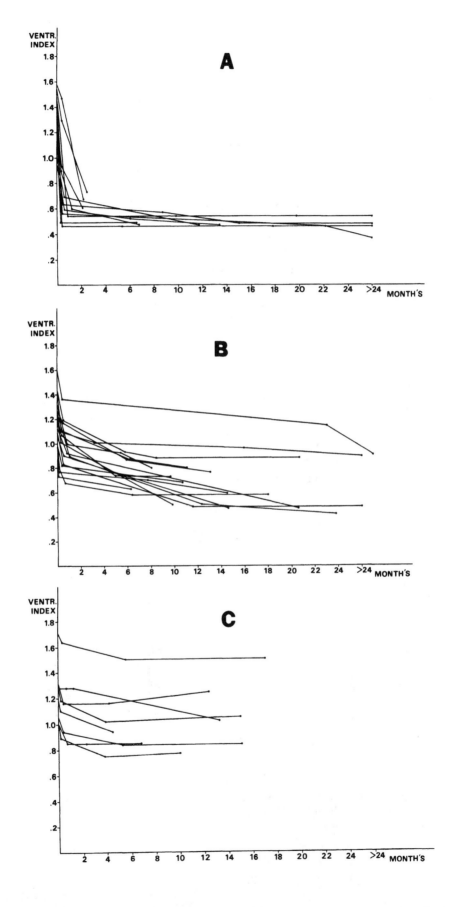

Results

No relationship was found between reduction of ventricular size and Rcsf. Regarding compliance, patients with marked ventricular reductions tended to have a small PVI. Since mild to moderate reductions did occur at all levels of compliance, linear regression analysis of RRm versus PVI yielded a coefficient of correlation of only −0.37. However, RRm represents magnitude of ventricular reduction. When also taking into account the rate of reduction, three groups could be distinguished:

1. A rapid and marked reduction followed by a stable or slightly decreasing ventricular volume (Fig. 1A). Mean RRm was 2.5±0.5, range 2.0–3.6. In this group A, consisting of 11 patients, maximum reduction was achieved within the first weeks after shunting or the first months at most.

2. A slow and moderate to marked reduction was seen in group B, comprising 16 patients (Fig. 1B). Mean RRm was 1.9±0.5, range 1.4–3.0. After a limited decrease in the first month, ventricular dimensions continued to decrease during the first year and even during the second year in a number of cases. The smallest ventricles in these patients were measured after a mean period of 18 months after surgery.

3. A minimal to mild reduction with a mean RRm of 1.2±0.1, range 1.1–1.3 (Fig. 1C). Some of the 8 patients of group C showed markedly disturbed csf dynamics and a good result of shunting, whereas in others Rcsf was mildly increased, the PVI high and the result of shunting poor.

As could be expected Rcsf values fell in the same range for groups A, B and C (Fig. 2). Although mean Rcsf was higher in group A the difference did not

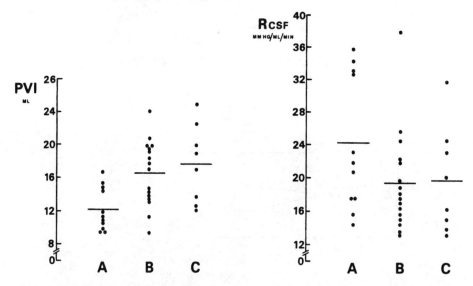

Fig. 2. PVI and Rcsf values in groups *A*, *B* and *C*. Analysis of variance: mean PVI of group *A* significantly different from that of groups *B* and *C*, $p < 0.005$; differences in mean Rcsf not significant

388

reach statistical significance. On the other hand it is clearly demonstrated in Fig. 2 that the lowest PVIs were found in group A. The mean PVI of 12.2 ml was also significantly different from that of groups B (16.5 ml) and C (17.6 ml). In group B, both Rcsf and PVI tended to be either high or low, whereas in group C, Rcsf and PVI were more or less inversely related.

Discussion

It is well known that the magnitude of ventricular reduction after shunting varies widely. This study revealed that the rate of reduction is also extremely variable with patients showing fast and very slow reductions. Therefore, studies relating the reduction of ventricular size to clinical improvement or other parameters should include CT scans taken one to two years after surgery.

No relation was found between ventricular size before shunting and Rcsf, PVI, or ventricular size after shunting. The magnitude of ventricular reduction did not correlate with Rcsf and rather weakly with PVI. Our most important finding was that a relationship exists between reduction of ventricular size and PVI when this reduction is classified on the basis of magnitude and rate. In patients exhibiting rapid and marked reduction after shunting, compliance before shunting was distinctly lower. Groups A and B mainly differed in the rate and groups B and C in the magnitude of reduction. Since the PVIs of A and B were different and that of B and C rather similar, compliance seems to affect primarily the rate of ventricular reduction.

CSF outflow resistance remains the key factor in the selection of patients for shunting, but PVI determinations could be of additional value for the prediction of ventricular reduction after shunting.

References

Børgesen SE (1984) Conductance to outflow of csf in normal pressure hydrocephalus. Acta Neurochir (Wien) 71:1–45

Kosteljanetz M (1986) CSF dynamics and pressure–volume relationships in communicating hydrocephalus. J Neurosurg 64:45–52

Shapiro K, Fried A, Marmarou A (1985) Biomechanical and hydrodynamic characterization of the hydrocephalic infant. J Neurosurg 63:69–75

Shenkin HA, Greenberg JO, Grosmann CB (1975) Ventricular size after shunting for idiopathic normal pressure hydrocephalus. J Neurol Neurosurg Psychiatry 38:833–837

Tans JTJ, Poortvliet DCJ (1983) Steady-state and bolus infusions in hydrocephalus. In: Ishii S, Nagai H, Broek M (eds) Intracranial pressure V. Springer, Berlin Heidelberg New York Tokyo, pp 636–640

Tans JTJ, Poortvliet DCJ (1985) CSF outflow resistance and pressure-volume index determined by steady-state and bolus infusions. Clin Neurol Neurosurg 87:159–165

Attempts to Predict the Probability of Clinical Improvement Following Shunting of Patients with Presumed Normal Pressure Hydrocephalus

D.J. Price

Department of Neurosurgery, Pinderfields Hospital, Wakefield WF1 4DG (UK)

With the advent of the CT scanner, hydrocephalus is more widely diagnosed and this imposes an increased need to discriminate between the very treatable condition of normal pressure hydrocephalus (NPH) from cerebral failure due to diffuse parenchymal atrophy or Alzheimer's disease. Such an ability to discriminate will hopefully prevent tragic, inappropriate relegation of dementing patients with a reversible condition to a life of misery or permanent residence in mental institution.

Although a CSF diversionary procedure is simple, it is not without risk and it is for this reason that it would be irresponsible to suggest indiscriminate surgery for all patients with radiological evidence of symmetrical pan-ventricular non-obstructive hydrocephalus.

The crucial distinction between NPH and atrophy was initially presumed to be a clinical one. The classical history was considered to be characterised by a gradual onset of symptoms over weeks and months with unsteadiness of gait, mild impairment of short term memory, a lack of attention and initiative, slowness and paucity of thought and action.

Methods of Measuring Outflow Resistance

The patient is anesthetized and maintained at a constant pCO_2 of between 3.5 kPa and 4 kPa. Two catheters are inserted into the right frontal horn of the ventricle through a burr hole and acrylic is used as a sealant. Normal saline is introduced through one catheter and the other is connected to a Gould P60 transducer. A Devices M19 recorder provides the means to recognize the achievement of steady state and estimate each mean ICP.

Method 1 – Constant Flow

A series of steady states relating to each infusion rate ranging from 0.3 up to a maximum of 5 ml per minute is carried out. The inflow rate is deduced by adding the presumed CSF formation rate of 0.3 ml/min to the infusion rate. For convenience the data are collected during the test on a lap-top computer and a simple graph is displayed on the screen to allow selection of the XY pairs. The linear

Eds.: J. T. Hoff and A. L. Betz
© Springer-Verlag Berlin Heidelberg 1989

regression for calculation of the slope of the graph is performed by a Hewlett Packard desk top computer.

Method 2 – Constant Pressure

For the last 11 patients, Børgesen's method (Børgesen et al. 1978), has been used to enable the two techniques to be compared. An outflow tube is connected and the infusion rate is maintained constant but the height of the orifice of the outflow tube is varied every 10 min with measurement of the volume of outflow during each second 5 min period. The same linear regression is used to calculate the outflow resistance.

Results

Preliminary Series

For a period from 1974–1980, I studied a series of 20 patients with symmetrical pan-ventricular non-obstructive hydrocephalus with 2 or 3 features of the clinical triad and a baseline ICP of less than 14 mm Hg. They were all treated with a

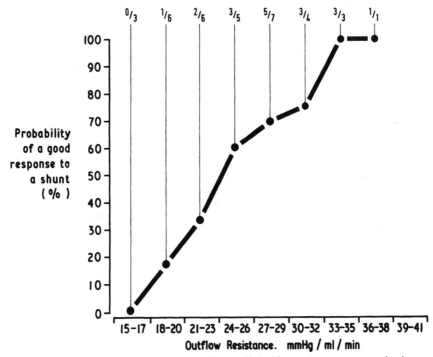

Fig. 1. The probability of a shunt causing a significant clinical improvement seems to be dependent on the outflow resistance

391

shunt. Initially I had the impression that the patients with atrophy had an outflow resistance below 10 mm Hg/ml/min and those with NPH had values above 15 mm Hg/ml/min (Price and Onabanjo 1976).

Main Series

On the basis of this very small series I decided to restrict shunt procedures to a second series of patients with the same clinical entrance criteria but only if the resistance exceeded 14 mm Hg/ml/min. Of 58 patients, 23 had resistances of less than 15 mm Hg/ml/min. The remaining 35 were treated with ventriculo-atrial shunts. None of the three patients with resistance values below 18 mm Hg/ml/min improved but as the resistance rose, the proportion of responsive patients in each small subgroup increased (Fig. 1). Of 52 linear regressions, 43 had R values in excess of 0.95.

When the two methods of measurement of resistance were compared in the last 11 patients, a very reasonable correlation was achieved ($Y = 0.29 + 0.96 X$, $R = 0.828$).

Comparison with Clinical and Radiological Presentation

Of the 23 patients with resistances of less than 15 mm Hg/ml/min, 7 had the full triad of clinical features. For those 35 patients with higher resistances, 21 had the full triad. The differences are insignificant. Of 6 patients with clear CT evidence of atrophy, all had outflow resistances below 15 mm Hg/ml/min. Eleven with most of the CT features of NPH all had resistances in excess of 14 mm Hg/ml/min. In the majority, however, features of atrophy and NPH were mixed and there was no correlation with outflow resistances.

Conclusion

I confirmed the findings of Gjerris et al. (1986), Tans and Poortvliet (1983) and Ekstedt (1978) that outflow resistance is a useful measurement for raising our suspicions of NPH and it is a more powerful predictor of a successful response to a shunt than any combination of clinical or radiological features.

References

Børgesen SE, Gjerris F, Sørensen SC (1978) The resistance to cerebrospinal fluid absorption in humans. A method of evaluation by lumbo-ventricular perfusion with particular reference to normal pressure hydrocephalus. Acta Neurol Scand 57:88–96

Ekstedt J (1978) CSF hydrodynamic studies in man. 2 normal hydrodynamic variables related to CSF pressure and flow. J Neurol Neurosurg Psychiatry 41:345–353

Gjerris F, Børgesen SE, Schmidt K, Sørensen PS, Gyring J (1986) Measurement of conductance to cerebrospinal fluid outflow by the steady-state perfusion method in patients with normal or increased intracranial pressure. In: Miller JD, Teasdale GM, Rowan JO, Galbraith SL, Mendelow AD (eds) Intracranial pressure VI. Springer, Berlin Heidelberg New York Tokyo, pp 411–416

Price DJ, Onabanjo (1976) A dynamic pressure profile in the management of patients with glioma. In: Beks JWF, Bosch DA, Brock M (eds) Intracranial pressure III. Springer, Berlin Heidelberg New York, pp 314–319

Tans JTJ, Poortvliet DCJ (1983) Steady-state and bolus infusion in hydrocephalus. In: Ishii S, Nagai H, Brock M (eds) Intracranial pressure V. Springer, Berlin Heidelberg New York, pp 636–640

Different Time Course of Clinical Symptoms and CSF Dynamics in Patients with Pseudotumor Cerebri

P. Soelberg-Sørensen, F. Gjerris, and J.F. Schmidt

University Department of Neurology and Neurosurgery, Rigshospitalet, DK-2100 Copenhagen (Denmark)

Introduction

Pseudotumor cerebri or benign intracranial hypertension is nearly uniformly reported to be a self-limiting disorder with an excellent long-term prognosis except for the occurrence of permanent visual loss in a minority of the patients (Corbett et al. 1982, Soelberg-Sørensen et al. 1988). In a number of cases pseudotumor may run a more protracted course with persisting or recurring symptoms or persistent increased intracranial pressure (ICP). In order to compare the clinical course of pseudotumor and the development of CSF dynamics, we followed 9 pseudotumor patients with neurological and ophthalmologic examinations and repeated measurements of ICP and resistance to CSF outflow (R_{out}) for an average of 25 months.

Material and Methods

Nine patients with pseudotumor were studied: 2 men and 7 women aged 13 to 66 years (median age 45 years). All fulfilled conventional criteria for pseudotumor cerebri: Increased intracranial pressure, papilledema, no mass lesion or hydrocephalus in CT, normal CSF composition, and no clinical suspicion of venous sinus thrombosis. Among possible predisposing factors, obesity was the most common finding: 5 of the 7 women were more than 25% overweight according to the ideal weight for Scandinavians. One patient had been treated with tetracycline for several years and 2 patients had arterial hypertension.

On admission and at each follow-up visit, all patients had a full neurological and ophthalmological examination. ICP was monitored by an epidural transducer for 24 h (2 patients) or via a lumbar cannula for 30–120 min (7 patients). The pressure during steady state was calculated and increments (plateau waves and B-waves) from this steady-state pressure were described. The resistance to CSF outflow (R_{out}) was measured by a lumbo-lumbar perfusion technique, which is a modification of the lumbo-ventricular perfusion method previously described (Børgesen et al. 1978). With the patient in the lateral recumbent position, a 1.2 mm cannula was inserted in the lumbar subarachnoid space, and when steady-state ICP was achieved, infusion of Ringer's lactate (V_{in}) was started at a rate of

Eds.: J. T. Hoff and A. L. Betz

0.92 to 1.82 ml per min. The outflow volume (V_{out}) from a tube connected with the lumbar cannula was collected and measured gravimetrically. The CSF formation rate (V_{for}) was assumed to be 0.4 ml per min. The absorbed CSF volume per min (V_{abs}) could then be calculated from the following formula: $V_{abs} = V_{in} + V_{for} - V_{out}$. The perfusion was performed at different steady-state pressure levels achieved by elevating the outlet of the outflow tube. The absorbed CSF volume was then plotted against the different obtained ICP values, and the slope of the resulting regression line expresses the conductance to CSF outflow, the reciprocal to R_{out} (Børgesen et al. 1978).

The patients were treated with acetazolamide and furosemide for up to 24 months or until cessation of symptoms. Follow-up visits including neurological, ophthalmologic and CT examinations took place with 3–6 months intervals, and the measurements of ICP and R_{out} were repeated after 12–48 months.

Results

On Admission. All patients had symptoms of increased ICP. Headache was the presenting symptom in 8 patients, of whom 7 complained of severe headache. Eight patients had experienced transient visual obscurations, two had permanent blurring of vision, and one had double vision. The symptoms had been present from 2 to 18 months, median 6 months. All patients had papilledema with disc hemorrhages and protrusion (1 to 3 diopters) and enlarged blind spots. The steady-state ICP was increased in all patients (18–35 mm Hg). Three patients had plateau waves of 5 to 20 min duration, with a peak pressure up to 60 mm Hg. All patients but one had B-waves (increments of ICP of one-half to two waves per min with an amplitude of 5 to 15 mm Hg) for more than 50% of the monitored time. In all patients, R_{out} was increased far beyond the upper limit of normal (12.5 mm Hg $\cdot$ ml^{-1} $\cdot$ min^{-1}). The median R_{out} was 29.4 mm Hg $\cdot$ ml^{-1} $\cdot$ min^{-1} (range 16.2–50.0). No significant correlation was found between ICP and R_{out} ($r = 0.23$; $p > 0.1$).

At the Last Follow-up Examination. Three patients still had headache as the only symptom that could be ascribed to increased ICP. In 4 patients, the papilledema had resolved completely; whereas 5 patients had developed chronic papillary changes with gliosis of the optic discs. The evolution in ICP and R_{out} is shown in Fig. 1. At the last examination only 3 patients had normal ICP and only one of these patient had normal R_{out}. The development of clinical symptoms and CSF dynamics appear in Table 1. Out of the 4 patients without symptoms and signs of increased ICP, 3 had normal ICP but only one of them also had normal R_{out}. Conversely, out of the 3 patients who still complained of headache, 2 had increased ICP but one had normal ICP and nearly normal R_{out}.

Table 1. Clinical symptoms, optic disc appearance, intracranial pressure (ICP), and resistance to CSF outflow (R_{out}) at first examination and at last examination

Patient	First examination					Last examination			
	Clinical symptoms	Optic disc appearance (diopters)	ICP (mm Hg)	R_{out} (mm Hg/ ml/min)	Interval (months)	Clinical symptoms	Optic disc appearance (diopters)	ICP (mm Hg)	R_{out} (mm Hg/ ml/min)
1	Headache	Edema (1.5)	20	24.4	18	0	Normal (0)	10	13.6
2	Headache Obscurations	Edema (1.0)	18	27.8	48	0	Normal (0)	8	7.1
3	Headache Obscurations	Edema (2.5)	35	29.4	30	Headache	Gliosis (1)	7	15.2
4	Headache Obscurations	Edema (3.0)	25	16.9	18	0	Normal (0)	20	19.2
5	Headache Obscurations	Edema (2.0)	26	47.6	24	Headache	Gliosis (1)	20	12.5
6	Headache Obscurations	Edema (3.0)	35	45.5	18	0	Gliosis (1)	20	30.3
7	Obscurations	Edema (3.0)[a]	22	21.7	24	0	Gliosis (0)	27	43.5
8	Headache Obscurations	Edema (2.0)	32	32.2	18	0	Normal (0)	25	23.2
9	Headache	Edema (3.0)	24	50.0	48	Headache	Gliosis (2)	32	35.7

[a] Unilateral papilledema; Normal ICP ≤15 mm Hg; Normal R_{out} ≤ 12.5 mm Hg/ml/min.

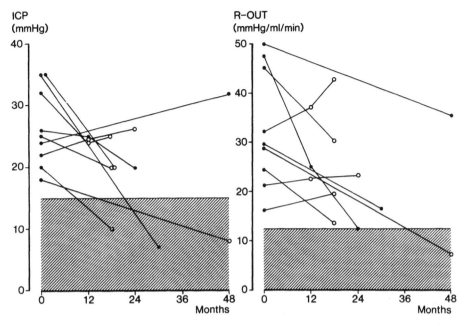

Fig. 1. Course of clinical symptoms, intracranial pressure (*ICP*), and resistance to CSF outflow (R_out) in patients with pseudotumor cerebri. *Closed circles* denote clinical symptoms and signs of increased ICP, *open circles* symptom-free patients. *Hatched area* indicate normal range

Discussion

The finding of increased R_{out} in patients with pseudotumor cerebri is in concordance with the findings of previous studies (Calabrese et al. 1978, Sklar et al. 1979, Gjerris et al. 1985) and support the hypothesis that a decreased bulk flow is of pathophysiological significance for this condition. This prospective study also demonstrates that symptoms and signs of intracranial hypertension disappear in the majority of patients, despite a sustained increased ICP in some and an apparently permanent or long-standing increased R_{out}. A few previous studies have reported a poor correlation between clinical symptoms and ICP (Corbett et al. 1982, Soelberg-Sørensen et al. 1988) and Foley (1977) and Rottenberg et al. (1980) have suggested that pseudotumor in some cases may be a chronic disease.

We propose the following hypothesis for the pathogenesis of pseudotumor cerebri. All patients with pseudotumor have an increased R_{out} as a common defect which may be caused by congenitally fewer arachnoid absorptive channels or by acquired structural changes of the arachnoid villi. Such individuals would be prone to develop clinical symptoms of intracranial hypertension in disorders with increased CSF formation, increased resistance to CSF absorption, or intracellular brain water accumulation. Changes in female sex hormone production, steroid withdrawal, pituitary-adrenal dysfunction, hypoparathyroidism, tetracycline and other unknown factors could be the precipitants provoking a rise in ICP. In some pseudotumor patients, ICP normalizes when the precipitating factor is eliminated, whereas in other patients the ICP is permanently stabilized at a higher level and the clinical symptoms and signs of intracranial hypertension resolve. In nearly all patients, however, an increased or high normal R_{out} value measured by the perfusion study will reflect the decreased absorption capacity at the arachnoid villi level.

In conclusion, monitoring of the lumbar pressure and measurement of R_{out} by the lumbo-lumbar perfusion method is of considerable diagnostic value. The examination can be repeated several times during the course of the disease to identify the different subgroups of pseudotumor patients: a group with remission of clinical symptoms and signs, normalization of ICP, and a decrease of R_{out} to normal or near normal values; a second group with clinical improvement but persistent increased ICP and R_{out}; and a third group with longstanding clinical symptoms and increased ICP and R_{out}.

References

Børgesen SE, Gjerris F, Sørensen SC (1978) The resistance to cerebrospinal fluid absorption in humans. Acta Neurol Scand 57:88–96

Calabrese VP, Selhorst JB, Harbison JW (1978) CSF infusion test in pseudotumor cerebri. Trans Am Neurol Assoc 103:146–150

Corbett JJ, Savino PJ, Thompson HS et al. (1982) Visual loss in pseudotumor cerebri: Follow-up of 57 patients from five to 41 years and a profile of 14 patients with severe visual loss. Arch Neurol 39:461–474

Foley KM (1977) Is benign intracranial hypertension a chronic disease. Neurology 27:388

Gjerris F, Soelberg-Sørensen P, Vorstrup S, Paulson OB (1985) Intracranial pressure, conductance to cerebrospinal fluid outflow, and cerebral blood flow in patients with benign hypertension (pseudotumor cerebri). Ann Neurol 17:158–162

Rottenberg DA, Foley KM, Posner JB (1980) Hypothesis: The pathogenesis of pseudotumor cerebri. Med Hypotheses 6:913–916

Sklar FH, Beyer CW, Ramanathan M (1979) Cerebrospinal fluid dynamics in patients with pseudotumor cerebri. Neurosurgery 5:208–216

Soelberg-Sørensen P, Krogsaa B, Gjerris F (1988) Clinical course and prognosis of pseudotumor cerebri. A prospective study of 24 patients. Acta Neurol Scand 77:164–172

Intracranial Pressure on Pre- and Post-Shunt Surgery in Patients with Normal Pressure Hydrocephalus (NPH)

K. Tanaka, H. Hayashi, K. Ohata, H. Sakamoto, and S. Nishimura

Department of Neurosurgery, Osaka City University Medical School, 1-5-7 Asahi-machi, Abeno-ku, Osaka 545 (Japan)

Introduction

Although shunt surgery is a generally accepted way of treating patients with NPH, there are only a few papers (Symon and Dorsch 1975) which report the changes in ICP after shunt. Without knowledge concerning ICP changes after shunt, we are apt to consider that the closing pressure of the shunt system which was installed was not low enough or that the patient was not a good candidate for the shunt surgery when it was not effective. In order to supplement the basic data, not only ICP changes but also changes in pressure volume index (PVI), outflow resistance (R_{out}) and the profile of B-waves after shunt were investigated.

Clinical Material and Methods

Fifteen patients with NPH underwent shunt surgery using Heyer-Schulte's on-off flushing reservoir with anti-siphon and low pressure Pudenz peritoneal catheter. A ventricular catheter was inserted into the lateral ventricle, opposite to the shunted side, for monitoring ICP and CSF manipulation. ICP was continuously monitored for 24 hr before and after opening the on-off valve. The highest and the lowest portions of the ICP fluctuation, except for the pressure waves, were sampled every 30 min throughout the period of ICP monitoring. The mean ICP ($mICP_{24}$) was arbitrarily defined as the mean pressure of all these pressure readings. Two prominent B-waves were sampled every 30 min and the peak pressure (BPp) and the trough pressure (BPo) of the B-waves were measured. The mean peak pressure and the magnitude of B-wave (Bmag = BPp − BPo) were calculated. PVI and R_{out} were measured periodically by Marmarou's bolus injection technique (Marmarou et al. 1975). All these measurements were obtained from a 24 hr period each of pre- and post-opening of the on-off valve. The patients were lying flat throughout the measurements and the reference point of the transducer for ICP monitoring was the external auditory meatus.

Results

Out of 17 shunt operations in 15 patients, the operation was effective symptomatically on 12 occasions (group E). On 5 occasions, the patients showed no change or an aggravation of symptoms (group N). Between these two groups, there were no statistical differences in terms of closing pressure of the entire shunt system, $mICP_{24}$, BPp and Bmag, PVI, or R_{out} in the pre-opening period of the on-off valve. The $mICP_{24}$ prior to the opening of the valve in groups E and N were 132.6 ± 28.6 (mean $\pm$ SD) and 113.8 ± 9.8 mm H_2O, respectively. In group E, $mICP_{24}$ decreased to 75.0 ± 25.8 mm H_2O after opening the valve and this change was statistically significant ($p < 0.01$). Even after the valve was opened, B-waves were still observed with less peak pressure and less magnitude. The BPp and the Bmag decreased from 19.9 ± 4.9 to 12.2 ± 3.4 mm Hg ($p < 0.05$), and from 4.6 ± 2.4 to 2.5 ± 1.3 mm Hg (not significant), respectively. PVI increased from 28.2 ± 12.8 to 45.9 ± 22.1 ml and R_{out} decreased from 5.95 ± 5.14 to $1.69 \pm 0,83$ mm Hg/ml/min and these changes were highly significant ($p < 0.01$). The % decrease of $mICP_{24}$ after the valve was opened, did not correlate with the % increase of PVI, but did correlate well with the % decrease of R_{out} ($p < 0.01$, $r = 0.7637$). In the patients of group N, shuntography was performed to test for any obstruction, there was no significant difference between pre- and post-opening periods in all of these parameters.

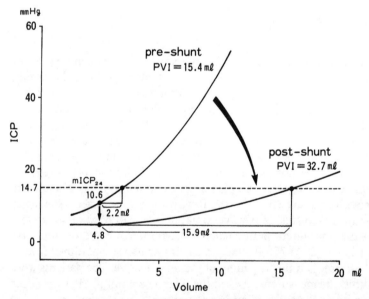

Fig. 1. After shunt surgery, PVI increased from 15.4 to 32.7 ml. R_{out} and $mICP_{24}$ decreased from 21.05 to 3.82 mm Hg/ml/min and from 10.6 to 4.8 mm Hg, respectively. On the pre-shunt pressure-volume curve, 2.2 ml of volume change in the intracranial cavity is enough to cause the ICP to rise above normal, but 15.9 ml will be needed post-shunt surgery. In this fashion, the shunt installation not only decreases the $mICP_{24}$ but also increases the CSF buffering capacity by increasing PVI and decreasing R_{out}

400

Discussion

After the on-off valve was opened, $mICP_{24}$ of the patients in group E decreased to 75.0 ± 25.8 mm H_2O. PVI increased by 72.3% from the pre-opening value of 28.2 ± 12.8 ml, and R_{out} decreased by 57.5% from the value of 5.95 mm Hg/ml/min. BPp also decreased from 19.9 to 12.2 mm Hg. It has been reported that the mICP correlates well with the R_{out} by several authors (Børgesen and Gjerris 1987, Kosteljanetz 1986). In addition to this fact, the % change of $mICP_{24}$ significantly correlated with the % change of R_{out} ($p < 0.01$). In this way, the shunt installation not only decreases the $mICP_{24}$ but also increases the CSF buffering capacity by increasing PVI and decreasing R_{out} (Fig. 1). It was our conclusion that we should appreciate the importance of Ro of the shunt system itself in decreasing the entire R_{out} of the patient after shunting. This concept will be discussed in detail in the other part of this volume (Tanaka and Nishimura, pp 368–373).

References

Børgesen SE, Gjerris F (1987) Relationships between intracranial pressure, ventricular size, and resistance to CSF outflow. J Neurosurg 67:535–539

Kosteljanetz M (1986) CSF dynamics and pressure–volume relationships in communicating hydrocephalus. J Neurosurg 64:45–52

Marmarou A, Shulman K, LaMorgese J (1975) Compartmental analysis of compliance and outflow resistance of the cerebrospinal fluid system. J Neurosurg 43:523–534

Symon L, Dorsch NWC (1975) Use of long-term intracranial pressure measurement to assess hydrocephalic patients prior to shunt surgery. J Neurosurg 42:258–273

Tanaka K, Nishimura S (1989) The importance of outflow resistance of the shunt system for elimination of B-waves. This volume, pp 368–373

CSF Hydrodynamics and CSF Flow Through a Shunt in Hydrocephalus

C. Kadowaki, M. Hara, M. Numoto, and K. Takeuchi

Department of Neurosurgery, Kyorin University School of Medicine, 6-20-2 Shinkawa, Mitaka, Tokyo 181 (Japan)

Introduction

Hydrodynamic studies of cerebrospinal fluid (CSF) were evaluated in eleven adult patients with communicating hydrocephalus. CSF flow through a shunt, measured with an inshunt CSF flowmeter developed by the authors, radioisotope (RI) cisternography, clearance of dye (phenolsulfonphthalein, PSP) administered intrathecally, and intracranial pressure (ICP) were compared with improvements in neurological symptoms and signs and changes in CT findings.

Materials and Methods

Eleven adult patients with communicating hydrocephalus in the present study included 4 females and 7 males with a mean age of 55 years (range 20–67 years). Six cases were due to ruptured aneurysm, 2 to cerebral contusion, one to hypertensive intracerebral hemorrhage and 2 to idiopathic hydrocephalus. All patients had some degree of mental deterioration from 7T (tracheostomy) to 14 on GCS. Ten of the 11 cases suffered from gait disturbance and all suffered from urinary incontinence. All patients were submitted to CT, RI (^{111}In-DTPA) cisternography and measuring CSF flow in a shunt with an inshunt flowmeter. Clearance tests of PSP administered intrathecally into urine within 24 hr were performed to clarify the degree of CSF absorption on 6 of the 11 cases, and ICP monitorings via either intraventricular or epidural pressure were also performed on 9 of the 11 cases. All had undergone ventriculo-peritoneal shunts with medium pressure catheters 7–120 days after diagnosis.

Results

Six of the 11 cases had clinical improvement in neurological symptoms and signs after shunting (Table 1).

Intracranial Pressure VII
Eds.: J. T. Hoff and A. L. Betz
© Springer-Verlag Berlin Heidelberg 1989

Table 1. Cases of hydrocephalus

Case	age/sex		Preoperative						Postoperative			
			CT Evans' ratio	RI cisternography		PSP clearance (%)	ICP		CSF flow		CT Evans' ratio	Neurology
				ventricular reflux	delayed circulation		mean (mmHg)	B	max/min (ml/min)	volume (ml/d)		
1	54	F	37	++	++	64	12/10	+	0.06/0.01	42	23	improved
2	64	F	42	+			12/8	+	0.07/0.01		42	no change
3	67	M	33	++	++	69	12/10	+	0.07/0.02	58	33	improved
4	52	F	40	++	-	72	10/8	-	0.09/0.01		35	improved
5	68	M	32	-	+	20	8/7	-	0.12/0.01	56	28	no change
6	63	M	39	++	-				0.13/0.01	115	32	improved
7	42	M	42	++					0.18/0.02		30	improved
8	60	M	40	++	-	28	15/7	+	0.23/0.02		23	improved
9	59	F	34	++	++	48	8/6	-	0.35/0.01		29	no change
10	53	M	35	+	-		5/4	+	0.64/0.01	278	32	no change
11	20	M	40	++	++		25/10	+	1.93/0.07	504	40	no change

CT

Preoperative CT revealed ventricular dilatation in all cases with a mean Evans' ratio of 37 (range 32–42). Ventricular sizes reduced postoperatively to an average of 32 (range 23–42) in 8 cases. Changes in ventricular size did not show a significant correlation with clinical response to shunting.

RI Cisternography

Scans of all cases yielded definitely positive results; ventricular reflux in 10, ventricular stasis in 8, convexity stasis in 5, and 6 patients favorably responded to shunting.

Dye Clearance Test

The dye clearance test revealed that 5 of the 6 cases had disturbed absorption with less than 70% secretion into urine within 24 hours. Four responded favorably.

ICP

Mean values in most of the 9 cases studied were lower than 15 mm Hg, 6 of them showed frequent B-waves and none showed A-waves. Only 3 of the 6 cases with B-waves responded to shunting. No correlation could be found between the appearance of B-waves and clinical improvement.

CSF Flow in Shunt

For all patients, CSF flow in the shunt fluctuated from 0.01 ml/min to 1.93 ml/min. Daily volumes of CSF flowing through the shunt were 42 ml–504 ml with peaks of 0.06 ml/min to 1.93 ml/min, and each had its own rhythmic pattern. Cases with peak CSF flow averaging 0.10 ml/min (range 0.06–0.23), for an average of less than 120 ml/day, showed improvements in neurological findings after shunting. However, in cases of moderately disturbed CSF absorption with 50% or less dye clearance within 24 hr, daily volume of CSF flowing through the shunt tended to exceed 115 ml.

Discussion

It is difficult to predict the benefits of a shunt procedure in NPH showing disturbances in CSF dynamics. Therefore, multiple clinical and laboratory features were evaluated with respect to any improvements in neurological status after shunting. Peterson et al. (1985) reported that typical NPH patients had about a 75% chance of some improvement after shunting, but reduction of ventricular size after shunting is not related to clinical improvement. Tamaki et al. (1983) found that the presence of B-waves in NPH is related to increased CSF malabsorption and provides a reliable indication of the shunt. Tans and Poortvliet (1988) reported that the most reliable predictive method for the benefit of shunting is to determine resistance to CSF outflow. However, the prognostic value of diagnostic tests is not yet clarified. Our results showed that clinical improvements after shunting could hardly be predicted on the basis of disturbed circulation of CSF in RI cisternography and dye clearance test, and reduction of ventricular size on CT.

Conclusion

The imaging diagnosis of serial CT and RI cisternography fall far short of adequately assessing the benefit of a shunt.

Clarification of CSF flow through a shunt can lead to an accurate calculation of the neurological changes.

References

Hara M, Kadowaki C, Konishi Y, Ogashiwa M, Numoto M, Takeuchi K (1983) A new method for measuring cerebrospinal fluid flow in shunts. J Neurosurg 58:557–561

Huckman MS (1981) Normal pressure hydrocephalus: Evaluation of diagnostic and prognostic tests. AJNR 2:385–395

Kadowaki C, Hara M, Numoto M, Takeuchi K (1986) CSF circulation in hydrocephalus. In: Miller JD, Teasdale GM et al. (eds) Intracranial pressure IV. Springer, Berlin Heidelberg New York Tokyo, pp 423–427

Peterson RC, Mokri B, Laws ER (1985) Surgical treatment of idiopathic hydrocephalus in elderly patients. Neurology 35:307–311

Tamaki N, Kusunoki T, Fujita K, Kose S, Noda S, Masumura M, Matsumoto S (1983) Hydrodynamics in normal pressure hydrocephalus – correlation between the incidence of B-waves, dynamics of cerebrospinal fluid circulation, and cerebral blood flow. In: Ishi S, Hagai H, Brock M (eds) Intracranial pressure V. Springer, Berlin Heidelberg New York, pp 669–674

Tans JTJ, Poortvliet DCJ (1988) Reduction of ventricular size after shunting for normal pressure hydrocephalus related to CSF dynamics before shunting. J Neurol Neurosurg Psychiatry 51:521–525

Normal Pressure Hydrocephalus in Children –
The State of Hypercompensation

J. Wocjan[1], L. Batorski[1], M. Czosnyka[2], P. Wollk-Laniewski[3],
and W. Zaworski[2]

[1] Clinic of Neurosurgery, Child's Health Centre, [2] Institute of Electronics Fundamentals,
[3] Department of Anesthesiology and Intensive Care, Child's Health Centre, Warsaw (Poland)

According to current knowledge, normal-pressure hydrocephalus (NPH) is characterized by the following biomechanical factors: normal or slightly elevated ICP level and increased resistance to absorption of cerebrospinal fluid (RCSF) (Bering and Sato 1963, Black 1980, Guidetti and Gagliardi 1972). However, little is known about the other biomechanical features of the cerebrospinal system which can also play a significant role in its pathomechanism. In some recent papers, suggestions that increased capability of CSF storage in the ventricular system may be a reason for its progressive enlargement despite normal ICP levels, have been presented (Kosteljanetz 1986).

Material and Methods

From a group of 80 children with an enlarged ventricular system examined in 1983–1987 in the Neurosurgical Clinic of Child's Health Centre using the constant-rate spinal infusion test, we chose twenty-two children with resting pressure considered to be "normal" i.e., below 11 mm Hg. Eleven patients from this group had RCSF within normal range – below 12 mm Hg/ml/min – forming a reference group; in another eleven the RCSF was found to be increased – above 12 mm Hg/ml/min, matching the criteria of NPH.

For the purpose of the statistical analysis, the following factors were compared: (1) Clinical: age, sex, duration of symptoms, head circumference (expressed as deviation from 50 percentile, in percents), history of infection of the central nervous system (CNS), the history of birth trauma, the presence of CNS malformations, history of epileptic seizures, results of funduscopic examination, results of psychometric tests (Psyche-Catell or Brunet-Lezine scale). (2) Factors describing cerebrospinal system: resting amplitude of the pulse wave (AMP), formation rate of CSF (If), the slope of the amplitude/pressure characteristic (AMP/p), elasticity (EI), pressure-volume index (PVI) calculated on the basis of EI (Avezaat and van Eijndhoven 1985). The hypothesis of zero difference between the average values in both groups was tested using the paired t-test.

Factors, listed in point 2, were calculated on the basis of the constant-rate spinal infusion test. The procedure of this optimized test was described previously (Wocjan et al. 1986). In brief: the child under general endotracheal anesthesia with N_2O_2 and 0.4 vol% Halothane, lies in left recumbent position. After the

Eds.: J. T. Hoff and A. L. Betz
© Springer-Verlag Berlin Heidelberg 1989

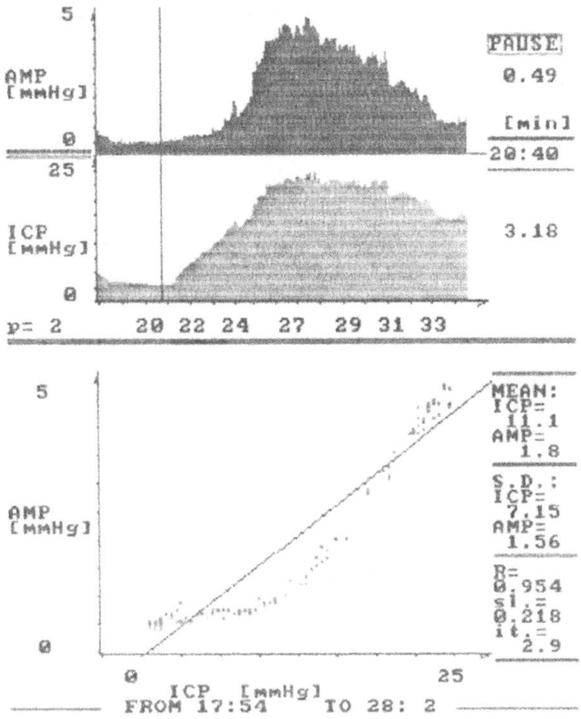

Fig. 1. The trends of amplitude of pulse wave (*AMP-upper*) and mean ICP registered during the constant rate infusion test. *Abscissa:* time in minutes from the start of registration. *Below:* amplitude/pressure statistical relationship. In the NPH children group, the relationship is commonly non-linear. Note that above the level of 13 mm Hg, the characteristic became steeper in this case, due to induced vasomotor responses, commonly observed (as for example B waves activity) in NPH

initial period of ICP stabilization (15 min on the average), infusion at a rate of 5 ml/min is started, until ICP increases by 10 mm Hg. Then the infusion is reduced to 1 ml/min and continued until ICP reaches a new steady-state level.

A computerized analysis was performed: both the ICP mean level and the amplitude of the pulse wave was calculated (sampling period about 9 sec) and stored in the form of the time-trends (Fig. 1). On the basis of these trends the amplitude/pressure characteristic was calculated.

The RCSF was estimated from the difference between the pressure level in the new steady-state and the resting pressure level, divided by the infusion rate (1 ml/min). Elastivity was derived by means of non-linear regression of ICP mean level versus time, according to the theoretical formulae expressing ICP rise during infusion (Avezaat and van Eijndhoven 1985), from the period of infusion at a rate of 5 ml/min. The above procedure allows us to obtain a formal correlation between RCSF and EI estimators.

The computerized analysis of the ICP signal was carried out using an IBM-PC XT computer with specialized software of our own design.

Results

No statistically significant differences in both the reference and NPH group were found in the clinical factors. The only statistically significant difference between

407

Table 1. P-probability of zero difference between two groups

Parameter	Reference group			NPH			p
	mean	SD	median	mean	SD	median	
Age (months)	51.0	49.0	27.0	19.5	16.3	12.0	0.06
Head circumference (%)	3.6	8.3	2.0	8.7	7.4	9.4	0.154
RCSF (mm Hg/ml/min)	8.9	2.3	10.0	17.5	3.1	17.0	<0.01
Resting ICP (mm Hg)	8.2	2.1	8.0	8.7	1.6	9.0	0.50
CSF formation rate (ml/min)	1.0	0.95	0.84	0.97	1.18	0.52	0.85
Resting AMP (mm Hg)	3.6	3.0	2.8	3.1	1.1	2.7	0.60
AMP/p (n.s.)	0.4	0.13	0.4	0.34	0.16	0.4	0.40
Elastivity (1/ml)	0.27	0.12	0.27	0.14	0.09	0.13	<0.01

parameters describing the cerebrospinal system in these two groups of patients (apart from RCSF ≤ the value on which the classification was made) was found in the mean value of an elastivity coefficients. Its mean value in the reference group was 0.27 (with 0.12 standard deviation [1/ml]), as compared to 0.14 (with 0.09 SD) in the group with the normal-pressure hydrocephalus ($p<0.01$). The mean values standard deviations and medians of the parameters of interest are presented in Table 1.

Discussion

The infusion test, apart from its practical meaning in the clinical diagnosis and selection of patients with hydrocephalus for surgical treatment, may provide information on this disease whose pathomechanism is still unknown. In this study, we used the results of this diagnostic procedure for the purpose of extending our knowledge on NPH in children.

On the basis of the presented results, we can conclude as follows: – differentiation between ex-vacuo and normal-pressure hydrocephalus in children (especially in the youngest group) is not possible on the basis of a clinical examination. – children with NPH have a significantly decreased cerebrospinal system elastivity (approximately by twofold in our material). This observation, in our opinion, is in accordance with those made by Shapiro et al. (1985) and Kosteljanetz (1986). Although the clinical significance of this phenomenon is still unclear, we would like to offer another hypothesis: as has been postulated in the work of Kosteljanetz (1986), the hydrocephalic process may, in some circumstances, begin with the phase of raised ICP and RCSF. The cerebrospinal system then reaches a new stabilization state. NPH could be considered as the late stage of such a process.

This consideration, in our opinion, can explain the significance and the paradoxical difference between the value of PVI found in adults and in children – a fact noted in many reports (Kosteljanetz 1986, Shapiro et al. 1985). It is well known that in children a natural compensatory mechanism exists with the possibility of head enlargement in response to increased ICP. If we agree with the dynamic nature of the hydrocephalic process, we must assume that the observed children with NPH must have undergone the acute stage with elevated ICP and RCSF. In this period, the above mentioned compensatory mechanism of accelerated head growth should have been activated. This thesis should be partially supported by the difference between the mean value of head circumference in the reference and NPH groups (however, it is statistically insignificant, $p=0.15$).

Here we postulate that increased PVI (or decreased elastivity) observed in children with NPH could be explained by the above discussed compensatory mechanism. The increased head circumference can be regarded as a remnant of the stage of increased ICP forming the state of hypercompensation. On the basis of presented materials the increased PVI seems to be an effect, not a cause, of NPH in children.

References

Avezaat CJJ, van Eijndhoven JHM (1984) Cerebrospinal fluid pulse pressure and craniospinal system. Doctor's Thesis, Erasmus University, Jongbloed and Zoon Publishers, The Hague
Bering EA Jr, Sato O (1963) Hydrocephalus: changes in formation and absorption of cerebrospinal fluid within the cerebral ventricles. J Neurosurg 20:1050–1060
Black PM (1980) Idiopathic normal pressure hydrocephalus. Results of shunting in 62 patients. J Neurosurg 52:371–377
Guidetti B, Gagliard FM (1972) Normal pressure hydrocephalus. Acta Neurochir (Wien) 27:1–9
Kosteljanetz M (1986) CSF dynamics and pressure–volume relationships in communicating hydrocephalus. J Neurosurg 54:45–52
Shapiro K, Fried A, Marmarou A (1985) Biomechanical and hydrodynamic characterization of the hydrocephalic infant. J Neurosurg 63:69–75
Wocjan J et al. (1986) Analysis of CSF dynamics by computerized pressure-elastance resorption test in hydrocephalic children. Childs Nerv Syst 2:98–99

CSF Pulsatile Flow on MRI and Its Relation to Intracranial Pressure

S. Ohara, H. Nagai, and Y. Ueda

Department of Neurosurgery, Nagaoya City University Medical School, 1 Kawasumi, Mizuho-cho, Mizuho-ku, Nagoya 467 (Japan)

Cerebral fluid (CSF) in the cranial cavity flows toward the spinal CSF space in a to and fro manner, responding to the pulsations of the brain. Therefore, the signal intensity of the CSF on magnetic resonance imaging (MRI) is affected and changed by the velocity of CSF flow (Bradley et al. 1986, Sherman and Citrin 1986). In general, the signal intensity of flowing fluid becomes less when the flow velocity is greater. Fluid flowing rapidly beyond some threshold value loses its signal on MRI. This is termed the signal void phenomenon (SVP).

In a retrospective examination of MRI, the authors noted some relationships between the SVP in CSF flowing in the ventricles and the state of the intracranial pressure (ICP). Using ECG-triggered MRI, we observed that the CSF in the ventricles changed its signal intensity with each cardiac cycle, responding to the brain pulsations. Also, the pattern of the intensity change with each cardiac cycle was altered by a change in the intracranial pressure. This is the first study of CSF intensity related to the ICP state using MRI.

Materials and Methods

MR images of 314 neurosurgical patients were studied in regard to the signal intensity of CSF in the ventricular system. Two-hundred-eighty-nine of these studies were performed without ECG triggered MRI and focused on whether or not the SVP in the aqueduct was observable. In the other 25 cases, the patterns of the signal intensity changes were examined in relation to the cardiac cycle by ECG-triggered MRI.

Nontriggered MR examinations were made with a double-echo eight multi-slice technique on a 0.5 tesla superconductive magnet (Gyroscan S5, Philips, Netherlands). All studies were done using both first and second spin-echo (SE) images, which were proton density (PD) weighted (Tr: 1500 ms, Te: 50 ms) and T2 weighted (Tr: 1500 ms, Te: 100 ms) pulse sequences respectively, with 10 mm slice thickness. The CSF appears slightly hypointensive relative to the brain on PD-weighted sequences and hyperintense on T2 weighted sequences. These show as gray and white respectively on a gray scale. The authors judged the relative to CSF in the lateral ventricles (i.e. black on gray scale) on PD-weighted and T2 weighted pulse sequences.

Eds.: J. T. Hoff and A. L. Betz
© Springer-Verlag Berlin Heidelberg 1989

On an ECG triggered MRI, 90 degree-rotation radiofrequency (RF) pulse was applied to a selectively excited planner volume with delay times of 20, 100, 200, 300, 400 and 500 msec from the R-wave of the subject's electrocardiogram. Changes of signal intensities resulting from each delay time were measured by setting ROI on the aqueduct or the third or fourth ventricle.

Result

Nontriggered MRI Study

In a study of MR images without ECG-triggering, a loss of the signal intensity (the signal void phenomenon, SVP) in CSF in the aqueduct was observed in 77 of 289 patients. This SVP was seen most frequently in patients suffering from communicating hydrocephalus (12 of 14) and in infants with chronic subdural hematoma (12 of 14). On the other hand, only seven of 50 patients with supraten-

Table 1. Relationship between pathologic diagnosis and the signal void phenomenon in patient examined with nontriggered MRI

	Number of cases	Number of SVP (%)
Intracranial tumor		
supratentorial	50	7 (14)
infratentorial	30	11 (37)
pituitary	17	4 (24)
Infarction		
supratentorial	21	6 (29)
infratentorial	3	1 (33)
Cerebral hematoma		
supratentorial	9	3 (33)
infratentorial	3	0 (0)
Vascular malformation		
supratentorial	11	1 (9)
infratentorial	10	1 (10)
Hydrocephalus		
communicating	14	12 (86)
non-communicating	9	0 (0)
Chronic subdural fluid		
collection (infant)	14	12 (86)
arachnoid cyst	13	3 (23)
Other malformation		
(cerebellar atrophy, Dandy-Walker Cyst)	3	1 (33)
Other disease	30	5 (17)
MR negative	52	10 (19)
Total	289	77 (27)

SVP: signal void phenomenon

torial tumors and none of 9 with noncommunicating hydrocephalus demonstrated the SVP (Table 1). The SVP was seen prior to surgery in only 11 of 30 patients with infratentorial tumors, but became clearly detected after suboccipital craniectomy and tumor resection in eight of the other 19.

The SVP was observed in 39 of 83 patients under 20 years of age and was noted even more frequently in children under 12 years of age (30 of 58 children). In adults, the SVP was seen in 13 of 72, 15 of 83 and 10 of 51 patients aged 21 to 40, 41 to 60 and over 61 years, respectively.

Intracranial pressure measurement revealed that there was no statistical difference between the pulse pressure of patients with communicating hydrocephalus and those of a control group.

The difference between the incidence of SVP in patients with supratentorial tumors and communicating hydrocephalus was statistically significant ($p < 0.01$) by Fisher's direct probability test and the change in the incidence of SVP in patients with infratentorial lesions before and after suboccipital craniectomy was also significant ($p < 0.05$) by the chi square test. From the point of view of the intracranial pressure state, these results seem to imply that the incidence of SVP is lower in patients with higher intracranial pressure and lower compliance of their craniospinal cavity. The converse would be true in patients with a low ICP.

ECG-Triggered MRI Study

The signal intensity of the CSF in the aqueduct was measured at each delay time after the R-wave on ECG-triggered MRI in 25 cases. It was difficult to interpret the meaning of the signal intensities in terms of their absolute values. Therefore, each intensity was converted to a percentile, in which the highest recorded intensity was defined as 100% and the lowest recorded intensity was defined as 0%. It was apparent that the maximum CSF flow velocity in the caudal direction occurred at the first point of the minimum intensity after the R-wave on the graph of signal intensity versus time after the R-wave. At the second point of the minimum intensity after the R-wave, the flow velocity was maximum in the rostral direction. CSF flow patterns in the 25 ECG-triggered MRI scans were divided into 6 groups based on the delay times after R-wave at which CSF flowed at maximum velocity. However, there was no specific relation between the underlying pathology and the CSF flow patterns.

Illustrative Case

A 59-year-old male with a complaint of gait disturbance was discovered to have dilated ventricles with the ventricular reflux of a contrast medium with stasis for over 48 hr in CT cisternography. Overnight monitoring of his intracranial pressure showed B-waves during sleep. A regional cerebral blood flow study showed about a 50% increase over baseline cerebral blood flow after CSF drainage via lumbar puncture. This patient was diagnosed as having normal pressure hydrocephalus.

412

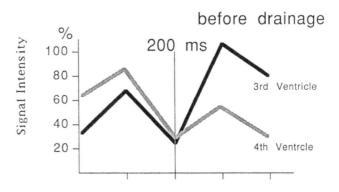

before drainage

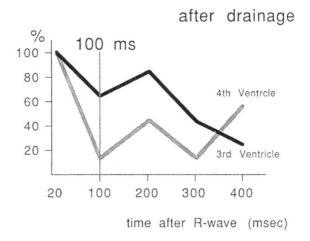

after drainage

Fig. 1. Relationship between CSF signal intensity and interval after R-wave on ECG-triggered MRI in a 59-year-old male with hydrocephalus. The delay time until the minimum intensity of CSF (the highest CSF flow velocity) decreased from 200 msec to 100 msec by decreasing the CSF pressure

On an ECG-triggered MRI, the signal intensity of CSF in the third and the fourth ventricles was measured before and after CSF drainage, which decreased the lumbar CSF closing pressure to one half of its opening pressure. The delay time until the detection of the first minimum intensity of CSF, which is the time after the R-wave at which the CSF flowed with the greatest velocity, was decreased from 200 msec to 100 msec following the reduction in the CSF fluid pressure (Fig. 1). This means that the intracranial CSF was more easily driven out into the spinal CSF space by the systolic expansion of the brain and its flow velocity reached its peak value with a shorter delay time after the beginning of systole. Thus, changes in the intracranial pressure state affected the pattern of CSF flow between the cranial and spinal cavities during a cardiac cycle.

Discussion

The velocity and direction of CSF flow changes during the cardiac cycle reflecting its pulsatile nature. In general, each MR image consists of 256 RF pulses from a planner volume resonant to each excitation RF pulse with two dimensional Fourier transformation techniques. Images from these 256 resonant pulses collected at random times during the cardiac cycle (non-triggered images) do not reflect the instantaneous velocity of CSF pulsatile flow, except for pseudo-triggering, but some flow velocity averaged over the cardiac cycle. So a SVP in a non-triggered MRI means that the amplitude of the to and fro movement of CSF pulsations is large enough to decrease the signal intensity, even after Fourier transmission of RF pulses collected randomly.

On the other hand, the signal intensity of CSF on an ECG-triggered MRI does reflect the instantaneous flow velocity of CSF during the cardiac cycle. When the timing of the signal acquisition coincides with the timing of the maximum velocity of CSF pulsatile flow, the signal intensity must be at its lowest. When the timing coincides with the minimum velocity, the signal must be at its highest. When the ICP and pulse pressure are normal, the craniospinal cavity is not tensely distended and the spinal CSF cavity can accommodate the influx of CSF forced out of the intracranial space easily.

Ridgway et al. (1986) reported that the peak velocity of caudal CSF flow was observed 200 msec after the R-wave in a normal volunteer with a heart rate of 75 beats per min. In our series, the heart rates of the 25 patients studied by ECG-triggered MRI were different from each other. So in order to compare the graphs of signal intensity, it may be necessary to convert the heart rate of each patient to some standard value. Nevertheless, the pattern of signal intensity after the R-wave as a function of time was changed by a decrease in the ICP and an increase in the compliance of craniospinal cavity by withdrawal of CSF. Thus it seems worthwhile to further study the relationship between ICP and CSF signal on ECG-triggered MRIs.

The pulsatile flow of CSF in the ventricular systems is affected by many factors: the brain pulsation transmitted from the cardiac pulsation, the compliance of the craniospinal cavity, the resistance to outflow of CSF from the fourth ventricle, the compressibility of the intracranial venous systems, the pulsation of the choroid plexus, the pulsation of large arteries at the base of the skull, the resistance to absorption of CSF by the arachnoid villi, as well as others. In the present study, we found that after those factors which directly cause CSF to flow (such as the brain's pulsations), the compliance of the cranial cavity and the spinal sac is the most important factor affecting the amplitude of the to and fro movement of CSF.

We wish to emphasize that both the brain's pulsations and the compliance of the craniospinal cavity are closely related to the presence of the SVP in CSF on MRI. As long as there is no mechanical obstruction to CSF flow, the SVP in CSF may reflect the pressure buffering capacity of the craniospinal cavity. If further investigations support our hypothesis, it may be possible to estimate intracranial pressure noninvasively by observation of the patterns of CSF signal intensity change on ECG-triggered MRIs.

References

Bradley WG, Kortman KE, Burgoyne B (1986) Flowing cerebrospinal fluid in normal and hydrocephalic states: appearance on MR images. Radiology 159:611–616

Ridgway JP, Turnbull LW, Smith MA (1986) A phase imaging technique and its use to measure low velocities in pulsatile CSF flow. In: Abstracts of annual meeting of society of magnetic resonance in medicine. Montreal, Radda GK (president), pp 108–109

Sherman JL, Citrin CM (1986) Magnetic resonance demonstration of normal CSF flow. AJNR 7:3–6

Changes of CSF Migration, Energy Metabolism and High Molecular Protein of the Neuron in Hydrostatic Intracranial Hypertension

N. Hayashi, T. Tsubokawa, T. Tamura, Y. Makiyama, and H. Kumakawa

Department of Neurosurgery, Nihon University School of Medicine, Itaboshi-ku, Tokyo 173 (Japan)

Introduction

In this paper, topographical changes of intraparenchymal CSF migration (Hayashi et al. 1987), microcirculation, and aerobic metabolism following acute and chronic hydrocephalus are presented. Ischemia sensitive dendrites and cell soma were studied with the specific high molecular protein; MAP 2 (microtubule associated protein) (Matus et al. 1981).

Method

The experiment was performed on 45 Sprague Dawley rats weighing 120–180 gm. The animals were anesthetized with nembutal (18 mg/kg IP). Acute intracranial hypertension was produced by injection of mock CSF into the cisterna magna and intracranial pressure (ICP) was increased to 30, 40 and 50 mm Hg over 20 min. Slowly progressive hydrocephalus (1, 2, 3 and 4 weeks) was produced by chemical meningitis (Kaolin (20 mg/0.1 ml)) in 30 rats. At the end of the experiment, measurement of intracranial pressure, immunohistochemical studies of MAP 2 (Hsu et al. 1981), topographical analysis of ATP, NADH, intraparenchymal CSF-Na fluorescein migration, and microcirculation (0.1 and 7 μ diameter fluoresbright microspheres single dye passage method) (Hayashi et al. 1987) were carried out using laser spectrophotometric analysis.

Results and Discussion

A) Acute Intracranial Hypertension: The critical ICP for changes of MAP 2 in the dendrite was 30–40 mm Hg. Intraparenchymal CSF migration was limited to the peri-ventricular tissue and cortical surface area (layer 1, 2). No direct correlation was observed between changes of MAP 2 and CSF migration except in the hippocampus. In the cortex, changes of MAP 2 were observed in layer 3 in the 30 mm Hg ICP and in layers 5 and 6 in the 40 mm Hg ICP (Fig. 1) with increased NADH at the zone of cortical perforating branches. Ischemic insults appeared

Eds.: J. T. Hoff and A. L. Betz
© Springer-Verlag Berlin Heidelberg 1989

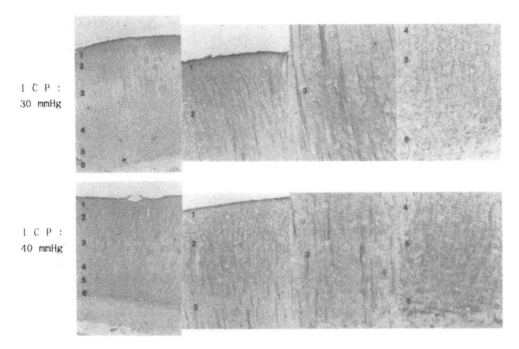

ICP: 30 mmHg

ICP: 40 mmHg

Fig. 1. Changes of microtubule associated protein 2 in the cortex following acute hydrostatic intracranial hypertension

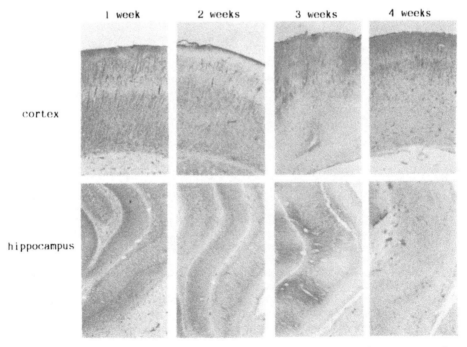

1 week   2 weeks   3 weeks   4 weeks

cortex

hippocampus

Fig. 2. Changes of the microtubule associated protein 2 in the cortex and hippocampus at the various stage in the slow progressed hydrocephalus

highly likely as a main cause of neuronal dysfunction in acute hydrocephalus. Otherwise, in the hippocampus, ischemic insult and hydrostatic edema could be speculated as the causes of MAP 2 changes.

B) Slowly Progressive Hydrocephalus (Chronic): In the early stage (1 week) of hydrocephalus, the changes of MAP 2 were limited to layer 3 in the cortex with microcirculatory disturbances and the highest ICP (9.6 + 0.8 mm Hg). Hydrocephalus at 2 weeks showed changes of MAP 2 that extended to CSF migration areas in layers 4, 5, 6 in the cortex (Fig. 2) and striatum orience in the hippocampus. After 3 weeks of hydrocephalus, changes of MAP 2 progressed more severely and correlated with intraparenchymal venous structures (Fig. 2). From these results, we can suggest that, in the late stage of chronic hydrocephalus, a mechanism involving the venous circulation which is outlet route of interstitial edema, will promote hydrocephalus-specific neuronal dysfunction.

Previous studies on the role of MAP 2 in the brain documented its involvement in dendrite sprouting, longterm cAMP-mediated effects on the electrical activity of the neuron, receptor regulation through actin and fodrin interaction of microtubules and the cell membrane, and cAMP-mediated growth and differentiation of dendrites (Bernhart and Matus 1982, Hsu et al. 1981, Matus et al. 1981). Therefore, changes of MAP 2 suggest a specific pattern of neuronal disturbances follow hydrocephalus.

Conclusion

The dendrite and cell soma specific high molecular protein, MAP 2, was sensitive to hydrostatic edema and changes of the microcirculation. The major effects on MAP 2 with disturbances in the microcirculation were observed in layer 3 in the cortex and with hydrostatic edema in CSF migration area (hioppocampus and layer 5–6 in the cortex). Specific patterns of dendrite changes in acute and chronic hydrocephalus were documented.

References

Bernhart R, Matus A (1982) Initial phase of dendrite growth. J Cell Biol 92:589–598
Hayashi N, Thsbokawa T et al. (1987) Alteration of cerebral energy metabolism and cytoskeletal protein with intraparenchymal routed CSF migration in the hydrocephalus. Childs Nerv Syst 12:11–17
Hsu SM, Raine L et al. (1981) The use of avidin-biotin-peroxydase complex (ABC) in immunoperoxydase technique. J Hist Cytol 29:577–580
Matus A, Bernhart R et al. (1981) HMWP proteins are preferentially associated with dendrite microtubules in the brain. Proc Natl Acad Sci USA 78:3010–3014

Increased Brain Water Self Diffusion Measured by Magnetic Resonance Scanning in Patients with Pseudotumor Cerebri

P. Soelberg-Sørensen, C. Thomsen, F. Gjerris, J.F. Schmidt, and O. Henriksen

University Departments of Neurology and Neurosurgery, Rigshospitalet, and Department of Magnetic Resonance, Hvidovre Hospital, DK-2100 Copenhagen (Denmark)

Introduction

The pathophysiology of the intracranial hypertension in pseudotumor cerebri is still an unsolved puzzle. Increased resistance to CSF outflow leading to an increased CSF volume (interstitial brain edema) (Johnston and Paterson 1975, Gjerris et al. 1985) and intracellular brain water accumulation (Sahs and Joynt 1956) are among the most frequently mentioned causative factors. The purpose of the present study was to characterize the increased brain water volume in pseudotumor cerebri by in vivo quantitative measurements of water diffusion in the brain tissue using magnetic resonance scanning.

Material and Methods

Seven patients fulfilling conventional diagnostic criteria for pseudotumor cerebri were studied. Five females aged 23–66 years and 2 males aged 53 and 58 years. All patients had increased intracranial pressure (ICP): mean steady-state pressure 23–40 mm Hg, and all had increased resistance to CSF outflow measured by a lumbo-lumbar perfusion study (Gjerris et al. 1985).

Magnetic resonance scanning was performed on a Siemens 1.5 Tesla whole-body scanner. All patients were imaged with a T_1-weighted and a T_2-weighted spin echo sequence. Quantitative diffusion measurements were obtained by using seven spin Hahn single echo sequences with pulsed gradients. The theoretical considerations and a detailed description of the method have been reported previously (Thomsen et al. 1987). Five slices were measured in each subject, and the diffusion coefficients measured in the patients with pseudotumor were compared with the findings in 7 healthy volunteers.

Results

All pseudotumor patients had normal spin echo images without focal lesions and normal sized ventricular systems. The diffusion images of the healthy subjects showed a regional difference with low diffusion coefficients in the white matter

Table 1. Measured water self diffusion coefficients in various regions of the brain in pseudo-tumor patients ($n=7$) and healthy controls ($n=7$)

Brain region	Diffusion coefficients ($10^{-9} \cdot m^2 \cdot s^{-1}$) median (range)		Mann-Whitney
	Pseudotumor	Controls	
Occipital cortex	2.24 (1.22 – 7.07)	1.73 (1.22 – 2.24)	$p < 0.01$
Occipital white matter	2.34 (1.73 – 3.54)	1.22 (0.25 – 1.73)	$p < 0.01$
Basal ganglia	3.54 (2.89 – 7.07)	2.24 (1.73 – 3.54)	$p < 0.01$
Central white matter	3.54 (1.99 – 3.54)	1.22 (0.25 – 1.73)	$p < 0.01$
Frontal white matter	3.54 (2.89 – 3.54)	1.73 (0.71 – 2.24)	$p < 0.01$
Frontal cortex	3.54 (2.24 – 7.07)	1.73 (1.22 – 2.24)	$p < 0.01$

and higher values in grey matter (Table 1). The diffusion in both white and grey matter was restricted. In white matter to 33% and in grey matter to 55% of water's self diffusion coefficient at 37°C ($4.0 \cdot 10^{-9}\ m^2 \cdot s^{-1}$). In all patients with pseudotumor the diffusion images showed an increased diffusion. Three patients had increased self diffusion localized in the periventricular regions, whereas 4 patients had equally increased diffusion in the whole brain. The median diffusion coefficients in the various brain regions of pseudotumor patients are shown in Table 1. In several patients the water self diffusion in some regions of the brain was equal to or above the self diffusion of water in water. In all areas examined the median diffusion coefficient was higher in pseudotumor patients than in controls.

Discussion

The findings of high brain water diffusion coefficients in the brain of patients with pseudotumor cerebri indicate a decreased overall viscosity of the brain tissue caused by an increased volume of free water intra- and/or extracellularly. The uneven distribution of enhanced water diffusion in some of the patients, being most predominant periventricularly where the diffusion coefficient was above the self diffusion of water in water, indicates a convective flow through the ependyma. This would be in agreement with the hypothesis of increased resistance to CSF outflow at the level of the arachnoid villi leading to an interstitial edema being responsible for the intracranial hypertension in pseudotumor (Johnston and Paterson 1975; Gjerris et al. 1985; Soelberg-Sørensen et al. 1988). However, an interstitial edema cannot alone explain the more widespread increased water self diffusion in the brain of some pseudotumor patients. The extracellular volume constitutes only 20% of the total water in the brain and even a substantial increase in extracellular volume cannot account for the measured difference in brain water self diffusion between controls and the pseudotumor patients. Hence, it can be concluded that the intracellular volume of free water is increased, supporting the theory of intracellular brain water accumulation in patients with pseudotumor cerebri (Sahs and Joynt 1956). In the future, measurements of brain water self diffusion may be of diagnostic value in patients with increase ICP of unknown origin.

References

Gjerris F, Soelberg-Sørensen P, Vorstrup S, Paulson OB (1985) Intracranial pressure, conductance to cerebrospinal fluid outflow, and cerebral blood flow in patients with benign hypertension (pseudotumor cerebri). Ann Neurol 17:158–162

Johnston I, Paterson A (1975) Benign intracranial hypertension. II Pressure and circulation. Brain 97:301–312

Sahs AL, Joynt RJ (1956) Brain swelling of unknown cause. Neurology 6:791–802

Soelberg-Sørensen P, Krogsaa B, Gjerris F (1988) Clinical course and prognosis of pseudotumor cerebri. A prospective study of 24 patients. Acta Neurol Scand 77:164–172

Thomsen C, Henriksen O, Ring P (1987) In vivo measurement of water self diffusion in the human brain by magnetic resonance imaging. Acta Radiol [Diagn] (Stockh) 28:353–361

Neuropsychological Testing in Normal Pressure Hydrocephalus

N.R. Graff-Radford[1], J.C. Godersky[2], D. Tranel[1], P.J. Eslinger[3], and M.P. Jones[4]

[1] Department of Neurology, [2] Department of Surgery, [4] Department of Preventive Medicine, The University of Iowa College of Medicine, Iowa City, Iowa. [3] Department of Psychology and Human Behavior, Brown University Providence, Rhode Island (USA)

There have been few systematic behavioral studies in normal pressure hydrocephalus despite the fact that cognitive decline is a characteristic feature. One study suggested that preoperative language deficits predicted a poor outcome with shunt surgery (DeMol 1985). Another indicated that dementia is usually irreversible in idiopathic NPH (Thomsen et al. 1986). We used serial neuropsychological tests to study 23 patients operated for NPH. Our aims were: (1) to look for behavioral predictors of surgical outcome; (2) to analyze the extent of improvement with surgery.

Methods

Patient Population

We operated on 23 patients for possible normal pressure hydrocephalus. Seventeen improved and 6 did not. All 23 patients had gait abnormalities, dementia, and urinary urgency or incontinence. CT showed hydrocephalus. Twenty had idiopathic NPH and three had NPH due to secondary causes.

Surgical Methods

Medium pressure Cardis-Hakim system shunts were used in all cases. Ventriculo-peritoneal shunts were performed on 20 and ventriculo-atrial on 3. Postoperatively all shunts were evaluated and found to be functioning.

Evaluation of Outcome

Preoperatively and 2 and 6 months postoperatively patients were evaluated with: (1) Ratings of serial videotapes of gait; (2) the Katz index of activities of daily living; and (3) neuropsychological test scores. If the patient improved on 2 or 3 of the outcome measures, we classified them as improved.

Intracranial Pressure VII
Eds.: J. T. Hoff and A. L. Betz
© Springer-Verlag Berlin Heidelberg 1989

The battery of neuropsychological tests sampled the areas of orientation, intelligence, memory, language, visuospatial functioning, and executive control. Criteria for cognitive improvement were a significant increase in test scores in 2 or more cognitive areas tested without a concomitant decline in any other area.

Statistical Methods and Results

To see which items predicted surgical outcome a logistic regression was performed on preoperative variables (Table 1). The only neuropsychological test item that reached significance was the Visual Naming Test from the Multilingual Aphasia Examination ($p=0.04$). Patients were classified into pass/fail groups based on preoperative performance on the Visual Naming test, and the linear regression showed this to be significantly related to improvement ($p<0.01$). We also per-

Table 1. Logistic regression results on each variable separately

Variable	n	# Respond	# Not respond	LRT[a]	p
Age	23	17	6	0.17	0.678
Gender	23	17	6	4.33	0.037
Years of education	23	17	6	0.55	0.458
Temporal orientation	23	17	6	0.56	0.453
Verbal IQ	22	17	5	1.50	0.220
Performance IQ	20	15	5	1.76	0.184
Verbal memory	23	17	6	0.32	0.572
VRT correct	22	16	6	1.00	0.316
VRT error	20	15	5	0.21	0.646
Visual naming score	19	14	5	4.21	0.040
Visual naming pass/fail	20	14	6	6.97	0.008
COWA	23	17	6	1.74	0.187
Visuospatial	23	17	6	0.41	0.521

Significant $p=0.05$; VRT = visual retention test; COWA = controlled oral word association
[a] Likelihood ratio test.

Table 2. Classification from logistic regression equation ($n=20$) based on visual naming (pass/fail score)

		Nonrespond	Respond	Subtotal
True	Nonrespond	5	1[a]	6
True	Respond	3*	11	14
	Total	8	12	20

Fisher's exact test p-value $=0.018$;   [a] Misclassifications.

formed Fisher's exact test looking at the improved and unimproved groups and the pass and fail groups on the Visual Naming Test. The results were significant (Table 2).

There was an 18 times greater chance of the patient improving with surgery if they had passed the Visual Naming tests.

While our data suggest that males have a worse prognosis than females, no other study that we know of has shown this. At this time we would treat this finding with reservation. Only 9 of the 23 patients improved significantly in 2 or more neuropsychological areas without concomitant decline in the other neuropsychological measures. Two patients had significant cognitive improvement at 2 months which was not maintained at 6 months. They were excluded from the improved neuropsychological group.

Conclusions

Patients suspected of having NPH and who have preoperative language deficits have a poor surgical prognosis. It is possible that these patients may have Alzheimer's disease alone or in combination with NPH. In fact, two patients who failed the Visual Naming Test have come to postmortem and had pathological characteristics of Alzheimer's and hydrocephalus.

In patients operated for NPH, neuropsychological parameters do not improve as often as gait and activities of daily living. Furthermore, even when patients improve on the neuropsychological tests, the recovery may be incomplete. We should point out that most of our patients have idiopathic NPH and that it has been reported that cognitive improvement is not often seen in this group (it occurred in only 2 of 19 patients in one report) (Thomsen et al. 1986). Eight of 9 patients who had significant cognitive improvement in our series had idiopathic NPH. The studies should not, however, be directly compared because different neuropsychological tests were given and criteria for improvement were different. Nonetheless, patients with idiopathic NPH may show definite cognitive improvement with surgery.

References

DeMol J (1985) Facteurs pronostiques du resultat therapeutique dans l'hydrocephalus a pression normale. Acta Neurol Belg 85:13–29
Thomsen AM, Børgesen SE, Bruhn P, Gjerris F (1986) Prognosis of dementia in normal pressure hydrocephalus after a shunt operation. Ann Neurol 20:304–310

^{123}I-IMP-SPECT and Lumbar Subarachnoid Pressure in Adult Hydrocephalus

O. Hirai, M. Nishikawa, M. Munaka, S. Watanabe, T. Kaneko, A. Fukuma, and H. Handa

Department of Neurosurgery, Hamamatsu Rosai Hospital, 25-Shogencho Hamamatsu (Japan)

Introduction

Despite many attempts, strict criteria for selection of patients with adult communicating hydrocephalus for shunting procedures are still far from established. The unexpectedly low success rates with shunting, in contrast to earlier reports (Adams et al. 1965), may be partly due to concomitant parenchymal damage or pre-existing degenerative brain diseases which can result in a progressive ventricular dilatation by means other than an impairment of CSF hydrodynamics (Hirai et al. 1988).

Either cerebral blood flow (CBF) measurement or continuous ICP monitoring used separately as predictors of successful shunting are controversial (Greitz et al. 1969, Grubb et al. 1977, Kushuner et al. 1984, Mathew et al. 1975). In the present study, topographical imaging of CBF by means of single photon emission computed tomography (SPECT) was used in conjuction with CT scan and CSF pressure measurement to predict shunt response.

Object and Methods

Eighteen patients with adult communicating hydrocephalus of various etiologies were investigated. Ventricular dilatation on CT was quantitatively evaluated by the bicaudate index (BCI); the ratio of bicaudate diameter to the distance between the inner skull tables along the same line. SPECT was carried out 20 min (early images) and 5 hr (late images) after intravenous injection of N-isopropyl-^{123}I-iodoamphetamine (IMP).

At the midventricular level of early images periventricular low perfusion was semiquantitatively estimated by dividing the maximum width of the area of reduced IMP uptake, including the no flow area in the lateral ventricle, by the maximum brain width. This was designated as the low perfusion index (LPI). All patients underwent continuous lumbar subarachnoid pressure (LSP) monitoring for 15 to 20 hr via an intrathecal indwelling catheter. Seven age-matched non-hydrocephalic patients served as controls for SPECT and CT.

A ventriculoperitoneal shunt was placed in 10 patients. Seven benefited from the shunting procedure and three failed. Eight patients were not shunted on clinical grounds. Subsequent observation in these patients revealed neither clinical deterioration nor further increase in ventricular size. Therefore, the values (SEM) were compared among control (7 cases), the improved group (7 cases) and the unchanged group (11 cases). The mean age in each group was 62.7 ± 2.9, 59.6 ± 3.5 and 67.9 ± 3.0, respectively. There were no statistically significant differences.

Results

Figure 1 presents early images in each group showing that the areas of reduced IMP uptake around the ventricle were apparently wider in hydrocephalus than in control, as might be expected. However, it should be stressed that the unchanged patients had a disproportionately more extensive reduction in perfusion compared with the improved patients. Additional reduction in IMP activity, other than in the paraventricular area, was found to be localized within the frontal region in the improved group, while it occasionally spread more widely to the temporal and/or the parietal regions in the unchanged group. Redistribution of IMP on late images was noted in all of the control and 6 of 7 improved patients but in only 6 out of 11 unchanged patients.

The above visual impressions were semiquantitatively substantiated in Fig. 2. In controls, the mean values of the BCI and LPI were $18.3 \pm 0.6\%$ and $33.4 \pm 1.0\%$. As the mean BCI increased to $29.9 \pm 1.0\%$ in the improved group, the LPI also significantly increased to $42.1 \pm 1.3\%$. A linear relationship with statistical significance was found in these values. However, the LPI values in the unchanged group scattered far above the regression line, with an average of $53.9 \pm 1.9\%$, despite a slightly smaller mean BCI of $27.3 \pm 0.9\%$.

The LSP measurements showed an opposite relation to the findings of SPECT, namely the mean resting pressure and peak pressure were 13.7 ± 1.5 mm Hg and 28.6 ± 1.4 mm Hg in the improved group, while they were 8.2 ± 1.1 mm Hg and 14.7 ± 1.4 mm Hg in the unchanged group. Statistically significant differences were also observed in these values ($P < 0.01$ and $P < 0.001$). These findings indicate that the extensively compromised periventricular perfusion, in the patients who were or will be refractory to shunting, was neither due to a rise in CSF pressure nor to the extent of ventricular dilatation, at least at the time of examination.

Discussion

The present study offers a new viewpoint on the pathophysiological mechanisms in adult hydrocephalus. As seen in the previous reports, CBF inevitably decreases and a postoperative increase in CBF seems to correlate with clinical improvement (Greitz et al. 1969, Mathew et al. 1975). However, preoperative evaluation of CBF is difficult since it is hard to determine a critical flow level in hydrocephalus,

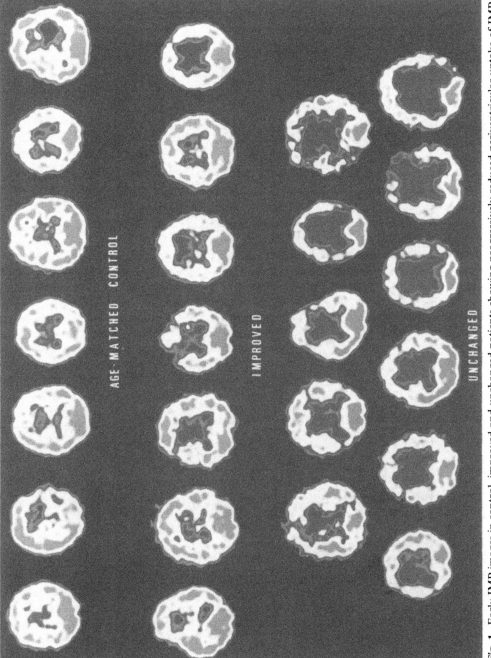

Fig. 1. Early IMP images in control, improved and unchanged patients showing progressively reduced periventricular uptake of IMP in this order

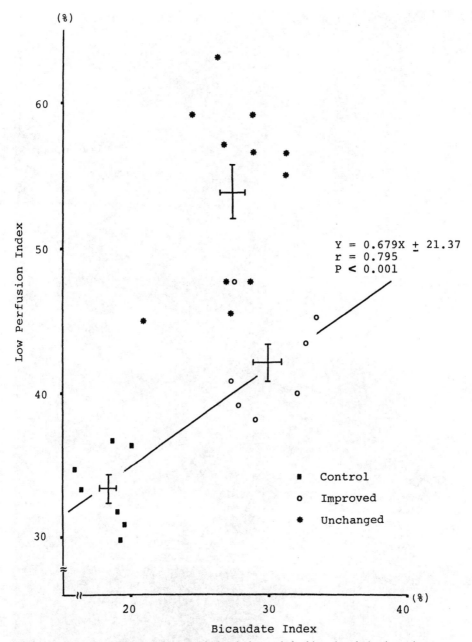

Fig. 2. Correlation between the low perfusion index and the bicaudate index in each group

and a temporary increase in CBF after lumbar puncture as an indicator of a good shunt response (Mathew et al. 1975), has not been substantiated by subsequent investigations (Grubb et al. 1977, Kushner et al. 1984). More importantly, analysis of periventricular perfusion, which may be more closely related to hydrocephalic compromise than the cortical flow, is limited by previously employed CBF

428

measurement techniques. Position emission tomography may provide useful information in terms of topographical patterns of blood flow, volume and oxygen metabolism as well as quantitative analysis (Powell et al. 1985), however, its contribution is limited because of cost and the need for a highly specialized apparatus.

Instead, IMP-SPECT has recently come into wide use mainly in ischemic brain disease, owing to its simplicity and images of diagnostic quality (Defer et al. 1987). Patterns of IMP uptake have been described for the various kinds of dementia (Sharp 1986), however, little is known about the features in hydrocephalus.

In this communication, particular attention was paid to the periventricular low perfusion area, in conjunction with ventricular size on CT and CSF pressure. As ventricles dilate with an elevated CSF pressure, periventricular uptake was necessarily compromised, but the degree was relatively mild where shunting procedures were effective since the causative factor in reducing CBF was mainly impaired CSF hydrodynamics. On the other hand, a large periventricular low perfusion disproportionate to the ventricular span without an elevation of CSFR pressure means that a primary parenchymal damage plays the major role, or that the condition has progressed to an irreversible state and therefore, refractory to a shunt. Mathew et al. (1975) also reported that the higher the preoperative mean CBF, despite some reduction as compared to normal individuals, the better the clinical recovery after shunting. In addition, as in the previous report (Mathew et al. 1975), most of our improved patients had exclusively frontal low perfusion, while various patterns of reduced uptake in IMP were observed in the unchanged group. Redistribution of IMP on late images, which is suggestive of viability of the brain (Defer 1987), was frequently seen in the improved cases.

Although, the possibility that this periventricular reduced activity of IMP might have been an artifact caused by no CBF in the ventricle should not be overlooked, the distinctive result demonstrated in this preliminary study, forecasts the usefulness of SPECT. Patients with an LPI of 50% or less and with a peak LSP of 25 mm Hg or more will benefit from shunting. Since hydrocephalic patients may present with various clinical and laboratory findings, shunting procedures should be decided after taking both the CSF hydrodynamics and underlying physiological state of the brain into account. It would be of no use to persist in "normal pressure" or classical criteria. That is the reason why the term "adult communicating hydrocephalus" was used here instead of "normal pressure hydrocephalus".

References

Adams RD, Fisher CM, Hakim S, Ojemann RG, Sweet WH (1965) Symptomatic occult hydrocephalus with "normal" cerebrospinal fluid pressure. A treatable syndrome. N Engl J Med 273:117–126

Defer G, Moretti JL, Cesaro P, Sergent A, Raynaud C, Degos JD (1987) Early and delayed SPECT using N-isopropyl-p-iodoamphetamine iodine 123 in cerebral ischemia. Arch Neurol 44:715–718

Greitz TVB, Grepe AOL, Kalmer MSF, Lopez J (1969) Pre- and postoperative evaluation of cerebral blood flow in low-pressure hydrocephalus. J Neurosurg 31:644–651

Grubb RL, Raichle ME, Gado MH, Eichling JO, Hughes CP (1977) Cerebral blood flow, oxygen utilization, and blood volume in dementia. Neurology 27:905–910

Hirai O, Handa H, Kikuchi H, Ishikawa M, Kinuta Y (1988) Continuous lumbar subarachnoid pressure monitoring as an indicator of shunt operation for so-called normal pressure hydrocephalus. Neurol Surg (Tokyo) (in press)

Kushner M, Youkin D, Weinberger J, Hurtig H, Goldberg H, Reivich M (1984) Cerebral hemodynamics in the diagnosis of normal pressure hydrocephalus. Neurology 34:96–99

Mathew NT, Meyer JS, Hartmann A, Ott EO (1975) Abnormal cerebrospinal fluid–blood flow dynamics. Implications in diagnosis, treatment, and prognosis in normal pressure hydrocephalus. Arch Neurol 32:657–664

Powell M, Brooks DJ, Crockard HA, Beaney RP, Leenders KL, Thomas DGT, Jones T, Marshall J (1985) Intracranial pressure (ICP) and positron emission tomographic (PET) studies in acute and chronic hydrocephalus. In: Miller JD et al. (eds) Intracranial pressure VI. Springer, Berlin Heidelberg New York, pp 451–456

Sharp P, Gemmel H, Cherryman G, Besson J, Crawford J, Smith F (1986) Application of iodine-123-labeled isopropylamphetamine imaging to the study of dementia. J Nucl Med 27:761–768

Concentrations of Neurotransmitters in Ventricular and Lumbar Cerebrospinal Fluid in Patients with Normal Pressure Hydrocephalus

A. Gjerris [1], P. Soelberg-Sørensen [2], and F. Gjerris [3]

[1] Department of Psychiatry, [2] Department of Neurology, [3] Department of Neurosurgery, Rigshospitalet, DK-2100 Copenhagen (Denmark)

Introduction

For several years concentrations of neurotransmitters and their metabolites in *lumbar* cerebrospinal fluid have been used for diagnostic purposes or to elucidate the pathophysiology of disorders in the central nervous system. In patients with normal pressure hydrocephalus (NPH) it would also be of interest to investigate a possible relationship between pathological features in NPH and concentrations of neurotransmitter substances in CSF. However, simultaneous measurements of various neurotransmitters in CSF obtained from lateral ventricles and the lumbar cistern have disclosed significant differences between the concentrations measured at the two sites (Moir et al. 1970, Jakupcevic et al. 1977, Bertilsson et al. 1982, Nordin et al. 1982, Tyce et al. 1986). These results have been interpreted differently, some advocating that a rostro-caudal gradient is an expression of the central origin of the transmitter substances; others suggesting that the differences in concentrations measured at different sites of the spinal canal depend on the concentrations in the adjacent spinal cord. The purpose of the present study is:

1. To investigate whether there is a relationship between the concentrations of transmitter substances measured and factors influencing CSF dynamics, i.e. the severity of cerebral atrophy indicated by Evans ratio and resistance to outflow of CSF in patients with NPH.
2. To investigate whether *lumbar* (L-CSF) concentrations of vasoactive intestinal polypeptide (VIP), cholecystokinin (CCK), noradrenaline (NA), dopamine (DA), 5-hydroxyindoleacetic acid (5-HIAA), 3-methoxy-4-hydroxy-phenylglycol (MHPG) and homovanillic acid (HVA) differ from concentrations measured in CSF collected from the *lateral ventricles* (V-CSF).
3. To investigate whether there is a correlation between concentrations measured in L-CSF and V-CSF.

Material and Methods

Material

Patients admitted to the Department of Neurosurgery, Rigshospitalet, Copenhagen, with the diagnoses of NPH were studied. All patients had progressive symp-

Table 1. Concentrations of neurotransmitters in CSF measured at the ventricular and at the lumbar level and correlations between concentrations measured at the two sites

Neurotransmitters	V-CSF	L-CSF	r_s
5-HIAA	448 nmol/l	124 nmol/l**	NS
MHPG	62 nmol/l	58 nmol/l	0,83**
HVA	1144 nmol/l	225 nmol/l**	NS
NA	0.8 nmol/l	1.5 nmol/l**	NS
DA	4.8 nmol/l	8.9 nmol/l*	0.94**
CCK	6 pmol/l	7 pmol/l	NS
VIP	9 pmol/l	14 pmol/l**	0.65*

* $p \le 0.05$; ** $p \le 0.01$.

toms of dementia, gait disturbances and/or urinary incontinence. In all patients, computerized tomography (CT) showed ventricular enlargement, i.e., Evans ratio above 0.30. No signs of multiple cerebral infarction were seen on CT. In all patients the intraventricular pressure was continuously monitored by a Statham P 23 transducer during a 24-hour period via a cannula introduced into the lateral ventricle. The intracranial pressure was normal (<12 mm Hg) in all patients, and the resistance to CSF outflow was increased in all but three patients (normal value $= <12.5$ mm Hg $\times$ ml^{-1} $\times$ min). At the end of a 24-hour period in which the intraventricular pressure was monitored, a lumbo-ventricular perfusion was performed to measure the resistance to CSF outflow. Before the perfusion study was performed, CSF samples were taken simultaneously starting with the collection of lumbar CSF and followed by the collection of ventricular CSF. A total of 16–20 ml CSF was collected from the patients.

Results

A significant negative correlation was found between L-CSF-VIP and Evans ratio ($r_s = -0.76$; $P \le 0.001$). V-CSF and L-CSF-CCK correlated negatively with resistance to outflow ($r_s = -0.73$; $P \le 0.05$).

In Table 1 the relationship between concentrations measured at the ventricular and the lumbar level is indicated.

Discussion

The significant correlations between Evans ratio and L-CSF-VIP and between V-CSF and L-CSF-CCK and resistance to outflow may suggest new ways for studying the pathophysiology of NPH. The study shows a significant difference between CSF concentrations measured at the two sites for all but two of the substances measured (MHPG and CCK). The difference takes two directions being higher at the lumbar level than at the ventricular level for NA, DA and VIP and lower for 5-HIAA and HVA. Our results are in accordance with reports from other groups (Moir et al. 1970, Sharpless et al. 1984, Tye et al. 1986) and add further information to the already existing knowledge of distribution of neurotransmitters in CSF (Gjerris et al. 1987, Gjerris et al. 1988). The lack of a consistent significant correlation between concentrations measured at the two levels emphasizes the necessity of further investigation before final conclusions can be drawn from CSF studies on concentrations of transmitter substances measured at the lumbar level.

References

Bertilsson L, Åsberg M, Lantto O, Scalia-Tomba G-P, Träskman-Bendtz L, Tybring G (1982) Gradient of monoamine metabolites and cortisol in cerebrospinal fluid of psychiatric patients and healthy controls. Psychiatry Res 6:77–83

Børgesen SE, Gjerris F (1982) The predictive value of conductance to outflow of CSF in normal pressure hydrocephalus. Brain 105:65–86

Gjerris A, Werdelin L, Gjerris F, Sørensen PS, Rafaelsen OJ, Alling C (1987) CSF-amine metabolites in depression, dementia and in controls. Acta Psychiatr Scand 75:169–628

Gjerris A, Gjerris F, Sørensen PS, Sørensen EB, Christensen NJ, Fahrenkrug J, Rehfeld JF (1988) Do concentrations of neurotransmitters measured in lumbar cerebrospinal fluid reflect the concentrations at brain level? Acta Neurochir (Wien) 91:55–59

Jakupcevic M, Lackovic Z, Stefoski D, Bulat M (1977) Non-homogeneous distribution of 5-hydroxyindoleacetic acid and homovanillic acid in the lumbar cerebrospinal fluid of man. J Neurol Sci 31:165–171

Moir ATB, Ashcroft GW, Crawford TBB, Eccleston D, Guldberg HC (1970) Cerebral metabolites in cerebrospinal fluid as a biochemical approach to the brain. Brain 93:357–368

Nordin C, Siwers B, Bertilsson L (1982) Site of lumbar puncture influences level of monoamine-metabolites. Arch Gen Psychiatry 39:1445

Sharpless NS, Thal LJ, Perlow MJ, Tabaddor K, Waltaz JM, Shapiro KN, Amin IM, Engel J, Brandall PH (1984) Vasoactive intestinal peptide in cerebrospinal fluid. Peptides 5:429–433

Tyce GM, Messick JM, Yaksh TL, Byer DE, Danielson DR, Rorie DK (1986) Amine sulfate formation in the central nervous system. Fed Proc 45:2247–2253

CSF Oxygen Tension and ICP

A.I.R. Maas [1], D.A. de Jong [1], and W.A. Fleckenstein [2]

[1] Department of Neurosurgery, University Hospital Rotterdam, Rotterdam (The Netherlands),
[2] Department of Physiology, Medical University of Lübeck (FRG)

One of the major factors leading to secondary brain damage in raised ICP is probably disturbed cerebral blood flow, metabolism and oxygenation secondary to raised ICP. Our hypothesis was that apart from measuring pressure it could be worthwhile to monitor cerebral oxygenation. The pO_2 in CSF can be regarded as a parameter that reflects the oxygen supply to the brain, the cerebral blood flow and the rate of cerebral oxygen metabolism. The aim of this study was to evaluate the possibility and clinical relevance of continuous CSF pO_2 monitoring.

Materials and Methods

The studies were performed in 6 cats and 5 beagle dogs, all anaesthetized and artificially ventilated. Catheters were inserted for continuous monitoring of arterial blood pressure, rectal temperature, ventricular fluid pressure, ventricular and cisternal pO_2. CSF pO_2 was recorded in the parietal subarachnoid space, cisterna magna and lateral ventricle. Subsequently, the animals were hypo- and hyperventilated and subjected to hypercarbic, hypoxic and hyperoxic ventilation. Each of the experiments was ended by returning to reference conditions. In three animals ICP was progressively raised by intraventricular injection of physiologic saline and cerebral perfusion pressure was further reduced by induction of hypotension with Trimetaphan. CSF pO_2 was measured with sterilizable, polarographic needle probes (low sensitive "licox" probe type, G.M.S. mbH, Kiel, FRG).

For positioning the pO_2 probes were fixed in stereotactic drives. When the probe tip, slowly driven forward, entered the CSF compartment, the signal increased suddenly from a low and variable pO_2 level to $60-80$ mm Hg.

Results

Control Conditions

The ventricular CSF pO_2 was 70.8 ± 6.5 mm Hg in the cats and 73.5 ± 4.5 mm Hg in the dogs. The cisternal pO_2 measured only in the cats was 60.8 ± 9.3 mm Hg.

Eds.: J.T. Hoff and A.L. Betz

In the subarachnoid space, the CSF pO_2 in cats was 41.2 ± 4.7 mm Hg and in the dogs 47.2 ± 4.9 mm Hg. The arterial pO_2 during controlled conditions in the cats was 124.7 ± 8.0 mm Hg and in the dogs 118.9 ± 7.7 mm Hg.

Ventilatory Experiments

Ventricular CSF pO_2 and cisternal CSF pO_2 were decreased markedly during hypoxia by almost the same extent. The response of the CSF pO_2 occurred rapidly after changing the inspiratory oxygen fraction: the first changes in CSF pO_2 were observed 17.4 ± 2.3 sec after decreasing FiO_2. The average maximal slope of CSF pO_2 was recorded at 31.4 ± 5.3 sec. During hyperventilation the ventricular CSF pO_2 and cisternal CSF pO_2 values were decreased significantly by 20.6 ± 4.3 mm Hg (29%) and 18.5 ± 3.9 mm Hg (28%). The results of the ventilation experiments are summarized in Table 1.

Reduction of Cerebral Perfusion Pressure

Raising ICP to levels of 30–40 mm Hg and reduction of cerebral perfusion pressure led to a significant decrease in ventricular CSF pO_2. The cisternal CSF pO_2, however, did not decrease but was increased, synchronous with a reflex blood pressure elevation.

Table 1. CSF pO_2 during ventilatory experiments

	VCSFpO$_2$ mm Hg ±SD	AVDpO$_2$ mm Hg ±SD	CCSFpO$_2$ mm Hg ±SD	ACDpO$_2$ mm Hg ±SD	paO$_2$ mm Hg ±SD	paCO$_2$ mm Hg ±SD
Reference conditions	70.8 6.5	53.9 12.4	65.8 9.3	58.9 10.3	124.7 8.0	37.8 3.1
Hypoxia (FiO$_2$ 0.15)	44.2 3.2	18.1 4.3	46.3 6.1	16.0 8.3	62.3 6.6	35.4 1.6
Hyperoxia (FiO$_2$ 0.5)	87.3 9.4	194.3 24.2	95.4 17.1	186.2 18.7	281.6 22.0	37.4 1.2
Hyperventilation	50.2 4.1	87.3 17.5	47.3 10.4	90.2 11.3	137.5 17.0	21.3 1.3
Hypoventilation	66.4 11.1	25.0 8.8	74.4 9.2	17.0 4.3	91.4 9.1	53.4 3.0
Hypercarbia	86.3 12.3	35.4 7.3	95.6 10.2	26.1 5.9	121.7 6.3	63.1 5.4

VCSFpO$_2$: ventricular CSF pO_2
AVDpO$_2$: arterioventricular pO_2 difference
CCSFpO$_2$: cisternal CSF pO_2
ACD pO$_2$: arterio-cisternal pO_2 difference
paO$_2$: arterial pO_2 value
paCO$_2$: arterial pCO_2 pressure

Discussion

The oxygen pressure of CSF in the lateral ventricle of the artificially ventilated cat and dog lay approximately at the same level.

Remarkably, before and after 3 hr of ventilatory experiments the CSF pO_2 was unchanged. The CSF pO_2 was stable and independent of small physiologic variations of intracranial and arterial pressures. The reproducibility and stability of the CSF pO_2 level in different species, after experimental disorder, and at physiologic variations of circulatory and ICP conditions suggests that the CSF pO_2 level is regulated.

The major influence on CSF pO_2 was exerted by the arterial pO_2 and pCO_2 levels. Only if the brain perfusion was lowered pathologically by extremely raised ICP or by arterial hypotension, is the CSF pO_2 level decreased markedly. This indicates that CSF pO_2 is not maintained if cerebral perfusion pressure is decreased below autoregulatory levels.

The observed fast CSF pO_2 changes are not easily explained if oxygen transport within the fluid compartments should only proceed by diffusion. An additional convectional oxygen transport in CSF must be assumed. The observed time course of CSF pO_2 changes cannot be explained by bulk flow of CSF. Hence, a multidirectional movement within the fluid must be considered. Most probably oscillations in intracranial pressure, due to heartbeat and respiration, are accompanied by convection in CSF. The marked decrease of ventricular CSF pO_2 and increase of AVD pO_2 during hyperventilation are findings of clinical interest, since the impairment of brain oxygen supply due to decrease of CBF during hyperventilation therapy can be determined directly by the technique demonstrated here.

Possible Physiological Role of the Cushing Response During Parturition

R.C. Koehler, A.P. Harris, M.D. Jones Jr., and R.J. Traystman

Departments of Anesthesiology/Critical Care Medicine, and Pediatrics, The Johns Hopkins Medical Institutions, Baltimore, Maryland 21205 (USA)

The Cushing response to elevated intracranial pressure (ICP) is often regarded as a defence mechanism of last resort when other mechanisms fail to maintain cerebral perfusion pressure. However, one physiological stress in which ICP may be commonly elevated is parturition. The fetus ordinarily is buoyed in amniotic fluid and uterine contractions produce equivalent increases in arterial pressure and ICP. However, once the head is engaged in the birth canal and begins to dilate the cervix, pressure on the skull is considerable. In the human fetus with its large, compliant skull, pressure on the equator of the skull may exceed amniotic fluid pressure by 50 mm Hg or more (Lindgren 1960), and this pressure appears to be nearly fully transmitted intracranially (Schwarcz et al. 1969). Because fetal arterial pressure is only 40–50 mm Hg greater than amniotic fluid pressure, cerebral ischemia might occur during intense labor. Even in non-human species with smaller skulls or closed fontanelles, the bone sutures usually are not fused and transient periods of elevated ICP are likely.

We examined how well a fetal animal maintains cerebral perfusion when ICP is elevated. The fetal circulation is at a disadvantage for increasing arterial pressure because cardiac output normally is relatively high under baseline conditions and may be unable to increase substantially (Rudolph 1986), and because 40% of cardiac output supplies the large, low resistance placental circuit, where vasoconstriction would impair oxygenation. We studied the circulatory response to elevated ICP in the chronically-catheterized fetal sheep preparation, which is a standard animal model for fetal circulatory studies (Rudolph 1985). First, we examined the steady state response to graded increases in ICP, and second, since uterine contractions are periodic, we investigated the dynamic response to cyclic oscillations in ICP.

Methods

Fetal sheep were studied at 0.9 gestational age. The ewe was anesthetized with halothane and a midline laparotomy was performed. Uterine incisions were made to expose fetal limbs and scalp for insertion of catheters into the inferior vena cava, abdominal aorta, brachiocephalic artery, sagittal sinus, and lateral ventricle (Cordis # 901302). All incisions were closed and the ewes recovered 48 hr before the experiment.

Arterial pressure and ICP were referenced to amniotic fluid pressure measured at fetal ear level. Fetal cerebral blood flow and peripheral organ blood flow were measured at six times by the radiolabelled microsphere technique adapted for fetal circulatory studies (Heymann et al. 1977). Cerebral O_2 uptake was calculated from the arterial-sagittal sinus O_2 content difference and blood flow to the cerebral hemispheres.

ICP was regulated by controlling the pressure in a reservoir of artificial cerebrospinal fluid connected to the lateral ventricular catheter. In ten animals, ICP was increased first to about 15 mm Hg, and then in four additional stepwise increments of about 6 mm Hg. Measurements were made 10 minutes after fixing the level of ICP. In twelve animals, ICP was cycled in a sinusoidal fashion ten times with a 3 min periodicity. The peak ICP was equivalent to each animal's baseline mean arterial pressure and the minimum ICP was equivalent to the animal's baseline ICP. In six of these animals, microspheres were injected at baseline and at 0, 0.75, 1.5, 2.25 and 3 min of the first 3 min cycle. In the remaining six animals, microspheres were injected at the corresponding times of the sixth ICP cycle. Values are presented as means $\pm$ SE.

Results

Cerebral hemodynamic data during stepwise elevation of ICP are shown in Table 1. As ICP was increased to 22 mm Hg, mean arterial pressure remained unchanged and cerebral perfusion pressure declined. With further elevations of ICP, mean arterial pressure rose by nearly equivalent increments, thereby minizing a further decline in cerebral perfusion pressure. Remarkably, cerebral blood flow and cerebral O_2 uptake remained at baseline levels.

The mechanism of the increase in arterial pressure involved peripheral vasoconstriction in selective organs with cardiac output unchanged. Significant decreases in renal and skin blood flow were detected at an ICP of 28 mm Hg and in gastrointestinal tract at an ICP of 34 mm Hg. At an ICP of 41 mm Hg, renal, gastrointestinal and skin blood flow decrased by 68 ± 8, 69 ± 7, and $65\pm9\%$, respectively. With a 33% increase in arterial pressure, vacular resistance qua-

Table 1. Cerebral hemodynamics during step elevations of ICP

ICP (mm Hg)	6	15	22	28	34	41
Mean arterial pressure (mm Hg)	50 ± 2	49 ± 2	52 ± 2	$56*\pm3$	$62*\pm2$	$67*\pm2$
Cerebral perfusion pressure (mm Hg)	44 ± 2	$33*\pm2$	$30*\pm2$	$28*\pm2$	$28*\pm2$	$26*\pm2$
Cerebral blood flow (ml/min/100 g)	117 ± 10	104 ± 8	92 ± 10	103 ± 10	122 ± 12	112 ± 19
Cerebral O_2 uptake (ml/min/100 g)	2.7 ± 0.2	3.0 ± 0.2	2.8 ± 0.3	3.3 ± 0.2	3.3 ± 0.2	3.0 ± 0.4

* $p < 0.05$ from baseline by analysis of variance and Dunnett's test

drupled in these three beds. Blood flow to the remaining carcass was unchanged. Most of the cardiac output was redistributed to the placenta. Placental blood flow increased in a passive fashion with the increase in arterial pressure. Arterial P_{O_2} was well-maintained (from 18 ± 1 to 21 ± 2 mm Hg).

In the second study, ICP was oscillated between a peak of 52 ± 1 mm Hg and a trough of 6 ± 1 mm Hg. During the first cycle, mean arterial pressure began to increase from its baseline value of 51 ± 1 mm Hg prior to the peak ICP, and it reached a peak of 61 ± 1 mm Hg at 30 sec after the ICP peak. During the subsequent ICP trough, arterial pressure partially recovered to 57 ± 1 mm Hg. Consequently, cerebral perfusion pressure never reached zero, but fell to a minimum of 4 ± 1 mm Hg at 10 sec prior to the ICP peak.

Microspheres were injected at quarter cycle intervals with the realization that the measured flows represent a time-weighted average over roughly 30 sec. Cerebral blood flow declined 65% at the ICP peak and returned to baseline at the ICP trough. Renal and intestinal blood flow decreased by 36 and 48%, respectively, at the ICP peak and returned to baseline at the ICP trough.

By the start of the sixth ICP cycle, mean arterial pressure was already elevated at 60 ± 2 mm Hg and it increased to a peak of 63 ± 2 mm Hg. Thus the phasic component of the blood pressure response was diminished. Instead arterial pressure remained elevated and renal and intestinal blood flow remained decreased throughout the cycle. Consequently, the minimum cerebral perfusion pressure achieved during the sixth cycle (10 ± 2 mm Hg) was not as low as the minimum obtained in the first cycle. Cerebral blood flow transiently fell by 43%. During the tenth cycle, the arterial pressure response remained unabated with a maximum of 67 ± 2 mm Hg and a minimum of 64 ± 2 mm Hg.

Discussion

These results indicate that near-term fetal sheep are capable of generating a potent Cushing response. With steady state elevations of ICP approaching baseline arterial pressure, cerebral blood flow and O_2 uptake were surprisingly well-maintained. These data contrast with postnatal lambs in which cerebral blood flow falls when cerebral perfusion pressure is reduced to 25 mm Hg by ventricular fluid infusion (Backofen et al. 1983). Moreover, in a similar model in adult sheep, increases in arterial pressure occur only when elevated ICP impairs cerebral O_2 uptake (Koehler et al. 1986). The observation that arterial pressure increases in fetal sheep without reductions in global cerebral O_2 uptake indicated that the response does not require profound ischemia. Perhaps pressure-stretch sensitive regions in the dorsal medulla are responsible for the response, as suggested by Hoff and Reis (1970) and Doba and Reis (1972). However, they elevated ICP with a supratentorial balloon which would be expected to cause more brainstem displacement than the ventricular fluid infusion method that we used. Another possible mechanism is that with low fetal P_{O_2}, discrete brain regions may be exquisitely sensitive to further tissue hypoxia imposed by elevated ICP. In support of this, we found that making postnatal lambs hypoxic appeared to lower the ICP threshold for increasing arterial pressure (Borel et al. 1987). Cerebral blood flow was likewise remarkably well-maintained.

As ICP approaches arterial pressure in postnatal sheep, cardiac output increases without profound visceral vasoconstriction (Koehler et al. 1983). In fetal sheep, baseline cardiac output is relatively high and did not increase with elevated ICP. Instead, the fetus relied on intense visceral vasoconstriction. Furthermore, because placental blood flow increased passively with arterial pressure, the fetus required disproportionately greater visceral vasoconstriction than postnatal animals. Whether less mature fetuses are capable of generating such profound vasoconstriction is unknown.

Our results with cyclic oscillations in ICP demonstrate that the fetal cardiovascular system can respond dynamically to periodic changes in ICP. Although the pressor response lagged about 30 sec behind the rise in ICP, it nevertheless responded with sufficient speed to prevent cerebral perfusion pressure and blood flow from falling to zero. Moreover, with repetitive cycles the pressor response became sustained throughout the cycle. Accordingly, the transient fall in cerebral perfusion pressure and blood flow was less on subsequent cycles.

Therefore, our data with ventricular fluid infusion in fetal sheep suggest that the Cushing response is capable of playing a prominent role during periodic ICP elevation associated with parturition. In addition to a generalized increase in cerebrospinal fluid pressure, external head compression during labor may cause displacement of the cerebrum and possibly brain stem. Brain stem displacement may enhance the pressor response more than fluid infusion alone. In either case, we speculate that the Cushing response may serve as an important mechanism for preserving cerebral viability during birth, and not simply as a last defense mechanism in adult life against a terminal event.

Acknowledgement. Supported by a grant from the National Institutes of Health (HL-38285).

References

Backofen JE, Koehler RC, Traystman RJ, Jones MD Jr, Rogers MC (1983) Importance of cerebral O_2 extraction reserve during elevated intracranial pressure in young lambs. In: Ishii S, Nagai H, Brock M (eds) Intracranial pressure V. Springer, Berlin Heidelberg New York, pp 333–341

Borel CO, Backofen JE, Koehler RC, Jones MD Jr, Traystman RJ (1987) Cerebral blood flow autoregulation during intracranial hypertension in hypoxic lambs. Am J Physiol 253:H1342–H1348

Doba N, Reis DJ (1972) Localization within the lower brainstem of a receptive area mediating the pressor response to increased intracranial pressure (the Cushing response). Brain Res 47:487–491

Heymann MA, Payne BD, Hoffman JI, Rudolph AM (1977) Blood flow measurements with radionuclide-labeled particles. Prog Cardiovasc Dis 20:55–79

Hoff JT, Reis DJ (1970) Localization of regions mediating the Cushing response in CNS of cat. Arch Neurol 23:228–240

Koehler RC, Backofen JE, Traystman RJ, Jones MD Jr, Rogers MC (1983) Peripheral organ blood flow distribution during raised intracranial pressure in young lambs. In: Ishii S, Nagai

H, Brock M (eds) Intracranial pressure V. Springer, Berlin Heidelberg New York, pp 880–884

Koehler RC, Backofen JE, McPherson RW, Rogers MC, Traystman RJ (1986) Relationships of regional cerebral blood flow, evoked potential responses, and systemic hemodynamics during intracranial hypertension. In: Miller JD, Teasdale GM, Rowan JO (eds) Intracranial pressure VI. Springer, Berlin Heidelberg New York, pp 365–368

Lindgren L (1960) The causes of fetal head moulding in labour. Acta Obstet Gynecol Scand 39:46–62

Rudolph AM (1985) Distribution and regulation of blood flow in the fetal and neonatal lamb. Circ Res 57:811–821

Schwarcz RL, Strada-Saenz G, Althabe O, Fernandez-Funes J, Caldeyro-Barcia R (1969) Pressure exerted by uterine contractions on the head of the human fetus during labor. In: Perinatal factors affecting human development. Pan Am Health Organ Sci Publ, pp 115–126

Electrocardiographic Changes are Associated with Elevated Blood Pressure Rather Than a Direct Effect of Raised Intracranial Pressure

C.P. McGraw, P.R. Palakurthy, and C. Maldonado

University of Louisville, School of Medicine, Louisville, Kentucky 40492 (USA)

The association between electrocardiographic abnormalities and elevated intracranial pressure (ICP) stemming from cerebrovascular accidents is well known. However, to our knowledge, no correlation has been made between specific electrocardiographic changes and the degree of measured ICP. In this study, the role of elevated ICP in the development of electrocardiographic changes and various cardiac arrhythmias was investigated.

Materials and Methods

Dogs ranging in weight from 14 to 36 kg were anesthetized using sodium pentobarbital (30 mg/kg). They were ventilated using a Harvard Pump Respirator via an endotracheal tube. A femoral vein was also catheterized for administration of drugs. Data from the multiple electrocardiographic leads (I, II, aVF and V5), arterial line and ICP (subarachnoid bolt) were displayed on an oscilloscope and stored. Every 10 minutes, the hydrostatic pressure column was elevated by 20 mm Hg increments until there was an acute drop in systemic blood pressure.

    The dogs were divided into four groups. The ICP in Group I dogs ($n = 11$), was elevated while monitoring the animal's blood pressure and electrocardiographic changes. Group II dogs ($n = 5$), were similarily handled, and a pharmacological autonomic blockade was achieved by intravenous propranolol hydrochloride 0.2 mg/kg administered at a rate of 1 mg/min, followed with atropine sulfate 0.2 mg/kg. Half doses were administered every 30 minutes to maintain blockade. Group III dogs ($n = 5$) were handled as Group I, however, arterial blood pressure was kept constant using continuous intravenous infusion of sodium nitroprusside (50 mg was added to 250 ml of isotonic fluids). Group IV dogs ($n = 5$) did not have ICP elevated, but arterial blood pressure was raised in increments using metaraminol infusion at a dose of 25 mg added to 250 ml of isotonic fluids. The mean arterial blood pressure increments for the Group IV dogs were similar to that of Group I. All dogs were euthanized with potassium while under sodium pentobarbital anesthesia and their hearts were examined.

Results

Group I Dogs

The most frequent T wave alteration was a change in polarity of the T wave ST-T changes. Bradyarrhythmia and the initial electrocardiographic changes were seen when the hydrostatic pressure column was equal to or greater than the mean arterial blood pressure. Electrocardiographic changes (both ST-T changes and rhythm disturbances) were reproducible. After the artificial ICP was decreased, electrocardiographic recordings returned to baseline. When the hydrostatic pressure was elevated to the previous increment, similar electrocardiographic changes were noted. Four dogs developed fresh subendocardial hemorrhages which were confined to the left ventricle. Hydrostatic pressure of 100 mm Hg resulted in fluid leaks from the dog's olfactory canal. Periorbital edema and pupillary dilatation were also seen at elevated ICP.

Group II Dogs

Baseline heart rate decreased following pharmacological blockage with propranolol and atropine. Elevation of the hydrostatic pressure column following pharmacological autonomic blockade did not result in significant elevation of arterial blood pressure. No electrocardiographic changes or subendocardial hemorrhages were seen in any of these dogs.

Group III Dogs

When baseline arterial blood pressure was maintained constantly in a normal range, there were no electrocardiographic changes or subendocardial hemorrhages even though ICP was elevated.

Group IV Dogs

When arterial blood pressure was elevated using continuous intravenous infusion of metaraminol, heart rate decreased in all dogs. Two dogs developed fresh subendocardial hemorrhages.

Discussion

Our study demonstrated a relationship between the elevation in the hydrostatic and the mean arterial blood pressure at which electrocardiographic changes were seen. These electrocardiographic changes occurred when the ICP was equal to or greater than the mean arterial blood pressure. The level of ICP needed to produce electrocardiographic changes in dogs is quite high and may be secondary to the decompression through the olfactory canal. In our study, electrocardiographic changes were seen in the majority of Group I dogs, in which no interventions were made to alter the arterial blood pressure. In Group II dogs, pharmacologic blockade resulted in a blunted blood pressure response and an absence of electrocardiographic changes. From this, we may assume that the autonomic nervous system is important in electrocardiographic changes associated with elevations in ICP. This indicates that electrocardiographic changes were secondary to sudden elevation in the arterial blood pressure, which may be the result of predominant sympathetic nervous system stimulation. Interestingly, similar electrocardiographic and rhythm changes were seen during sudden elevations in blood pressure without altering ICP. Since catecholamine blockade eliminated acute rises in blood pressure and the electrocardiographic changes, this suggests that catecholamines were responsible for the electrocardiographic changes in this study. Subendocardial hemorrhages were seen in Group I dogs, in which blood pressure was not controlled. Similar hemorrhages were also noted when arterial blood pressure alone was elevated using metaraminol. Interestingly, these hemorrhages were confined to the left ventricle.

In conclusion, electrocardiographic changes were seen when the artificial ICP was nearly equal to mean arterial blood pressure. The electrocardiographic changes were reproducible and are the result of marked arterial blood pressure elevation secondary to elevated ICP.

Session IV: Control of ICP

Chairmen: D.P. Becker and S. Cotev

445

Effect of Mannitol on Experimental Infusion Edema

S. Inao [1], P.P. Fatouros [2], and A. Marmarou [1]

[1] Richard Reynolds Neurosurgical Research Laboratories, Division of Neurosurgery, Medical College of Virginia, Richmond, Virginia 23298 (USA)
[2] Department of Radiology, Medical College of Virginia, Virginia Commonwealth University, Richmond, Virginia (USA)

Introduction

The effect of mannitol in reducing brain water has been under considerable scrutiny since the work of Takagi et al. (1983) who reported that mannitol reduced ICP but did not reduce tissue water measured gravimetrically. These results directly contradicted earlier findings by other workers. Further controversy arose with the reports by Muizelaar et al. (1983) which showed that the pressure reducing properties of mannitol act primarily through a vasoconstrictive effect and not by water reduction. This study was designed to document the acute and chronic effects of mannitol in reducing ICP, measuring tissue water by MRI and specific gravity methods.

Materials and Methods

Surgical Preparation

Twenty eight 2.2–5.7 kg adult cats were anesthetized with α-chloralose, intubated, and allowed to breath spontaneously. Cannulation of a femoral vein catheter was placed for drug administration. In one group of animals an additional arterial cannula was placed for blood sampling and pressure monitoring. All animals had stereotactic infusions of serum (0.25 cc/136 minutes) into the central white matter (Marmarou et al. 1982). One group of animals had cisterna magna catheters placed for ICP and pressure volume index (PVI) measurements.

MR Imaging

Magnetic Resonance Imaging was performed on all animals in a clinical MRI unit (Siemens Magnetom, 1.0 Tesla) using a standard orbital surface coil. Axial scans 2–4 mm thick at the central semiovale level were performed. For T_1 calculation, inversion recovery (IR) images at different inversion times (TI = 250, 600, 1000, 1700 msecs) were obtained using a repetition time (TR) of 4 seconds. T_2 values of the brain were calculated from the spin echo (SE) images with differing echo times (TE = 100, 150, 200, 250 msecs) using the same TR.

Mannitol Administration

In all animals, a mannitol bolus was administered (2 g/kg) over a three minute period at the end of the edema infusion, after control MRI (T-1 and T-2) scans were acquired. Mannitol was then continuously infused at a rate of 2 g/kg/hour, beginning thirty minutes after bolus injection and continued for either twenty or ninety minutes.

Blood Sampling

Arterial blood was analyzed for arterial blood gases, osmolarity, and hematocrit at regular intervals for the duration of the experiment.

Protocol

Five experimental groups were studied. The first group was a control ($n=7$) in which MRI was imaged after edema infusion and without mannitol treatment (T_1 and T_2). Group 2 (Acute-MRI; $n=6$) was given infusion edema and a mannitol bolus. MRI was acquired ten minutes after the bolus, for the next forty minutes (T_1). During the imaging, thirty minutes post bolus, mannitol was infused continuously for twenty minutes, to study the acute effects of mannitol on brain edema. The animal was then sacrificed at fifty minutes. Group 3 (Chronic-MRI; $n=5$) was given infusion edema and a mannitol bolus. MRI was then acquired ten minutes after bolus, for 40 minutes (T_1) and then for 70 minutes (T_1 and T_2) until sacrifice at 120 minutes. During the imaging, thirty minutes post bolus, mannitol was infused continuously for ninety minutes hence, studying delayed effects of mannitol on brain edema. The fourth group (Acute-no MRI; $n=2$) was given bolus mannitol after infusion edema and then sacrificed thirty minutes later. Group 5 (Chronic-no MRI; $n=8$), was given infusion edema and a mannitol bolus, then continuous infusion of mannitol for 120 minutes, then sacrificed. Blood pressure, heart rate, ICP, hematocrit, and osmolarity were also measured.

In all groups brain water content was determined by gravimetric techniques. In summary, the above groups provided MRI and gravimetric tissue water at 30, 50, and 120 minutes post bolus mannitol.

All values were expressed as mean ± standard error of the mean.

Results

Relaxation Time-Water Content Correlation

In groups 1–3, comparisons were made between relaxation times (T_1 and T_2) and water content measurements obtained in identical brain areas. 27 pair of T_1-water content and 22 pair of T_2-water content data were obtained in our MRI series with cats. These data indicate a good correlation between relaxation time (T_1, T_2) and tissue water content ($r=0.95$ for T_1-water, $r=0.91$ for T_2-water).

Acute and Delayed Effects of Mannitol on Tissue Water Content

In group 2, water content decreased in normal (non-infused hemisphere) white matter (1.0%, $p < 0.01$ respectively). No significant decrease was found in non-infused grey matter. Edematous (infused hemisphere) white and grey matter water content also decreased (1.6%, $p < 0.01$, and 0.8%, $p < 0.05$ respectively).

In group 3, water content decreased more than in group 2 in all tissue groups. In non-infused white matter, water content dropped 2.6% ($p < 0.01$). In non-infused grey matter, water dropped 2.2% ($p < 0.01$). In infused white matter, 2.7% ($p < 0.01$), and in infused grey matter water dropped 3.1% ($p < 0.01$).

In group 4, no significant change was observed in water content in animals sacrificed at 30 minutes post bolus.

Acute and Delayed Effects of Mannitol on Relaxation Times

In group 2, neither T_1 nor T_2 changed significantly in normal or edematous white matter.

In group 3, T_1 decreased 36 msec. in normal ($p < 0.01$) and 52 msec. in edematous white matter. T_2 did not change significantly in either normal or edematous tissue.

Acute and Delayed Effects of Mannitol on ICP, PVI, and Osmolarity

In group 4, ICP increased immediately following the mannitol bolus ($9.3 \pm .6$ to $12.7 \pm .9$, $p < 0.05$) then dropped below control values within 10 min. ($p < 0.01$), and remained low for the remainder of the experiment.

PVI increased from 1.0 ± 0.2 to 1.8 ± 0.3 ($p < 0.05$) 30 min. following the mannitol bolus then decreased to 1.5 ± 0.3 at 120 min. post-bolus.

Mean arterial blood pressure decreased significantly immediately following the bolus, then returned to normal within 10 min., similar to the time course of the ICP change seen.

Serum osmolarity was maintained above control, and hematocrit was lower than control at all times during post mannitol period. Arterial blood gas measurements remained unchanged throughout the experiment.

Discussion

This study demonstrates that bolus mannitol followed by continuous infusion effects an osmolarity gradient of 25 mOSM for a two hour period, resulting in a 2.6% reduction of tissue water in both edematous and normal brain. At 90 min., water reduction is at the 1% level. At 30 min. post bolus no water reduction was evident. The observation that ICP was significantly reduced in the absence of water reduction at 30 min. supports the contention that ICP reduction in the acute phase of mannitol action is not by water removal from brain tissue. This is in agreement with studies of Takagi et al. (1983). Moreover, the observation that PVI is increased during periods when brain tissue water remained at control levels, suggests that other factors, perhaps vascular, are operational in effecting a rise in PVI and slackening of brain (Muizelaar et al. 1983). Although the PVI changes, which are thought to reflect increased venous volume, suggest a vascular mechanism, the results by Takagi indicate that CSF surrounding the large surface vessels may be responsible for the acute ICP reduction and cannot be ruled out by this study. At 50 min., although the reduction of water is small (1%), our calculations show that the equivalent brain volume is significant and contributes to ICP reduction. Thus, beyond 30 min. the mechanisms responsible for the reduction of ICP in the presence of a sustained osmolarity gradient are multifactorial.

Finally, we have shown that MRI is a useful method for non-invasive measure of tissue water which can detect small changes in tissue on the order of 1.0%.

Acknowledgements. This work was supported by NIH Grants 5RO1NS19235 and 5RO1NS12587 and the Richard Roland Reynolds Neurosurgical Research Fund.

References

Marmarou A, Tanaka K, Shulman K (1982) The brain response to infusion edema: Dynamics of fluid resolution. In: Hartmann A, Brock M (eds) Treatment of cerebral edema. Springer, Berlin Heidelberg New York, pp 11–18

Muizelaar JP, Wei EP, Kontos HA et al. (1983) Mannitol causes compensatory cerebral vasoconstriction and vasodilation in response to blood viscosity changes. J Neurosurg 59:822–828

Takagi H, Saitoh T, Kitahara T et al. (1983) The mechanism of ICP reducing effect of mannitol. In: Ishi H, Nagai H, Brock M (eds) Intracranial pressure V. Springer, Berlin Heidelberg New York, pp 729–733

Immediate and Long-term Effects of Mannitol and Glycerol: A Comparative Experimental Study

R. García-Sola, F. Gilsanz, and D. Chillón

Department of Neurosurgery, Hospital de la Princesa; Department of Experimental Surgery, Clínica Puerta De Hierro, Autonomous University, Madrid (Spain)

There is an apparent discrepancy between the advantages attributed to glycerol and the more frequent use of its "rival", mannitol. This has led us to perform this study for the purpose of producing an experimental model of intracranial hypertension, a medium in which to compare the immediate and long-term effects of the repeated administration of the two hyperosmotic agents in conditions more similar to those of the human clinic.

Material and Methods

The experimental conditions have been described previously (García-Sola et al. 1980) and consist basically of the implantation into 18 goats of two small epidural balloons for measuring the intracranial pressure (ICP), a flowmeter around both internal maxillary arteries for determination of cerebral blood flow (CBF), and femoral catheters for the measurement of blood pressure (BP) and intravenous infusion (IV). After determination of BP and bilateral ICPs and CBFs in basal conditions in the conscious goat, the animal was subjected to a focal cold injury (CI). From then on, these parameters were determined every four hours for three consecutive days.

Three groups of 6 experiences each were performed; C, control; M, mannitol (24 hours after CI, an IV solution of 20% mannitol was administered every 12 hours at a dose of 1 g/kg body weight for 10 min); and G, glycerol (a solution of 10.1% glycerol was administered at the same rate as in group M, at a dose of 0.5 g/kg body weight).

Results and Discussion

Immediate Postinfusion Effects (Fig. 1 a)

ICP. Both hyperosmotic agents produce the greatest decrease in ICP at 20 min postinfusion ($p < 0.01$). Four hours postinfusion, the ICP in group M increases significantly with respect to the minimum values registered at 20 min postinfusion ($p < 0.05$), slightly surpassing basal values, an event which does not occur with glycerol.

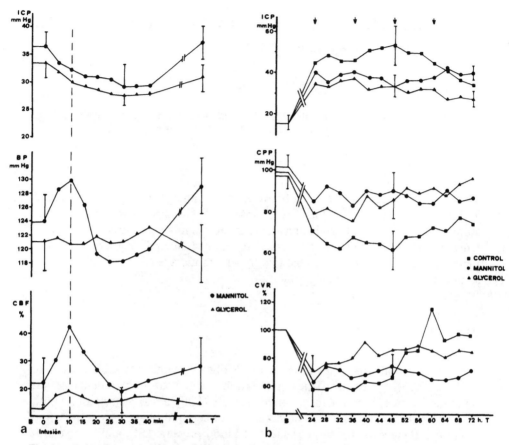

Fig. 1. a Immediate postinfusion effects of Mannitol and Glycerol on ICP, BP and CBF.
b Long-term effects of Mannitol and Glycerol infusions (↓) on ICP, CPP and CVR

CBF. Once the infusion of mannitol is finalized, there is an increment in CBF ($p<0.05$) which is associated with an increase in the BP. However, in group G, CBF increases less rapidly and is more stable. In human clinics, it has been seen that glycerol administration also produces an increase in the CBF (Meyer et al. 1974). One explanation, aside from the expansive effect of the blood volume, is the increase in the cerebral perfusion pressure (CPP) observed with glycerol ($p<0.05$ at 20–30 min).

Long-term Effects (Fig. 1 b)

ICP. With mannitol, ICP remains lower than that of group C ($p<0.05$ from 48 to 56 h) except in the last 12 hours. In contrast, with glycerol, the ICP is found at all times to be lower than in group C, this difference being even greater when compared with the mannitol group ($p<0.01$).

This net difference can be attributed to the fact that glycerol provokes no rebound phenomena or a very slight one, due to metabolization of it by the brain

(Meyer et al. 1974), compard to the progressive loss of the capacity to lower the ICP observed with repeated infusion of mannitol. This will determine the appearance of a "long-term rebound phenomenon".

CVR. The phenomenon of compensating vasodilation associated with elevation of ICP, which serves to prevent vascular collapse (García Sola et al. 1980), is observed in all groups, being most pronounced in the control group (from 24 to 48 h). The subsequent tendency toward spontaneous diminution of ICP in this group produces a tendency toward the normalization of CVR. Nevertheless, in groups M and G, with similar and higher CPPs than group C, there is greater vasodilation (more pronounced with mannitol and associated with a larger increase in the CBF).

To explain these discrepancies, it may be necessary to advocate the direct effect of these hyperosmotic agents on the increase in CBF by their rheological qualities, which decrease the viscosity of the blood (Kassell et al. 1981).

Acknowledgements. This work has been financed by the FIS and the CAICYT.

References

García-Sola R, Vaquero J, Cabezudo J, Bravo G (1980) Evolution of intracranial pressure and cerebral blood flow in cryogenic cerebral edema. In: Shulman K et al. (eds) Intracranial pressure IV. Springer, Berlin Heidelberg New York, pp 268–271
Kassell N, Baumann KW, Hitchon PW et al. (1981) Influence of continuous high dose infusion of mannitol on cerebral blood flow in normal dogs. Neurosurgery 9:283–286
Meyer JS, Shamizu K, Ohuchi T et al. (1974) Cerebral metabolic effects of glycerol in fusion in diabetics with stroke. J Neurol Sci 21:1–22

Effects of Mannitol on Spontaneous Tone of Intracerebral Arterioles

M. Takayasu and R.G. Dacey Jr.

Division of Neurological Surgery, University of North Carolina, 148 Burnett Womack Building, Chapel Hill, North Carolina 27599-7060 (USA)

Introduction

The direct effects of hyperosmolar solutions such as mannitol on vascular smooth muscle, which have been reported mostly in the peripheral vessels, are controversial. Authors who used preconstricted vessels demonstrated vasodilation effects of hyperosmolar solution (Krishnamurty et al. 1977), whereas the other authors who used non-preconstricted vessels demonstrated vasoconstriction effects (Andersson et al. 1974, Kent et al. 1983). Sasaki et al. (1986), however, reported vasodilation by hyperosmolar solutions not only under condition of preconstriction but also with resting tension in a cerebral arterial ring preparation. This study was undertaken to clarify the effects of mannitol on vascular smooth muscle in the cerebral microcirculation. For this purpose, spontaneously developed tone in rat cerebral parenchymal arterioles in vitro was examined in vessels with different tone state by changing the pH of organ bath solution.

Methods

Methods for isolation and cannulation techniques are described by Dacey and Duling in 1982. Briefly, intracerebral penetrating arterioles of 30 to 70 µm in diameter were surgically isolated from the first (M-1) portion of the middle cerebral artery from rat brains. The vessel segments were transferred to a temperature controlled chamber on the stage of a Nikon inverted microscope and were cannulated using glass pipettes. Vessel diameters were monitored using a video-dimensional analysis system (modified Colorado Video, Model 321) under constant transmural pressure of 60 mm Hg applied via the cannulating pipette. Control vessel diameter was defined as the diameter to which vessels spontaneously contracted during the equilibration period of approximately 45 minutes in modified Ringer's solution (PSS) of pH 7.3 at 37°C. The vessel diameter was expressed as percent of the control vessel diameter thereafter. Drugs were applied to the vessel extraluminally by changing organ bath solution.

In the first experiment, the dose-response curve of mannitol (0.1, 0.5, 1 and 2%) was obtained in control tone state at pH 7.3. The results were compared to those with another hyperosmolar solution, sucrose (0.2, 1, 2 and 4%) in nearly equal osmolarity.

Next, mannitol dose-response curves were determined in vessels with different tone state by changing the pH of organ bath solution to pH 6.8 and pH 7.6. Since vasoconstriction is reported in non-preconstricted peripheral vessels, the effects of the highest concentration (2%) of mannitol were examined in maximally dilated parenchymal arterioles, which can be induced with Ca^{2+}-free solution containing 0.5 mM EGTA.

Basic parameters, such as control vessel diameters, pH responses to pH 6.8 and pH 7.6, were compared with one way analysis of variance (ANOVA), in order to determine whether these parameters were homogenously distributed in each of the four groups (mannitol groups at pH 7.3, pH 6.8 and pH 7.6 and sucrose group at pH 7.3). Correlation between the diameter of the vessel and the osmolarity of mannitol or sucrose solutions was investigated by least squares regression after log conversion of the vessel diameter (Morrison 1967). In order to determine whether the dose response curves are parallel, a growth curve analysis was performed (Grizzie and Allen 1969). Comparison of control and mannitol response in Ca^{++}-free solution was done using Student's t-test. Values were considered to be significantly different at $p < 0.05$.

Results

The control vessel diameter was 49.4 ± 3.4 μm ($n = 19$, M $\pm$ SE). Vessels dilated to $120.1 \pm 1.2\%$ of control diameter when extraluminal solution pH was lowered to 6.8 and constricted to $81.4 \pm 0.8\%$ of control diameter when pH was raised to 7.6. These basic parameters of vessel were not significantly different in each of four groups (p values ranged from 0.33 to 0.64).

Effects of Mannitol and Sucrose Solutions in Control Tone State at pH 7.3

At a bath solution pH of 7.3, mannitol and sucrose solutions released spontaneously developed arteriolar tone in a dose-dependent manner (Fig. 1). The degree of vasodilation was similar between mannitol and sucrose solutions in nearly equal osmolarity. Linear regression analysis was done with vessel diameter (percent of control) as dependent variables and osmolarity of PSS as the independent variable. Correlation coefficients (r) ranged from 0.96 in mannitol and 0.95 in sucrose. Both were statistically significant ($p < 0.0001$). The slopes for these two dose-response curves were not significantly different from each other ($p = 0.14$), and therefore, these dose-response curves did not appear to be significantly different.

Effects of Mannitol Solutions in Different Tone State

Either in increased tone state at pH 7.6 or in decreased tone state at pH 6.8, vessels dilated significantly with mannitol in a dose-dependent manner. Vessel diameters

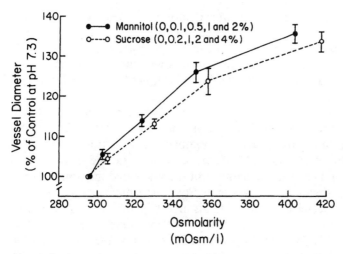

Fig. 1. Effects of mannitol and sucrose solutions on vessel diameters in control tone state at pH 7.3. Results are expressed as mean ± SEM

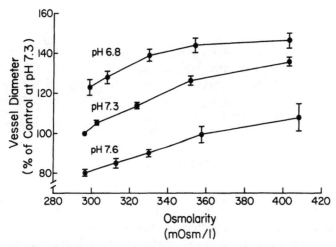

Fig. 2. Effects of mannitol solutions on vessel diameters in increased tone state at pH 7.6 and in decreased tone state at pH 6.8. Results are expressed as mean ± SEM

correlated well with osmolarity of organ bath at both pH ($r = 0.93$ at pH 7.6 and 0.95 at pH 6.8, $p < 0.05$) (Fig. 2). The slopes for these dose-response curves were not significantly different from each other ($p = 0.49$).

Ca^{2+}-free solution containing 0.5 mM EGTA induced vasodilation to 149.5 ± 3.9% ($n = 4$). Even in this maximally reduced tone state, 2% mannitol solution did not induce any vasocontraction and showed the same degree of vasodilation to 149.9 ± 3.9% ($n = 4$) ($p = 0.95$).

Discussion

The mechanism through which hyperosmolar solutions such as mannitol lowers intracranial pressure is not fully understood yet. The traditional theory is osmotic dehydration of the brain (Shenkin et al. 1962, Wise et al. 1963). However, Muizelaar et al. recently hypothesized autoregulatory vasoconstriction secondary to increased cerebral blood flow (CBF) from decreased blood viscosity (Muizelaar et al. 1983). Intravascular infusion of hyperosmolar solutions is mostly reported to increase CBF in vivo studies (Meyer et al. 1972, Johnson and Harper 1973, Hardebo and Nilsson 1980). However, the direct effects of hyperosmolar solutions on vascular smooth muscle in vitro studies are controversial.

The present study demonstrated vasodilation effects of mannitol and sucrose on spontaneously developed tone of intracerebral arterioles at pH 7.3. The degree of vasodilation correlated well with osmolarity, irrespective of hyperosmolar agents. The results suggest that hyperosmolarity per se produces a dilation effect on the vessels. Mannitol also induced vasodilation in vessels with different tone state, that is, increased tone state at pH 7.6 and reduced tone state at pH 6.8. The mannitol dose-response curves in vessels with different tone state were parallel to each other, suggesting that vasodilation effects of mannitol are essentially constant irrespective of tone state of vessels. No vasoconstriction effects of mannitol were noted even in vessels with maximally reduced tone in Ca^{2+}-free solution containing 0.5 mM EGTA. This result contrasted with that reported by Kent et al. who demonstrated that hyperosmolar solutions induced vasoconstriction in rat aortic strips under resting tension mainly due to intracellular calcium mobilization (Kent et al. 1983).

In the present experiment, hyperosmolar solutions were applied to the vessels extraluminally instead of intraluminal administration for technical reasons. This is different from the clinical situation, where hyperosmolar solutions are administered exclusively intraluminally. Although intraluminal application could produce some different effects through endothelium, extraluminal application of the solutions does not appear to be an unreasonable way to study the direct effect of hyperosmolar solutions on vascular smooth muscle.

Extrapolation of the present data to the entire cerebral vascular system may not be justified because longitudinal variation of responsiveness to vasoactive agents is well known in cerebral vessels (Dacey and Dulin 1984, Takayasu et al. 1988). Therefore, the present study indicates that mannitol has vasodilation effects at least on intracerebral arterioles in any tone state of the vessels which are the most distal resistance vessels in the cerebral circulation and are responsible for a significant part of total cerebrovascular resistance.

Acknowledgments. We thank Mitchell Dyer for technical assistance and Lynn Thomas for preparation of the manuscript.

References

Andersson C, Helstrand P, Johansson B, Ringberg A (1974) Contraction in venous smooth muscle induced by hypertonicity. Calcium dependence and mechanical characteristics. Acta Physiol Scand 90:451–461

Dacey RG, Duling BR (1982) A study of rat intracerebral arterioles: methods, morphology and reactivity. Am J Physiol 243:H598–H606

Dacey RG, Duling BR (1984) Effect of norepinephrine on penetrating arterioles of rat cerebral cortex. Am J Physiol 246:H380–H385

Grizzle JE, Allen DM (1969) Analysis of growth and dose response curves. Biometrics 25:357–381

Hardebo JE, Nilsson B (1980) Hemodynamic changes in brain caused by local infusion of hyperosmolar solutions, in particular relation to blood-brain barrier opening. Brain Res 181:49–59

Johnston IH, Harper A (1973) The effect of mannitol on cerebral blood flow. An experimental study. J Neurosurg 38:461–471

Kent RL, Sheldon RJ, Harakal C (1983) The effects of hyperosmolar solutions on isolated vascular smooth muscle examined with verapamil. Pharmacology 26:157–163

Krishnamurty VSR, Adams HR, Smitherman TC, Templeton GH, Willerson JT (1977) Influence of mannitol on contractile responses of isolated perfused arteries. Am J Physiol 232:H59–H66

Meyer JS, Fukuuchi Y, Shimazu K, Ohuchi T, Ericsson AD (1972) Abnormal hemispheric blood flow and metabolism in cerebrovascular disease. II. Therapeutic trials with 5% CO_2 inhalation, hyperventilation and intravenous infusion of THAM and mannitol. Stroke 3:157–167

Morrison DF (1967) Multivariate statistical methods. McGraw-Hill Book Company, New York, pp 216–222

Muizelaar JP, Wei EP, Kontos HA, Becker DP (1983) Mannitol causes compensatory cerebral vasoconstriction and vasodilation in response to blood viscosity changes. J Neurosurg 59:822–828

Sasaki T, Kassell NF, Fujiwara S, Torner JC, Spallone A (1986) The effects of hyperosmolar solutions on cerebral arterial smooth muscle. Stroke 17:1266–1271

Shenkin HA, Goluboff B, Haft H (1962) The use of mannitol for the reduction of intracranial pressure in intracranial surgery. J Neurosurg 19:897–901

Takayasu M, Bassett JE, Dacey RG Jr. (1988) Effects of calcium antagonists on intracerebral penetrating arterioles in rats. Neurosurg 69. In press

Wise BL (1963) Effects of infusion of hypertonic mannitol on electrolyte balance and on osmolarity of serum and cerebrospinal fluid. J Neurosurg 20:961–967

Experimental Cerebral Edema, Isotonic Intravenous Infusions, Mannitol, Serum Osmolality, Electrolytes, Brain Water, Intracranial Pressure, and Cerebral Blood Flow

H.E. James, S. Schneider, S. Bhasin, and T.G. Luerssen

Division of Neurosurgery/Surgery and the Department of Pediatrics, School of Medicine, University of California, San Diego, California 92123 (USA)

Introduction

Mannitol and intravenous fluid resuscitation are therapies that are commonly employed in multiple trauma. Much discussion exists as to the correct dosage of mannitol, but the concomitant fluid resuscitation, mannitol and response to this agent, has received limited attention (James 1980). The current study addressses isotonic saline hydration, mannitol, ICP and CBF.

Materials and Methods

Two groups of albino rabbits were the primary structure of this study: one, with a 90 second cryogenic lesion over the left hemisphere cortex (dura intact) and the other was sham-operated animals (James and Laurin 1981). In turn, subgroups were created in whom during the 3 hour experimental trial they were administered either "maintenance" or "above maintenance" intravenous isotonic saline. A subset was created that received mannitol. The animals were anesthetized with halothane (2%), their scalps infiltrated with marcaine (1%), following a left parieto-occipital freeze lesion or sham operation, 24 hours to the experimental run. For the experimental trial, the animals were intubated with halothane anesthesia, mechanically ventilated with a mixture of oxygen (50%), nitrous oxide (45%), halothane (0.5%) and paralyzed with pancuronium (1 mg/dose). Arterial and venous femoral catheters were placed and continuous monitoring of blood gases was performed to maintain a $PaCO_2$ of 37–43 torr. A cisternal 19-gauge catheter recorded ICP, bilateral EEG monitoring with platinum subdermal electrodes was recorded; bilateral platinum CBF probes were placed 2 mm into the frontal lobes, 1.5 mm from the sagittal suture, with stereotactic technique. Control CBF runs were performed in each animal prior to the experimental trial, so that all subgroups had their own baseline studies, with 8 to 12 animals in each subgroup and 8 to 12 CBF studies were performed per subgroup. After 3 hours all animals were sacrificed for studies of brain water (gravimetry), extravasation of previously administered Evans blue dye and location of CBF electrodes. Samples of serum osmolality, sodium and potassium were taken prior to infusion and at 60, 120, 180 min. into the experiment. The animals that were in the "maintenance" IV fluid subgroup received a minimum of 41 ml to a maximum of 58 ml 3 hours; the "above maintenance" from 63 to 83 ml/3 hours (isotonic saline). Mannitol (20%) was infused by pump at a rate of 1 g/kg/hour for 3 hours, in lesioned and unlesioned animals.

Results

Serum Osmolality and Sodium

The initial serum osmolality was 287 ± 8 and 293 ± 6 mOsm/L in the sham-operated and the cryogenic subgroups respectively. There was no statistical difference at 60, 120 and 180 min. into the trials with that initial value. No statistical difference was noted in the "above maintenance" initial osmolality with the subsequent values during the trials. Following mannitol 1 g/kg/hour there was an increase in serum osmolality. No significant change in serum sodium or potassium was seen in the "maintenance" or in the "above maintenance" groups that did not receive mannitol. In the subgroup that received mannitol following cold injury, animals with maintenance isotonic saline had a significantly higher serum osmolality than the above maintenance group ($p < 0.005$); a significant decrease of serum sodium from that of controls was noted in the animals with cold injury following mannitol and above maintenance isotonic saline ($p < 0.005$) (Table 1).

Brain Gravimetry

As expected there was a significant increase in the water content of the white matter of the group with the cryogenic insult in the left hemisphere, when compared to controls ($p < 0.005$), but there was no difference between the equivalent subgroups when comparing the maintenance against the above maintenance fluid subgroups. In the cryogenic injury and mannitol subset, there was a significant reduction of water content in the animals that received maintenance IV saline, when compared to that group that received mannitol with above maintenance saline ($p < 0.005$) (Table 1).

Intracranial Pressure

The ICP values are listed in Table 2. There was no statistical difference between the various subgroups of the maintenance and the above maintenance IV saline, or between themselves, except for the expected rise following the cryogenic injury, when compared to the sham-operated. After mannitol infusion a decreasing trend was noted in the cold lesioned only.

Table 1. Experimental groups and results[a]

		Serum osmolality[b] (mOsm/l)	Serum sodium[b] (mEq/L)	Brain gravimetry Left hemisphere		Right hemisphere	
				Gray	White	Gray	White
Controls		287±8	146±11[e]	1.0415±0.0009	1.0404±0.0009	1.0418±0.0036	1.0406±0.001
Maintenance fluids:	Lesion	287±6	148±9.8	1.0400±0.0008	1.0360±0.0036[c]	1.0415±0.0004	1.0385±0.0023[e]
	No lesion	280±8	151±8.8	1.0415±0.009	1.0404±0.0009[d]	1.0418±0.0036	1.0406±0.001[f]
Above maintenance fluids:	Lesion	280±7	130±9.0	1.0399±0.008	1.0360±0.0030[c]	1.0419±0.0002	1.0413±0.0019
	No lesion	294±8	137±8.4	1.0414±0.0009	1.0401±0.0008[d]	1.0419±0.0033	1.0412±0.0023
Mannitol 20% (1 g/kg/hour/3 hrs)	Maintenance	308±7	138±8.8	1.0424±0.0001	1.0418±0.002	1.0416±0.0023	1.0414±0.0011
	Above maintenance	315±8	136±9.8	1.0423±0.0007	1.0413±0.001	1.0430±0.002	1.0396±0.004
Mannitol 20% with cryogenic lesion (1 g/kg/hour/3 hrs)	Maintenance	329±9[c]	130±6.9	1.0419±0.002	1.0398±0.002[c]	1.0435±0.0024	1.0390±0.0003
	Above maintenance	298±8[d]	128±8.4[f]	1.0419±0.0001	1.0381±0.002[d]	1.0428±0.0021	1.0392±0.002

[a] Values expressed in mean and standard deviation; [b] At 180 min. of the experimental trial; [c] See (4); [d] $p < 0.005$ from (3) [e] See below; [f] $p < 0.025$ from (5).

Table 2

	CBF[a] (ml/100 g/min)		ICP[b] (torr)		SAP (torr)	PaCO$_2$[c] (torr)
	Left	Right	Initial	Final		
Controls (means ± SD)	64.4 ± 20.4	66.6 ± 21.9		1.96 ± 2	102 ± 14.9	39.7 ± 1.6
Mannitol 20% (1 g/kg/hour)	47.8 ± 22.5	48.7 ± 14.6	1.96 ± 1.2	1.7 ± 2.0	114.2 ± 9.8	40.7 ± 2.2
Mannitol 20% (1 g/kg/hour) with cold lesion	64.7 ± 19.8	44.1 ± 17.8	5.2 ± 3.0	3.1 ± 2.3	103.8 ± 8.8	38.7 ± 1.3

[a] Mean of 11 to 22 CBF runs during study period, per subgroup; [b] Mean ICP values; [c] Mean PaCO$_2$ of experimental runs.

Cerebral Blood Flow

Mannitol infusions created in this model a decrease in CBF over both hemispheres, though this was not statistically significant when compared to controls. In those with cold lesion over the left hemisphere there was similar CBF values to the controls, but in the contralateral (uninjured) hemisphere the previously noted decrease with mannitol, was also seen (Table 2).

Discussion

A CBF decreasing trend was noted during the mannitol infusion, except over the injured left hemisphere, where vasoconstriction could be impaired. Isotonic saline IV challenges in the current acute phase of this study did not produce elevations of ICP, but those animals that with mannitol received higher volumes of IV fluids did have an increase in the water content of the white matter of the injured hemisphere, when compared to the mannitol and lower IV saline group. The effectiveness of mannitol in extracting brain water can be impaired by the volume of IV fluid that is simultaneously administered (Javid et al. 1964).

References

James HE (1980) Methodology for control of intracranial pressure with hypertonic mannitol. Acta Neurochir (Wien) 51:161–172

James HE, Laurin RA (1981) Intracranial hypertension and brain edema in albino rabbits. Part 1. Experimental models. Acta Neurochir (Wien) 55: 213–226

Javid M, Gilboe D, Cesario T (1964) The rebound phenomenon and hypertonic solutions. J Neurosurg (Wien) 21:1059–1066

Effects of Mannitol-Induced Hemodynamic Changes on Intracranial Pressure Responses in Dogs

N. Abou-Madi[1], J. Katz[2], M. Abou-Madi[1], and D. Trop[1]

[1] Department of Neuro-Anesthesia, Montreal Neurological Institute, McGill University, Montreal, Quebec H3A 2B4 (Canada)
[2] Department of Medical Sciences, University of Florida, Gainesville, Florida (USA)

Introduction

Rapid administration of mannitol in individuals with normal intracranial pressure (ICP) causes an initial increase in ICP (Cottrell et al. 1979). In contrast, it has recently been demonstrated that a mannitol bolus rapidly reduces ICP in animals with intracranial hypertension (Abou-Madi et al. 1987). In both situations, mannitol's initial impact on ICP appeared to derive from its vascular rather than its osmotic effect. This study compares the relationship between ICP and hemodynamic changes following bolus administration of mannitol: 1 – In dogs with normal ICP. 2 – In dogs with experimentally induced intracranial hypertension.

Methods

Sixteen unmedicated mongrel dogs, weighing 18–22 kg, were studied. Anesthesia was induced with a single IV dose of thiopentene $12 \, \mathrm{mg \cdot kg^{-1}}$. The dogs were intubated and ventilated using compressed air. $PaCO_2$ was adjusted to $40 \pm 2 \, \mathrm{mm \, Hg}$. Anesthesia was maintained with increments of fentanyl and metocurine given IV as needed. Normothermia was afforded by the use of a heating blanket. ICP was continuously transduced and recorded from the cisterna magna. A 20-gauge catheter was placed in the femoral artery to permit the continuous recording of the mean systemic arterial blood pressure (MAP). A flow-directed pulmonary artery thermodilution cardiac output catheter was inserted via the right internal jugular vein to measure the central venous pressure (CVP) the mean pulmonary artery pressure (PAP), the pulmonary capillary wedge pressure (PCWP), and the cardiac output (CO). The total peripheral resistance (TPR) and the pulmonary vascular resistance (PVR) were calculated from the following formulae: $\mathrm{TPR = MAP - CVP/CO \times 80}$ and $\mathrm{PVR = \overline{PAP} - PCWP/CO \times 80}$ $(\mathrm{dynes \cdot sec \cdot cm^{-5}})$. The dogs were randomly divided into 3 groups. In group A (six dogs): after a stabilization period of 30 min, baseline measurements of ICP, heart rate (HR), MAP, CVP, PAP, PCWP, and CO were obtained and a 20 percent solution of mannitol: $2 \, \mathrm{g \cdot kg^{-1}}$, was rapidly infused over a 3-minute period. Data were collected at the end of the infusion and at 2, 5 and 10 minutes post-infusion. In group B (six dogs): an epidural balloon was inserted and gradu-

Table 1. Mean changes in ICP (mm Hg), HR (beats/min), MAP (mm Hg), CVP (mm Hg), PAP (mm Hg), PCWP (mm Hg), CO (L/min), TPR (dynes · sec · cm^{-5}) and PVR (dynes · sec · cm^{-5}) ±SEM, following mannitol infusion 2 g/kg

	Group A (without brain compression) n=6			Group B (with brain compression) n=6		
	Baseline	End of infusion	Ten-minutes post-infusion	Baseline	End of infusion	Ten-minutes post-infusion
ICP	8.2±0.5	12.3±0.7*	8.0±0.7	24.5±2.5	20.0±1.8*	15.6±2.1*
HR	60.0±3.8	112.7±4.9*	87.8±3.9*	80.0±8.3	124.5±12.2*	110.0±11.3*
MAP	75.1±2.3	114.2±4.3*	92.6±4.3*	111.5±2.4	83.2±2.0*	114.7±2.7
CVP	4.8±0.5	8.3±0.3*	6.7±0.6*	6.1±0.3	11.2±0.8*	7.5±0.4*
PAP	13.4±0.3	21.7±0.8*	16.3±0.3*	16.2±0.7	27.7±1.5*	21.0±1.3*
PCWP	6.3±0.3	10.0±0.7*	7.8±0.4*	8.3±0.3	14.0±1.2*	11.0±0.9*
CO	2.0±0.1	5.1±0.2*	2.4±0.1*	2.4±0.1	6.1±0.4*	4.1±0.3*
TPR	2796±84	1674±37*	2806±118	3530±141	966±87*	2213±223*
PVR	266±8	183±10*	279±23	263±23	177±10*	203±21

* $p < 0.05$.

ally inflated with 3 ml of air. Once a 30-minute sustained elevation of ICP was secured, mannitol was infused following the same protocol as in group A dogs. Group C: Consisted of 4 control dogs that received no mannitol despite the inflation of the epidural balloon. Data were analysed using analysis of variance and Dunnett's modified t-test. P values <0.05 were considered significant.

Results

Results are detailed in Table 1. Data are expressed as the mean ± SEM. In group A: Mannitol caused a significant initial rise in ICP, HR, MAP, CVP, PAP, PCWP and CO, in contrast TPR dropped and PVR decreased. In group B dogs: Mannitol caused an immediate decline in ICP and MAP, and a greater drop in TPR and PVR compared to group A. HR, CVP, PAP, PCWP, and CO closely correlated with group A results.

Discussion

Our study has shown an initial rise of ICP in normal dogs given mannitol. In contrast an initial decrease of ICP was seen when mannitol was given to dogs with intracranial hypertension. There were significant hemodynamic changes in these two groups that were similar in most respects. The HR, cardiac filling pressures and CO responded in an equivalent manner. The effects on TPR and MAP however significantly differed between the groups. There was a modest fall of TPR in the normal dogs given mannitol. The group B dogs demonstrated a precipitous fall of TPR in response to mannitol. This reduction in TPR induced by mannitol has been shown to be largely due to histamine release (Findlay et al. 1981). It is therefore not surprising that this vasodilatory action results in a greater decrease of resistance in the already constricted vessels of the dogs with increased ICP. In dogs with no mass lesion, mannitol in addition to its direct cerebral vasodilating properties, augmented plasma volume, increased CO, and raised MAP. A transient increase in cerebral blood flow and volume may have caused the initial rise in ICP. On the other hand, intracranial hypertension eliminates the cerebral vasculature's capacity to autoregulate and any change in MAP is reflected in ICP (Ikeyama et al. 1978). MAP itself is affected by changes in CO and TPR. Knowing that both groups enjoyed a similar rise in CO, there was a greater fall in TPR in group B dogs caused by mannitol. This allowed the MAP to fall rather than to rise and therefore caused the ICP to drop.

In conclusion, our data support the safety of rapid administration of relatively large doses of mannitol in the setting of intracranial hypertension. Furthermore, we suggest that the drug's initial effect derives in large part from hemodynamics.

References

Abou-Madi M, Trop D, Abou-Madi N, Ravussin P (1987) Does a bolus of mannitol initially aggravate intracranial hypertension? A study at various $PaCO_2$ tensions in dogs. Br J Anaesth 59:630–639

Cottrell JE, Robustellio A, Post K, Turndorf H (1977) Furosemide and mannitol-induced changes in intracranial pressure and serum osmolality and electrolytes. Anesthesiology 47:28–30

Findlay SR, Dvorak AM, Kagey-Sobotka A, Lichtenstein LM (1981) Hyperosmolar triggering of histamine release from human basophils. J Clin Invest 67:1604–1613

Ikeyama A, Maeda S, Ito A, Banno K, Nagai H, Furuse M (1978) The analysis of the intracranial pressure by the concept of the driving pressure from the vascular system. Neurochirurgia (Stuttg) 21:43–53

The Effect of Rapid Mannitol Infusion on Cerebral Blood Volume

P.A. Roberts, J.E. Moragne, G. Williams, B. Pendleton, J. Smith, P. Tompkins, and M. Pollay

OUHSC Division of Neurosurgery, P.O.-Box 26307, Oklahoma City, Oklahoma (USA)

Introduction

Mannitol therapy has been well documented to be effective in reducing elevated intracranial pressure (ICP) (Pollay et al. 1983, Wise and Chater 1962). This reduction in ICP is dependent on reversal of the blood/brain osmotic gradient. However, it has been observed that too rapid an infusion rate may give rise to an early transient increase in ICP prior to a subsequent decrease (Ravussin et al. 1986, Roberts et al. 1987). This study was undertaken to evaluate the possible mechanism(s) by which this transient increase in ICP occurs.

Materials and Methods

Adult dogs (20–35 kg) were used for this study. Anesthesia was induced, arterial and venous catheters placed and after intubation, respiration was maintained with mechanical ventilation. A needle placed in the cisterna magna allowed continuous measurement of ICP using a Camino pressure monitor. In some animals a Swan-Ganz catheter was placed in the pulmonary artery for measurement of cardiac output by the thermo-dilution technique. The temporalis musculature was removed bilaterally to the level of the zygomatic arch, and the underlying cranium was devascularized. One group of animals received rapid intravenous infusion of mannitol (1 mg/kg at a rate of 2 ml/kg/min). Another group received an equivalent volume of isotonic saline at the same rate. Cardiac outputs in response to rapid infusions of either mannitol or saline were determined in two additional groups. Red blood cells withdrawn from the animal were labeled with Technicum 99m and infused into the animal. Following a 30 min. equilibration period, changes in cerebral blood volume (CBV) were monitored using an external Na-I detector placed adjacent to the devascularized cranium. Systemic blood samples drawn at 30 min. intervals were used to construct a calibration curve taking into account both radioactive and biological decay. The response at the Na-I detector was recorded and CBV determined using the calibration curve.

Results

In the animal group receiving rapid mannitol infusion mean arterial blood pressure (MBP) briefly decreased and then transiently peaked, stabilizing at a pressure 13% higher than baseline. ICP in this group showed a transient increase at the same time as the increase in MBP. This increase was prior to the anticipated decrease in ICP resulting from mannitol infusion. CBV was also transiently increased during the time of MBP and ICP increase. The saline infused group showed no early decrease or transient peak but an overall increase in MBP of 7% above baseline. This group showed no changes in ICP or CBV. In both mannitol and saline infused groups, cardiac output increased in response to the bolus infusion. These responses occurred in the same time frame and were of similar magnitude (Fig. 1).

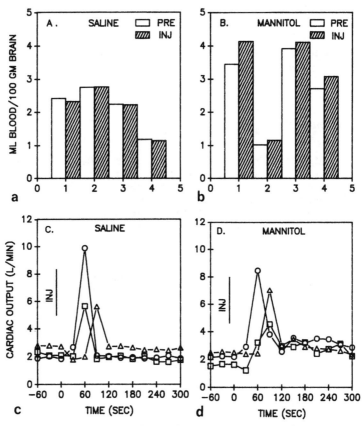

Fig. 1. a, b Cerebral blood volume, saline and mannitol respectively. *Open bar* represents pre-injection volume, *hatched bar* represents post-injection volume, 4 animals in each group. **c, d** Cardiac output, saline and mannitol respectively

Discussion

The rate of infusion of mannitol resulting in the most favorable reversal of the blood/brain osmotic gradient may bring about a transient elevation prior to the expected decrease in ICP (Ravussin et al. 1986, Roberts et al. 1987). Both mannitol and saline caused similar changes in cardiac output. Mannitol caused a brief increase in ICP in association with an increase in CBV while saline infusion caused no change in either ICP or CBV. These observations would imply that an additional mechanism, other than increased cardiac output, must be involved in the resultant elevation in ICP seen with mannitol. It has been shown that hyperosmotic mannitol administration induces vascular dilation (Sasaki et al. 1986). The observations in this study indicate that this is true, particularly regarding the cerebral vasculature, as shown by the observed increase in CBV with mannitol administration. The results of this study show that the transient increase in ICP resulting from rapid mannitol infusion is primarily due to an increase in CBV which is not solely caused by an increase in cardiac output. It is felt that a certain degree of cerebral vasodilatation occurs with the administration of isotonic saline. In clinical situations, although rapid mannitol administration is more effective in establishing the greatest blood/brain osmotic gradient, and hence the most effective lowering of ICP, one should be aware of the potential consequences of too rapid an infusion, which may result in a transient increase in CBV and thus a brief undesirable increase in ICP.

References

Pollay M, Fullenwider C, Roberts PA et al. (1983) Effect of mannitol and furosemide on blood-brain osmotic gradient and intracranial pressure. J Neurosurg 59:945–950
Ravussin P, Archer DP et al. (1986) Effects of rapid mannitol infusion on cerebral blood volume: A positron emission tomographic study in dogs and man. J Neurosurg 64:104–113
Roberts PA, Pollay M et al. (1987) Effect on intracranial pressure of furosemide combined with varying doses and administration rates of mannitol. J Neurosurg 66:440–446
Sasaki T, Kassell NF et al. (1986) The effects of hyperosmolar solutions on cerebral smooth muscle. Stroke 17:1266–1271
Wise BL, Chater N (1962) The value of hypertonic mannitol solution in decreasing brain mass and lowering cerebrospinal-fluid pressure. J Neurosurg 19:1038–1043

A Study of the Concentration of Mannitol for the Treatment of Raised ICP

M. Tanaka, Y. Yoshiyama, R. Kondo, T. Kobayashi, T. Ohwada, F. Tomonaga, and H. Takagi

School of Pharmaceutical Sciences, Kitasato University, Kitasato Emergency Center, Kitasato University Hospital, Department of Neurosurgery, Yamato City Hospital, Kanagawa (Japan)

Introduction

Mannitol is a well known hypertonic agent for the control of raised intracranial pressure (ICP). However, the most effective method of administration of mannitol has not yet been established. In this paper, the authors made 10%, 20%, and 30% of mannitol and set volume and rate of administration of mannitol, in an attempt to clarify the most effective method of mannitol administration to obtain the lowest and the longest reduction of raised ICP.

Materials and Methods

Fifteen adult cats, average weight 3.7 kg, were anesthetised with intraperitoneal administration of pentobarbital (30 mg/kg), intubated and mechanically ventilated with room air using a Harvard respirator. Mean arterial blood pressure (BP) and central venous pressure (CVP) were monitored continuously. Arterial blood gases were examined and $PaCO_2$ was maintained at 30 torr.

The cats were placed on a stereotaxic head holder and bilateral frontal burr holes were opened. Small balloons filled with sterile water were inserted epidullary, one of which was used for elevation of ICP and the other for monitoring ICP. The cisterna magna was cannulated by a 21 gauge needle for measuring cisterna magna pressure as a reference of epidural pressure.

The cats were divided into 3 groups (5 cats in each group), 10%, 20%, 30% mannitol administration groups. The volume and rate of mannitol administration was set at 0.667 ml/kg/min in each group. This made 10%, 20%, 30% mannitol administration equal to 1 g/kg, 2 g/kg, 3 g/kg mannitol with 15 minutes infusion, respectively. In each group, mannitol concentration (mg/ml), serum osmolality (mOsm/kg), Glucose (mg/dl), BUN (mg/dl), Creatinine (mg/dl), Na (mEq/L), K (mEq/L), Cl (mEq/L) were sequentially (every 5 min) examined for 120 min.

Intracranial Pressure VII
Eds.: J. T. Hoff and A. L. Betz
© Springer-Verlag Berlin Heidelberg 1989

Results

ICP Changes

The initial ICP was raised to 20 mm Hg by inflating the epidural balloon. In group 1 (10% mannitol administration), ICP slowly decreased and reached a minimum at 17 min after beginning mannitol infusion. The rate of ICP reduction was 37%. Then, the ICP gradually elevated and reached the initial ICP level 37 min later. The ICP continued to increase and reached twice the initial ICP 120 min later. In group 2 (20% mannitol administration), the ICP rapidly decreased and reached a minimum 23 min. later. The rate of ICP reduction was 64%. Then, the ICP gradually elevated and reached the initial ICP 100 min later. In group 3 (30% mannitol administration), the ICP more rapidly decreased and reached a minimum 39 min later. The rate of ICP reduction was 70%. Then, the ICP slowly elevated, but remained lower than initial ICP over 120 min. (Fig. 1).

Mannitol Concentration

In each group, the concentration of mannitol was rapidly elevated during mannitol administration and reached maximums of 5.3 mg/ml, 11.2 mg/ml, 18.7 mg/ml in groups 1, 2, and 3, respectively at the time of termination of mannitol administration. Then, it gradually decreased in an exponential curve, reaching 0.35 mg/ml, 1.59 mg/ml, 4.71 mg/ml in groups 1, 2, and 3, respectively (Fig. 2).

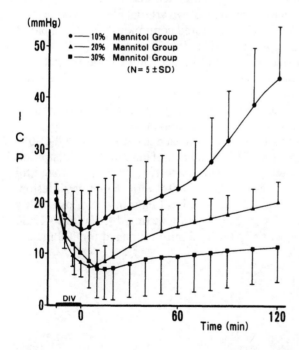

Fig. 1. Time course of ICP after the administration of 10%, 20%, 30% of mannitol at a rate of 0.667 ml/kg/min, DIV: duration of mannitol infusion

470

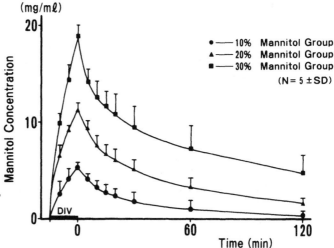

Fig. 2. Time course of mannitol concentration, DIV: duration of mannitol infusion

Serum Osmolality

Effective serum osmolality was calculated by subtracting the calculated osmolality from actual serum osmolality, which reflected the effect of mannitol itself. In each group, it reached a maximum at the end of mannitol administration, 20 mOsm/kg, 47 mOsm/kg, 79 mOsm/kg groups 1, 2, and 3, respectively, then gradually decreased in an exponential curve like the mannitol concentration curve (Fig. 3). The correlation coefficients with mannitol were 0.8942, 0.9748, 0.9758 in groups 1, 2, and 3, respectively.

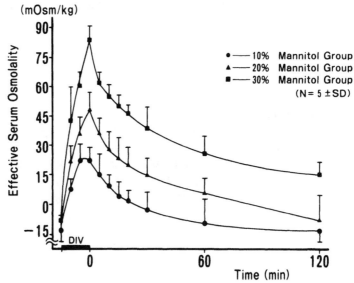

Fig. 3. Time course of effective serum osmolality effective serum osmolality = actual serum osmolality − {1.86 Na (mEq/L) + glucose (mg/dl)/18 + BUN (mg/dl)/2.8}, DIV: duration of mannitol infusion

Discussion

In this experiment, the rate of infusion volume of mannitol was set at 0.667 ml/kg/min., the infusion time was set at 15 min. and only concentration (g/ml) was varied. Consequently only the effect of mannitol concentration on reduction of raised ICP needed to be examined.

Results showed that ICP reduction potential depended on osmotic gradient, which was created at the end of mannitol infusion. The higher the mannitol concentration was, the more profound and prolonged the ICP reduction observed. This finding supported the report of Roberts (1987), that a greater decrease in ICP occurred followed more rapid mannitol administration. Marshall (1978) reported even 0.25 g/kg 25% mannitol, given at the rate of 20 ml/min (5 g/kg), was sufficient to show an ICP reduction.

However, group 1 (10% mannitol administration), that is 1 g/kg of mannitol administration in 15 min., showed a marked rebound phenomenon. The difference lay in the difference of volume/kg/minute, the administered volume was twice as large in this experiment.

The speed of mannitol infusion (ml/min. or g/min.) as well as the total dosage or volume used are the great factors in achieving an effective osmotic gradient for reduction of raised ICP, Shenkin (1962).

Group 2 (20% mannitol administration) showed sufficient reduction of ICP for 100 min without disturbing vital signs, serum electrolytes or other parameters. However, in group 3 (30% mannitol administration), although a profound and prolonged ICP reduction was observed, transient but significant lowering of BP and a decrease of urinary output were noticed in 2 cases out of 5. This finding indicates that a high concentration of mannitol may induce an abrupt shift of water into circulation and may cause cardiac and renal dysfunction.

Summary

The authors conclude that the greater the concentration of mannitol administered, the higher the effective osmolality developed. In addition, greater concentration of mannitol, causes more profound and prolonged ICP reduction. However, the total volume and the rate of mannitol administration have great influence on the effectiveness of ICP reduction and the maintenance of circulation and renal function. In clinical practice, a small dose of 20% mannitol is recommended, administered in a bolus or at least within 15 min. for the control of raised ICP.

References

Marshall LF, Smith RW, Rausher LA, Shapiro HM (1978) Mannitol dose requirements in brain-injured patients. J Neurosurg 48:169–172

Roberts PA, Pollay M, Engles C, Pendleton B, Reynolds E, Stevens FL (1987) Effect on intracranial pressure of furosemide combined with various doses and administration rates of mannitol. J Neurosurg 66:440–446

Shenkin HA, Goluboff B, Haft H (1962) The use of mannitol for the reduction of intracranial pressure in intracranial surgery. J Neurosurg 19:897–901

Paired Comparison of Hypnotic and Osmotic Therapy in the Reduction of Intracranial Hypertension After Severe Head Injury

N.M. Dearden and J.D. Miller

Department of Clinical Neurosciences, Western General Hospital, University of Edinburgh (UK)

Introduction

Enthusiasm for barbiturate therapy to control post-traumatic intracranial hypertension has been curbed by the failure of two controlled studies to show benefit over mannitol therapy (Schwartz et al. 1984, Ward et al. 1985). Situations may exist however, in which barbiturate therapy proves superior to other treatments for raised intracranial pressure (ICP).

After severe head injury cerebral metabolism is reduced in the absence of seizure activity or hyperthermia. Two patient groups may be identified from measurement of the difference in oxygen content between arterial and jugular bulb venous blood ($ajdO_2$). In the first group cerebral blood flow (CBF) and metabolism remain coupled with a reduction in CBF and normal $ajdO_2$ (commonly seen after focal brain injury with mass lesion formation). Elective hyperventilation of such patients may result in global ischaemia ($ajdO_2 > 9$ mls O_2 per 100 mls). In the second group deranged autoregulation is associated with relative or absolute hyperaemia and a low $ajdO_2$ (< 4 mls O_2 per 100 mls blood); this is often seen after diffuse brain injury (Obrist et al. 1984).

Experimental barbiturate therapy is more effective at reducing ICP while preserving cerebral perfusion pressure (CPP) when ICP elevation is associated with cerebral hyperaemia, than when the cause is a mass lesion. In the latter case CPP is reduced by barbiturate therapy with a risk of cerebral ischaemia (Bricolo and Glick 1981).

Hypnotic agents appear to have greater efficacy for reduction of ICP when cerebrovascular reactivity to carbon dioxide is preserved (Messeter et al. 1986, Nordstrom et al. 1988).

Mannitol given experimentally induces compensatory cerebral vasoconstriction in response to changes in blood viscosity (Muizelaar et al. 1983). In human head injury the efficacy of bolus dose mannitol at reducing raised ICP is significantly greater when pressure autoregulation is preserved (Muizelaar et al. 1984) and where pretreatment CPP is below 70 mm Hg (Rosner and Coley 1987). The efficacy of mannitol may be enhanced by concomitant administration of loop diuretics (Pollay et al. 1983).

Methods

This continuing study compares the magnitude and duration of reduction of ICP and preservation of CPP following paired hypnotic and mannitol therapy after severe head injury.

A group of 17 head injured patients were managed according to a standard regime including artificial ventilation with sedation using phenoperidine and paralysis with pancuronium. Ventilator adjustments were standardised with respect to inspiration, pause, expiration ratio (25/10/65 percent respectively), respiratory rate and peak inflation pressure to provide standard conditions in which it was possible to analyse ICP waveform. This was done using the ratio of height of ICP trace attributable to arterial pulsation divided by amplitude of the ICP due to respiration, the P/R ratio. PaO_2 was maintained above 16 kPa and $paCO_2$ between 3.0–4 kPa in adults (3.0–3.5 kPa in children). In all patients ICP (subdural catheter with or without Camino catheter), CVP (subclavian line), BP (radial artery), brain electrical activity by Cerebral Function Monitor (CFM) and arterial and jugular venous bulb blood samples were measured. (Jugular blood samples were obtained from a catheter advanced in retrograde manner via the R internal jugular vein to the jugular bulb after radiological verification of the catheter tip position.) If ICP rose above 25 mm Hg during the first 24 hours post injury or 30 mm Hg thereafter, *once remediable causes were excluded,* patients were given thiopentone 5 mg per kg over 5 min via a central venous line. Subsequent rises in ICP were treated with gamma hydroxybutyrate 60 mg per kg iv over 10 min or mannitol 0.5 g per kg iv over 15 min. Paired arterial and jugular bulb gases were measured before each therapy and at the point of maximum reduction of ICP. ICP, BP, CVP and CFM were recorded continuously during the study. The time from the end of drug administration to the time of maximum reduction of ICP and the time for ICP to return to treatment threshold levels (duration of action) was recorded. CPP was documented before treatment and at the point of maximum reduction of ICP. Intracranial pathology was classified as focal (haematoma and/or unilateral contusion or swelling) or diffuse injury.

Results

Based on the response of ICP, CPP and duration of action of each treatment 4 response groups were identified from the 17 patients studied. One agent was considered superior if ICP was reduced below 20 mm Hg with preservation or improvement of CPP by that agent only. In each response group the pretreatment values of $ajdO_2$, CPP, CFM lower border voltage and P/R ratio of the ICP waveform together with intracranial pathology were recorded in an effort to identify predictive factors favouring either hypnotic (thiopentone or gamma hydroxybutyrate) or mannitol treatment (Table 1).

In 2 patients mannitol therapy was superior. Pretreatment CPP was below 60 mm Hg in one patient (JM, Table 2). Mannitol reduced ICP and elevated CPP above 60 mm Hg in both patients. The times to maximum reduction of ICP from the end of infusion of mannitol were 10 min and 17 min and the durations of reduction of ICP below the treatment threshold were correspondingly 57 and 76 min. In both patients pretreatment ajdO$_2$ levels were within normal limits (4−9 vol%) and remained so after mannitol. Hypnotic therapy failed to reduce ICP or improve CPP. After hypnotic therapy ajdO$_2$ values were ischaemic (>9 vol%) in both patients. The CFM lower border voltage was 3−4 µV before treatment, compared to a "normal" range of 6−12 µV. Pretreatment P/R ratio of the ICP waveform was 0.50 and 0.61 and below the 95% confidence limits of 0.8−1.4 (Table 2).

In 3 patients, all of whom had suffered diffuse cerebral swelling associated with multiple intracerebral contusions, hypnotic therapy proved superior to mannitol. Patient DG had sustained elevation of ICP while the other 2 (WG and CG) had plateau waves (Table 2). Prior to therapy CPP was below 60 mm Hg in all patients. Hypnotics reduced ICP and improved CPP above 60 mm Hg in all 3 patients whereas in the same cases mannitol failed to reduce ICP below threshold treatment values. The time to maximum reduction of ICP with hypnotic was 37 min in patient DG and 6 min in the other 2. After hypnotic therapy the durations of reduction of ICP were 67 min in patient DG, 42 min in patient WG and 29 min in patient CG. Pretreatment ajdO$_2$ was low in patient DG, normal in patient WG and ischaemic in patient CG. After hypnotic therapy ajdO$_2$ was unchanged in patient DG and with normal limits in the other 2. In contrast ajdO$_2$

Table 1. Details of patients in study

Response to therapy	Patient initials	Age	Day of pathology		Admission Glasgow Coma Score				Glasgow Outcome Score 6 months post injury
			study	focal diffuse	E	M	V	Total	
Mannitol superior	GM	24	2	F	1	2	1	4	Moderately disabled
	(JM)	14	5	F	1	2	1	4	dead
Hypnotic superior	DG	10	4	D	3	1	1	5	Moderately disabled
	CG	3	1	D	1	4	2	7	Moderately disabled
	WG	25	3	D	2	3	1	6	Good recovery
Agents similar	(JM)	14	3	F	1	2	1	4	Dead
	CS	8	2	F	1	4	2	7	Good recovery
	HW	22	3	F	1	5	1	7	Good recovery
	HM	54	3	F	2	3	2	7	Dead
	JR	41	2	F	1	3	2	6	Severely disabled
	KL	21	1	F	3	5	1	9	Moderately disabled
	JB	31	3	F	1	2	2	5	Severely disabled
	GM	44	2	F	4	5	2	11	Dead
	DM	17	2	F	1	2	1	4	Dead
Neither effective	CG	62	4	F	1	3	1	5	Dead
	FS	43	1	D	1	1	1	3	Dead
	LP	24	2	F	1	2	1	4	Dead

( )=Same patient

values were unchanged by mannitol. Pretreatment lower border CFM voltage was between 8 and 9 μV and the P/R ratio was high (2.1–5.7) in all patients before therapy (Table 2).

In 9 patients, all of whom had suffered focal brain injury, both methods of treatment appeared to have similar efficacy. CPP was below 60 mm Hg in 5 patients before hypnotic and in 7 patients before mannitol treatment. After hypnotic therapy CPP rose above 60 mm Hg in 3 and fell below 60 mm Hg in 4 patients. Mannitol raised CPP above 60 mm Hg in 4 patients. Overall hypnotic raised CPP in 5 patients and mannitol in 8 patients. The time to maximum reduction of ICP was 18 min (range 4.5–26 min) with hypnotic therapy and 23.7 (range 1–55 min) afer mannitol. Durations of ICP reduction were 31.8 min (range 1–104 min) and 58.9 min (range 14–116 min) respectively. Prior to therapy $ajdO_2$ was normal in all patients and remained so in 8 patients after either therapy. In patient GM $ajdO_2$ was ischaemic after hypnotic while in patient CS it was hyperaemic after mannitol (Table 2). Pretreatment CFM lower border voltage was 4–7 μV and the P/R ratio was low in 1 normal in 6 and high in 2 patients before therapy.

In 3 patients neither therapy reduced ICP or elevated CPP above 60 mm Hg. Pretreatment $ajdO_2$ was normal in 2 patients and ischaemic in the third, in whom ICP elevation was associated with a Cushing response. These values were unchanged by either treatment. Pretreatment CFM lower border voltage was 2.4–4.0 μV while the P/R ratio was low (0.6) in 1 patient and high in 2 patients (2 and 6) (Table 2).

The data of the 14 responsive patients was analysed to establish any relationship between the ICP or CPP response and pretreatment values of $ajdO_2$, CFM voltage and P/R ratio in either treatment group. There was significant correlation between the percentage ICP change from pretreatment value and the CFM lower border voltage but in opposite directions in both groups (hypnotic $r = -.833$, $p < 0.001$, mannitol $r = .614$, $0.02 > p > 0.01$). The change in CPP correlated with pretreatment CFM lower border voltage after hypnotic ($r = .657$, $0.01 > p > 0.001$) but not after mannitol. The duration of reduction of ICP did not correlate with CFM lower border voltage prior to treatment with hypnotic but did with mannitol ($r = -.675$, $0.01 > p > 0.001$). There was no correlation between the percentage change in ICP or the change in CPP and pretreatment $ajdO_2$. In contrast pretreatment P/R ratio correlated with the percentage change of pretreatment ICP before hypnotic ($r = -.638$, $0.01 > p > 0.001$) but just failed to each significance with mannitol ($r = .462$). There was no correlation between the duration of ICP reduction, the percentage change in ICP or the change in CPP and the pretreatment CPP in either group.

Discussion

The results of this study endorse the case for considering selective therapy for raised ICP after head injury. The 17 patients studied represent only 9% of the severely head injured patients treated with artificial ventilation and ICP monitor-

Table 2. Paired comparisons of hypnotic and mannitol therapy

Response to therapy	Patient initials		ICP mm Hg		CPP mm Hg		CFM and Volts pretreatment	P/R ratio pretreatment	AJDO$_2$ mls O$_2$/100 mls blood	
			Pretreatment	Posttreatment	Pretreatment	Posttreatment			Pretreatment	Posttreatment
Mannitol superior	GM	hypnotic	41	34	64	63	4	0.5	5.93	9.09**
		mannitol	36	18	77	97	4	0.55	5.76	4.73
	(JM)	hypnotic	42	37	41	43	3	0.61	7.21	10.11**
		mannitol	44	19	57	77	2	0.69	7.57	4.77
Hypnotic superior	DG	hypnotic	45	20	47	65	9	2.1	0.90*	0.57*
		mannitol	47	42	54	61	7	1.7	0.87*	0.55*
	CG	hypnotic	33	7	44	67	9	5.7	13.20**	8.88
		mannitol	40	33	39	49	9	4.7	13.69**	13.02**
	WG	hypnotic	50	16	49	73	8	2.4	7.24	6.63
		mannitol	47	26	59	77	8	2.3	6.28	5.76
Agents similar	(JM)	hypnotic	35	28	60	58	4	1.25	5.21	6.23
		mannitol	40	26	56	84	4	1.25	5.00	4.12
	CS	hypnotic	26	12	41	50	5	1.3	8.23	5.38
		mannitol	28	19	42	54	7	1.0	6.24	3.62*
	HW	hypnotic	34	20	58	69	6	1.1	6.36	6.13
		mannitol	37	22	54	72	6	0.97	6.59	4.48
	HM	hypnotic	39	22	54	64	7	1.0	6.82	6.55
		mannitol	44	24	44	66	6	0.86	6.14	5.04
	JR	hypnotic	30	19	56	47	5	1.78	5.18	6.29
		mannitol	32	27	51	48	2	1.75	5.07	4.83
	KL	hypnotic	25	16	45	46	5	1.0	7.98	8.62
		mannitol	27	17	51	60	5	1.75	6.50	6.24
	JB	hypnotic	29	18	63	49	5	2.3	4.13	4.11
		mannitol	28	19	65	72	4	1.3	5.07	5.23

GM	hypnotic	62	27	60	55	5	0.57	8.04	11.20**
	mannitol	54	29	56	82	4	0.6	8.83	6.07
DM	hypnotic	32	19	76	96	6	1.09	6.04	6.33
	mannitol	35	27	68	81	5.5	0.51	5.39	5.63
Neither effective									
CG	hypnotic	59	33	56	47	2.5	6.0	6.11	5.37
	mannitol	60	33	50	59	2.5	7.0	5.40	5.16
FS	hypnotic	82	83	58	55	4	0.6	17.36**	17.26**
	mannitol	84	73	58	56	4	0.6	13.28**	13.89**
LP	hypnotic	54	48	37	46	2	2.4	6.14	4.62
	mannitol	59	44	41	57	2	2.4	4.80	4.00

( ) Same patient; * Hyperaemic values; ** Ischaemic values

ing over a two and a half year period. Although ICP was raised in over 40% of these patients at some stage during intensive care, in the majority of cases alleviation of a simple primary cause was the mainstay of management. Thereafter most patients were responsive to hyperventilation further reducing paCO$_2$ by 0.5 kPa. The patients in this study therefore represent a select group in whom these measures had proved inadequate to control ICP.

Thirteen patients had focal head injury and 4 diffuse head injury. Of the patients responsive to treatment, 11 had focal and 3 diffuse brain injury. Although 2 of the patients with focal head injury subsequently developed bilateral cerebral swelling in all 11 patients mannitol was the preferred agent. Hypnotic proved superior in the 3 patients with diffuse injury.

After the study, further therapy to reduce ICP in the 14 responsive patients was selected by analysis of the effects of either treatment on ICP and CPP. In 11 patients mannitol was selected while in the other 3 hypnotic infusion was preferred.

The correlation between CFM lower border voltage and ICP response to hypnotics endorses the results of Bingham et al. 1985. However, this study also reports a negative correlation between CFM lower border voltage and the efficacy of mannitol. These results suggest that unless the CFM lower border voltage exceeds 4–5 µV mannitol should be considered the agent of choice for reduction of ICP.

The significant correlation between P/R ratio and ICP response to hypnotic endorses the view that ICP waveform analysis may be a useful guide to selection of ICP reduction in therapy.

There was no correlation between the absolute or percentage change in ICP, the change in CPP or the duration of ICP reduction with the pretreatment CPP after mannitol. These results do not therefore support the conclusions of Rosner and Coley 1987 that mannitol is most effective at reducing ICP when pretreatment CPP is low.

Conclusions

1. ICP reduction therapy must be more selective.
2. In the majority of head injured patients with raised ICP a simple remediable cause is present. This must be detected and eliminated prior to instituting more aggressive measures.
3. If ICP remains high, if the P/R ratio is above 1.5, and if the CFM lower border voltage exceeds 5 µV then hypnotic therapy should be tried, taking appropriate measures to avoid hypovolaemia and arterial hypotension, and continued if ICP is reduced while CPP is preserved or elevated above 60 mm Hg.
4. In other cases of raised ICP resistant to simple measures, however, mannitol will prove more effective and safer to use, in particular when P/R ratio is below 0.8, CFM border is lower than 4 µV and the cause of elevated ICP is related to focal brain injury or swelling.

References

Bingham RM, Procaccio F, Prior PF, Hinds CJ (1985) Cerebral electrical activity influences the effects of etomidate on cerebral perfusion pressure in traumatic coma. Br J Anaesth 57:843–848

Bricolo AP, Glick RP (1981) Barbiturate effects on acute experimental intracranial hypertension. J Neurosurg 55:397–406

Messeter K, Nordstrom C-H, Sundbarg G et al. (1986) Cerebral hemodynamics in patients with acute severe head trauma. J Neurosurg 64:231–237

Muizelaar JP, Wei EP, Kontos HA, Becker DP (1983) Mannitol causes compensatory cerebral vasoconstriction and vasodilatation in response to blood viscosity changes. J Neurosurg 59:822–828

Muizelaar JP, Lutz HA, Becker DP (1984) Effect of mannitol on ICP and CBF and correlation with pressure autoregulation in severely head injured patients. J Neurosurg 61:700–706

Nordstrom C-H, Messeter K, Sundbarg G et al. (1988) Cerebral blood flow, vasoreactivity, and oxygen consumption during barbiturate therapy in severe traumatic brain lesions. J Neurosurg 68:424–431

Obrist WD, Langfitt TW, Jaggi JL et al. (1984) Cerebral blood flow and metabolism in comatose patients with acute head injury. (Relationship to intracranial hypertension.) J Neurosurg 61:241–253

Pollay M, Fullenwider C, Roberts A, Stevens FA (1983) The effect of mannitol and furosemide on blood-brain osmotic gradient and intracranial pressure. J Neurosurg 59:945–950

Rosner MJ, Coley I (1987) Cerebral perfusion pressure: A hemodynamic mechanism of mannitol and the post mannitol hemogram. Neurosurgery 21 (2):147–156

Schwartz ML, Tator CH, Rowed RW et al. (1984) The University of Toronto head injury treatment study: A prospective, randomised comparison of pentobarbital and mannitol. Can J Neurol Sci 11:434–440

Ward JD, Becker DP, Miller JD et al. (1985) Failure of prophylactic barbiturate coma in the treatment of severe head injury. J Neurosurg 62:283–388

The Level of ICP Modifies the CSF Pressure Response to Changes in MAP and CVP After Mannitol

P. Ravussin[1], M. Abou-Madi[3], D. Archer[3], R. Chiolero[1], D. Trop[3], J. Freeman[1], and N. deTribolet[2]

Departments of Anesthesia[1] and Neurosurgery[2], Centre Hospitalier Universitaire Vaudois, University of Lausanne, 1011 Lausanne (Switzerland), and Department of Anesthesia[3], Montreal Neurological Institute, McGill University, Montreal, Quebec H3A 2B4 (Canada)

Introduction

Transient rises in cerebro-spinal fluid pressure (CSFP) and cerebral blood volume (CBV) occur after mannitol infusion in patients with brain tumors and normal CSFP (Cottrell et al. 1977). This increase could be detrimental in patients with an already elevated CSFP. The effect of mannitol on CSFP was therefore studied in two populations of patients with similar intracranial pathology, those with a normal CSFP and those with an elevated CSFP.

Material and Methods

With institutional approval and informed consent, 49 consecutive, adult, ASA grade 3 patients scheduled for intracranial surgery, tumor resection (36) and aneurysm clipping (13), were studied. No patient had any pathology judged likely to obstruct the CSF pathways between the intracranial and lumbar spaces, and so lumbar CSFP was considerd to accurately reflect ICP. After induction with midazolam (0.1–0.4 mg/kg), fentanyl (2–6 µg/kg), and pancuronium (0.1 mg/kg), anesthesia was maintained with midazolam 0.1–0.3 mg/kg/h and N_2O 66% in O_2 with increments of fentanyl and pancuronium. Slight hypocarbia was maintained ($PaCO_2$ 32–36 mm Hg). Lumbar CSFP, through a 20 G malleable spinal needle, mean arterial pressure (MAP), and central venous pressure (CVP) were recorded on a two-channel Model 78342 A Hewlett-Packard System (Hewlett-Packard Inc., Palo Alto, California, USA) before (baseline, T_0), and 2, 5, 10, 20 and 45 min after the beginning of a rapid infusion of 20% mannitol (1 g/kg) infused over a 10 min period. Prior to mannitol infusion, patients were assigned to two groups: Group I with a baseline CSFP$\leq$15 mm Hg ($n=24$, 47.4$\pm$2.4 yrs and 65.7$\pm$2.6 kg) and Group II with a baseline CSFP$>$15 mm Hg ($n=25$, 57.3$\pm$2.7 yrs and 66.7$\pm$2.3 kg). Mean values $\pm$ SEM are reported. Student's paired t-test was used to compare data between groups; $p<0.05$ was considered significant.

Intracranial Pressure VII
Eds.: J. T. Hoff and A. L. Betz
© Springer-Verlag Berlin Heidelberg 1989

Results

There was no significant difference in the demographic data or baseline cardio-vascular values between the two groups except for age. Table 1 summarises our results. Mean baseline CSFP values were 10.5 ± 0.53 mm Hg in Group I and 20.8 ± 1.1 in Group II. During the infusion of mannitol, CSFP increased significantly in Group I up to a maximal increase of 29% at 5 min, whereas it decreased rapidly and immediately in Group II. CSFP values between groups were significantly different 2 and 5 min after mannitol had been started. In both groups MAP fell 7% ($p < 0.05$) and CVP increased 10% and 88% respectively (NS between groups).

Discussion

This study confirms in humans what has recently been demonstrated in a canine model of intracranial hypertension (Abou-Madi et al. 1987): although mannitol is a vasodilator (Coté et al. 1979) and may cause an increase in CBV directly and/or indirectly (autoregulation mediated) (Ravussin et al. 1986), it can be used safely to promote brain dehydration in patients with raised CSFP. One explanation for the early opposing effect of mannitol on CSFP seen in Groups I and II with similar hemodynamic responses may be found by analysing the concept of transmission of arterial and venous pressures to CSFP (Ikeyama et al. 1978) in which "n" represents the transmission rate of MAP and CVP to CSFP and is defined by equation (1):

$$n = CSFP - CVP/MAP - CVP \qquad (1)$$

The effects on CSFP of rapid changes of MAP and CVP between baseline (T_0) and x min (T_x) after the beginning of mannitol infusion can thus be estimated using equation (2):

$$\delta CSFP_{T_0 - T_x} = n_{T_0} \cdot (MAP_{T_0} - MAP_{T_x}) + (1 - n_{T_0}) \cdot (CVP_{T_0} - CVP_{T_x}) \qquad (2)$$

where $\delta CSFP_{T_0 - T_x}$ is the change in CSFP between T_0 and T_x due solely to the MAP and CVP changes between T_0 and T_x. From equation (1), if CSFP is close to CVP, "n" is very small and $(1 - n)$ approximates 1. Therefore, as in Group I, an increase in CVP will transiently increase CSFP, thus counteracting the osmotic brain dehydrating effect of mannitol, whereas the concomitant decrease in MAP will have little repercussion on CSFP. However, if CSFP is increased as in Group II, "n" increases and therefore a decrease in MAP will accentuate the rapid dehydrating effect of mannitol and further decrease CSFP whereas the concomitant increase in CVP will have relatively less effect on CSFP; "n" = 1 at the limit of extreme intracranial hypertension (CSFP = MAP). Thus in Groups I and II we can correct the observed CSFP at T_x for the hemodynamically related changes in MAP and CVP which occurred between T_0 and T_x by substracting $\delta CSFP_{T_0 - T_x}$ from $CSFP_{T_x}$ and thus obtaining the corrected $CSFP_{T_x}$ ($CSFP_{T_x}$, Table 1), which is the value of CSFP at T_x if vascular pressures had not changed.

Table 1. Effect of rapid infusion of mannitol (1 g/kg over 10 min) on CSFP, MAP, and CVP and values of n** and CSFPc*** in groups I and II ($\bar{x} \pm$ SEM)

Parameters	Groups	Baseline (T_0)	2 min	5 min	10 min	20 min	45 min
			after the beginning of mannitol infusion				
CSFP	Group I	+10.5±0.53	+12.8±0.67*	+13.5±0.78*	12.5±0.99*	9.5±0.67*	7.5±0.56*
	Group II	+20.8±1.1	+18.6±0.89*	16.5±0.82*	14.4±0.80*	11.1±0.82*	9.0±0.63*
CSFPc	Group I	+10.5±0.53	+10.9±0.6	+12.2±0.9*	11.9±0.9	10.3±0.7	8.4±0.6*
	Group II	+20.8±1.1	+18.4±1.0*	+15.5±1.0*	12.5±0.8*	12.0±0.8*	9.5±0.6*
MAP	Group I	89±2.8	83±2.6*	84±3.5*	91±3.5	92±3.3	92±3.3
	Group II	90±2.7	84±2.6*	85±2.8*	89±3.0	92±2.7	95±2.8*
CVP	Group I	3.9±0.53	6.6±52*	7.8±0.6*	8.2±0.73*	6.6±0.66*	4.7±0.63
	Group II	5.1±0.78	6.9±0.76*	7.9±0.72*	9.6±0.76*	7.4±0.72*	5.5±0.78
n**	Group I	+0.081±0.009	+0.083±0.009	+0.076±0.013	0.055±0.013*	0.034±0.008*	0.032±0.007*
	Group II	+0.185±0.015	+0.155±0.014*	+0.113±0.013*	0.06 ±0.01*	0.043±0.008*	0.04 ±0.007*

* = significant at $p < 0.05$ within groups I and II, + = significant at $p < 0.05$ between groups I and II;

** n = transmission rate of arterial and venous pressures to CSFP (see text for explanation);

*** CSFPc = corrected CSFP using "n" (see text for explanation).

In conclusion, mannitol can be given safely to patients with raised CSFP. Analysis of the vascular driving pressures (MAP and CVP) which contribute to CSFP suggests that the early opposing effect of mannitol on CSFP seen in Groups I and II may be due partly to the intracranial hypertension itself.

References

Abou-Madi M, Trop D, Abou-Madi N, Ravussin P (1987) Does a bolus of mannitol initially aggravate intracranial hypertension? A study at various PaCO$_2$ tensions in dogs. Br J Anaesth 59:630–639

Coté CJ, Greenhow DE, Marshall BE (1979) The hypotensive response to rapid intravenous administration of hypertonic solutions in man and in the rabbit. Anesthesiology 50:30–35

Cottrell JE, Robustelli A, Post K, Turndorf H (1977) Furosemide- and mannitol-induced changes in intracranial pressure and serum osmolality and electrolytes. Anesthesiology 47:28–30

Ikeyama A, Maeda S, Ito A, Banno K, Nagai H, Furuse M (1978) The analysis of the intracranial pressure by the concept of the driving pressure from the vascular system. Neurochirurgia (Stuttg) 21:43–53

Ravussin P, Archer DP, Tyler JL, Meyer E, Abou-Madi M, Diksic M, Yamamoto L, Trop D (1986) Effects of rapid mannitol infusion on cerebral blood volume. A positron emission tomographic study in dogs and man. J Neurosurg 64:104–113

Lidocaine Can Reduce Intracranial Pressure Associated with Intracranial Space-Occupying Lesions

E. Arbit, G.R. DiResta, M. Khayata, N. Lau, and J.H. Galicich

Neurosurgical Research Laboratory, Department of Surgery, Memorial Sloan-Kettering Cancer Center, Cornell University Medical College, New York City, New York 10021 (USA)

Introduction

Recent reports indicate that lidocaine hydrochloride may attenuate surges in intracranial pressure (ICP) produced experimentally by air embolism and clinically resulting from surgical stimulation during craniotomy or endotracheal suctioning and intubation. This study was undertaken to examine the role of lidocaine hydrochloride in reducing raised intracranial pressure produced by an intracranial space-occupying lesion. Our results indicate that intracranial pressure (ICP) is reduced consistently by an average of 26% with a concomitant increase in cerebral perfusion pressure of 13%.

Methods and Results

Fifteen adult male Sprague-Dawley rats with an average weight of 367 grams were studied. Anesthesia was induced with halothane/oxygen mixture and maintained with alphachlorolose 30–40 mg/kg. The two femoral arteries, one vein, and the trachea were cannulated with polyethylene tubes. The animals were mounted in a stereotactic head holder (KOPF), connected to a rodent respirator (Harvard Apparatus), and paralyzed with pancurarium bromide (0.1 mg/kg initially and then with 0.05 mg/kg hourly). Three cranial openings were made in the left frontal, right frontal, and left parietal areas. An ICP probe (Camino, San Diego, California, USA) was inserted into the subdural space in the left parietal region and laser-Doppler flowmetry (LDF) probe (T.S.I., Inc., St. Paul, Minnesota, USA) was placed on the frontal cortex for a continuous cerebral blood flow measurement. A catheter with a balloon attached to its tip (Pediatric Swan-Ganz) was introduced into the epidural space at the right parietal site. All cranial openings were sealed with dental cement. Blood pressure, heart rate, temperature, intracranial pressure, and cerebral blood flow were continuously recorded on a multichannel recorder (Grass, Quincy, Mass.) and arterial blood gases were monitored (Corning, Medfield, Mass.) at frequent intervals. The animals were kept hyperoxemic, normocapneic, and normothermic throughout the experiments. After initial preparation the animals were left undisturbed for 30 min at which point their intracranial pressure was 10 ± 1.1 mm Hg. The intracranial

Eds.: J. T. Hoff and A. L. Betz

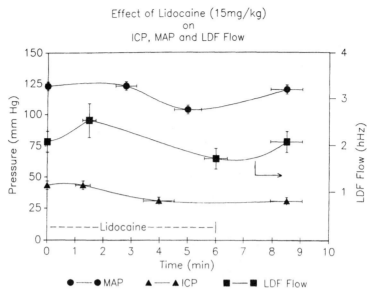

Fig. 1. Histogram showing the relation between mean arterial blood pressure (*MAP*), intracranial pressure (*ICP*), cerebral perfusion pressure (*CPP*), and cerebral blood flow measured by laser Doppler flowmetry (*LDF*), before and after lidocaine infusion

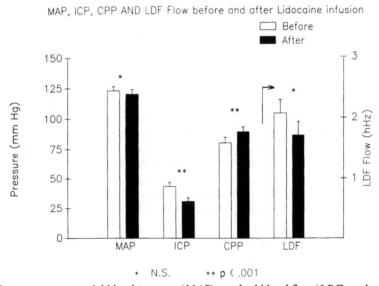

Fig. 2. Relation between mean arterial blood pressure (*MAP*), cerebral blood flow (*LDF*), and intracranial pressure (*ICP*), relative to time of lidocaine infusion. Note that during LH infusion MAP and CBF dropped but returned to baseline by about 9 min, while ICP continued to be reduced (up to 2 hours, not shown)

pressure was then gradually increased by inflating the epidural balloon (infusion pump) with saline at a rate of 0.1 ml/min. The preparation was allowed to stabilize at a mean of 47.5 ± 5.65 mm Hg, a pressure increment found to be devoid of cardiovascular changes. Lidocaine was then administered intravenously at a rate of 0.015 ml/min to a total dose of 15 mg/kg. The animals were monitored for at least two hours after termination of LH infusion. As control, five animals received normal saline at the same infusion rate to an equivalent volume as the lidocaine, and only after a period of 30 min lidocaine was administered.

The mean resting arterial pressure (MAP) was 129.1 ± 3.73 mm Hg. During LH infusion, MAP dropped to 100.0 ± 4.00 mm Hg and five minutes after infusion, it stabilized at 127.3 ± 4.00 mm Hg, a mean net drop of 1.8 ± 1.43 mm Hg ($2.9 + 0.6\%$). Figure 1: arterial blood gases during the experiment were as follows: $pCO_2 = 36.5 \pm 1.6$, $paO_2 = 331.1 \pm 33.4$, and $pH = 7.42 \pm 0.019$. Heart rate and temperature were unaffected. The resting ICP prior to balloon inflation was 10.0 ± 1.1 mm Hg, and after inflation it was 47.5 ± 5.65 mm Hg. Following LH infusion, ICP consistently decreased by $25.7\% \pm 3.95$ ($p < 0.001$). ICP after saline infusion (controls) remained unaffected.

Cerebral blood flow, as measured by LDF was 1.92 ± 0.56 hectaherz (hHz) pre-infusion, and 1.6 ± 0.56 hHz during infusion, a decrease of 17% ($p < 0.001$) and quickly (within minutes) returned to baseline when infusion was complete. Figure 2: cerebral perfusion pressure, as calculated by the standard formula ($CPP = MAP - ICP$), was 81.6 ± 6.74 preinfusion, and increased to 92.2 ± 5.91 postinfusion, a net increase of 13%, with $p < 0.001$.

Discussion

The local anesthetic and antiarrhythmic drug lidocaine hydrochloride has been shown to possess the capability to reduce intracranial pressure associated with surgical stimulation, endotracheal stimuli, and in an experimental model of increased intracranial pressure produced by air embolism (Bedford et al. 1980, Donegan 1980, Evans et al. 1984, 1987; Yano et al. 1986). In this study, lidocaine was tested for its capability to reduce increased intracranial pressure associated with an intracranial space-occupying lesion simulated by an inflatable balloon. In addition to monitoring cardiovascular parameters, we also monitored continuously cerebral blood flow by laser-Doppler flowmetry. Our results show that elevated intracranial pressure in the rat may be effectively reduced by about 26% following lidocaine hydrochloride infusion. The reduction of ICP did not correspond to a decrease in blood pressure nor was it associated with a decrease in cerebral blood flow. Cerebral perfusion pressure was increased by 13%. In the control group whereby lidocaine was substituted with saline intracranial pressure remained unaffected. The mechanism whereby lidocaine reduced intracranial pressure is unclear. From the rapidity of onset of the effect on intracranial pressure, it is unlikely to be related to decreased production or increased resorption of CSF but rather related to cerebral blood volume and compliance. The most likely explanation for the observed reduction of ICP seemingly would have been the result of decrease in cerebral metabolisms and, hence, cerebral blood flow (Sakabe et al. 1947). However, our study showed that cerebral blood flow remained unchanged during and after lidocaine administration. Evans et al. entertained the possibility that the protective effect of lidocaine on cerebral blood vessels could be instrumental in the ability of the drug to attenuate elevations of intracranial pressure (Evans 1987).

If lidocaine was found to be effective in reducing intracranial pressure in humans, it would have distinct therapeutic advantage over barbiturates because it does not have the undesirable side effects of sedation and cardiovascular depression. Lidocaine is metabolized in the liver but unlike barbiturates, has a non-restrictive clearance limited by liver-blood flow only. Less than 20% of lidocaine is excreted unchanged in the urine. The elimination half-life of lidocaine following a bolus infusion is typically $1-1\frac{1}{2}$ hours; after infusion period of 24 hours, it is approximately 3 hours. The optimal dose required to suppress EEG activity without inducing seizures has yet to be determined. However, it has been shown that a single bolus of lidocaine of 160 mg/kg abolished EEG activity but only for 45 min (Astrup et al. 1981). The dose of lidocaine used in this experiment of 15 mg/kg is tenfold higher than the conventional dose recommended for patients with cardiac arrhythmias. In experimental animals including the rat this amount seems to be well tolerated and has minimal hemodynamic effects while its effects on ICP is immediate and long lasting. Our results suggest that lidocaine may be a useful agent for reducing intracranial hypertension associated with intracranial space-occupying lesions.

References

Astrup J, Skorsted P, Gjerris F et al. (1981) Increase in extramedullary potassium in the brain during circulatory arrest: effects of hypothermia, lidocaine, and thiopental. Anesthesiology 55:256–262

Bedford RF, Persing JA, Poberskin L et al. (1980) Lidocaine or thiopental for rapid control of intracranial hypertension. Anesth Analg 59:435–437

Donegan MF, Bedford RF (1980) Intravenously administered lidocaine prevents intracranial hypertension during endotracheal suctioning. Anesthesiology 52:516–518

Evans DF, Kobrine AI, LeGrays DC et al. (1984) Protective effect of lidocaine in acute cerebral ischemia induced by air embolism. J Neurosurg 60:257–263

Evans DE, Kobrine AI (1987) Reduction of experimental intracranial hypertension by lidocaine. Neurosurgery 20:542–547

Sakabe T, Naekawa T, Ishikawa T et al. (1947) The effects of lidocaine on canine cerebral metabolism and circulation related to the electroencephalogram. Anesthesiology 40:433–444

Yano M, Nishiyama H, Yokota H et al. (1986) Effects of lidocaine on ICP response to endotracheal suctioning. Anesthesiology 64:651–653

ICP Reduction by Lidocaine:
Dose Response Curve and Effect on CBF and EEG

M. Khayata, E. Arbit, G.R. DiResta, N. Lau, and J.H. Galicich

Neurosurgical Research Laboratory, Department of Surgery, Memorial Sloan-Kettering Cancer Center, Cornell University Medical College, New York City, New York 10021 (USA)

Introduction

Management of elevated intracranial pressure is a common problem in neurosurgical patients presenting with a mass effect due to tumors, hemorrhage, or hydrocephalus. There are cases where intracranial hypertension persists despite conventional therapy. There are also circumstances where rapid control of the ICP is needed without the delay of onset required by some of the presently available agents. Most of the presently acutely used agents (i.e. mannitol, hyperventilation) act through their effect on reducing cerebral blood volume.

Lidocaine, a widely used local anesthetic and anti-arrhythmic drug, has been shown to dampen the elevations in intracranial pressure associated with intubation and suctioning. We have previously shown that Lidocaine Hydrochloride (LH) is effective in lowering the elevated intra-cranial pressure associated with a mass lesion using a rat epi-dural balloon model. The ICP consistently dropped by 26% using 15 mg/kg with only a transient effect on mean arterial pressure (MAP) and local cerebral blood flow (l-CBF).

The mechanism by which the ICP is reduced is unclear. Vasoconstrictor effects, hemodynamic effects, decreased CSF production, and metabolic etiologies are postulated.

The aim of the study was to investigate the effect of LH on ICP, l-CBF, EEG, and MAP at various doses (5, 10, and 15 mg/kg) given intravenously (IV). This would provide information regarding the effectiveness of more conventional doses of LH on the above parameters. We also sought to know whether the reduction in ICP is produced by the transient hemodynamic effect (decrease in MAP and l-CBF) or by some other mechanism such as the induction of a preconvulsive state. To determine the time of onset of the reduction of ICP by LH and its duration of action we tested the different concentrations of LH in a rat model with an epidurally placed balloon simulating a mass lesion.

Materials and Methods

Surgical Procedures

Eighteen male, Sprague-Dawly rats with a mean weight of 383 gm were used in the experiments. Anesthesia was induced with halothane 2% (in 100% O_2) and the rats were maintained with an intra-muscular injection of alpha-Chloralose at a dose of 40 mg/kg dissolved in warm normal saline. A maintenance dose of 20 mg/kg was given at three hours. Bifemoral cut-downs were performed with cannulation of one femoral vein for drug injection an two femoral arteries for blood pressure monitoring and arterial blood gas (ABG) determinations. The vessels were cannulated with heparinized poly-ethylene PE-50 tubing and the blood pressure line was connected to a pressure transducer. After tracheostomy, the rats were placed on a Kopf stereotactic holder and ventilation was supported by a rodent respirator. The animals were paralyzed with tubocurarine chloride (0.1 mg/kg IV initially, then 0.05 mg/kg/1 hr) as needed to control respiration. Arterial blood gas measurements of pH, pCO_2, and pO_2 were taken. These parameters were maintained within physiologic range using respiratory settings. Continuous temperature monitoring was done using a rectal probe and the temperature was maintained at 37 °C using a heating pad and an infra-red heating lamp.

The skull was then sharply exposed and three 2 mm burr holes were placed. A right parietal burr hole just anterior to the lamdoid suture was used to carefully introduce a small epidural balloon anteriorly. A left parietal hole allowed stereotactic epidermal placement of the needle probe of the laser Doppler flowmeter. Probe placement was monitered microscopically to ensure that the brain surface was not compressed. An ICP optical transducer-probe was tightly placed in the left frontal region anterior to the coronal suture in a subdural position. Three subdermal silver chloride EEG electrodes were placed over the parietal regions and they were connected to an AC amplifier for continuous EEG recording.

The system was allowed to stabilize after placement of the monitoring devices. We tested the reactivity of the cerebral vasculature to hypercapnia prior to l-CBF measurements. The ICP was then increased from a baseline of 7 mm Hg by slowly inflating the epidural-balloon with normal saline at a rate of 0.1 cc/min. The ICP was allowed to equilibrate at a level of 40 ± 4 mm Hg (mean $\pm$ standard error of the mean). Once the ICP stabilized, a continuous infusion of LH (at 5, 10, and 15 mg/kg) was administered at a rate of 0.015 cc/min given IV. Blood pressure, heart rate, temperature, ICP, l-CBF, and EEG were continuously recorded. The measurements were performed at the beginning of the infusion and at the end of it. The animals were then followed for a variable amount of time extending from 10 min up to one hour. In six of the rats (three at 5 mg/kg and three at 10 mg/kg) the monitoring was extended up to at least one hour after lidocaine infusion.

Local Cerebral Blood Flow Measurement

Cerebral blood flow was continuously and non-invasively measured using an infra-red laser Doppler flow (LDF) meter. The mean Doppler shift frequency is linearly related to blood flow but has units of hectaHertz (hHz) (Bonner 1981). This output can be converted into conventional flow units using the combination LDF-Hydrogen clearance probe (DiResta 1987). Experiments conducted with a combination probe demonstrated that the two techniques were highly correlated. The LDF probe used has a measurement volume of approximately 1 mm³. We followed the time-flow dynamics for this tissue volume in our studies and the results are reported as percent change from baseline which is taken to be the beginning of the infusion of the drug.

Statistics

Statistical analysis was done using the mean, standard error, and Students' *t*-test (paired and unpaired). Results were expressed as mean ± standard error (SE) of the mean. A *p* value less than 0.05 was considered significant unless otherwise specified.

Results

The physiologic parameters between the different groups prior to the infusion of LH were not statistically different. The overall arterial blood prior to inflation of the balloon was pH 7.42, the pCO_2 was 37.2, and the pO_2 was 330. The body temperature was maintained at an overall mean of 37.1 C.

LH at a dose of 15 mg/kg resulted in a significant drop in the ICP from a value of 40 ± 1.6 mm Hg down to 26.7 ± 1.85 mm Hg ($n = 7$, $p < 0.001$). This 33.3% (see Fig. 1) decrease in the ICP was accompanied by a drop of the MAP from 113 ± 4.64 mm Hg down transiently to 91.25 mm Hg during the infusion and then by recovery back up to 105.5 ± 1.66 mm Hg at the end of infusion. The LH infusion was at a continuous rate and lasted 6.3 minutes. The laser Doppler flow meter showed a 19.7% drop in the CBF from a baseline value of 2.03 ± .24 hHz down to 1.63 ± .23 hHz ($n = 7$; $p < 0.1$). This was also a transient decrease which recovered once the lidocaine was stopped. The EEG was not changed during the entire period of infusion of LH. No flattening of the EEG was seen nor was there any spike-and-wave pattern at this dose of LH.

The lower doses of LH were also effective in reducing the ICP. The 10 mg/kg of LH resulted in a drop from 29.7 ± 1.87 mm Hg to 20.8 ± 1.05 mm Hg. This 30% decrease in the ICP was associated with only a 3% drop in the CBF (Fig. 1). The MAP was not affected by this dose of LH and remained stable at 122.3 mm Hg.

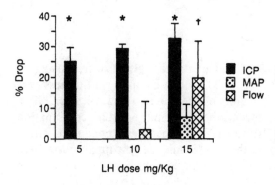

Fig. 1. B- or graph representation of the effect of lidocaine on ICP, CBF, and MAP. * Means there is a significant drop with $p < 0.05$. + Significant at $p < 0.1$

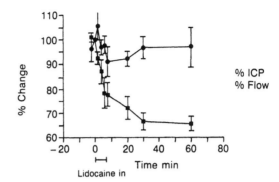

Fig. 2. Line curve representation of the effect of 5 mg/kg of lidocaine on ICP and l-CBF. The flow changes minimally while the ICP is decreased up to one hour

Similarly, the 5 mg/kg dose was effective in producing a reduction in the ICP by 25.2% ($n = 5$, $p < 0.002$) but did not affect the l-CBF or MAP despite its effectiveness in lowering the ICP (Fig. 1). Specifically, there were no transient changes in the MAP as seen with the higher doses of lidocaine.

The onset of action of the lidocaine was within the first six minutes of its administration and its effect lasted throughout the one hour observation period (Fig. 2). In one case a repeat infusion of 5 mg/kg of lidocaine was given at 2 hours and a prompt decrease of 22% of the ICP was obtained.

When comparing the percent decrease in the different groups using multiple t-tests, there was no significant difference between the various dosage groups in their ability to drop ICP. Thus, even though the percent drop in ICP is greater with the larger dose of LH (33.3% with 15 mg/kg LH vs. 26% for the 5 mg/kg dose), the difference is actually not statistically significant. This is despite the fact that at higher doses of LH we see some of the hemodynamic effects on the systemic circulation. There was also a drop in the laser Doppler flowmeter readings at the 15 mg/kg dose which seems to have paralleled the changes in the MAP, i.e. returning to pre-infusion value once the arterial pressure normalized. These changes probably reflected the hemodynamic effects of LH on the systemic circulation.

Discussion

In our experimental model where an intracranial balloon was used to simulate a mass lesion lidocaine at 15 mg/kg rapidly decreased the ICP by 33% while only transiently affecting MAP and l-CBF. Similarly, Malkinson (1985) showed that a 1.5 mg i.v. bolus of LH decreased the ICP in the anesthetized rat without any mass effect. In the work by Evans and Kobrine, using a dog ischemic model, LH (5 mg/kg) greatly attenuated the intracranial hypertension caused by vertebral artery air embolisation. Lidocaine, 1.5 mg/kg i.v., was also used by Bedford to induce rapid control of the ICP in ten neurosurgical operations (1980). It has also been found to suppress the cough reflex and the elevation in the ICP associated with endotracheal suctioning (Yano 1986).

The onset of action of LH on ICP was within five minutes of its infusion which is quick and its duration of action was of at least one hour. This may be related to the fact that LH has been shown (DeBoer 1980) to attain peak levels in the CSF within six minutes of intravenous infusion and that there is a negligible blood brain barrier for this drug. The effects of LH did not become attenuated when the drug was being cleared out of the circulation (2–3 half lives); thus it seems to act indirectly, through a mechanism, obscure as yet, rather than directly as a vaso-constrictor effect. Also, since different doses of LH had an effect of similar magnitude on the ICP, it seems to be acting through a mechanism with saturable kinetics at the concentrations used in our experiments.

There are several possible mechanisms that one can invoke to explain the drop in the ICP that we have observed. These include hemodynamic effects leading to hypotension and a drop in the ICP, cerebral electrical activation causing changes in CBF, inhibition of metabolism (CMR), and a decrease in the production rate of CSF by the choroid plexus.

In the hemodynamic effects, the MAP decreases – even transiently – thereby resulting in an associated drop in l-CBF and ICP. We did not observe a change in the CBF in the 5 and 10 mg/kg groups nor was there any influence on the MAP despite a definite reduction in the ICP in these animals making this a highly unlikely possibility.

Another potential mechanism includes cerebral electrical activation causing a change in the CBF or in the metabolic rate resulting in an ICP drop. Tommasino et al. (1981) showed that, in rats, larger doses (over 20 mg/kg) than the ones used in these experiments were required to produce seizures. This was accompanied by a lowered l-CBF (32%) in certain regions of the brain. Forty mg/kg was the concentration necessary to produce a pre-convulsive electroencephalogram (EEG) in rats and was associated with a decrease in the local cerebral metabolic rate for glucose (CMR-g) of a similar magnitude to that in flow. In our experiment, LH did not affect the EEG at the 15 mg/kg dose given over six minutes nor did it affect the local CBF. There was no change in the amplitude or the frequency of the EEG activity and this makes the possibility that modification of electrical activity is producing the ICP drop highly unlikely. Since no convulsive pattern was observed in our animals but the ICP was reduced, the changes in metabolism and blood flow accompanying the seizure activity that are present with the higher doses of lidocaine do not seem to be important in its ability to reduce the ICP.

LH could be exerting its effect by decreasing CBF thereby decreasing cerebral blood volume and reducing ICP. The l-CBF in our model did not decrease with the infusions of LH except for a transient drop with the 15 mg/kg dose where a hemodynamic factor was probably the cause. Takeshita (1974), in dogs, showed no changes in the CBF at 3 and 15 mg/kg, which is consistent with our findings. $CMRO_2$ was reduced, however, by 10% for 5 min at 3 mg/kg and by 30% for one hour with the 15 mg/kg. The CBF was directly measured by the sagittal sinus cannulation and use of square-wave electromagnetic flowmeter. DiFazio (1981) showed a 44% decrease in the CBF using microspheres at 3 mg/kg of LH. Johns (1985) studied the effect of LH on systemic rat arterioles. He showed that 8 mg/kg LH produces vasoconstriction in the systemic rat arteriole, while higher doses of the drug resulted in vasodilatation. If there is a similar effect on the cerebral circulation, then one would expect a drop in the cerebral blood volume (CBV). The CBF could even be maintained at a near normal value as we measured, but at the expense of a higher intravascular resistance. Thus, a decrease in the CBV, accounting for a drop the ICP, remains as a possibility but it is important to appreciate that the local CBF is maintained nonetheless as demonstrated by our experiments.

Lidocaine has long been thought of as being able to inhibit cerebral metabolism. Geddes (1956) demonstrated that LH (5 mM) was able to inhibit only the potassium induced oxygen consumption of rat brain cortex by 48%. Astrup (1981, 1982, 1987) has shown that massive doses of LH IV (160 mg/kg) in dogs can inhibit cerebral oxygen metabolism to a greater degree when administered with pentobarbital than can pentobarbital alone. He showed that the drug was effective in abolishing synaptic transmission and inhibiting cerebral metabolism (by an extra 35% over barbituates). He hypothesized that LH decreased metabolism by two means: suppression of cortical electrical activity and stabilization of neuronal membranes thereby blocking the leak of ions from the cells and saving on the enegy required for maintaining the membrane potentials. As mentioned earlier, Tommasino reported a 30% drop in CMR-g with over 20 mg/kg of LH. Whether the inhibition of the cerebral metabolic rate, if present at our doses of LH, is effective in lowering the ICP can not be obtained from the present data and without measuring CMR directly. However, a medication which might also affect cerebral metabolism would have a valuable role in the combined treatment of intracranial hypertension.

Another possible mechanism of action of LH which can explain the drop in ICP is the inhibition of the production of cerebrospinal fluid (CSF). Effectively, LH has been shown to reduce the cerebral adenosine tri-phosphate (ATP) concentration (Milde 1987). Haschke (1975) reported a 50% inhibition of electron transport in the brain mitochondria by LH. This was done by reversibly uncoupling oxidative phosphorylation and thereby producing inhibition of oxygen consumption. This may explain the decreased ATP concentration as observed by Milde as well as the ability of LH to inhibit the sodium channel. LH has also been shown to inhibit the Na-dependent glucose transport of ions across the renal brush-border membrane (Wright 1987). Similarly, in the choroid plexus, LH produced a 26% inhibition of the active accumulation of nicotine in the CSF (Spector 1982). Thus if transport mechanisms are inhibited by LH in a manner similar to that seen with ouabain, CSF production may decrease and so does the ICP. A similar effect would have been expected with Diamox where CSF production is also inhibited. However, Diamox, being a carbonic anhydrase inhibitor, causes an initial dilatation in the blood vessels and a one hour increase in the ICP prior to its onset of action.

LH is rapidly metabolized in rats. The total body clearance of LH is nine times greater in this species than in man. LH is rapidly removed by the liver and is then extensively recirculated in the biliary circulation. The half life of LH in rats is 33 min (DeBoer 1980) while in man it is 96 min.

In conclusion, lidocaine quickly reduced ICP even with the 5 mg/kg dose in rat for at least one hour. At this dose, it did not affect MAP, EEG, or CBF as measured in our experiments and therefore promises to be a useful tool in our attempts at controlling intracranial hypertension. Its possible mechanisms of actions include: inhibition of CSF production, a drop in the cerebral blood volume, and a decrease in the cerebral metabolic rate. Further studies are needed to assess the optimal dose of the drug in primates and to further clarify its mode of action. Its applications are wide spread in the usually difficult task of controlling the raised intracranial pressure associated with cerebral trauma.

Acknowledgement. This work has been in part supported by the Whitman fund in memory of their daughter Devon.

References

Astup J (1982) Energy-requiring cell functions in the ischemic brain. J Neurosurg 56:482–497

Astrup J (1988) Lidocaine and cerebral metabolism. Anesthesiology 68:470–471

Bedford RF, Persing JA, Pobereskin L, Butler A (1980) Lidocaine or thiopental for rapid control of intracranial hypertension. Anesth Analg 59 (6):435–437

Bonner R, Nossal R (1981) A model for laser-Doppler measurements of blood flow in tissue. Appl Optics 20:2097–2107

DeBoer AG, Breimer DD, Pronk J, Gubbens JM (1980) Rectal bioavailability of lidocaine in rats. Absence of significant first pass elimination. J Pharmacol Sci 69:804–807

DiFazio CA, Lescanic ML, Miller ED (1981) The effects of lidocaine on the whole body distribution of radioactively labeled microspheres in the conscious rat. Anesthesiology 55:269–272

DiResta et al. (1987) Hybrid blood flow probe for simultaneous H_2 clearance and laser-Doppler velocimetry. Am J Physiol 254:G573–G581

Evans DE, Kobrine AI (1987) Reduction of experimental intracranial hypertension by lidocaine. Neurosurgery 20 (4):542–547

Geddes IC, Quastel JH (1955) Effects of local anaesthetics on respiration of rat brain cortex in vitro. Anesthesiology 17 (5):666–671

Haschke RH, Fink BR (1975) Lidocaine effects on brain mitochondrial metabolism in vitro. Anesthesiology 42 (6):737–740

Johns RA, DiFazio CA, Longnecker DE (1985) Lidocaine constricts or dilates rat arterioles in a dose-dependent manner. Anesthesiology 62:141–144

Malkinson TJ, Cooper CE, Veale WL (1985) Induced changes in intracranial pressure in the anesthetized rat and rabbit. Brain Res Bull 15:321–328

Milde LN, Milde JH (1987) The detrimental effect of lidocaine on cerebral metabolism measured in dogs anesthetized with isoflurane. Anesthesiology 67:180–184

Sakabe T, Maekawa T, Ishikawa T, Takeshita H (1974) The effects of lidocaine on canine cerebral metabolism and circulation related to the electroencephalogram. Anesthesiology 40 (5):433–441

Spector R, Goldberg MJ (1982) Active transport of nicotine by the isolated choroid plexus in vitro. J Neurochem 38:594–596

Tommasino C, Maekawa T, Shapiro HM (1986) Local blood flow during lidocaine-induced seizures in rats. Anesthesiology 64:771–777

Wright EM, Scell RE (1987) Effects of lidocaine on transport properties of renal brush-border membranes. Biochem Biophys Acta 896:256–262

Yano M, Nishiyama H, Yokota H, Kato K, Yamamoto Y, Otsuka T (1986) Effect of lidocaine on ICP response to endotracheal suctioning. Anesthesiology 64:651–653

The Effect of Superimposed High-Frequency Auxiliary Ventilation on Intracranial Pressure

A. Korn, A. Aloy, T. Czech, K. Ungersböck, H. Schuster, and B. Plainer

Neurochirurgische Universitätsklinik und Universitätsklinik für Anästhesie
und Allgemeine Intensivmedizin, Währinger Gürtel 18–20, 1090 Wien (Austria)

Introduction

Conventional treatment of elevated intracranial pressure (ICP) includes various medications and physical measures of proven merit. Timely intubation and moderate hyperventilation, accompanied by adequate sedation and relaxation might certainly be mentioned as a first step in dealing with critical patients. Further important measures which have become established in clinical routine include raising of the head of the patient's bed, intermittent osmotherapy and various types of medications.

Different methods of mechanical ventilation have been examined as to their effects upon elevated ICP. No consistent results have been reported for high-frequency ventilation (Hurst et al. 1984, Rubio et al. 1987). For this reason, and also because of the technical and mechanical difficulties involved, high frequency ventilation has attained practically no clinical relevance in the treatment of high ICP.

Unlike other authors, we use a combined method with a simple economical system (*Logic Air CliniJet*) for superimposed high-frequency ventilation. This supplementarily ventilation technique was originally used for pulmonary support but we often observed it to have a distinct ICP-reducing secondary effect on ICP-monitored patients. In the meantime this ICP-reducing effect has become an important indication for the superimposed high-frequency ventilation technique described below.

The goal of our study was to describe this ICP-reducing effect and to show, that it does not appear to be due solely to arterial P_aCO_2's effect on the cerebral vasculature.

Methods and Patients

We present here a series of measurements on 17 patients (aged 14–72), admitted to the neurosurgical intensive care unit for intracranial pressure monitoring. Twelve patients were under observation post-operatively (6 after neurysm clipping after subarachnoid hemorrhage, 4 with intracerebral bleeding, 1 after removal of a right occipital glioblastoma, 1 with acute subdural hematoma) and five patients had suffered severe head trauma accompanied by diffuse brain edema without localized intracranial space-occupying lesions.

All patients received conventional (*Dräger UV 2*) controlled ventilation (continuous positive pressure ventilation (CPPV), inspiration/expiration ratio 1:2, moderate hyperventilation with an arterial P_aCO_2 of 30 mm Hg, PEEP at 5–8 mbar). In addition to routine monitoring of ECG, intraarterial blood pressure and epidural pressure (*Gaeltec Ict/b*), the pulmonary artery pressure, wedge pressure and cardiac output were measured using a Swan-Ganz catheter. Resistance values for both pulmonary and systemic circulations were calculated.

The high-frequency ventilation was superimposed intermittently for 10–15 minutes per hour. The Jet ventilation was applied as a supplement via a special connector, the tidal volume of the conventional CPPV, while under close P_aCO_2 monitoring, being first reduced and then increased after the supplementary ventilation cycle in such a way that no change in the arterial P_aCO_2 occurred.

Circulatory and intracranial-pressure readings, blood gas parameters, cardiac output and calculated resistance values were evaluated fifteen minutes before, during and fifteen minutes after each Jet application.

The operating principle of the Jet is to add short bursts of gas to the inspired air at a high frequency. The FiO_2 of the Jet is set to match that of the respirator. The effect in terms of both oxygenation and ICP reduction seems greatest when the gas pulse curve is approximately rectangular. The patient himself feels no individual pulses, merely a vibration which is often experienced as pleasant.

The apparatus employed is volume-cycled. A cylinder which is opened via a magnetic valve delivers constant stroke volumes in accordance with the discharge pressure setting. Variable parameters on this device include frequency (continuously adjustable between 1 and 12 Hz, the maximum effect on ICP being at approximately 6–10 Hz (360–600/minute), air-burst pressure (adjustable between 0.5 and 5 bar, our standard setting for adults being 2.5 bar, which corresponds to a stroke volume of 15 ml), and the FiO_2. In contrast to other models where, among other things, the rate of pressure increase is adjustable, this model seems especially suitable for routine clinical practice mainly because it is so simple to use (Fig. 1).

Results

In stable, normovolemic patients, changes in heart rate, arterial blood pressure and pulmonary artery pressure were insignificant during Jet ventilation. Although we did observe drops in blood pressure by up to 20 mm Hg in individual cases, they were invariably attributable to hypovolemia, and systemic blood pressure recovered within half a minute after the end of Jet ventilation. Fluid deficits were then corrected, and after subsequent Jet applications blood pressure remained stable.

Similarly (Sladen et al. 1984), in agreement with other authors, no significant changes in systemic and pulmonary vascular resistance were observed.

Inflating pressures, both peak and mean, were slightly reduced. With regard to oxygenation we did not observe any real improvement in Jet ventilation in this

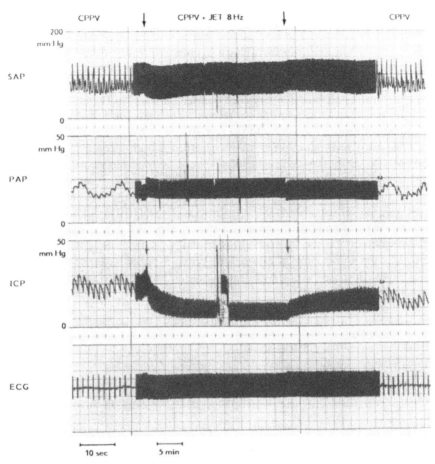

Fig. 1. Intracranial (*ICP*), pulmonary (*PAP*) and systemic pressure (*SBP*), heart rate (*HR*); before, during and after superimposed high frequency ventilation (*SHFV*)

Table 1. Intracranial (ICP) and systemic (SBP$_{mean}$) pressure, blood gas parameters, cardiac index (CI), calculated pulmonary (PVRI) and systemic (SVRI) resistance values and heart rate (HR); fifteen minutes before, during and fifteen minutes after superimposed high frequency ventilation (SHFV); average values ± standard deviation of seventeen patients

	Before SHFV CPPV	CPPV + Jet	15 min. after SHFV CPPV
ICP (mm Hg)	34.7 ± 14.2	17.9 ± 10.1 *	17.2 ± 10.9 *
p$_a$O$_2$ (mm Hg)	117.4 ± 26.7	118.8 ± 28.2	140.8 ± 29.8 *
p$_a$CO$_2$ (mm Hg)	31.2 ± 1.8	30.8 ± 2.3	30.7 ± 2.0
CI (l min^{-1} m^{-2})	3.4 ± 0.7	3.2 ± 0.7	3.3 ± 0.8
SVRI (dyn s cm^{-5} m^{-2})	1899 ± 492	2023 ± 554	2229 ± 609
PVRI (dyn s cm^{-5} m^{-2})	142 ± 118	139 ± 96	132 ± 80
SBP$_{mean}$ (mm Hg)	89.7 ± 15.3	89.3 ± 14.7	87.2 ± 14.0
HR (min^{-1})	95.5 ± 18.2	96.4 ± 17.4	92.7 ± 23.0

* $p < 0.01$.

499

group of patients. However, 15 minutes after the end of superimposed high-frequency ventilation, the P_aO_2 values were found to be slightly but significantly (Students t-test, $p < 0.01$) elevated, as compared with initial values. Although these results seem not to agree with the literature (Murray et al. 1987), they may be explained by the fact that our patients were all free of pulmonary disease (the oxygen saturation was in every case greater than 99% (Table 1).

In any event, CO_2 elimination remained unchanged during and after superimposed Jet ventilation owing to the adjustment technique mentioned previously.

The most prominent effect of superimposed high-frequency ventilation was on pathologically elevated intracranial pressure: in about two-thirds of patients, an appreciable reduction in pressure began immediately upon commencing Jet ventilation. This reduction usually continued on even after the end of supplementary ventilation for about 45–90 minutes. If the ICP began to rise again, Jet therapy was resumed with practically the same results. No rebound effect taking the form of an ICP rise to levels above initial pressures immediately following the end of application was observed. One-third of patients were refractory to this treatment. In these cases the conventional methods with their known complications would be used.

Discussion

We have been studying the phenomenon of ICP reduction during superimposed high-frequency ventilation for two years (in over 150 patients altogether, but in the cases described here there was an indication for pulmonary artery catheterization), yet we can only attempt a hypothetical explanation.

We have observed no hemodynamic effects of supplementary Jet ventilation.

On the one hand, superimposed high-frequency ventilation could achieve its lowering effect on ICP through the mechanism of hyperventilation; on the other hand, we have observed a reduction in elevated ICP even when we attempted to adjust the arterial P_aCO_2 during Jet to the same level as before Jet; thus a possible further mechanism, additional to the CO_2 effect on arterial vasculature must be assumed to exist.

Only the inflating pressures were reduced. The venous return from the cerebral circulation might thus be facilitated, causing the ICP to decrease, but this is merely speculative at present.

In any case, we now regard elevated intracranial pressure as an additional indication for superimposed high-frequency ventilation, alongside it's better-known applications for improving pulmonary gas exchange (Rouby et al. 1985). We consider an epidurally measured ICP of over 35 mm Hg in an intubated and sedated patient to be an absolute indication for this therapy. However, where the ICP shows a steady tendency to rise from a low initial value (around 10 mm Hg), we would recommend beginning therapy even earlier, at about 20 mm Hg. The clearest pressure reductions were seen in these instances, that is – before a plateau was reached.

So, in our opinion the reasons for superimposed Jet ventilation are to: a) improve oxygenation, b) eliminate atelectases, c) mobilize secretions and d) reduce elevated ICP.

Contraindications for high-frequency ventilation taken from the literature (Rouby 1985) are: a) hypovolemia and b) cardiac decompensation.

We believe we have found an additional therapeutic option in intermittent superimposed high-frequency ventilation which, if negative effects on hemodynamics and lung can be ruled out, can already be employed, even though it's theoretical basis as an intracranial pressure lowering therapy has not yet been proven. The great advantage of this form of therapy appears to be that it is minimally invasive and has no lasting negative side effects upon discontinuation. A simple and user-friendly apparatus seems indispensable for routine clinical practice.

References

Hurst JM et al. (1984) Use of high frequency Jet ventilation during mechanical hyperventilation to reduce intracranial pressure in patients with multiple organ system injury. Neurosurgery 4:530–534

Murray IP et al. (1987) Pulmonary embolism: High frequency jet ventilation offers advantages over conventional mechanical ventilation. Crit Care Med 2:114–117

Rouby JJ et al. (1985) Factors influencing pulmonary volumes and CO_2 elimination during high-frequency jet ventilation. Anesthesiology 63:473–482

Rubio JJ et al. (1987) Effects of high-frequency jet ventilation on intracranial pressure and cerebral elastance in dogs. Crit Care Med 6:602–605

Sladen A et al. (1984) High-frequency jet ventilation versus intermittent positive-pressure ventilation. Crit Care Med 9:788–790

Does Increased FiO$_2$ Alter NADH Redox State and Protect Brain Cells from Intracranial Pressure Change in Rabbits?

B. Bissonnette[1], P.E. Bickler[2], G.A. Gregory[2], and J.W. Severinghaus[2]

[1] Department of Anaesthesia and the Research Institute, The Hospital for Sick Children, Toronto, Ontario, M5G 1X8 (Canada)
[2] Department of Anesthesia and Cardiovascular Research Institute, University of California, San Francisco, California (USA)

Introduction

Elevated intracranial pressure is an important pathophysiologic feature of head injury, post ischemic reperfusion, and a variety of diseases states including cerebral edema, infection, and hemorrhage. Reduced blood flow to the brain and brain stem and an imbalance between oxygen supply and demand are viewed as the key mechanisms of injury due to elevated intracranial pressure. Despite the importance of these mechanisms, there is little information concerning the relationship of intracranial pressure to brain tissue oxygenation. Therefore, we designed this study to examine the effect of progressive changes in intracranial pressure on cerebrocortical oxygenation and cerebral blood volume and also to determine if increased inspired oxygen concentration would protect the brain cells against the deleterious effect of raised intracranial pressure changes.

Methods

With the approval of the Committee on Animal Research, we continuously recorded systemic arterial pressure, central venous pressure and intracranial pressure in 6 male New Zealand White rabbits, weighing 2.8–3.5 kg, who were anesthetized with urethane and paralyzed with pancuronium. Body temperature was recorded and maintained at 39°C by a servocontrolled heat lamp. All animals were mechanically ventilated to maintain normocarbia. The level of inspired oxygen concentration was adjusted over a range of 0.21 to 1.0. End-tidal gas samples were analyzed by a mass spectrometer. The head was fixed in a stereostatic apparatus and two burr holes were drilled. The dura-meter was left intact. Intracranial pressure was measured from an epidural bolt and also a short lumbar puncture needle positioned in the cisterna magna. The 22 gauge needle was connected to a Y-connector to allow injection of artificial cerebrospinal fluid to increase intracranial pressure. The intracranial pressure bolt was sealed in place with 8% cyanoacrylate dental cement to avoid any pressure leak. Through the second burr hole, cerebrocortical nicotine-amide-adenosine dinucleotide (NADH) fluorescence and ultraviolet reflectance were measured by a fiberoptic microfluororoflectometer (Chance et al. 1962, Jobsis et al. 1971) (Johnson Re-

Intracranial Pressure VII
Eds.: J.T. Hoff and A.L. Betz

search Foundation, University of Pennsylvania). A 50 watt air cooled mercury arc lamp was used as the source light. The light, after passing through the primary filter, illuminated the brain cortex via a fiberoptic cable applied directly to the dura-mater. The NAD/NADH redox state and relative cerebrocortical blood volume were determined from these measurements. The emitted NADH fluorescent (450 nm wavelength) and the reflected light (366 nm wavelength) were conveyed to the photomultiplier tubes by the fiberoptic cable. The light incident on the photomultiplier tubes was first filtered (for NADH fluorescence Kodak-Wratten 2C and 47 gelatine filters; for reflectance, Corning 5874 glass filter). NADH fluorescence measurement in vivo is based on the fact that only the reduced nicotine-amide-adenosine dinucleotide fluorescence when it is illuminated at 366 nm (Chance et al. 1962). The reflected light (the sum of reflected and scattered light), measured at 366 nm, was used to indicated changes in tissue blood volume. The increase in the cerebral blood content (vasodilation) results in an increase in the absorbance of the light and therefore a decrease in the intensity of the reflected light conversely with diminished blood volume the intensity increase (Jobsis et al. 1971). The reflected light is proportional to blood flow since there is a close relationship between cerebral vascular volume and blood flow. Changes in the blood content of the cortex but not the oxygenation of the blood can cause alterations in the detection of NADH fluorescence (Chance et al. 1962). To compensate these changes in NADH concentration, the correction factor described by Jobsis et al. (1971) was used. The method of transient dilution of brain blood by injection of $0.3-0.7$ cc of saline into the carotid artery increases the intensity of the fluorescence and reflected light. Finally, the correction factor (k) is defined by the ratio of the hemodilution induced between fluorescence and reflectance. The true variation in tissue NADH concentration is equal to the equation $\Delta CF = F - k (\Delta R)$, where the F and R are the changes recorded at 450 and 366 nm. Corrected NADH fluorescence, ΔCF, represented the real changes in [NADH]. O_2 utilization was then estimated by the change in relative [NADH]. Relative vascular volume was estimated by measuring changes in reflected light (the sum of reflected and scattered light). Multiple analysis of variance was used and $p < 0.05$ was considered statistically significant.

Results

In all 6 animals, [NADH] increased when intracranial pressure was greater than 18 ± 2.2 cm H_2O. Above this threshold, the rate of [NADH] increase was inversely proportional to the inspired oxygen concentration increase. When the concentration of inspired oxygen was raised from 0.21 to 0.5, a linear decrease in NADH concentration was observed. This indicates that oxygen was consumed by the mitochondrial respiratory chain and NAD/NADH redox state was adequately maintained. However, when the inspired oxygen concentration was increased above 0.5 little additional benefit in cerebrocortical oxygenation was achieved (Fig. 1). Capillary blood volume, which is proportionate to cerebrocortical blood volume, increased as intracranial pressure increased until the pressure exceeded 30 ± 1.8 cm H_2O and then capillary blood volume decreased.

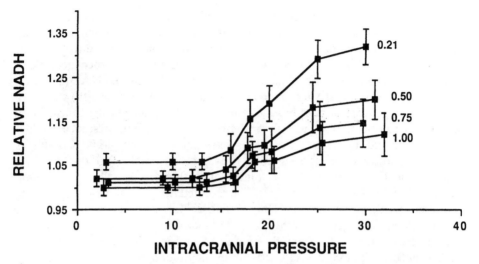

Fig. 1. NADH concentration increased when intracranial pressure was greater than 18 ± 2.2 cm H_2O. Above this treshold, the rate of [NADH] increase was inversely proportional to the FiO_2 increase. Raising the FiO_2 above 0.5 gave little additional benefit in cerebrocortical oxygenation

Discussion

These results indicate that high intracranial pressure definitely decreases cellular oxygen supply. Moreover, another indication of this decrease in cellular oxygenation is the measured increase in cerebrocortical blood volume; this increase in blood volume is acutely determined by an increase in cerebrocortical blood flow in response to hypoxia. Others have shown that any increase in cerebrocortical blood flow produces improved cellular oxygenation and that this is a cellular defense mechanism. However, this increase in cerebrocortical volume could have been the result of venous return alteration by the increase intracranial pressure. The pressure applied to the intracortical venules would trap blood and finally dilate the vessels upstream. On the other side, the pressure applied by the tip of the fluorometry probe which could have been great enough to mechanically decrease capillary blood flow once the intracranial pressure was very high $(30 \pm 1.8$ cm $H_2O)$ could suggest that the obstruction produced by increased intracranial pressure was not only applied to the venous circulation, but also to cortical arterial supply.

Conclusion

In summary, we have shown that with elevated intracranial pressure: 1) Increased oxygenation of blood gives greater cellular protection against changes in intracranial pressure and 2) little additional benefit to cerebrocortical oxygenation is achieved by increasing the inspired oxygen concentration above 0.5. This should be an important consideration in neurological intensive care units where it has been common practice to deliver high concentration of inspired oxygen to patients with high intracranial pressure even though pulmonary oxygen toxicity may result. Therefore we recommend limiting the inspired oxygen in these patient to 0.5 or less.

References

Chance B, Cohen P, Jobsis F, Shoener B (1962) Intracellular oxidation-reduction states in vivo. Science 137:499–508

Jobsis FF, O'Connor MJ, Vitale A, Vreman H (1971) Intracellular redox changes in functioning cerebral cortex. J Neurophysiol 34:735–749

Risberg J, Ancri D, Ingvar H (1969) Correlation between cerebral blood volume and cerebral blood flow in the cat. Exp Brain Res 8:321–326

Treatment of Increased Intracranial Pressure Using Oncodiuretic Therapy: Combined Albumin and Furosemide

L.M. Klebanoff, M. Kliot, M. Fink, and K.D. Post

Departments of Neurology and Neurosurgery, The Neurological Institute, 710 West, 168th Street, New York City, New York 10032 (USA)

Elevated intracranial pressure (ICP) is a common complication of severe head injury, intracranial hemorrhage, cerebral infarction, intracranial neoplasms, and some toxic and viral encephalopathies. Although the ability to normalize ICP does not guarantee a good recovery, aggressive management of elevated ICP has been shown to significantly decrease mortality (Marshall et al. 1979).

Several treatment modalities are currently in use for controlling increased ICP (Quest 1985). These include osmotic diuretics such as glycerol, urea, and mannitol as well as potent loop diuretics such as furosemide. Diuretics are associated with serious side effects such as hypotension, due to rapid intravascular volume depletion, serum electrolyte disturbances, and, in the case of mannitol, rebound increases in ICP. To minimize these side-effects, we have recently employed a protocol of using furosemide in combination with a concentrated colloid solution of 25% albumin (Albright et al. 1984). The rational is to increase plasma oncotic pressure thereby drawing extravascular fluid from edematous brain tissue into the intravascular space making this excess fluid available for diuresis. This combined oncodiuretic therapy has the advantage of lowering elevated ICP by dehydrating edematous brain. It avoids the complications of hypotension and electrolyte disturbances of standard osmotic diuretics by producing normovolemic dehydration.

In the setting of documented intracranial hypertension measured with an epidural (Ladd) monitor, our treatment protocol is to rapidly infuse 1 gram per kilogram of a 25% albumin solution with simultaneous intravenous bolus administration of 0.5 milligram per kilogram of furosemide. Supplemental doses of furosemide are given as necessary to achieve a urine output of approximately 250 cc per 12.5 grams of albumin given. Serial ICP measurements are recorded. Serum albumin and total protein, serum electrolytes, serum and urine osmolarities, and urine outputs are measured. Blood pressure and respiratory status are kept as constant as possible. Care is taken to note simultaneous therapies such as sedative administration, adjustment of head position, and pulmonary care.

Preliminary results in patients with increased ICP secondary to intraparenchymal hemorrhage, head trauma, and intracranial neoplasm have shown this oncodiuretic regimen to be effective in significantly reducing elevated ICP. Increases in plasma albumin and volume of diuresis correlated with reduction in ICP (see Table 1). No episodes of hypotension nor serum electrolyte disturbances were encountered. In addition, despite repeated trials of the protocol over many days, there was no decrement of effect nor rebound intracranial hypertension.

Table 1

Subject	Diagnosis	Intracerebral pressure (mm Hg)			Albumin (mg/dl) pre/post	Urine output (ml)
		Pre-Rx.	Post-Rx.	% change		
23 y/o M	Head trauma	37	31	16	4.4/5.9	2075
DS	s/p MVA	55	41	25	5.9/6.5	1500
27 y/o F	Cerebellar	35	11	69	2.7/4.0	475
BL	ICH	35	20	43	3.5/4.4	400
30 y/o M	Head trauma	35	10	71	3.3/4.7	1500
RL	s/p MVA	22	13	41	4.6/5.1	760
40 y/o F	Basal ganglia	29	19	34	4.0/5.3	1000
EH	ICH – left					
50 y/o M	Par-temp GBM	30	21	30	3.1/4.4	1100
JV	surg X 3-left					
65 y/o F	Occipital ICH	41	31	24	4.7/5.7	1000
MP	Right	33	22	27	4.8/6.3	700
82 y/o F	Fronto-par	34	26	24	3.7/5.1	950
RH	ICH – right	35	28	20	4.8/5.7	550
		44	20	55	4.1/4.7	700

This treatment may be particularly useful in settings where hypotension is to be avoided, in nutritionally depleted patients with low plasma albumin, and in patients who require prolonged treatment for intracranial hypertension.

References

Albright AL, Latchaw RE, Robinson AG (1984) Intracranial and systemic effects of osmotic and oncotic therapy in experimental cerebral edema. J Neurosurg 60:481–489

Marshall LF, Smith RW, Shapiro HM (1979) The outcome with aggressive treatment in severe head injuries. Part 1: The significance of intracranial pressure monitoring. J Neurosurg 50:20–25

Quest D (1985) Increased intracranial pressure, brain herniation, and their control. In: Wilkens RH, Rengachary SS (eds) Neurosurgery, Volume 1. McGraw-Hill, New York, pp 332–342

Induced Arterial Hypertension in the Treatment of High ICP

J.P. Muizelaar

Division of Neurosurgery, Medical College of Virginia, P.O.-Box 631, Richmond, Virginia 23298-0631 (USA)

Although hyperventilation is the best known means of reducing ICP by cerebral vasoconstriction, there are alternative ways to effect vasoconstriction. The effect of mannitol is in part due to vasoconstriction, be it secondary to blood viscosity changes (Muizelaar et al. 1984, Muizelaar et al. 1983) or to blood pressure increase (Rosner and Coley 1986/87). Moreover, Rosner has shown that increasing cerebral perfusion pressure by lowering the head can lead to vasoconstriction with ensuing decrease in ICP (Rosner and Coley 1986). We had shown that increasing blood pressure in patients with intact autoregulation can lead to a decrease in ICP (Muizelaar et al. 1984). In three patients, in whom we had observed ICP to decrease with higher blood pressure during tests of autoregulation, arterial hypertension was induced to treat otherwise uncontrollable ICP.

Patients

Patient A was a 21-year-old male, admitted with GCS of 3 and an epidural hematoma (Table 1). ICP problems were constant, requiring hyperventilation and frequent mannitol administration. On day 3, during tests of autoregulation, his ICP was noted to decrease from 36 to 32 torr with raising of his blood pressure from 114 to 135. During this manipulation, however, his PVI decreased from 8 to 6. He was kept on phenylephrine for 12 hours, but then his ICP rose again and his phenylephrine was stopped after 20 hours. The patient was brought in barbiturate coma, but this, too, could not control his ICP and he died on day 6.

Patient B was an 8-year-old boy, admitted with GCS 7, and an acute subdural hematoma, whose ICP rose from 8 to above 25 mm Hg 24 hours post-injury. This could not be controlled by hyperventilation to a $PaCO_2$ of 19 mm Hg, CSF

Table 1. Changes during tests of autoregulation

Patient	MABP (mm Hg)	ICP (mm Hg)	PVI (ml)	CBF ml/100 g/min	AVDO vol %
A	114–135	36–31	8–6	31–33	1.8–1.9
B	85–115	38–19	–	41–38	6.7–6.9
C	100–130	30–24	9–17	22–30	7.0–6.9

drainage or mannitol. Raising his MABP from 85 to 115 mm Hg brought his ICP down to just below 20 mm Hg. He was kept on phenylephrine for 10 hours, at which time is MABP remained around 100 mm Hg with no further ICP problems. He made a good recovery.

Patient C was a 12-year-old boy who was admitted with GCS of 6 and normal CT scan. In the ensuing 5 days, he had constant ICP problems, requiring CSF drainage, hyperventilation, and mannitol. His PVI hovered around 10 ml, indicating a very stiff brain. On days 4 and 5 post-injury, he had received 20 doses of 100 ml of mannitol and when his osmolality rose above 320, it was decided to induce hypertension as earlier tests of autoregulation had shown a good decrease in ICP with administration of phenylephrine. He was kept on the drug for 3 days, during which time he needed only five doses of mannitol, the first of which was given only 24 hours after the initiation of the hypertension therapy. His PVI was around 17 during those days. After three days, his blood osmolality had decreased sufficiently to allow using mannitol alone. Five months later, while recovering but still severely disabled, he suddenly died of unknown cause.

Discussion

This paper shows that autoregulatory vasoconstriction to reduce CBV can possibly be used to control rising ICP. Pressure autoregulation is intact in severely head injured patients in 67% (Muizelaar et al. 1984). The mean ICP change with higher blood pressure was +0.4 mm Hg with a range of −8 to +11 mm Hg (Muizelaar et al. 1984). Thus, although in general, the ICP changes are certainly not spectacular, in certain cases they may be. Normally, the vasoconstriction obtainable by raising blood pressure from a normal level is rather small (maximal 10%). But, it is possible that because of the trauma, the curve in Fig. 1 has shifted to the right because of vasospasm in the conducting arteries. Under those circumstances, vasoconstriction of 20–30% is easily obtained, resulting in considerable decrease in CBV and ICP.

Although we have shown that it is possible to control ICP by raising blood pressure, the question of safety remains unresolved as yet. There is a concern that hypertension increases cerebral edema after head injury. Theoretically, this should not happen when autoregulation is intact: The arteriolar vasoconstriction "blunts" the increased blood pressure so that, at the level of the capillaries, transmural pressure remains the same. Nevertheless, this novel therapy to control ICP must be considered experimental and be used only as a last resort or as a possible alternative for barbiturate-coma.

References

Muizelaar JP, Lutz HA, Becker DP (1984) Effect of mannitol in ICP and CBF and correlation with pressure autoregulation in severely head-injured patients. J Neurosurg 61:700–706

Muizelaar JP, Wei EP, Kontos HA et al. (1983) Mannitol causes compensatory cerebral vaso-constriction and vasodilation in response to blood viscosity changes. J Neurosurg 59:822–828

Rosner MJ, Coley IB (1986) Cerebral perfusion pressure, intracranial pressure, and head elevation. J Neurosurg 65:636–641

Rosner MJ, Coley IB (1987) Cerebral perfusion pressure: a hemodynamic mechanism of manni-tol and postmannitol hemogram. Neurosurgery 21:147–156

Intracranial Pressure in Preterm Infants: Effects of Nursing and Parental Care

B.A. Osband (Foerder), S. Blackburn, R. Zuill, L. Casey, D. Fahey, and P. Mitchell

Department of Parent and Child Nursing SC-74, School of Nursing, University of Washington, Seattle, Washington 98195 (USA)

Periventricular-intraventricular hemorrhage (PVH-IVH) is a major cause of both short and long term morbidity and increased mortality in small (<1500 gm) preterm (<34 wks G.A.) infants (Papile et al. 1978). The etiology of PVH-IVH in the preterm remains unclear. The incidence of PVH-IVH is increased in the presence of events that lead to changes in cerebral vascular hemodynamics. The preterm is also vulnerable because of impaired vascular autoregulatory mechanisms and the fragility of the highly vascular periventricular germinal matrix (Brann 1985). Changes in cerebral hemodynamics are reflected in changes in intracranial pressure (ICP) which can be measured non-invasively using a transfontanel pressure monitor (Bada 1983). Various activities, many related to nursing care, are associated with transient or sustained changes in ICP in adults and children (Mitchell 1986), but have not been studied in preterm infants.

The purpose of this study was to examine the effects of nursing and parental care activities on the ICP in preterm infants. Specific activities included sensory stimulation, feeding, routine caregiving, all with respect to infant state of arousal. ICP variation with time of day was also examined.

Methods

Informed consent was obtained from parents. A convenience sample of eight preterm infants, admitted to the neonatal intensive care unit who were between 3–21 days formed the sample. These infants were physiologically stable at the time of data collection. Data were collected during two four hour periods on each infant, one in the A.M. and one in the P.M. ICP was measured with an epidural fiberoptic sensor (Ladd ICP m1000) from the anterior fontanel according to the method of Hill and Volpe (1981). ICP data were collected every 30 sec and stored in a computerized data acquisition system (Thomas and Brengleman 1986). Simultaneously data regarding nursing care, infant state, tactile stimulation and feeding were also collected by two research assistants with interobserver reliability ranging from 79% (feeding) to 88% (tactile stimulation).

Intracranial Pressure VII   511
Eds.: J.T. Hoff and A.L. Betz
© Springer-Verlag Berlin Heidelberg 1989

Results

Mean ICP values, calculated for each infant using 30 sec intervals, were generally in the range reported by Bada (1983) of 6.0–7.5 mm Hg.

Diurnal Variation

Data were analyzed twice, with and without caregiving. The Wilcoxon non-parametric signed ranks test for related samples was calculated between morning and evening mean ICP values for each infant, with and without caregiving. There were no significant differences between the means of the morning and the means of the evening.

Patterns of ICP over time were evaluated graphically, using mean ICP values for 30 min intervals. There did not appear to be any distinct diurnal patterns however, three infants demonstrated "trough" patterns, a similar gradual decrease in ICP followed by a gradual increase over time; two other infants exhibited a "flat" pattern and the remaining three a "seesaw" pattern marked by up/down fluctuations over time.

Sensory Stimulation

Data on parental sensory contact, nurse contact, parental caregiving, nurse caregiving and no sensory stimulation for each infant state and for all states combined were collected every 30 sec. For all states of arousal combined, ICP was significantly higher during nursing sensory contact ($XR^2 = 8.1$, $p < .02$, Friedman analysis of variance by ranks), with no significant differences between parental sensory stimulation and periods of no contact. ICP was higher during parental physical care than during nursing caregiving in in 3 of 4 infants in whom this comparison was possible (range of means for parents 4.5–8.8 mm Hg, for nurses 2–6.8 mm Hg).

No significant differences were found in ICP values with change in infant state (light sleep, drowsy, quiet alert) compared with no sensory contact, and between parental and nurse contact.

Feeding/Non-nutritive Sucking

There were no significant differences in mean ICP values for feeding intervals and intervals independent of caregiving (Wilcoxon signed ranks test and T test for related measures). Mean ICP values for non-caregiving intervals in all states ranges from 3.43–7.06 mm Hg, while mean ICP values for feeding intervals ranged from 2.90–8.04 mm Hg. Mean ICP values for gavage feeding ($n=3$) ranged from 4.00–9.32 mm Hg, for nipple feeding ($n=8$) from 1.07–8.33, for breast feeding ($n=8$) from 2.28–6.50 mm Hg. Though these differences were not statistically significant they provide suggestive evidence that during breast feeding ICP is lower than during either gavage or nipple feeding. Mean ICP with non-nutritive sucking across all infants was 5.65 mm Hg for pacifier and 4.43 mm Hg for finger sucking. Visual analysis of changes in ICP with non-nutritive sucking reveals a marked decrease in ICP when a crying infant whose ICP is elevated is given a pacifier.

Summary

Normal nursing caregiving activities do not pose a threat to intracranial dynamics for medically stable preterm infants. Although variability was evident among behavioral states and some caregiving activities, ICP rarely exceeded normal limits in these medically stable preterm infants. ICP response to parental contact was not significantly different from no contact, but was higher during parent caregiving than nurse caregiving. Non-nutritive sucking reduced and stabilized ICP following crying. The trend toward lowest ICP with breast feeding suggests that there may be benefits to breast feeding in the preterm that extend beyond nutrition.

References

Bada HS (1983) Intracranial monitoring – Its role and application in neonatal intensive care. Clin Perinatol 10 (10):223–236

Brann AW (1985) Factors during perinatal life that influence brain disorders. In: Prenatal and perinatal factors associated with brain disorders (pp 273–284). NIH Publication 85-1149

Hill A, Volpe J (1981) Measurement of ICP using the Ladd intracranial pressure monitor. J Pediatr 98:974–976

Mitchell P (1986) Intracranial hypertension: Influence of nursing care activities. Nurs Clin North Am 231 (4):563–576

Papile LA et al. (1978) Incidence and evolution of subependymal and intraventricular hemorrhage: A study of infants with birth weights less than 1500 gm. J Pediatr 92:529–534

Thomas KA, Brengleman G (1986) Computerized data acquisition systems: An innovation in the study of human response patterns. International nursing research conference. Edmonton, Alberta

Intracranial Pressure Controlled Therapy of Brain Edema in Cerebrovascular Disease

A. Haass, R. Kloss, G. Hamann, P. Krack, and K. Schimrigk

Department of Neurology, Neurologische Universitätsklinik, D-6650 Homburg/Saar (FRG)

Introduction

In subarachnoid hemorrhage (SAH), in intracerebral hematoma (ICH) and in large ischemic stroke, there may be a critical increase in intracranial pressure (ICP). Intubation, hyperventilation and correct positioning of the head often are not sufficient to control ICP. Thus hyperosmolar substances such as glycerol, mannitol and sorbitol need to be administered.

To give reliable therapeutic guidelines, we studied the intensity and duration of the ICP reducing effect of sorbitol (i.v.) and glycerol (p.o.), and the time dependent serum and cerebrospinal fluid (CSF) concentrations of glycerol. A pressure transducer was implanted epidurally to measure intracranial pressure and to quantify the therapeutic antiedemic effects of glycerol and sorbitol. ICP, systemic arterial pressure (SAP), and cranial perfusion pressure (CPP) were continuously monitored by a Dr. Weiss Neuromonitor.

Patients and Methods

The investigations included 13 patients with SAH, 15 patients with ICH and 8 patients with ischemic stroke. ICP was measured after epidural implantation of a Gaeltec pressure transducer. ICP and SAP were recorded by a Gaeltec (ICP) and a Siemens (SAP) amplifier respectively. A neuromonitor (Dr. Weiss Neuromonitor, Berlin GFR) was used for calculating CPP and continuous monitoring of ICP, SAP and CPP. When a critical ICP level of 25–30 mm Hg was reached, we administered either 50 g sorbitol (125 ml Tutofusin S 40) as a short i.v. infusion or 50 g glycerol (125 ml of a 40% solution) as a bolus via a gastric tube. The serum and CSF glycerol concentrations were measured with a modified triglyceride assay (Boehringer, Mannheim).

Results

The efficacy of the hyperosmolar substances depended on the ICP intensity. We differentiated a phase of low (20–25 mm Hg), medium (25–35 mm Hg) and high

Intracranial Pressure VII
Eds.: J. T. Hoff and A. L. Betz
© Springer-Verlag Berlin Heidelberg 1989

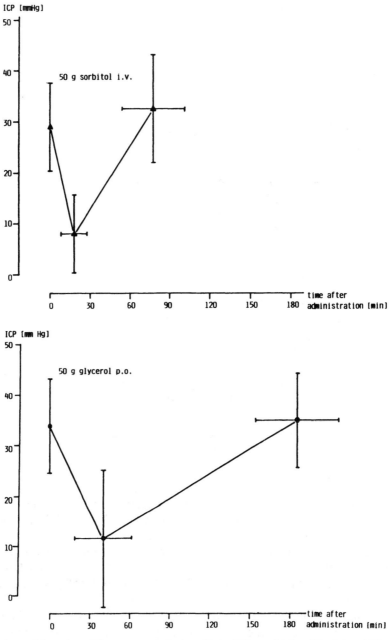

Fig. 1. Intensity and duration of the pressure reducing effect of 50 g sorbit i.v. (90 min) and 50 g glycerol p.o. (180 min) during the phase of high intracranial pressure intensity in subarachnoid hemorrhage

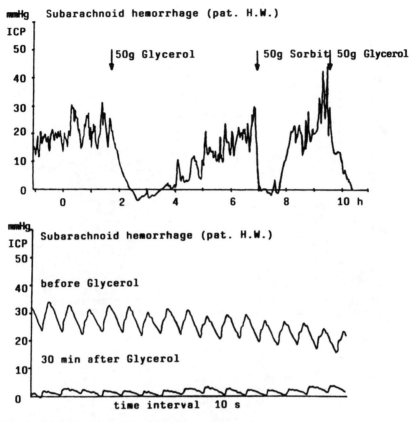

Fig. 2. Original registration of ICP by a "Dr. Weiss Neuromonitor" showing the pressure reducing effect of glycerol and sorbitol during the phase of medium intracranial pressure intensity in subarachnoid hemorrhage

(>35 mm Hg) ICP intensity. In ICH and in stroke the ICP increased constantly during the first days and reached a maximum after 4–13 days. This phase of maximal pressure lasted 3–6 days according to the severity of the disease. In SAH on the other hand, onset, duration and intensity of the ICP increase were much more variable. The consumption of hyperosmolar drugs depended on ICP intensity. The amount varied from 2×50 g glycerol to 4×50 g glycerol along with 4×50 g sorbitol per day.

The duration of the pressure reducing effect of a single dose of glycerol or of sorbitol varied depending on ICP intensity. In the phase of high pressure intensity, the effect of glycerol (50 g) and sorbitol (50 g) lasted 3 h and 1.5 h respectively (Fig. 1).

In the phasae of medium ICP increase, glycerol and sorbitol acted 6–8 h and 3–4 h respectively (Fig. 2). The pressure reducing effect of glycerol consistently lasted twice as long as that of sorbitol in each of the different ICP intensity phases.

After administration of 50 g glycerol p.o., serum glycerol concentration rapidly increased to approx. 120 mg/dl and decreased to 50 mg/dl after 180 min. CSF

516

glycerol concentrations however only gradually increased to maximal values around 30 mg/dl.

Discussion

Glycerol and sorbitol are suitable drugs for hyperosmolar therapy in raised intracranial pressure (Haass et al. 1987, Hase and Reulen 1980, Michalik et al. 1983, Rottenberg et al. 1977). In a phase of high intracranial pressure the effect of sorbitol only lasts for a period of approximately 90 min, whereas glycerol acts for as long as three hours. In phases of medium or low pressure, the therapeutic effect lasts much longer, with glycerol consistently acting twice as long as sorbitol.

The varying duration of the pressure reducing effect of hyperosmolar substances in the therapy of intracranial pressure highlights the need for continuous measuring of ICP in order to control therapy effectively. Moreover onset, duration and intensity of ICP vary interindividually and according to the pathogenetic mechanism of the respective disease. A strict regimen of hyperosmolar drugs does not take into account the varying course of intracranial pressure. As the different pressure phases cannot sufficiently be differentiated on clinical grounds, only an exact monitoring of the ICP allows an adequate dosage of hyperosmolar substances.

We obtained comparable results in SAH, in ICH and in stroke, so the same therapy probably is applicable to cerebrovascular disease in general.

After oral administration of glycerol, the serum glycerol concentration rapidly raises and thus leads to a therapeutic increase in serum osmolality. The combination of glycerol and sorbitol at the dosage indicated, allows an effective therapy of ICP without exceeding the respective elimination rates. In CSF there is only a slight increase in glycerol concentration. Thus with this dosage (maximally 4×50 g/day), even when applied for a longer period, there is no considerable crossing of glycerol from blood into CSF and the blood-brain-barrier seems to be relatively impermeable for glycerol. So generally there must be no fear of a rebound effect. Nevertheless on one single occasion we measured a glycerol concentration of 113 mg/dl in the CSF of a female patient. The dosage of glycerol and sorbitol should not exceed 4×50 g for each hyperosmolar drug. If higher doses are used, the blood-brain-barrier should be controlled for permeability.

References

Haass A, Kloss R, Brenner M, Hamann G, Harms M, Schimrigk K (1987) ICP-gesteuerte Hirnödembehandlung mit Glycerin und Sorbit bei intracerebralen Blutungen. Nervenarzt 58:22–29

Hase U, Reulen HJ (1980) Wirkung von Sorbit und Mannit auf den intrakraniellen Druck. Neurochirurgia (Stuttg) 23:205–211

Michalik M, Schulz W, Järisch M, Zschenderlein R, Schulze HAF (1983) Orale Glycerintherapie bei intrakranieller Drucksteigerung. Dtsch Gesundh-Wesen 38:494–501

Rottenberg DA, Hurwitz BJ, Posner JB (1977) The effect of oral glycerol on intraventricular pressure in man. Neurology 27:600–608

Cerebro-Spinal Fluid Pressure Changes and Rate of Recovery After Propofol for Elective Craniotomy

P. Ravussin, J.P. Guinard, D. Thorin, and J. Freeman

Department of Anesthesia, Centre Hospitalier Universitaire Vaudois, University of Lausanne, 1011 Lausanne (Switzerland)

Introduction

Propofol in its aqueous formulation has many of the properties required for total intravenous anesthesia particularly a short recovery time (Coates et al. 1986). However, its effect on cerebro-spinal fluid pressure (CSFP), cerebral perfusion pressure (CPP) and rate of recovery is unknown in patients scheduled for intracranial surgery lasting several hours. We evaluated therefore both the effect of propofol alone on CSFP and CPP, and the rate of recovery in patients undergoing elective craniotomy.

Methods

With ethical committee approval and informed consent, 23 consecutive, adult, ASA grade 3 patients (54 ± 3.6 yrs, 67 ± 2.4 kg) scheduled for elective intracranial surgery, tumor resection (15), aneurysm clipping (6), trigeminal neuralgia (1) and CSF fistula (1), were studied. No patient had any pathology judged likely to obstruct CSF pathways between the intracranial and lumbar CSF spaces, thus lumbar CSFP was considered to accurately reflect intracranial pressure (Takizawa et al. 1986). All patients received midazolam (0.1 mg/kg) intramuscularly and metoprolol (1 mg/kg) orally 1 hour before induction of anesthesia. Lumbar CSFP, mean arterial pressure (MAP), and heart rate (HR) were recorded on a two-channel Model 78342A Hewlett-Packard System (Hewlett-Packard Inc., Palo Alto, California, USA) just before induction (baseline, T_0), at 0.5, 1, 1.5, 2, 3, and 4 min after an induction dose of propofol 1.5 mg/kg injected over 30 sec, and at intubation, application of the skull-pin head-holder and incision. A continuous infusion of propofol was started initially at 100 µg/kg/min at the same time as the induction dose. Fentanyl 2 µg/kg and pancuronium 0.1 ml/kg were injected after 2 min and controlled ventilation performed to maintain the $PaCO_2$ between 32–35 mm Hg. Patients were left unstimulated prior to tracheal intubation. Anesthesia was maintained with a continuous infusion of propofol and N_2O 50% in O_2 with increments of fentanyl and pancuronium. At the end of the procedure, N_2O and propofol were stopped, pancuronium reversed, and recovery assessed using the Glasgow Coma Scale (GCS) score and by noting the times to (1) spontaneous ventilation, (2) eye-opening, (3) extubation, (4) obey orders, (5) speak, and (6) orientation in time and space. Mean values ± SEM are reported. Baseline and post-propofol data were compared using Student's paired t-test with the Bonferroni correction for multiple comparisons; $p < 0.05$ was considered significant.

Results

All 23 patients had a GCS score of 15 preoperatively and the morning following surgery. Propofol infusion lasted 333 ± 21.5 min. Mean total doses and rates of propofol and fentanyl were 1486 ± 92 mg (69.8 ± 3.6 µg/kg/min) and 661 ± 40 µg (1.89 ± 0.12 µg/kg/h) respectively. Mean values of each variable at each time interval during induction are shown in Table 1 A. CSFP was decreased significantly from 0.5 to 2 min after propofol alone (maximal decrease 37%) but approached baseline values by 4 min. The CPP (MAP-CSFP) remained above 70 mm Hg. Heart rate did not change. Intubation, application of the skull-pin head-holder and incision did not cause a significant rise in CSFP and MAP. Maintenance of anesthesia was uneventful. Recovery was rapid (Table 1 B).

Table 1
A Effect of an induction dose of propofol 1.5 mg/kg on CSFP, MAP, CPP and HR (mean values ± SEM, mm Hg and cpm)

Baseline (T$_0$) values		Minutes after the induction dose of propofol					
		0.5	1	1.5	2	3	4
CSFP	11.9 ± 1.4	$9.0 \pm 1.3*$	$8.1 \pm 1.2*$	$7.5 \pm 1.0*$	8.1 ± 1.0	9.7 ± 1.5	11 ± 1.8
MAP	97 ± 2.3	97 ± 2.8	92 ± 2.4	87 ± 2.4	87 ± 3.1	85 ± 2.6	$84 \pm 2.8*$
CPP	85 ± 2.3	88 ± 2.8	84 ± 4.4	79 ± 2.7	79 ± 3.1	76 ± 3.1	73 ± 3.2
HR	63 ± 2.2	65 ± 3.0	65 ± 2.3	64 ± 2.5	64 ± 2.4	64 ± 2.1	66 ± 2.5

* $p < 0.05$

B Recovery from anesthesia

	Times					
	(1)	(2)	(3)	(4)	(5)	(6)
Minutes	2.2	8.3	8.8	10.7	12.5	19.2
± SEM	± 0.6	± 1.7	± 1.5	± 2.4	± 2.5	± 2.8

	Minutes after the end of propofol infusion					
	0 min	2 min	5 min	10 min	20 min	30 min
GCS scores 13–15 (%)	0	4.3	21.7	52.1	73.9	87

Times (1)–(6): see "methods". GCS = Glasgow Coma Scale

Discussion

In this study of 23 patients, an induction dose of propofol of 1.5 mg/kg significantly decreased CSFP by 37%. As propofol has already been shown to increase cerebro-vascular resistance (Stephan et al. 1987), this decrease in CSFP may thus be due to a decrease in cerebral blood volume, as previously suggested for barbiturates (Shapiro et al. 1973). As with barbiturates, this effect is transient, demonstrating the rapid redistribution and metabolism of propofol. With the induction dose used in this study, the maximal decrease in MAP was only 10% (14% after fentanyl administration) which is less pronounced than described by Coates et al. (1987). When associated with fentanyl, propofol obtunded the usual CSFP and MAP responses to intubation and noxious stimulations as reported recently by Van Aken et al. (1988). Recovery was rapid, with a GCS score of 13–15 in 20/23 patients at 30 min. Thus propofol appears to be a suitable short-acting intravenous agent for induction and maintenance of general anesthesia in neurosurgery, and the use of volatile agents can be avoided.

References

Coates DP, Monk CR, Prys-Roberts C, Turtle MJ (1987) Hemodynamic effects of infusions of the emulsion formulation of propofol during nitrous oxide anesthesia in humans. Anesth Analg 66:64–70

Shapiro HM, Galindo A, Wyte SR, Harris AB (1973) Rapid intraoperative reduction of intracranial pressure with thiopentone. Br J Anaesth 45:1057–1062

Stephan H, Sonntag H, Schenk HD, Kohlhausen S (1987). Einfluß von Disoprivan (Propofol) auf die Durchblutung und den Sauerstoffverbrauch des Gehirns und die CO_2-Reaktivität der Hirngefäße beim Menschen. Anaesthesist 36:60–65

Takizawa H, Gabra-Sanders T, Miller JD (1986) Analysis of changes in intracranial pressure and pressure volume index at different locations in the craniospinal axis during supratentorial epidural balloon inflation. Neurosurgery 19:1–8

Van Aken H, Meinshausen E, Prien T, Brüssel T, Heinecke A, Lawin P (1988) The influence of fentanyl and tracheal intubation on the hemodynamic effects of anesthesia induction with propofol/N_2O in humans. Anesthesiology 68:157–163

Influence of Single Bolus of Propofol on Cerebrospinal Fluid Pressure and Cerebral Blood Flow Velocity

A. Parma [1], R. Massei [1], D. Mulazzi [1], C. Ferrari da Passano [2], G. Granata [2], G. Tomei [2], P. Rampini [2], and R. Trazzi [2]

[1] Department of Anaesthesiology, University of Milan, and [2] Department of Neurosurgery, University of Milan, 20122 Milan (Italy)

Introduction

There are many experiences with Propofol for induction and maintenance in neuroanaesthesia (Siani et al. 1986). A wide range of clinical and experimental results on cerebrospinal fluid (CSF) pressure (McDowall et al. 1985, Zattoni et al. 1988), cerebral blood flow (Ravussin et al. 1988, Stephan et al. 1987), systemic arterial pressure (Parma et al. 1988, Coates et al. 1987), $CMRO_2$, reactivity of cerebral circulation to CO_2, cerebral blood flow and cerebral vascular resistance (Stephan et al. 1987), were presented during recent years.

Flow velocity in the middle cerebral artery can be detected continuously using an easy non-invasive method proposed by Aaslid et al. (1982): the Transcranial Doppler (TCD). A decrease of flow velocity under 10 cm/sec can be a risk factor for neurological disease (Cabrini et al. 1987). The TCD can be used to evaluate changes of the flow velocities associated with the cerebral vasospasm following subarachnoid hemorrhage (Aaslid et al. 1984), cerebral vascular disease (Cabrini et al. 1987), head injuries and cerebral death (Ringelstein 1986).

In this study, modification of flow velocity, following a single bolus of Propofol for induction in neuroanaesthesia, has been evaluated by TCD.

Material and Methods

This study has been approved by the Hospital Ethical Committee and all the patients gave their informed consent. Twenty patients (12 females and 8 males, ASA class 1 or 2), with intracranial tumors have been recruited. All patients had normal cardiac, hepatic, renal, hemopoietic and endocrine function.

Premedication consisted of atropine sulphase 0.007 mg/kg i.m. 45' before induction of anaesthesia.

Lumbar and ventricular cerebrospinal fluid (CSF) pressure, mean arterial blood pressure (MABP), using a 20 gauge catheter inserted into a radial artery before the Allen test were all measured at baseline (before induction) and at 1, 2, 3, 4, and 5 minutes after induction with Propofol 2.5 mg/kg i.v. over 30 seconds.

MABP and cerebrospinal fluid (CSF) pressure were recorded in the supine position using calibrated transducers connected to a two channel monitor.

The velocity of cerebral blood flow was measured using a TC2-64 Transcranial Doppler with an ultrasound signal of 2 MHz. The depth of signal varied between 25 and 135 mm.

Pancuronium bromide 0.08 mg/kg was administered after induction and ventilation was controlled by face mask at normocapnia. All patients were intubated and mechanically ventilated.

Statistical Analysis

Analysis of variance (ANOVA) was used to evaluate the effect of time. For multiple comparison of means at time points, the least-significant-difference (LSD) test was used, while comparisons versus baseline values were assessed by the Dunnet test. $P < 0.05$ was considered to indicate statistical significance. All values were expressed as mean $\pm$ (SD). The correlations between CSF pressure-MAP, MAP-cerebral flow velocity, CPP-cerebral flow velocity were studied through the regression lines.

Results

The mean age and weight of the patients were 40.4 years and 68.15 kg respectively. The intracranial pathology included 14 tumors of the supratentorial region and 6 tumors of the subtentorial region.

Patients have been retrospectively stratified into two groups, according to the CSF pressure basal values: lower than 10 mm Hg (8 patients), and higher than 10 mm Hg (12 patients).

Cerebrospinal Fluid Pressure (CSF) (Fig. 1)

CSF pressure and MABP decreased in both groups, significance ($P < 0.05$) at 2' and 3' for CSF pressure and at 1', 2', 3' for MABP in the group with higher baseline CSF pressure; in the group of patients with baseline value of CSF pressure lower than 10 mm Hg only MABP reached significance at 1'.

Cerebral Perfusion Pressure (Fig. 2)

A fall, within the physiological range, of CPP was detected at 2' only in patients with baseline CSF pressure greater than 10 mm Hg. CPP decreased also in the other group, but not significantly.

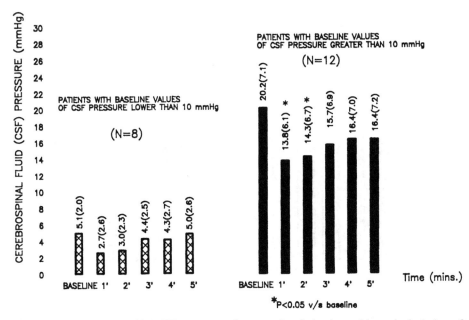

Fig. 1. Cerebrospinal fluid (CSF) pressure changes after induction with a single bolus of 2.5 mg/kg of Propofol given over 30″ – Mean values (SD)

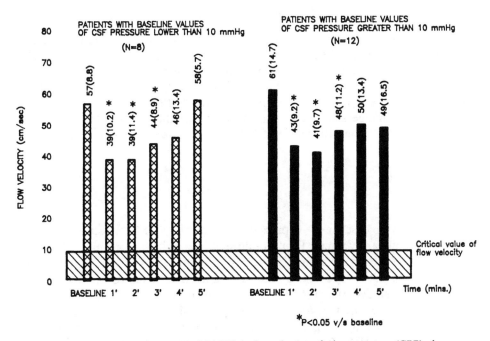

Fig. 2. Mean arterial blood pressure (MABP) and cerebral perfusion pressure (CPP) changes after induction with a single bolus of 2.5 mg/kg of Propofol given over 30″ – Mean values (SD)

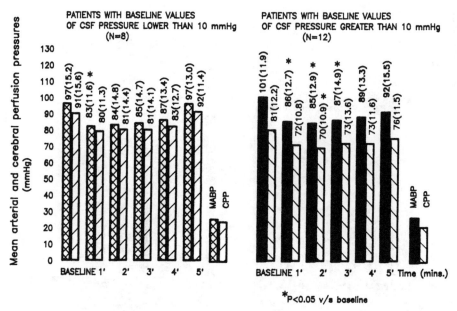

Fig. 3. Cerebral blood flow velocity modifications assessed using Transcranial Doppler (TCD), after induction with a single bolus of 2.5 mg/kg of Propofol given over 30″ – Mean values (SD)

Cerebral Blood Flow Velocity (Fig. 3)

The middle cerebral arteries were found in all patients at a depth between 45 mm and 55 mm. The normal flow velocity before induction was 60 ± 12 cm/sec. The cerebral blood flow velocity decreased significantly in both groups at 1′, 2′, 3′ after the induction dose of Propofol, but the flow velocity remained over a critical value of 10 cm/sec. All values returned to normal with 4′ after induction. Heart rate did not change significantly at any time in either group. There were no significant correlations after a single bolus of Propofol (2.5 mg/kg over 30″).

Discussion

In patients with baseline CSF pressure >10 mm Hg, CSF pressure and CPP, decrease significantly after a Propofol dose of 2.5 mg/kg, according to Ravussin et al. (1988). CSF pressure and CPP return to basal values within 3′ after induction, showing that Propofol is a short acting intravenous anaesthetic (Hartung et al. 1987). The decrease of CSF pressure after Propofol is probably due to an increase of cerebrovascular resistance (Stephan et al. 1987). The decrease of CSF pressure after Propofol is probably due to an increase of cerebrovascular resistance (Stephan et al. 1987), with a concomitant decrease in cerebral blood volume (Giffin et al. 1984); as already explained for barbiturates (Shapiro et al. 1972), etomidate (Milde et al. 1985), althesin (Bendtsen et al. 1985) and midazolam (Forster et al. 1982, Massei et al. 1985).

The MABP decrease, observed in all patients, is caused by the decrease in systemic vascular resistance and cardiac output (McCollum and Dundee 1986, Coates et al. 1987). The fall of MABP does not induce a dangerous fall of CPP.

Our results demonstrate that the lower values of CPP, reached at 2' in patients with baseline CSF pressure >10 mm Hg, were within safety limits. As regards TCD, cerebral flow velocity fell in both groups of patients at 1', 2' and 3' due to the MABP decrease; in both groups it never reached the critical value of 10 cm/sec, considered to be the value under which ischemic diseases or EEG alterations appear (Cabrini et al. 1987).

At 5' after induction the TCD mean value returned to baseline in patients with baseline CSF pressure <10 mm Hg, while in the other group the value was lower. This is probably due to a better response of the cerebral autoregulation in the first group.

In conclusion, Propofol decreases increased CSF pressure without causing dangerous falls of CPP and cerebral blood flow velocity.

Acknowledgements. The authors would like to express their gratitude for the valuable help and good cooperation to A. Canavesi, P. Cedroni (Statistical and Safety Group of ICI-Pharma, Italy).

References

Aaslid R, Markwalder TM, Nornes H (1982) Non invasive transcranial doppler ultrasound recording of flow velocity in basal cerebral arteries. J Neurosurg 57:769–774

Aaslid R, Huber P, Nornes H (1984) Evaluation of cerebrovascular spasm with transcranial doppler sonography. J Neurosurg 60:37

Bendtsen A, Kruse A, Madsen JB, Astrup J, Rosenorn J, Blatt-Lyon B, Cold GE (1985) Use of continuous infusion of althesin in neuroanaesthesia. Changes in cerebral blood flow, cerebral metabolism, the EEG and plasma alphaxolone concentration. Br J Anaesth 57:369–374

Cabrini GP, Granata G, Ferrari da Passano C (1987) Valutazione pre ed intraoperatoria dei circoli di compenso della carotide interna con doppler transcranico in 40 pazienti sottoposti a disatuzione carotidea. In: Monduzzi (ed) XXXVI Congresso Nazionale della Società Italieana di Neurochirurgia. Maratea, pp 393–399

Coates DP, Monk CR, Prys-Roberts C, Turtle M (1987) Hemodynamic effects of infusion of the emulsion formulation of propofol during nitrous oxide anaesthesia in humans. Anesth Analg 66:64–70

Forster A, Judge O, Morel D (1982) Effects of midazolam on cerebral blood flow in human volunteers. Anesthesiology 56:453–455

Giffin P, Cottrell JE, Shwiry B, Hartung J, Epstein J, Lim K (1984) Intracranial pressure, mean arterial pressure and heart rate following midazolam or thiopental in humans with brain tumours. Anesthesiology 60:491–494

Hartung HJ (1987) Beeinflussung des intrakraniellen Druckes durch Propofol (Disoprivan). Erste Ergebnisse. Anaesthesist 36:66–68

Massei R, Baratta P, Beretta L, De Silva E, Tomei G, Gaini SM, Rampini B (1985) Variazioni della pressione intracranica durante induzione con midazolam. Minerva Anestesiol 51:537–542

McCollum JSC, Dundee JW (1986) Comparison of induction characteristics of four intravenous anaesthetic agents. Anaesthesia 41:995–1000

McDowall DG, Morris PJ, Dearden NM, Hashiba M, Gilsanz S (1985) Propofol on cerebral blood flow and intracranial pressure. Abstract, 6th international symposium on intracranial pressure, 9–13 June 1985. Glasgow, Scotland

Milde LN, Milde JH, Michenfelder JD (1985) Cerebral functional, metabolic and hemodynamic effects of etomidate in dogs. Anesthesiology 63:371–377

Parma A, Cristofori G, Massei R, Cenzato M, Sironi VA, Giuliani R, Trazzi R (1988) Propofol for induction and maintenance by continuous infusion of anaesthesia in disk herniation. Submitted to Anesth Analg

Ravussin P, Guinard JP, Ralley F, Thorin D (1988) Effect of Propofol on cerebrospinal fluid pressure and cerebral perfusion pressure in patients undergoing craniotomy. Anaesthesia [Suppl] 43:37–41

Ringelstein EB (1986) Transcranial doppler monitoring. In: Aaslid R (ed) Transcranial Doppler sonography. Springer, Wien New York, pp 147–163

Shapiro HM, Galindo A, Wyte SR, Harris AB (1973) Rapid intraoperative reduction of intra-cranial pressure with thiopentone. Br J Anaesth 45:1057–1062

Siani C, Zattoni J, Verardo T, Dolcini G, Balestrero MA, Santini M, Della Rocca M (1986) Risposta pressoria intracranica ed emodinamica sistemica a 0.35, 0.80 e 2.5 mg/kg ev di Diprivan in pazienti neurochirurgici coscienti e normoventilati. Abstract, III Riunione Italo-Francese di Neuroanestesia e Rianimazione, Capri 16–17, Maggio 1986

Stephan H, Sonntag H, Schenk HD, Kohlhausen S (1987) Einfluß von Disoprivan (Propofol) auf die Durchblutung und den Sauerstoffverbrauch des Gehirns und die CO_2-Reaktivität der Hirngefäße beim Menschen. Anaesthesist 36:60–65

Zattoni J, Siani C, Rossi A, Campora D, Bozzo N, Guiducci G, Mescola P (1986) Effetti pressori intracranici e arteriosi sistemici di 0.80 mg/kg di Diprivan e di 1.6 mg/kg di thiopentene ev in pazienti neurochirurgici. Abstract, III Riunione Italo-Francese di Neuroanestesia e Riani-mazione, Capri 16–17, Maggio 1986

Zattoni J, Siani C, Rossi A, Balestrero MA, Ardizzone G, Rivano C (1988) Propofol by continuous infusion for anaesthesia in major neurosurgery. Anaesthesia [Suppl] 43:Sum-maries

Impact of Sufentanil on ICP in Patients with Brain Tumors

C. Long, N. Shah, W. Marx, E. Arbit, J.H. Galicich, and R. Bedford

Departments of Anesthesiology and Neurological Surgery, Memorial Sloan-Kettering Cancer Center, Cornell University Medical College, New York City, New York 10021 (USA)

Introduction

Most opioid anesthetics have been shown to have negligible or salutary effects on ICP as long as hypercarbia is avoided (Dubois 1987, Shupak and Har 1985). Accordingly, narcotic-based anesthetic techniques combined with hyperventilation are often regarded as the standard for operations on patients with brain tumors and other space-occupying lesions. Recently, however, a canine study has documented that Sufentanil causes profound increases in cerebral blood flow (CBF) without evidence of an increase in cerebral metabolic rate for oxygen. The authors concluded that Sufentanil was acting as a cerebral vasodilator and that it may be contraindicated in patients with compromised intracranial compliance (Milde and Milde 1987). Because of the importance of these observations in clinical practice, we initiated the following study to examine the effects of Sufentanil on CSF pressure in well-compensated patients with brain tumors.

Methods

The subjects were 10 adult patients undergoing elective excision of supratentorial tumors. All were awake and cooperative preoperatively. General anesthesia was induced with a thiopental-N_2O-vecuronium sequence and mechanical ventilation was instituted to maintain a constant end-tidal CO_2 tension. With the patients in lateral decubitus position, a lumbar 18 gauge spinal needle was inserted into the subarachnoid space and CSF pressure was continuously monitored via a calibrated transducer referenced to the midline. Mean arterial pressure was recorded via a radial artery catheter, and cerebral perfusion pressure (CPP) was calculated by subtracting CSF pressure from mean arterial pressure. After obtaining control CSF pressure, hemodynamic values and blood gas tensions (mean $PaCO_2$ = 35.2 mm Hg ± 1.5 S.E.), the level of anesthesia was deepened with a bolus injection of Sufentanil, 1 µg/kg, IV. CSF pressure and hemodynamic parameters then were recorded for 10 minutes. Throughout the study period external sensory stimuli were carefully avoided.

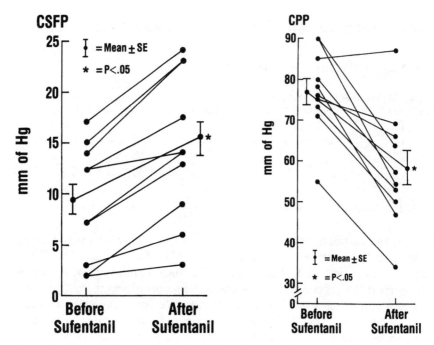

Fig. 1. Baseline CSFP and CPP during N_2O-O_2 vecuronium anesthesia and the peak values recorded in response to Sufentanil 1 µg/kg IV during the 10 minute observation period

Results

The peak changes recorded for each individual during the 10-minute observation period are summarized in Fig. 1. We observed a mean CSF pressure increase of 58%, and a mean decrease in CPP of 25%, both being significant at the $P < .05$ level

Discussion and Conclusion

We believe these clinical findings are compatible with the results of the canine study described above. The fact that ICP increases even as arterial pressure is decreasing suggests that Sufentanil acts as a cerebral vasodilator in humans. Although more vigorous hyperventilation or concomitant administration of agents known to reduce ICP might ameliorate the impact of Sufentanil, the efficacy of these maneuvers in this situation remains unknown at this time.

In contrast to the results of this study, it has been our observation that Fentanyl, when given in combination with N_2O according to the same protocol, has no impact on CSF pressure in patients with brain tumors. Because of the striking difference in response between Fentanyl and Sufentanil, we can only conclude that: 1) Sufentanil probably should be avoided in patients with known or suspected compromised intracranial compliance, and 2) that Fentanyl should remain as one of the mainstays of anesthetic management in this situation.

References

Dubois M (1987) Pharmacokinetics of alfentanil continuous infusion in neurosurgical patients. Anesth Analg 66:544

Milde LN, Milde JH (1987) The cerebral hemodynamic and metabolic effects of Sufentanil in dogs. Anesthesiology 67:A570

Shupak RC, Har JR (1985) Comparison between high-dose Sufentanil-oxygen and fentanyl-oxygen for neuroanesthesia. Br J Anaesth 57:375

Effects of Antihypertensive Drugs on Intracranial Hypertension

S. Hirose, Y. Handa, M. Hayashi, N. Shirasaki, H. Kobayashi, and H. Kawano

Department of Neurosurgery, Fukui Medical School, Matsuoka-cho, Yoshida-gun,
Fukui 910-11 (Japan)

Systemic hypertension is frequently observed in patients with cerebrovascular
disease, such as hypertensive intracerebral hemorrhage and subarachnoid hemorrhage, which is often associated with intracranial hypertension. Continuing systemic hypertension might not only augment the risk of rebleeding but also might
increase the blood flow and blood volume, resulting in more marked increase in
intracranial hypertension. On the other hand, it has been reported that some
antihypertensive drugs can produce an increase in intracranial pressure (ICP). In
this study, we examined the effects of some antihypertensive agents that are
commonly used in neurosurgical practice, on systemic arterial blood pressure
(ABP), ICP and cerebral perfusion pressure (CPP) in patients with both increased
ICP and systemic hypertension, and attempted to clarify the risks and benefits of
these agents when used in patients with raised ICP.

Materials and Methods

Thirty-eight patients were studied: 22 patients with hypertensive intracerebral
hemorrhage and 16 with subarachnoid hemorrhage due to rupture of intracranial
aneurysm. The ICP was recorded with an indwelling ventricular catheter connected with a pressure transducer. The ABP was recorded from a catheter inserted
into the femoral artery or the dorsalis pedis artery. The CPP was determined as
the difference between the APB and the ICP. Patients were assigned to two groups
on the basis of their mean ICP. Group I comprised 20 patients with a mean ICP
of 20 to 40 mm Hg (moderately increased ICP group), and group II consisted of
18 patients with a mean ICP of more than 40 mm Hg (severely increased ICP
group). The effect of following antihypertensive drugs on ABP, ICP and CPP
were studied; nifedipine, chlorpromazine, reserpine, furosemide and thiopental.
Nifedipine (20 mg) was administered sublingually, chlorpromazine (20 mg) and
reserpine (2 mg) intramuscularly, and furosemide (20 mg) and thiopental
(20 mg/kg) intravenously. The mean values of ABP, ICP and CPP in both groups
in each study were calculated every 20 minutes after administration of drugs to
180 minutes and compared to the mean values before drug administration.

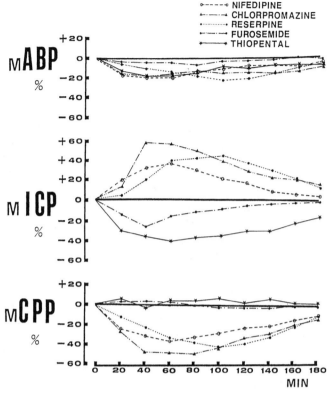

Fig. 1. Changes in mean arterial blood pressure (*mABP*), mean intracranial pressure (*mICP*) and cerebral perfusion pressure (*mCPP*) after administration of antihypertensive drugs in group II (severely increased ICP group). *Ordinate:* mean increases in mABP, mICP and mCPP compared with values observed before drug administration. The values are expressed as percentages of those before drug administration

Results (Fig. 1)

Administration of nifedipine, chlorpromazine and reserpine reduced the mean ABP by 18–20% in both groups ($p < 0.05$ in each). In group I, these agents raised the mean ICP by 10–35% and decreased the mean CPP by 20–32% ($p < 0.01$ for both), whereas in group II these agents more markedly increased the mean ICP by 38–64% and decreased the mean CPP by 40–54% ($p < 0.01$ for both). Furosemide produced no significant ($p < 0.05$) reduction in mean ABP, but a slight reduction in the mean ICP in each group. Thiopental reduced both mean ABP and ICP in both groups. The effect on ICP was pronounced in group II, in which mean ABP fell by 18% ($p < 0.05$) and mean ICP decreased 50% ($p < 0.01$), whereas in group I mean ABP was reduced by 16% and mean ICP dropped 23% ($p < 0.05$ in each). The CPP did not change from the preadministration value, because mean ABP and ICP showed parallel decrease.

Discussion

Nifedipine, which is one of the calcium channel blockers, and chlorpromazine and reserpine acting as the alpha-adrenergic blocker are described to have not only systemic vasodilating action, but also potential vasodilating action on the cerebral blood vessels (Giffin et al. 1983). In this study, it is suspected that the increase in ICP caused by these vasodilating drugs was produced by increase of the cerebral blood volume. The more marked increase in ICP in group II than in group I was thought to be caused by the greater reduction of the compliance in the cranial cavity in the severely increased ICP group. This rise in ICP by these drugs is suspected to create the potential risk of herniation as claimed by the previous report (Bauer et al. 1987). It is believed that barbiturates can produce general depression of the central nervous system and also decreases ICP. The decrease in ICP is thought to be caused by the reduction of cerebral blood volume by direct vasoconstrictive action and decrease of the cerebral metabolic demand. Hayashi et al. (1987) suggested that the reduction of ICP might result from alleviation of the cerebral vasomotor instability by depression of the medullary vasomotor center. In this study, administration of thiopental caused a parallel decrease in ICP and ABP, the decrease in ICP was more pronounced in the severely increased ICP group. These results suggest that barbiturates are preferable to agents with calcium channel and alpha-adrenergic blocking actions in the treatment of systemic hypertension in patients with intracranial hypertension, especially when the increase in ICP is severe and compliance in the intracranial cavity becomes fairly small.

References

Bauer JH, Reams GP (1987) The role of calcium entry blockers in hypertensive emergencies. Circulation [Suppl V] 75:174–181

Giffin JP, Cottel JE, Hartung J, Shwiry B (1983) Intracranial pressure during nifedipine-induced hypotension. Anesth Analg 62:1078–1080

Hayashi M, Kobayashi H, Kawano H, Handa Y, Kabuto M (1987) The effects of local intraparenchymal pentobarbital on intracranial hypertension following experimental subarachnoid hemorrhage. Anesthesiology 66:758–765

ICP- and IOP-Effects of Deliberate Hypotension Using Urapidil

T. Wallenfang[1], H.J. Hennes[2], J.P. Jantzen[2], and G. Fries[1]

Departments of Neurosurgery[1] and Anaesthesiology[2], Johannes-Gutenberg-University, Medical School, D-6500 Mainz (FRG)

Deliberate hypotension is an accepted method to facilitate certain neurosurgical and intraocular procedures. The rationale is to reduce transmural pressure on arterial vessels and thus to facilitate preparation of cerebrovascular aneurysms and malfunctions – or in ophthalmology to reduce the risk of expulsive bleeding (Jantzen and Earnshaw 1988).

Classical hypotensive agents are known to increase intracranial pressure (ICP) which adversely effects cerebral perfusion pressure (CPP) until the dura is open (Sicking et al. 1986).

We have investigated effects of the new sympatholytic Urapidil (Ebrantil®, Byk Gulden Konstanz, FRG) on hemodynamics, ICP, IOP and pulmonary function.

Methods

Ten German landrace piglets (bw $\bar{x}$ 26 kg [23–29]) were premedicated (azaperone 8 mg/kg i.m.), anesthetized (piritramide; induction: 1 mg/kg i.v.; maintenance: 2 mg/kg/h p. inf.), intubated and instrumented (arterial line, Swan-Ganz catheter, ventricle catheter, anterior chamber cannula). Ventilation was controlled by end tidal capnometry (volume controlled ventilator, 60% N_2O in O_2). Control measurements were performed and repeated when a reduction of mean arterial pressure (MAP) by 50% was achieved or when the maximum dosage of 4 mg/kg was administered. Derived parameters were calculated using standard formulae. Statistical evaluation utilized the t-test.

Results

MAP could be reduced to ≥ 50 mm Hg, irrespective of baseline; indicating that a reduction by 50% was not achieved in all pigs. ICP and IOP did not increase clearly, cardiac output (CO) increased (+15%), systemic vascular resistance (SVR −10%) and central venous pressure (CVP) decreased. In contrast pulmonary artery pressure (PAP +21%) and pulmonary vascular resistance (PVR +24%) increased (Table 1). All measures returned to baseline ≤ 10 min following

Table 1. Results ($\bar{x} \pm$ SD)

	Control	Hypotension
MAP:	87.2±19	77.7±21
ICP:	14.1±4.7	15.4±6.0
Elastance:	17.2±8.7	16.0±5.0
CPP:	73.1±22	64.1±24
IOP:	14.7±4.4	15.3±3.5
PAP:	19.8±3.9	24.0±6.4
CVP:	8.4±2.7	8.0±2.2
PCWP:	7.7±2.5	8.1±1.3
SVR:	2012±515	1823±543
PVR:	326±70	406±152
CO:	3.00±0.2	3.44±0.6
HR:	104±32	105±17
etpCO$_2$:	4.5±0.4	4.8±0.6
Pulmonary		
– compliance	20±7.1	20±8.2
– resistance	13.5±7.8	14.7±8.4
S$\bar{v}$O$_2$	56.6±11	60.6±11
SaO$_2$	98.1±1.4	97.8±1.1

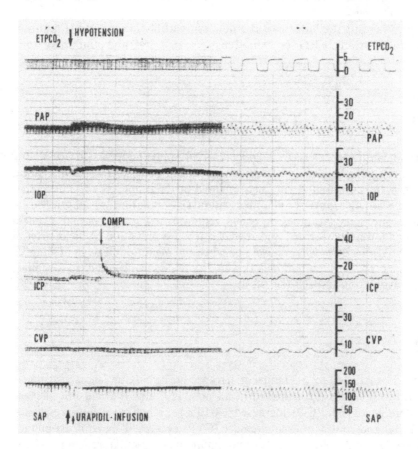

Fig. 1. Hypotension using Urapidil-infusion

534

discontinuation of Urapidil infusion. No undesired degree of hypotension and no compensatory hypertension were observed.

Conclusion

Urapidil reduces MAP (but not PAP) when administered at a dosage of 2–4 mg/kg to anesthesized pigs (Fig. 1). Myocardial performance is improved, pulmonary function is not affected. Arterial hypotension is short-lived, easily controlled and not associated with a rise in ICP or IOP. Urapidil appears to be a suitable agent when moderate and short lasting arterial hypotension is indicated and when an increase in ICP/IOP (or uncontrolled hypotension) are to be avoided. This could apply to patients with brain injury and intracerebral hemorrhage (Wallenfang et al. 1988) that are at risk of hypertension.

References

Jantzen JP, Earnshaw G (1988) Effects of anesthetic agents and muscle relaxants on intraocular pressure. Semin Anesth 7:67
Sicking K, Puchstein C, van Aken H (1986) Loweing of elevated blood pressure with urapidil – Influence on cerebral perfusion. Anasth Intensivther Notfallmed 27:147
Wallenfang T, Fries G, Jantzen JP, Bayer J, Trautmann F (1988) Pathomechanism of brain oedema in experimental intracerebral mass hemorrhage. Acta Neurochir (Wien) [Suppl] 43 (in press)

No Effect on ICP of ACE-Inhibition During Induced Hypotension

J.F. Schmidt, A.R. Andersen, F. Gjerris, and O.B. Paulson

Department of Neurosurgery and Neurology, Rigshospitalet, University of Copenhagen, DK-2100 Copenhagen (Denmark)

Introduction

Experimental studies in rats have demonstrated that the angiotensin converting enzyme (ACE) inhibitor Captopril shifts the lower and upper limits of autoregulation of cerebral blood flow (CBF) towards lower blood pressure levels (Barry et al. 1984). Studies in patients with severe cardiac failure, hypertension and normal volunteers suggest a similar effect in man (Paulson et al. 1988). The present study was undertaken in order to further evaluate the effect of Captopril on cerebral autoregulation, the intracranial pressure (ICP) and the cerebral perfusion pressure.

Methods

Eight patients with normal pressure hydrocephalus (24 to 77 years) were studied. The resting *mean arterial blood pressure* (MAP) was 100 mm Hg (65–131 mm Hg) and the *intracranial pressure* was 10 mm Hg (4–13 mm Hg). ICP was continuously measured intraventricularly during the study. *Regional cerebral blood flow* (rCBF) was measured by xenon-133 inhalation and single photon emission computerized tomography (SPECT) using TOMOMATIC 64. The rCBF was measured at normal and at low MAP. *Global CBF* was in addition estimated from the reciprocal arterio-venous oxygen difference of the brain. All CBF values were corrected for changes in $PaCO_2$ with 4% pr. mm Hg (Olesen et al. 1971). The MAP was measured continuously intra-arterially. MAP was lowered stepwise by approximately 40 mm Hg using a combination of ganglion blockade (trimetaphane-camsylate, Arfonad, Roche) and vacuum application on the lower abdomen and the legs. MAP was increased approx. 35 mm Hg by norepinephrine. Hypo- and hypertension was induced in a control period and 1 hour after 50 mg Captopril perorally.

Statistics

To evaluate autoregulation each CBF value was plotted to the corresponding perfusion pressure. The lower limit was calculated on a computer by repeated

Table 1. The lower limit of CBF autoregulation. The influence of 50 mg Captopril

Subject	Perfusion pressure (mm Hg) (MAP − ICP)		
	Before treatment	1 hour after treatment	Difference
NPH 1	89	68	−21
NPH 2	95	79	−16
NPH 3	55	77	22
NPH 4	86	49	−37
NPH 5	105	102	−3
NPH 6	66	51	−15
NPH 7	64	59	−5
NPH 8	78	53	−25

The shift in the lower limit (mean: −12 mm Hg) is significant $p < 0.05$.

fitting of two regression lines: a horizontal curve was drawn through the mean CBF value of the measurements of the highest two perfusion pressures, and a sloped regression line was drawn through the remaining data sets below the given perfusion pressure. The combined sum of squares for the two lines was calculated. Similar calculations were performed successively by including the next data set one at the time in the horizontal curve and omitting it from the sloped curve. The two lines yielding the minimum sum of squares were chosen as optimal and drawn through the plot. The lower limit of CBF autoregulation was defined as the perfusion pressure at the intersection of the two lines. The Wilcoxon matched-pairs signed ranks test was used for statistical analysis.

Results

In 7 of 8 patients with normal pressure hydrocephalus Captopril lowered the lower limit of cerebral autoregulation of CBF (Table 1). The median shift was significant ($p < 0.05$). No changes in the ICP values were found either after administration of Captopril or under induced hyper- or hypotension. No changes were seen in the regional distribution of CBF during hypotension, but the mean CBF was lower.

Comments

The study supports that the angiotensin-I converting enzyme inhibitor Captopril shifts the lower limit of cerebral autoregulation of CBF towards lower blood pressure levels in man leaving the intracranial pressure unaffected. This shift is possibly mediated by a direct effect on the larger resistance vessels of the cerebral vasculature (Strandgaard and Paulson 1984). Thus patients would be expected to benefit from Captopril at hypotensive anesthesia with respect to CBF.

References

Barry DI, Jarden JO, Paulson OB, Graham DI, Strandgaard S (1984) Cerebrovascular aspects of converting enzyme inhibition. I. Effects of intravenous captopril in spontaneously hypertensive and normotensive rats. J Hypertens 2:589–597

Olesen J, Paulson OB, Lassen NA (1971) Regional cerebral blood flow in man determined by the initial slope of the clearance of intra-arterially injected 133-xenon. Stroke 2:519–540

Paulson OB, Waldemar G, Andersen AR, Barry D, Petersen EV, Schmidt JF, Vorstrup S (1988) Role of angiotensin in cerebral blood flow autoregulation. Circulation (In print)

Strandgaard S, Paulson OB (1984) Cerebral autoregulation. Stroke 15:413–416

Propofol and Intracranial Pressure

B. Mazzarella [1], P. Mastronardi [1], T. Cafiero [1], G. Gargiulo [1], and L. Stella [2]

[1] II. School of Medicine and Surgery, II. Department of Anesthesiology and Reanimation,
[2] Institute of Neurosurgery, 80131 Naples (Italy)

Introduction

Increase in intracranial pressure (ICP) is one of the most common complications in patients with intracranial pathology. In neuroanesthesia the necessity of avoiding drugs which have the potential to increase ICP is well known. This study was designed to evaluate the effects of Propofol (P) on ICP in patients, in comparison with Thiopentone (TPS), in order to assess the suitability of this new intravenous anesthetic agent in neuroanesthesia.

Materials and Methods

Thirty patients with a mean age of 49.5 ± 2.6 years, 19 males and 11 females, ASA class I to III were studied. Patients with severe cardiac or hepatic impairment were not studied. The intracranial pathology was: vascular malformation (8 cases), hydrocephalus (10 cases), and brain tumor (12 cases). Consciousness was present in all cases. The patients were studied in the supine position with the ICP zero reference at the midcranial level. ICP monitoring was performed in all cases for diagnostic or therapeutic indications via a ventricular catheter connected to a pressure transducer (Statham) and recorded on a polygraph. Patients were premedicated with atropine 0.5 mg intravenously and randomly allocated to receive P $2.5 \text{ mg} \cdot \text{kg}^{-1}$ and then TPS $4 \text{ mg} \cdot \text{kg}^{-1}$ or "vice versa". In all cases the successive anesthetic agent was injected after complete recovery from the effects of the other one. BP, ECG and $ETCO_2$ were also monitored. Ventilation was spontaneous or assisted in case of apnea with oxygen 100% by facemask. Based on ICP baseline values patients were divided into two groups: group A with ICP below 15 mm Hg (13 cases) and group B with ICP above 15 mm Hg (17) cases. CPP was calculated as the difference between MAP and ICP. Statistical analysis of data was carried out using Student's t-test.

Results

The results are summarized in the following tables (1 A, B). In Table 1 A the ICP changes after P or TPS administration in normotensive patients (group A) are

Table 1A, B. ICP, MAP and CPP changes after an induction dose of Thiopentone (TPS) or Propofol (P) in patients with ICP baseline value below 15 mm Hg. Group A (13 cases)

A	Baseline value	1 min.	2 min.	5 min.
		after TPS		
ICP mm Hg	11.5±2.0	9.9±1.5	9.0±1.6	9.5±1.7
MAP mm Hg	97.0±2.2	90.3±2.5	88.0±2.3	82.1±2.0
CPP mm Hg	85.1±1.8	80.1±1.9	79.1±1.8	73.0±1.9

B	Baseline value	1 min.	2 min.	5 min.
		after P		
ICP mm Hg	1.5±2.0	8.9±2.1	7.0±1.7*	9.9±1.9
MAP mm Hg	97.0±2.2	81.1±2.5*	80.1±2.2*	80.2±1.7*
CPP mm Hg	85.1±1.8	72.0±2.1	73.0±1.9	70.1±1.8

* $p < 0.05$.

shown. In this group a decrease in ICP was achieved with both drugs, but a significant decrease in ICP at 2 min was obtained only after P administration. A significant reduction in MAP at 1, 2 and 5 min was noted after P injection. No significant changes in CPP were recorded. In Table 1 B the ICP changes in hypertensive patients (group B) are shown. In this group a reduction in ICP was successfully achieved at 1, 2 and 5 min with both drugs. A significant decrease in MAP at 5 min after TPS and at 1, 2 and 5 min after P administration. No significant change in CPP was noted. No significant changes in HR and ECG were recorded in both groups.

Conclusions

An ideal anesthetic for neuroanesthesia must not increase ICP. Of the drugs currently used in clinical anesthesia the volatile agents are potent vasodilators (Drummond et al. 1983, Mazzarella et al. 1985) and can increase ICP. TPS and benzodiazepines do not raise ICP, nevertheless they do not have a pharmacokinetic profile which makes them suitable (Giffin et al. 1984, Mastronardi et al. 1984) for maintenance of anesthesia. P can be used both for (Cafiero et al. 1987, De Grood et al. 1985) induction and maintenance allowing a short and complete recovery from anesthesia. In this study we showed that P has a similar action on ICP compared to TPS and does not affect CPP. In fact, even if CPP decreases, it remains within safe limits. In conclusion, P can be considered a suitable anesthetic in neuroanesthesia.

References

Drummond JC, Todd MM, Toutant SM, Shapiro HM (1983) Brain surface protrusion during enflurane, halothane and isoflurane anesthesia in cats. Anesthesiology 59:288–293

Mazzarella B, Mastronardi P, Cafiero T, Gargiulo G, Frangiosas A, Tommasino C, Stella L, De Chiara A (1985) Isoflurane and intracranial pressure. In: Miller JD, Teasdale GM (eds) Intracranial pressure VI. Springer, New York, pp 732

Giffin JP, Cottrell SE, Shwiry B, Hartung J, Epstein J, Lim K (1984) Intracranial pressure, mean arterial pressure and heart rate following midazolam or thiopental in humans with brain tumors. Anesthesiology 60:491–494

Mastronardi P, Gargiulo G, Cafiero T, Carideo P, Stella L, Falivene R (1984) Effetti sulla pressione intracranica di una nuova benzuodiazapina idroscolubile: il Midazolam. Minerva Anestesiol 50:173–176

Caiero T, Gargiulo G, Mastronardi P, Stella L, De Vivo P (1987) Nuovi anestetici e pressione intracranica. In: Cucciniello B (ed) Attualita in Neurochirurgia. XXXVI Congr Naz Soc Ital. Neurochir, pp 253–257

De Grood PMRM, Ruys AHC, Van Egmond J et al. (1985) Propofol (Diprivan) emulsion for total intravenous anesthesia. Postgrad Med J [Suppl 3] 61:65–69

Session V: Trauma, Hemorrhage and Inflammation

Chairmen: M. Brock, J.T. Hoff, H.M. Eisenberg, P. Reilly, L.F. Marshall, and H.J. Reulen

Biochemical and Biophysical Parameters Under Thiopental Infusion
in Severe Head Injured Patients
F. Della Corte, P. Carducci, A. Clemente, M. Sciarra, R.S. Brada, C. Anile,
and R. Proietti

ICP-Course After Weaning from Artificial Ventilation in Patients
with Severe Brain Trauma
R. Schedl, G. Ittner, R. Jaskulka, F. Kiss, N. Mutz, and W. Thurner

Evaluation of Medical Management for Severe Head Injury
M. Shigemori, T. Moriyama, T. Tokutomi, K. Harada, N. Nishio,
and S. Kuramoto

Intracranial Pressure Changes in Response to Deep Brain Stimulation
in Traumatic Prolonged Coma Patients
T. Tsubokawa, Y. Katayama, and S. Miyazaki

The Use of Narcotics and Hyperventilation for the Treatment of Posttraumatic
Brain Swelling: Theoretical Basis and Clinical Experience
A. Yabuki, M. Maeda, and S. Ishii

Relationship Between Attenuation Changes on CT and Posttraumatic CSF-CKBB-
Activity in Severely Head-Injured Patients
L. Rabow, D. Cook, A. DeSalles, M.H. Lipper, H.D. Gruemer, A. Marmarou,
and D.P. Becker

ICP and Biomechanical Responses After Closed Impact Injury to the Spinal Cord
M. Albin and L. Bunegin

Intracranial Pressure in Experimental Subarachnoid Haemorrhage
N. Dorsch, N. Branston, L. Symon, and J. Jakubowsky

Cortical Tissue Pressure in Injured Brain After Subarachnoid Hemorrhage
J. Chen, S. Hatashita, and J.T. Hoff

Experimental Hypertensive Putaminal Hemorrhage: Part 1. Physiological Study
S. Waga, Y. Morooka, A. Morikawa, M. Sakakura, and T. Kojima

Experimental Hypertensive Putaminal Hemorrhage: Part 2. Pathological Study
S. Waga, H. Tochio, Y. Morooka, A. Morikawa, K. Knamaru, and T. Kojima

Estimation of Intracranial Pressure in Acute Subarachnoid Hemorrhage
Based on CT
C. Kadowaki, M. Hara, M. Numoto, and K. Takeuchi

Intracranial Pressure (ICP) and Cerebral Blood Flow Velocity (BFV) in Patients
with Subarachnoid Hemorrhage Under Treatment with Nimodipine
K.E. Richard, P. Sanker, and M. Alcantara

ICP in the Diagnosis of Acute Hydrocephalus After Aneurysmal Subarachnoid
Hemorrhage
H.-P. Stoiber, J.-P. Castel, P. Dabadie, and H. Loiseau

The Traumatic Coma Data Bank: Monitoring of ICP

A. Marmarou, R. Anderson, J.D. Ward, H.M. Eisenberg, J.A. Jane,
L.F. Marshall, H.F. Young, and the NIH TCDB Writing Group

Richard Reynolds Neurological Research Laboratories, Division of Neurosurgery,
Medical College of Virginia, Richmond, Virginia 23298 (USA)

Aggressive treatment of raised ICP following traumatic injury is considered essential for reduction of mortality and improvement of neurological outcome. Strong evidence in support of this concept has been provided by several investigators (Narayan et al. 1981, Miller et al. 1977, Saul and Ducker 1982). However, the complex and mutually interactive processes triggered by mechanical brain injury precludes a more exact determination of the direct influence of raised ICP upon outcome. The problem is further confounded by the lack of a defined set of ICP descriptors and a well defined treatment threshold which is universally acceptable. Moreover, age and injury severity (GCS), have been shown to be strong predictors of outcome (Choi et al. 1988) and the influence of these parameters places further demand on the numbers of patients required to clearly delineate the relationship of a single factor, such as ICP, upon outcome from severe head injury. As a result of the multifactorial nature of the problem, it is understandable that with limited study populations, some investigators show a close relationship of raised ICP to outcome while others question the emphasis placed on treatment of raised intracranial pressure (Smith et al. 1986, Stuart et al. 1983). The objective of this study was to determine the relationship of ICP to outcome (GOS) utilizing the Traumatic Coma Data Bank (TCDB) where ICP data from relatively large numbers of patients were considered adequate to address this important issue.

Methods

This study is based upon data obtained from 1030 patients admitted to the TCDB. Excluded from analysis were patients who died before resuscitation ($n = 137$); had penetrating missile injury ($n = 167$); were not ICP monitored (319); or had less than 4 hours monitoring ($n = 17$). Of the remaining 658 patients, 428 patients were monitored for a minimum duration of 42 hours, beginning before 18 hours post injury and not ending before 60 hours post injury. For purposes of analysis the 24 hour day was subdivided into 4 hour "blocks". The ICP average bedside monitor reading at the "end hour" was documented at each center and recorded along with the ICP therapy administered during each 4 hour block. The time series of ICP for each patient was summarized in increasing units of time reduction which included four hour blocks, days and the full course of measurement. A stepwise logistic regression procedure was used to select a subset of the candidate ICP descriptors that best explained 6 month GOS outcome. The candidate regressors included: Gender; ICP mean, maximum, variance; TIL mean, maximum, variance; CPP mean, maximum, variance; Presence of intracranial lesion; and Surgery for intracranial lesion. As all patients were aggressively treated for ICP elevation, time spent at elevated pressure was considered to be an important parameter and was also included as a candidate regressor. This was accomplished by determining the "proportion of time greater than X where X was varied from 5 mm Hg to 80 mm Hg in increments of 5 mm Hg". A similar procedure was used for regressing "time at elevated TIL greater than X" as X was varied from 1 to the maximum therapy intensity of 14. As stated earlier, previous reports have indicated that factors of age, admission motor score and admission pupillary response are good predictors of outcome. Therefore, in order to isolate and test for ICP effect, we forced these variables into each putative model considered by the stepwise logistic regression procedure.

Results

Among the candidate regressors, age, admission motor score and admission pupillary response were each highly significant in explaining outcome in this sample ($p < .0001$). Beyond these variables, the proportion of time above 20 mm Hg was next selected and was also highly significant in explaining outcome ($p < .0001$). With these four regressors modeled, no other variable significantly reduced the model residuals. The likelihood ratio statistic for this model was 136.5 (4 degress of freedom; $p < .0001$) indicating that the model was highly significant. The outcome probability as a function of the proportion of time spent

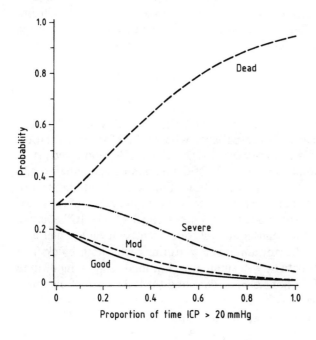

Fig. 1. Outcome vs proportion of time $ICP > 20$ at gms $= 3$, pupil resp $= 1$, and Age $= 30$

above 20 mm Hg is shown in Fig. 1. These probability curves were based on the median values of Glasgow motor score, Age, and Pupillary response for the population under study. At time zero intercept, the outcome probability is governed solely by admission GCS, Age, and pupillary response. As time above 20 mm Hg increases, the probability of a Good or Moderate outcome decreases monotonically and the probability of death as an outcome increases monotonically. Similarly, the probability of severe disability also decreases with increasing time above 20 mm Hg.

Discussion

These data indicate that mortality and morbidity resulting from traumatic injury is strongly related to the time duration of elevated ICP above 20 mm Hg. It is the first data to our knowledge that has isolated the deleterious effect of ICP from other strong prognostic factors such as Age, Admission Motor Score and pupillary response. The critical ICP threshold of 20 mm Hg evolved as a product of regression studies which scanned a wide range of pressure to determine the level of ICP which was maximally related to outcome as indexed by GOS. Interestingly, therapy intensity level did not emerge as a strong prognostic factor. We attribute this to the fact that a uniform management protocol for ICP was not adopted during the course of this study. We would expect that with a uniform ICP treatment protocol for all centers, the TIL time and duration factor correlation would bear a stronger relation to outcome and ICP level as shown in previous studies (Maset et al. 1987). In summary, a study of the TCDB population has revealed that the proportion of time at elevated ICP is a strong predictor of outcome (GOS) and the level of 20 mm Hg has been identified as a critical ICP threshold ($P < .0001$).

Acknowledgements. This research was supported in part by the Grant NO1-NS3-2341 from the National Institutes of Health. Additional facilities and support were provided in part by the Richard Roland Reynolds Neurosurgical Research Laboratories.

References

Choi SC, Ward JD, Becker DP (1983) Chart for outcome prediction in severe head injury. J Neurosurg 59:294–297

Maset L, Marmarou A, Ward JD et al. (1987) Pressure-volume index in head injury. J Neurosurg 67:832–840

Miller JD, Becker DP, Ward JD (1977) Significance of intracranial hypertension in severe head injury. J Neurosurg 47:503–516

Narayan RK, Greenberg RP, Miller JD et al. (1981) Improved confidence of outcome prediction in severe head injury. J Neurosurg 54:751–762

Saul TG, Ducker TB (1982) Effects of intracranial pressure monitoring and aggressive treatment on mortality in severe head injury. J Neurosurg 56:498–503

Smith HP, Kelly DL Jr, McWhorter JW et al. (1986) Comparison of mannitol regiments in patients with severe head injury undergoing intracranial monitoring. J Neurosurg 65:820–824

Stuart GG, Merry GS, Smith JA et al. (1983) Severe head injury managed without intracranial pressure monitoring. J Neurosurg 59:601–605

Head Injury: Outcome in 4 Regional Head Injury Centers – Preliminary Report

L.F. Marshall and TCDB Writing Group

Neurological Surgery H-893, University of California Medical Center, 225 Dickinson Street, San Diego, California 92103 (USA)

On January 1, 1984, four neurosurgical centers, in cooperation with the Biometry and Field Studies Branch of the National Institute of Neurological and Communicative Disorders and Stroke, began a prospective study of traumatic coma. The major objective of this study was to gather a large body of time-oriented data on patients suffering severe head injury. Basic issues such as the importance of prehospital care, the nature and types of complications occurring during the critical-care phase, and overall outcome from head injury in these regions were studied.

Patients admitted to the hospital with a Glasgow Coma Scale (GCS) score of 8 or less, or those who deteriorated to a GCS of 8 or less within 48 hours of admission were included. Intracranial pressure (ICP) monitoring was carried out and a CT scan was obtained for all patients who were felt to be salvageable. In addition to the data which has been collected during the pilot phase (Marshall et al. 1983), data for the full-phase Traumatic Coma Data Bank (TCDB) included information on the ICP course utilizing the concept of therapy intensity level (TIL) as described by Marmarou (Mafet et al. 1987), as well as a narrative summary prepared by the attending neurosurgeon. Patient accrual for the full-phase TCDB ended on September 30, 1987. At that time more than 1000 patients suffering severe head injury had been entered. Outcome is based on the patient's last evaluation (Mean time = 313 days post injury).

Results

Outcome is described for 746 prospectively studied patients who suffered *closed* head injury and who were admitted to the hospital alive. Table 1 demonstrates the types of brain injuries that the patients suffered, and introduces a CT based diagnostic schema. The categories described are new ones and represent a major change in our thinking about "diffuse" injury. The diagnostic categories include: "diffuse brain injury with no visible pathology" (a patient who has a normal scan); "diffuse injury" (a patient with normal cisterns who may have contusions or hemorrhages <25 cc within the parenchyma of the brain): "diffuse swelling" (a patient whose scan indicates absent or compressed cisterns and a shift of 0–5 mm); and "diffuse injury with shift" (a patient who has absent or compressed cisterns and a shift of greater than 5 mm). Mass lesions were categorized in the usual fashion.

Table 2 demonstrates outcome as it relates to these diagnostic categories. Note the progressive increase in mortality as evidence of increasing intracranial volume is demonstrated on the CT scan.

Table 3 illustrates a predictive model utilizing linear regression which analyzes factors important in outcome in patients with diffuse swelling. The major importance of elevated ICP in such patients is striking, and the relatively diminished importance of age and best motor exam support previous observations in the pilot TCDB that patients with absent or compressed cisterns have outcomes relatively independent of motor score and age (Toutant et al. 1984). This strongly suggests that success or failure of treatment of elevated ICP in such patients is the major factor in determining outcome.

Table 4 illustrates the outcome in patients with intracranial hematomas. Outcome appears somewhat improved over other reports. Only 20 of 159 patients with acute subdural hematomas were not unconscious at the scene. Age was a major factor in determining outcome. Patients over 40 with an intracranial hemorrhage fared much more poorly.

Some intercenter differences in outcome were observed. Several analyses were performed using logistic regression to test for these intercenter differences in patients with good or moderate outcomes at last contact (Table 5). Additional covariates utilized in the model were age, length of coma, and length of follow-up. Center differences were still marginally significant ($p < 0.011$), whereas the other factors were highly significant ($p < 0.006$). This indicates that much of the out-

Table 1. Intracranial diagnosis × center (exclude GSW and brain dead)

Table of D4 by center

D4 (Intracranial DIAG)	Center (Center)				Total
Frequency COL PCT	1	2	3	4	
Unknown	8	2	4	3	17
	5.93	0.77	2.15	1.81	
Dif nvp	2	20	18	12	52
	1.48	7.72	9.68	7.23	
Diff inj	26	58	53	40	177
	19.26	22.39	28.49	24.10	
Dif swel	42	46	26	39	153
	31.11	17.76	13.98	23.49	
Dif shif	6	18	4	4	32
	4.44	6.95	2.15	2.41	
Evac mas	44	94	79	59	276
	32.59	36.29	42.47	35.54	
Non-evac	7	18	2	9	36
	5.19	6.95	1.08	5.42	
Brainste	0	3	0	0	3
	0.00	1.16	0.00	0.00	
Total	135	259	186	166	746

Table 2. GOS at discharge × intracranial diagnosis (exclude GSW and brain dead)

Table of D21 by D4

D21 (Glasgow Outcome Scale)	D4 (intracranial DIAG)								Total
Frequency ROW PCT COL PCT	Un-known	Dif nvp	Diff inj	Dif swel	Dif shif	Evac mas	Non-evac	Brainstem	
Good	0	14	15	5	1	14	1	0	50
	0.00	28.00	30.00	10.00	2.00	28.00	2.00	0.00	
	0.00	26.92	8.47	3.27	3.13	5.07	2.78	0.00	
Moderate	1	18	46	20	1	49	3	0	138
	0.72	13.04	33.33	14.49	0.72	35.51	2.17	0.00	
	5.88	34.62	25.99	13.07	3.13	17.75	8.33	0.00	
Severe	0	10	72	41	6	72	7	1	209
	0.00	4.78	34.45	19.62	2.87	34.45	3.35	0.48	
	0.00	19.23	40.68	26.80	18.75	26.09	19.44	33.33	
Vegetat	0	5	20	35	6	34	6	0	106
	0.00	4.72	18.87	33.02	5.66	32.08	5.66	0.00	
	0.00	9.62	11.30	22.88	18.75	12.32	16.67	0.00	
Dead	16	5	24	52	18	107	19	2	243
	6.58	2.06	9.88	21.40	7.41	44.03	7.82	0.82	
	94.12	9.62	13.56	33.99	56.25	38.77	52.78	66.67	
Total	17	52	177	153	32	276	36	3	746

Table 3. Predictors in patients with CT diagnosis of diffuse swelling

$n = 117$	Mortality $= 33\%$	
High ICP	<0.001	0.038
Eye react	<0.001	0.61
Low ICP	0.023	0.93
Best motor	0.51	0.97
Age	0.68	0.97

come differences between centers can be explained by variations in the population, but that there are still some small differences which require further study.

Table 6 demonstrates the relationship between excessive alcohol use and mortality in patients who have reactive pupils following resuscitation, a group which normally has a known favorable outcome.

Table 4. GOS at discharge by type of evacuated mass lesion by age (exclude GSW and brain dead)

Type	GOS	Age		Total
		≤ 40	> 40	
EPI	Good	6	0	6
	Moderate	13	2	15
	Severe	10	0	10
	Vegetat	5	1	6
	Dead	5	3	8
	Total	39	6	45
SUB	Good	4	0	4
	Moderate	14	4	18
	Severe	31	10	41
	Vegetat	12	4	16
	Dead	39	41	80
	Total	100	59	159
INTRA	Good	4	0	4
	Moderate	14	1	15
	Severe	18	3	21
	Vegetat	7	5	12
	Dead	10	9	19
	Total	53	18	71

Total of the observed frequency table is: 275. All cases had complete data for this table

Table 5. GOS at last contact × center (exclude GSW and brain dead)

Table of J19 by center

J19 (last GOS)	Center (Center)				Total
Frequency COL PCT	1	2	3	4	
Good	22	89	36	51	198
	16.30	34.36	19.35	30.72	
Moderate	25	48	32	17	122
	18.52	18.53	17.20	10.24	
Severe	25	30	41	20	116
	18.52	11.58	22.04	12.05	
Vegetat	5	14	7	13	39
	3.70	5.41	3.76	7.83	
Dead	58	78	70	65	271
	42.96	30.12	37.63	39.16	
Total	135	259	186	166	746

Table 6. Alcohol history and outcome in patients with reactive pupils post resuscitation

Hx of alcohol use	% Mortality	n
None	6.7	135
Occasional	2.5	80
Regular	10.0	80
Excessive	24.1	54

Discussion

The present report summarizes the outcome in 746 prospectively studied, consecutively entered patients. The utilization of an entirely new series of diagnostic categories in patients with diffuse injury represents an improvement on previous diagnostic schema. The emphasis on the association of the CT evaluation with progressive elevations of ICP should allow for the earlier recognition of patients who are at higher risk for intracranial hypertension, but in whom the clinical examination would tend to predict a good or a moderate outcome.

The relationship between increasing alcohol use and increasing mortality in patients with a predicted good or moderate outcome is important and deserves further study. Preliminary analyses, comparing for age, mechanism of injury, and complications, either related to neurosurgical procedures or separate, failed to reveal an explanation.

A mortal or vegetative outcome can be expected in approximately 40% of patients with severe head injury cared for in centers comparable to those described here. Given the fact that a large number of patients who had a fatal outcome died within the first few hours, we appear to be approaching the limit in reducing the mortality from head injury. Further therapeutic trials must focus on changing the morbidity of this very common affliction of a modern society.

Acknowledgements. This work was supported by the Pilot Traumatic Coma Data Bank under Contracts NO1-NS-9-2306, 2307, 2308, 2309, 2313, 2340 and the Traumatic Coma Data Bank (TCDB) under Contracts NO1-NS-3-2339, NO1-NS-3-2340, NO1-NS-3-2341, NO1-NS-3-2342, NO1-NS-6-2305 from the National Institute of Neurological and Communicative Disorders and Stroke (NINCDS). The TCDB Manual of Operations which includes the TCDB data forms is available from the National Technical Information Service (NTIS), U.S. Department of Commerce, 5285 Port Royal Road, Springfield, VA 22161 (NTIS Accession No. PB87 228060/AS).

References

Mafet AL, Marmarou A, Ward JD et al. (1987) Pressure volume index in head injury. J Neurosurg 67:832–840

Marshall LF, Becker DP, Bowers SA, Cayard C, Eisenberg H, Gross CR, Grossman RG, Jane JA, Kunitz SC, Rimel R, Tabaddor K, Warren J (1983) The national traumatic coma data bank – Part 1: Design, purpose, goals, and results. J Neurosurg 59:276–284

Toutant SM, Klauber MR, Marshall LF, Toole BM, Bowers SA, Seelig JM, Varnell JB (1984) Absent or compressed basal cisterns on first CT scan: ominous predictors of outcome in severe head injury. J Neurosurg 61:691–694

CT Scan Findings in 683 Patients with Severe (GCS ≤ 8) Closed Head Injury: A Report from the NIH Traumatic Coma Data Bank

H.M. Eisenberg[1], H.E. Gary Jr.[1], B. Turner[1], J.A. Jane[2], A. Marmarou[3], L.F. Marshall[3], H.F. Young[4], and the NIH TCDB Writing Group[3]

[1] Division of Neurosurgery, The University of Texas Medical Branch, Galveston, Texas 77550 (USA); [2] Department of Neurological Surgery, University of Viriginia School of Medicine, Charlottesville, Virginia (USA); [3] Division of Neurosurgery, Medical College of Virginia, Richmond, Virginia (USA); [4] Division of Neurosurgery, University of California San Diego, San Diego, California (USA)

CT scans are available on virtually all patients admitted to the hospital with severe closed head injury, and this method of examination can therefore be considered the least biased way of reviewing the gross pathology in this population of patients. In this report we present our preliminary CT findings on 683 patients admitted to the NIH Traumatic Coma Data Bank, a four-centered prospective study involving the Medical College of Virginia, the University of California San Diego, the University of Texas Medical Branch and the University of Virginia. The study began as a pilot during which data were collected on almost 600 patients (Eisenberg et al. 1983, Marshall et al. 1983 a, Marshall et al. 1983 b). The full phase of the study has now completed its accrual period during which data were entered on an additional 1030 patients. The major admission criterion is a head injury producing a Glasgow Coma Scale score ≤ 8 after basic (nonsurgical) resuscitation or deterioration to this level within 48 hours of injury. While data on 1030 patients have been entered into this study, this report deals with the analysis of the 955 patients whose data had been completely edited at the time of this report (93% of the total data set). The data are undergoing continued analysis and this report must be considered preliminary.

For these analyses, we use data derived only from the initial CT scans. Data from subsequent CT scans will be analyzed for later reports. However, since there were no absolute criteria for obtaining follow-up scans, data from sequential scans must be considered biased. While there may be some question about the clinical validity of very early CT scans, particularly with regard to occurrence of delayed hematomas, delayed mass lesions were very uncommon in this series, involving less than 5% of cases. The CT scans were analyzed using methodology developed and tested for the pilot phase and revised for the full phase of the study. Inter-observer reliability was continuously evaluated among the centers. Further, only designated readers, usually one per center, abstracted the data from the CT scans.

The CT scans were evaluated according to many features including the quality of the CT scan; whether contrast agents were used; the volume of high and/or mixed density mass lesions; the location of intraparenchymal mass lesions; the position of midline structures; the size of the lateral ventricles; the condition of the mesencephalic cisterns; the presence of blood in the ventricles and in the sub-arachnoid spaces; and the presence of atrophy. The volume of an intraparen-chymal or extraaxial mass lesions was estimated by measuring the area of high or mixed density abnormalities (contusions or hematomas) for each contiguous scan slice; multiplying the area by the height of the slice (usually 10 mm) and then summing the volumes for the contiguous slices. We recognize that this method overestimates volume, and that more accurate estimates might have been achieved by using formulas that smooth out the sides (the height) of the lesion. However, we opted for simplicity and believe it unlikely that a more complex method would have contributed importantly to the clinical significance of the findings. The volume of hypodense tissue (edema) surrounding the high or mixed density areas was calculated separately. We did not, however, measure purely hypodense lesions. We believe that large hypodense lesions without contusions or hematoma are uncommon in the first few hours after injury. The volumes of lesions (high or mixed density) estimated at less than 15 cc were not recorded, and these were considered as "small lesions". Volumes greater than 15 cc were consid-ered potentially operable and were classified as "large lesions". We recognize that this classification is arbitrary and that clearly some of the large lesions were not removed. Nonetheless, our goal was to capture as much information as possible about mass lesions without making the task impossibly labor intensive. The locations of both small and large intraparenchymal mass lesions were classified according to site: frontal, fronto-temporal, temporal, temporo-parietal, parietal and occipital.

The patients were divided according to the following mutually exclusive groups:

1) Normal CT Scan – the CT scans were totally normal.
2) Mass Effect – midline shift > 3 mm and/or the presence of a large mass lesion (high or mixed density abnormality > 15 cc). This group was then subdivided according to whether the mesencephalic cisterns were abnormal or normal.
3) Diffuse Swelling – small lateral ventricles and/or absent or compressed mesen-cephalic cisterns. These patients did not have features of mass effect; that is, their midline structures were within 3 mm of the midpoint of the skull and no "large lesions" (> 15 cc) were present.
4) Other Abnormalities.

Of the 955 patients whose data were available and edited at the time of this report, 272 were excluded from this analysis for the following reasons: 1) dead on arrival to ER ($n = 131$); 2) gunshot wound ($n = 109$); and 3) no CT scan ($n = 32$), leaving 683 initial CT scans for these analyses.

Only 42 (6%) patients had normal CT scans. It should not be surprising that the risk of dying was significantly less in this subset than in the group as a whole. What is more interesting perhaps is that the risk of dying for the 21% of patients classified as "Other Abnormalities" is similar to that for the "Normal CT Scan" group. This leads us to suggest that some findings seen on initial scans, such as the presence of "small lesions" and blood in the ventricles or subarachnoid space, do not predict mortality. The risk of dying was significantly greater for the group categorized as "Mass Effect" than for the group "Diffuse Swelling". It was noted, however, that those patients classified as "Mass Effect" were more likely to have absent or compressed mesencephalic cisterns than those classified as "Diffuse Swelling". After further classifying these two groups of patients as having either normal or compressed-absent cisterns, we found that mortality was the same for those with mass effect and those with diffuse swelling within each of the two cistern categories. Furthermore, patients with absent or compressed cisterns were approximately three times as likely to die as those with normal cisterns for both the "Mass Effect" and "Diffuse Swelling" groups. Despite the important predictive power of abnormal cisterns, the presence of small ventricles clearly contributed to the prediction of mortality in the "Diffuse Swelling" group so that patients with both abnormalities were more likely to die than those with only abnormal cisterns. When the individual features used to categorize the group defined as "Mass Effect" were studied separately, both the volume of a mass and the degree of shift were associated with increased risk of dying.

Of the CT features that are predictive of early elevations of intracranial pressure here defined as > 20 mm Hg during the first 72 hours, the volume of high and/or mixed density lesions, the degree of midline shift and the status of the mesencephalic cisterns were all statistically significant ($p < .01$) in a model that included all of the features. The volume of the edematous tissue surrounding a mass lesion, however, did not have predictive value. Lastly, we found that elevated ICP (> 20 mm Hg) after removal of either an intraparenchymal or extra-axial mass lesion was common and seemed unrelated to the size of the lesion that prompted the operation. This finding then supports the validity of monitoring intracranial pressure after removal of lesions in patients initially comatose.

Acknowledgements. This work was supported by the Traumatic Coma Data Bank (TCDB) under Contracts NO1 NS 3-2339, NO1 NS 3-2340, NO1 NS 3-2341, NO1 NS 3-2342, NO1 NS 6-2305 from the National Institute of Neurological and Communicative Disorders and Stroke (NINCDS). The TCDB Manual of Operations which includes the TCDB data forms is available from the National Technical Information Service (NTIS), U.S. Department of Commerce, 5285 Port Royal Road, Springfield, VA 22161 (NTIS Accession No. PB87 228060/AS). We are grateful to Liz Zindler for assistance in manuscript preparation.

References

Eisenberg HM, Cayard C, Papanicolaou AC, Weiner RL et al. (1983) The effects of three potentially preventable complications on outcome after severe closed head injury. In: The Vth International Symposium on Intracranial Pressure. Springer, Berlin Heidelberg New York, Chapter 93, pp 549–553

Marshall LF, Becker DP, Bowers SA, Cayard C, Eisenberg HM et al. (1983a) The national traumatic coma data bank. Part 1: Design, purpose, goals, and results. J Neurosurg 59: 276–284

Marshall LF, Toole BM, Bowers SA (1983b) The national traumatic coma data bank. Part 2: Patients who talk and deteriorate: Implications for treatment. J Neurosurg 59:285–288

Brain Swelling in Fatal Head Injuries

G.M. Teasdale[1], D.I. Graham[2], and A. Lawrence[1]

[1] University Department of Neurosurgery; [2] University Department of Neuropathology,
Institute of Neurological Sciences, Southern General Hospital, Glasgow (UK)

Introduction

Brain swelling is considered to be common in severe head injuries and is the focus of much intensive management (Bruce et al. 1978, Snook et al. 1984, Obrist et al. 1984). Brain swelling however, can be simply a reaction to brain damage and its true frequency, causes, and significance remain in doubt. We have analysed data from a series of fatal cases, each subjected to a full neuropathological study. Our aims were to discover the incidence of brain swelling and to relate its occurrence to features of primary damage and to other secondary complications such as hypoxia and raised intracranial pressure.

Methods

During the 15 year period 1968–1982 a full necropsy, including comprehensive histological examination, was performed on 434 non missile head injured patients who had been treated in the Regional Neurosurgical Unit in Glasgow. The series was not consecutive, the majority of patients being drawn from 1968–1972 and 1981–1982, during which time 80–85% of fatal cases were examined. There were 342 males (79%) and 92 females (21%). Their ages ranged between 3 months and 89 years with a mean of 38 years; 87 (20%) were children < 14 years old. The median survival was 4–7 days and ranged from 2 hours to 14 years. 241 (55%) of injuries were due to a road traffic accident. Details of the neuropathological techniques have been reported previously (Adams et al. 1980). In the present study, the occurrence of three features was analysed: a) ischaemic brain damage as determined by the finding of either diffuse cortical change or focal ischaemic damage either in an arterial territory, or in the boundary zones between arterial territories, the basal ganglia or the hippocampus (Graham et al. 1978). b) Pressure necrosis in the parahippocampal gyrus was taken as an index that intracranial pressure (ICP) had been raised during life (Adams and Graham et al. 1976, Graham DI 1987). c) Brain swelling was graded as unilateral when a space-occupying effect resulted in enlargement of part or all of a cerebral hemisphere, usually in association with shift in the midline; bilateral swelling was determined from assessment of enlargement of both hemispheres with reduction of ventricular size out of proportion to the patient's age. In the detection of

Eds.: J. T. Hoff and A. L. Betz

swelling account was taken of post mortem changes (Sarwar and McCormick 1978). When brain swelling was present, the pathologist determined if it could be related to cerebral contusions, to hypoxic/ischaemic lesions, to an intracranial haematoma or to other causes.

Results

Frequency of Swelling. Brain swelling was detected in 218 cases (50%). It was more commonly unilateral (123) cases than bilateral (95 cases). Brain swelling was present in 61% of cases dying within a week of injury and in 23% of later deaths.

Association of Swelling with Features of Primary Damage

Table 1 shows that cerebral contusions were detected in more than 90% of cases, irrespective of the presence or absence of swelling. An intracranial haematoma was common in patients with unilateral brain swelling but was also found in almost half the cases with no swelling even in those dying in the first week.

The classical features of severe diffuse axonal shearing (DAI) injury were found in a minority of cases and commonly were found without bilateral swelling. Of the deaths in the first week 45% of cases with DAI did not have swelling, and after this period none with DAI had bilateral swelling.

Secondary Damage

Evidence of either hypoxic ischaemic damage (378, 87% of cases) or of raised intracranial pressure (324, 79% of cases) was found more commonly than brain swelling. Evidence of raised ICP was found in 60% of patients without swelling

Table 1. Occurrence of brain swelling and features of brain damage in 434 fatal head injuries

	Brain swelling			p value
	Absent $n=218$	Unilateral $n=123$	Bilateral $n=95$	
Primary lesions				
Contusions	196 (90%)	120 (98%)	91 (96%)	$0.025 < p < 0.05$
Diffuse axonal jnjury	55 (25%)	10 (8%)	17 (18%)	$p < 0.001$
Intracranial haematoma	105 (48%)	91 (74%)	21 (22%)	$p < 0.001$
Secondary damage				
Hypoxia/ischaemia	180 (83%)	14 (93%)	84 (88%)	$0.25 < p < 0.05$
Raised ICP	130 (60%)	114 (93%)	80 (84%)	$p < 0.001$

Table 2. Factors judged by neuropathologist to be responsible for brain swelling

	Brain swelling	
	Unilateral	Bilateral
Total	173	95
Contusions/Haematoma	74 (60%)	19 (20%)
Hypoxia/Ischaemia	13 (11%)	30 (32%)
Combination of lesions	34 (28%)	19 (20%)
Other/unknown	–	25 (27%)

but was more common in patients with swelling, especially unilateral. Hypoxia occurred in more than 80% of cases with or without brain swelling. Brain swelling alone was an extremely uncommon finding: 2 cases in 310 first week deaths.

Causes of Brain Swelling (Table 2)

In the great majority of cases in which brain swelling was detected, the neuropathologist was able to identify the cause. Of the small number of cases in whom it was not possible to identify a causitive lesion, most were children and most were judged to have sustained a significant primary injury. There was only one patient who had spoken after the injury, and hence did not have diffuse primary damage, but who showed bilateral brain swelling as the principal post mortem feature.

Conclusions

Several points can be deduced from these data. In 40% of a series of cases dying in the first week after injury, death occurred without evidence of brain swelling. By contrast, raised intracranial pressure and hypoxia were common findings in such cases. There was little in these data that supports the concept that diffuse shearing injury commonly interferes with vascular integrity and leads to a specific traumatic oedema; indeed in 40% of cases dying in the first week with severe diffuse axonal shearing, brain swelling was absent. In the majority of cases in which brain swelling was detected, a preceeding cause could be identified. These facts point to the conclusion that brain swelling per se was rarely the primary mechanism of brain damage in these fatally head injured patients. Nevertheless, there remained a small number of fatal cases, one or two per year in a population of 2.7 million, in whom brain swelling appeared to be the major intracranial lesion. Most of these cases were children and had been injured severely from the start. Much more needs to be learned about the mechanisms of such swelling and how it is best managed but the rarity of such cases will hinder systematic study.

References

Adams JH, Graham DI (1976) The relationship between ventricular fluid pressure and the neuropathology of raised intracranial pressure. Neuropathol Appl Neurobiol 2:323–332

Adams JH, Graham DI, Scott G, Parker LS, Doyle D (1980) Brain damage in non-missile head injury. J Clin Pathol 33:1130–1145

Bruce DA, Alavi A, Bilanuk L et al. (1978) Diffuse cerebral swelling following head injury in children: The syndrome of 'malignant brain oedema'. J Neurosurg 48:679–688

Graham DI, Adams JH, Doyle D (1978) Ischaemic brain damage in fatal non-missile head injuries. J Neurol Sci 39:213–234

Graham DI, Lawrence AE, Adams JH et al. (1987) Brain damage in non-missile head injury secondary to high intracranial pressure. Neuropathol Appl Neurobiol 13:209–217

Obrist WD, Langfitt TW, Jaggi JL et al. (1984) Cerebral blood flow and metabolism in comatose patients with acute head injury: relationship to intracranial pressure. J Neurosurg 61:241–253

Sarwar M, McCormick WF (1978) Decrease in ventricular and sulcal size after death. Radiology 124:409–411

Snook JE, Minderhoud JM, Wilminde JT (1984) Delayed deterioration following mild head injury in children. Brain 107:15–36

The Significance of Intracerebral Hematoma Location on the Risk of Tentorial Herniation and Clinical Outcome

B.T. Andrews and L.H. Pitts

Department of Neurological Surgery, University of California at San Francisco and the San Francisco General Hospital, San Francisco, California 94143-0870 (USA)

Introduction

Intracrebral hematomas (ICH) may occur following head trauma (Diaz et al. 1979, Soloniuk et al. 1986), or spontaneously, due to as variety of mechanisms (Ojemann and Heros 1983, Ott et al. 1974, Paillas and Alliez 1973, Ropper and Davis 1980). The clinical presentation of ICH usually includes the sudden onset of headache, focal neurological deficits and depression of the level of conscious- ness (Fisher et al. 1965, Ojemann and Heros 1983, Ott et al. 1974, Paillas and Alliez 1973, Ropper and Davis 1980). A small number of patients with either post-traumatic or spontaneous (Diaz et al. 1979, Fisher et al. 1965, Ojemann and Heros 1983, Ott et al. 1974, Soloniuk et al. 1986). ICH may develop signs of brainstem compression, which markedly worsens the prognosis for recovery (Fisher et al. 1965, Ojemann and Heros 1983, Ott et al. 1974, Soloniuk et al. 1986).

While it is well known that ICH within the cerebellum may rapidly lead to brainstem compression and a poor outcome (Fisher et al. 1965, Ojemann and Heros 1983, Ott et al. 1974, Pozzati et al. 1981), previous reports do not suggest a similar concern toward hematomas in specific supratentorial locations. We have reviewed our series of patients with supratentorial intracerebral hematomas, and determined a high incidence of brainstem compression when the hematoma is localized to the temporal and temporoparietal region (Andrews et al. in press).

Materials and Methods

The records and cranial computerized tomograms (CT scans) of all patients with supratentorial ICH admitted between 1983 and 1987 were reviewed. Those with a major neurological deficit or in coma prior to the development of ICH were excluded to avoid confounding clinical deficits due to direct axonal or brainstem injury, as were those with pathology other than supratentorial ICH localized primarily to a single lobe. CT scans were performed upon admission or at the time of clinical deterioration; ICH volume was estimated on serial axial CT sections, and maximal midline shift was measured and recorded. Surgical evacuation of the hematoma by craniotomy was performed for focal neurological deficit (including

Table 1. Outcome at the time of hospital discharge

	Frontal $(n=18)$	Parieto-occipital $(n=10)$	Temporal $(n=17)$	Temporal with signs of herniation $(n=7)$
Good:	8 (44%)	6 (60%)	3 (18%)*	0 (0%)
Moderately disabled:	3	0	7	2
Severely disabled:	3	0	2	2
Vegetative:	0	0	0	0
Dead:	4 (22%)	4 (22%)	5 (29%)	3 (43%)

* Significantly worse than for the parieto-occipital group: $p < 0.05$.

clinical signs of brainstem compression), or neurological deterioration. Outcome was determined using the Glasgow Outcome Scale (Jennet and Bond 1975) at the time of hospital discharge.

Results

There were 18 patients with hematomas limited to the frontal region, 17 with hematomas in the temporal or temporoparietal region, and 10 with hematomas in the parieto-occipital region. No patient with hematomas in the frontal or parieto-occipital regions developed clinical signs of tentorial herniation on admission or during the later hospital course. In contrast, 3 of 17 patients with hematomas in the temporal or temporoparietal region had signs of herniation at the time of admission, and 4 developed these signs during the subsequent 12 hours; the overall incidence of brainstem compression (41%) was significantly greater than for the other two groups ($p < 0.05$).

The mean hematoma volume for the three groups was no different (frontal 47 ± 28 cc's; occipital 53 ± 26 cc's; temporal 41 ± 21 cc's). No patient with a temporal hematoma smaller than 30 cc's in volume developed signs of brainstem compression; in contrast 7 of 11 (64%) patients with hematomas larger than 30 cc's did develop such signs ($p < 0.05$). There was no correlation between the hematoma size and maximal midline shift among patients with frontal or parieto-occipital hematomas, however, among patients with temporal or temporoparietal hematomas there was strong correlation between the two (correlation coefficient 0.829).

Outcome at the time of hospital discharge is shown in Table 1. Patients with temporal hematomas had a worse outcome than those in the other two groups; no patient with signs of brainstem compression had a good outcome.

Discussion

Patients with intracerebral hematomas of 30 cc's or larger, located in the temporal or temporoparietal region appear to be at much greater risk for anatomical midline shift and the early development of clinical signs of upper brainstem compression than patients with hematomas in the frontal or parieto-occipital lobes. Such patients should be considered for prompt surgical evacuation of these lesions before the development of tentorial herniation, to improve the outcome in these patients.

References

Andrews BT, Chiles BW, Pitts LH (1988) The significance of intracerebral hematoma location on the risk of tentorial herniation and clinical outcome. J Neurosurg (in press)

Diaz FG, Yock DH, Larson D, Rockswold GL (1979) Early diagnosis of delayed posttraumatic intracerebral hematomas. J Neurosurg 50:217–223

Fisher CM, Picard EH, Polak A, Dalal P, Ojemann RG (1965) Acute hypertensive cerebellar hemorrhage: Diagnosis and surgical treatment. J Nerv Ment Dis 140:38–57

Jennett B, Bond M (1975) Assessment of outcome after severe brain damage: A practical scale. Lancet I:480–484

Ojemann RG, Heros RC (1983) Spontaneous brain hemorrhage. Stroke 14:468–475

Ott KH, Kase CS, Ojemann RG, Mohr JP (1974) Cerebellar hemorrhage: Diagnosis and treatment: A review of 56 cases. Arch Neurol 31:160–167

Paillas JE, Alliez B (1973) Surgical treatment of spontaneous intracerebral hemorrhage: Immediate and long-terms results in 250 cases. J Neurosurg 39:145–151

Pozzati E, Piazza G, Padovani R, Gaist G (1981) Neurosurgery 8:102–103

Ropper AH, Davis KR (1980) Lobar cerebral hemorrhages: Acute clinical syndromes in 26 cases. Ann Neurol 8:141–147

Soloniuk D, Pitts LH, Lovely M, Bartkowski HJ (1986) Traumatic intracerebral hematomas: Timing of appearance and indications for operative removal. J Trauma 26:787–793

Outcome After Diffuse Head Injuries and ICP Elevations

B.P. Uzzell [1, 2] and C.A. Dolinskas [3]

[1] Division of Neurosurgery, Hospital of the University of Pennsylvania, Philadelphia, Pennsylvania 19104 (USA) and [2] Present address: Department of Neurology, University of Pittsburgh, 325 Scaife Hall, Pittsburgh, Pennsylvania 15261 (USA); [3] Department of Radiology, Pennsylvania Hospital, Philadelphia, Pennsylvania 19107 (USA)

The effects of ICP elevations on outcome after diffuse lesions after head injury have been ignored until recently. The outcome measure most often used has been the GOS with ratings that are often insensitive to the state of conscious survivors.

In order to obtain a better understanding of outcomes, this study examined: 1) the relationship between six-month postinjury GOS scores and diffuse CT lesions, 2) the relationship between six-month postinjury GOS scores and intracranial hypertension and diffuse CT lesions, and 3) the neuropsychological outcome in conscious survivors of diffuse CT lesions and intracranial hypertension.

Methods

Subjects

A total of 95 consecutively hospitalized head injured patients with DAI and DS CT lesions (Zimmerman et al. 1978 a, b) were included in this study. Fifty-five of these patients who received continuous ICP monitoring were assigned to one of two groups: ICP ≥ 20 mm Hg or ICP < 20 mm Hg. Twenty-four conscious survivors of DAI or DS lesions and the presence or absence of acute ICP elevations received neuropsychological tests within nine months following injury.

Procedure

All patients were hospitalized and intracranial hypertension was treated when necessary with hyperventilation, supplemented by mannitol and pentobarbital infusion. Judgments for a patient's inclusion in either the DAI or DS CT group was based on a review of the entire series of CT scans. GOS ratings were made at six months postinjury, and neuropsychological measurements of intelligence, memory, and learning were completed within nine months postinjury.

Results and Conclusions

A significant difference ($\chi^2 = 15.75$, $p < .01$) between GOS scores and percent of DAI and DS cases was obtained. Poorer outcomes (Deaths 37%, Persistent

Table 1. Neuropsychological measures: results from ICP and CT groups[a]

Measure	ICP groups			CT groups		
	ICP ≥ 20 mm Hg (n=12)	ICP < 20 mm Hg (n=12)	p[b]	DAI (n=12)	DS (n=12)	p[b]
Intelligence						
Full scale IQ	75.1±4.7	91.3±5.8	0.04	81.7±6.0	84.9±5.6	NS
Verbal IQ	82.5±4.8	98.4±5.5	0.04	89.6±5.6	91.3±5.7	NS
Performance IQ	68.8±4.7	83.1±4.8	0.05	73.3±6.4	78.6±4.8	NS
Memory						
Memory quotient	65.8±4.3	80.0±5.0	0.05	70.0±3.8	75.8±7.0	NS
Verbal recall (%)						
Immediate	11.7±3.7	28.5±5.9	0.02	18.2±5.1	22.0±5.8	NS
Delayed	13.3±6.5	36.4±5.9	0.02	18.1±6.0	31.6±8.3	NS
Verbal learning digits correct						
Forward	6.3±0.7	6.5±0.4	NS	6.3±0.7	6.5±0.3	NS
Backward	3.5±0.5	4.2±0.4	NS	3.8±0.4	4.0±0.4	NS
Associate learning						
Easy	9.1±1.4	11.5±1.2	NS	9.0±1.1	11.6±1.5	NS
Hard	2.6±0.9	3.2±1.1	NS	1.4±0.8	4.4±1.0	0.03

[a] Results are means ± SEs; IQ = Intelligence Quotient.
[b] Significance levels from t-tests.

Vegetative States 8%, Severe Disability 16%) occurred more often after DAI lesions, than after DS lesions (Deaths 18%, Persistent Vegetative States 0%, Severe Disability 5%). In contrast, good outcomes (Good Recovery 56%, Moderate Disability 21%) were more frequent after DS lesions, than after DAI lesions (Good Recovery 29%, Moderate Disability 10%).

Differences between GOS scores of patients with and without intracranial hypertension were nonsignificant, suggesting the combination of intracranial hypertension and diffuse lesions did not influence outcomes. However, data trends suggested more Deaths (49%) and fewer Good Recoveries (15%) in patients with acute ICP elevations, than in patients without ICP elevations (Deaths 25% and Good Recovery 31%).

Table 1 shows more intellectual and verbal recall impairments (both immediately and delayed) at the time of the neuropsychological examination in patients with histories of acute intracranial hypertension and diffuse lesions. Such intellectual losses correlate with a diffuse injury, while memory impairments have been associated with hippocampal damage during the initial stages of herniation following raised intracranial pressure (Uzzell et al. 1986).

No neuropsychological differences were obtained between the DAI and DS patients, except for learning hard paired-associate words, which were more difficult for the DAI than for the DS group. These learning deficits suggest the axonal disruption and degeneration of white matter associated with DAI lesions may undermine storage and retrieval processing of new information. Further study is needed to support this conclusion.

Interestingly, reciting increasing lengths of digits both forward and backward (which are included on almost every mental status examination) was performed equally well by both diffuse CT lesion and ICP groups, making this measure nondiagnostic in distinguishing these groups.

References

Uzzell BP, Obrist WD, Dolinskas CA, Langfitt TW (1986) Relationship of acute CBF and ICP findings to neuropsychological outcome in severe head injury. J Neurosurg 65:630–635

Zimmerman RA, Bilaniuk LT, Bruce D, Dolinskas CA, Obrist WD, Kuhl D (1978a) Computed tomography of pediatric head trauma; acute general cerebral swelling. Radiology 126:403–408

Zimmerman RA, Bilaniuk LT, Gennarelli TA (1978b) Computed tomography of shearing injuries of the cerebral white matter. Radiology 127:393–396

ICP in the Elderly Head Injury Population

A.M. Ross, S. Kobayashi, and L.H. Pitts

Department of Neurosurgery, University of California, San Francisco, California 94143 (USA)

Introduction

In 1979, Jennett et al. reported that age and Glasgow Coma Score (GCS) independently influence outcome of head injured patients. Pitts et al. (1980) reported
a linear relationship between ICP measured between 6–24 hours after severe head
injury and outcome. Teasdale (1986) suggests that ICP measurement is useful in
all patients with mass lesions, occult hematoma, postoperative swelling and in
patients with a normal CT scan and any of the following risk factors: an abnormal
motor response, hypotension, or over 40 years old. Although age was not reported, Seelig et al. (1986) found that patients with an $ICP \geq 30$ torr within
72 hours of head injury and were also hypotensive (systolic $BP \leq 90$ mm Hg) had
a mortality rate of 79%. Luerssen et al. (1988) reported that an increasing mortality rate in head injury patients correlated with age in the adult population and
with severity of admission GCS. ICP monitoring in head injured patients has been
studied extensively, but little specific information is available concerning ICP
monitoring in the elderly. This study was done to explore the relationship of ICP
to outcome in the elderly head injured population.

Method

A retrospective review of 1066 cases of patients with significant head injuries was
conducted. Seventeen percent ($n = 181$) of the patients with head injury were over
65. Of these, 63% ($n = 114$) had ICP monitoring. These charts were reviewed and
categorized into 2 groups. Group I ($n = 54$) had frequent peaks of, or a sustained
ICP above 20 mm Hg within the first 96 hours after injury and Group II ($n = 60$)
consistently had an ICP less than 20 mm Hg. The charts were reviewed for admission GCS, cause of head injury, incidence of concurrent multitrauma, initial ICP,
ICP peak values at various times (0–28 days after head injury), results of CT
scans, type of operation and findings, occurrence of reoperation, presence of
shock (systolic blood pressure below 90 mm Hg), presence of apnea, cause of
death, time to death, and outcome at 1, 3, 6, and 12 months after head injury.

Results

Group I comprised 47% of the head injury population over 65 with ICP monitoring and 5% of the total head injury population. Group II comprised 53% of the head injury population over 65 with ICP monitoring and 6% of the total head injured population. The summary of demographic data including etiology of head injury, incidence of concurrent multitrauma (i.e., trauma to limb, chest or trunk) and admission GCS is in Table 1.

The mean of the initial ICP for Group I and II was determined to be 22 and 6 mm Hg, respectively. These values were found to be significantly different ($p < .001$) using a two-tailed t-test. In Group I ($n = 54$), 52% had an initial ICP < 20 mm Hg, 31% had an initial ICP of 20–40 mm Hg, and 17% had an initial ICP > 40 mm Hg. In Group II ($n = 60$), 5% had an initial ICP of 15–20 mm Hg, 18% had an initial ICP of 10–14 mm Hg, 65% had an initial ICP < 10 mm Hg, and 12% had missing data for this variable. At 24 hours, ICP could not be maintained < 20 mm Hg with the use of controlled ventilation and osmotic diuretics in 85% of Group I patients. At 2–3 days, 54% of Group I patients continued to have uncontrolled intracranial hypertension (ICP > 20 mm Hg). A summary of the incidence of ICP monitoring in both groups is included in Table 1.

CT scans were reviewed for presence of herniation, type of mass lesion and brain shift. CT scans were available in 70% of Group I and in 85% of Group II patients. Herniation was present in 21% ($n = 8$) of Group I and in 16% ($n = 8$) of Group II patients with CT scans. The most common CT findings present in order for Group I and Group II observations are: SDH 50% ($n = 19$) and 53% ($n = 27$), ICH 42% ($n = 16$) and 33% ($n = 17$), bilateral lesions (i.e., EDH, SDH and ICH) both 32% ($n = 12$) and 25% ($n = 13$), contusions 16% ($n = 6$) and 20% ($n = 10$), and EDH 8% ($n = 3$) and 2% ($n = 1$), respectively. Brain shift was present in 68% ($n = 26$) of Group I and in 59% ($n = 30$) of Group II patients. Of this, 31% ($n = 8$) of Group I and 20% ($n = 6$) of Group II had persistent shift on serial CT scans. Brain shift data was missing in 30% of Group I and in 18% of Group II patients.

Operation performed and operative findings varied little between groups. *Reoperation* was more common in Group I patients, almost significantly so. In Group I, 22% ($n = 12$) came to reoperation as compared to 8% ($n = 5$) in Group II ($p < .10$). Operations performed were significantly different in the two groups. Eleven patients underwent craniotomy for unilateral mass lesion in Group I, versus 2 patients in Group II ($p < .025$). In Group I, there was 1 V-P shunt placed, and 2 of the 11 patients with craniotomy also underwent lobectomy and 1 of the 11 also had debridement. In Group II, there were 2 craniotomies for hygromas and 1 for abscess. A summary of these findings are included in Table 1.

Presence of shock and episodes of apnea were significantly higher in Group I than in Group II. Systolic BP > 90 mm Hg was present in 59% of Group I patients and in 77% of Group II patients. However, shock was present in 41% ($n = 22$) of Group I and in 15% ($n = 9$) of Group II patients in the first 72 hours after head injury ($p < .005$). Episodes of apnea were present in 13 patients of Group I and in 6 of patients of Group II ($p < .05$).

Table 1. Summary of demographic data

	Group I (n = 54)	Group II (n = 60)
Mean age (years)	77	76
Men/Women (n)	34/20	38/22
Etiology (%)		
Fall	54	58
Pedestrian vs. motor vehicle	24	18
Assault	6	8
Motor vehicle accident	6	3
Gunshot wound	2	3
Other	7	7
Admission GCS (%)		
3–8	54	47
9–11	15	13
12–15	32	40
Initial ICP (mean)	22 mm Hg	6 mm Hg ($p < 0.001$)
ICP monitored (%)		
1 day	98	93
3 days	87	87
7 days	33	33
8–12 days	14	5
Presence of shock (n = 54)	22	9 ($p < 0.005$)
Episodes of apnea (n = 59)	13	6 ($p < 0.05$)
Incidence of multitrauma (n)	10	9
Operations and findings (%)		
Unilateral mass lesion (SDH, EDH, ICH)	50	57
Combined lesions	15	12
Bilateral mass lesions	9	7
Bur hole for ICP	11	9
No operation	2	12
Reoperation	n = 12	n = 5 ($p < 0.10$)
Unilateral mass lesion	n = 11	n = 2 ($p < 0.025$)
V-P shunt	n = 1	
Hygroma		n = 2
Abcess		n = 1

Cause of death and time to death were reviewed for 52 patients in Group I and for 39 patients in Group II. To compare the clinical course of the groups, Group I had a higher mortality rate and earlier time to death, and Group II had more extracranial complications and a later time to death.

Outcome was classified using the Glasgow Outcome Score (GOS). Death was significantly more frequent in Group I than in Group II ($p < .005$). In Group I, 96% were dead by 12 months, 2% were severely disabled, and 2% were lost to follow up. In Group II, GOS at 12 months revealed that 65% were dead, 2% were vegative, 13% had a severe disability, 5% were moderately disabled, 12% had a good recovery, and 3% were lost to follow-up. Outcome data is summarized in Table 2.

Table 2. Outcome at 12 months

Glascow Outcome Score (%)	Group I	Group II
Death	96	65 ($p < 0.005$)
Vegetative		2
Severe disability	2	13
Moderate disability		5
Good recovery		12
Lost to follow up	2	3

Discussion

Many of the variables reviewed were not significantly different between the groups (i.e., age, etiology of injury, admission GCS, days ICP monitored, CT scan findings, incidence of multitrauma, and findings at first operation). We presume that the significantly higher incidence of shock, apnea, and the presence of traumatic lesions at reoperation found in Group I patients adversely elevated ICP. The higher incidence of shock and apnea may be due to the significance of the other injuries. However, on further evaluation, both groups had a similar incidence of multitrauma. The two survivors (1 severely disabled and 1 lost to follow-up at 12 months) in Group I both had an admission GCS of 14 and were younger (68 and 69 years of age) than the mean age.

The long term management of the elderly with elevated intracranial pressure may have dictated the cause of death and time to death. These patients may have been supported less aggressively (i.e., no clinical intervention for infections) or may have been allowed to expire as per family wishes.

Conclusion

The findings in this review confirm that an ICP greater than 20 mm Hg has an adverse affect on outcome. An overall mortality in this review of 80% at 6 months in these elderly patients affirms the adverse affect of age on outcome after head injury.

References

Jennett B, Teasdale GM, Braakman R, Minderhoud J, Heiden J, Kurze T (1979) Prognosis of patients with severe head injury. Neurosurgery 4(4):283–289

Luerssen TG, Klauber MR, Marshall LF (1988) Outcome from head injury related to patient's age – A longitudinal prospective study of adult and pediatric head injury. J Neurosurg 68:409–416

Pitts LH, Kaktis JV, Juster R, Heilbron D (1980) ICP and outcome in patients with severe head injury. In: Shulman K, Marmarou A, Miller JD, Becker DP, Hockwald GM, Brock M (eds) Intracranial pressure IV. Springer, Berlin Heidelberg New York

Seelig JM, Klauber MR, Toole BM, Bowers-Marshall S (1986) Increased ICP and systemic hypotension during the first 72 hours following severe head injury. In: Miller JD, Teasdale GM, Rowan JO, Galbraith SL, Mendelow AD (eds) Intracranial pressure VI. Springer, Berlin Heidelberg New York Tokyo

Teasdale GM, Mendelow AD, Galbraith S (1986) Causes and consequences of raised intracranial pressure in head injuries. In: Miller JD, Teasdale GM, Rowan JO, Galbraith SL, Mendelow AD (eds) Intracranial pressure VI. Springer, Berlin Heidelberg New York Tokyo

Isolated Stimulation of Glycolysis Following Traumatic Brain Injury

B.J. Andersen and A. Marmarou

Richard Reynolds Neurosurgical Research Laboratories, Division of Neurosurgery, Medical College of Virginia, Richmond, Virginia 23298 (USA)

Introduction

Clinical investigators have postulated that head trauma causes cerebral metabolic derangement, as evidenced by the presence of CSF lactate and brain acidosis (DeSalles et al. 1986). Work in our laboratory (Unterberg et al. 1988) reported decreased tissue pH within 15 minutes following trauma that eventually normalizes. Post traumatic tissue acidosis has been reported to correlate tightly with increased brain lactate (McIntosh et al. 1987). We have also found (Inao et al. 1988) increased cerebrospinal fluid and brain tissue lactate at 15 minutes post-trauma. We hypothesized from these studies that the metabolic derangement responsible for cerebral lactic acidosis occurs within minutes of trauma. To investigate this hypothesis, we focused our investigation on the first 15 minutes following trauma and measured global cerebral blood flow, cerebral metabolic rate of oxygen utilization, cerebral metabolic rate of glucose utilization, and performed ^{31}P magnetic resonance spectroscopy in traumatized, ventilated cats. Data was obtained immediately following trauma and serially for the first hour post-trauma.

Materials and Methods

Anesthesia was provided by intravenous α-chloralose (40 mg/kg/8 hours). Animals were paralyzed and artificially ventilated. Once surgical preparation was completed, control measurements of global cerebral blood flow (using microsphere method), arterial oxygen and glucose contents, and sagittal sinus oxygen and glucose contents were made in Group 1 ($n=9$), and control measurements of pH_i, PCr, Pi, and ATP were made using ^{31}P MR spectroscopy in Group 2 ($n=8$). Both groups of animals were then subjected to 3.2 ± 0.1 atmosphere lateral fluid percussion trauma. Following trauma, the parameters described above were obtained in their respective groups at predetermined times for the first 60 minutes post-trauma. After the last measurements were obtained, all animals were sacrificed by lethal injection of potassium chloride. The brains of the animals in Group 1 were then removed and fixed in aldehyde fixatives for 48 hours for cerebral blood flow calculation. The brains of animals in Group 2 were removed and inspected for gross neuropathology.

Results

Cerebral Blood Flow, Oxygen, and Glucose Utilization

Immediately following trauma (5 minutes) there was a 52% increase in global cerebral blood flow (35.3 ± 2.7 to 51.3 ± 8.9 ml/100 g/min, $p < 0.01$) which returned to control values by 15 minutes post-trauma. This is similar to the post-traumatic blood flows reported by DeWitt (DeWitt et al. 1986) and represents pressure passive hyperemia due to traumatic loss of vasoreactivity (Lewelt et al. 1980). The cerebral metabolic rate of oxygen utilization did not vary statistically from the control value of $0.98 \pm .13$ μmoles/g/min during the experiment. However, the cerebral metabolic rate of glucose utilization increased 243% ($0.28 \pm .03$ to $0.96 \pm .19$ μmoles/g/min, $p < 0.001$) as early as 5 minutes post-trauma, then gradually returned to normal by 2 hours post-trauma.

Tissue pH and High Energy Phosphates

Following trauma, intracellular pH dropped from the control value of $7.04 \pm .02$ to $6.89 \pm .05$ ($p < 0.001$) at 30 minutes, then returned to essentially normal values by 90 minutes. The ratio of phosphocreatine to inorganic phosphate (PCr/Pi) was chosen as an indicator of energy stores. The control value for this ratio was $1.52 \pm .28$ and did not change statistically throughout the experiment.

Discussion

These data show that glycolysis is stimulated soon after trauma without a concomitant increase in oxidative phosphorylation. The findings of increased glucose utilization and simultaneous acidosis, coupled with other studies in our laboratory that show brain lactate increasing after similar levels of fluid percussion trauma (Inao et al. 1988), support this conclusion. These data prompted us to ask two basic questions concerning post-traumatic cerebral energy metabolism; why does trauma appear to stimulate only glycolysis, and why does lactate appear in the absence of ischemia?

The explanation for increased glycolysis centers about the energy supply required for membrane pump activity. Many types of cerebral insults, including seizures (Lothman et al. 1975), intracerebral bleeding (Hubschmann and Nathanson 1985), mechanical stimulation (Julian and Goldman 1962), and cerebral (Takahashi et al. 1981, Katayama et al. 1988, Milito et al. 1988) or spinal cord trauma (Young and Koreh 1986) cause membrane depolarization and disruption of ionic concentration gradients. Re-establishment of normal intra-cellular ionic concentrations is mainly accomplished through active, energy dependent ionic pumps located in cellular membranes (Howse et al. 1974, Lewis and Schuette 1975).

It has been reported from various cell types that membrane ionic pumps depend on glycolysis for high energy phosphates whereas oxidative metabolism supplies energy for non-membrane activity (Weiss and Hiltebrand 1985, Benjamin and Verjee 1980, McDonald et al. 1971, Hellstrand et al. 1984, Bricknell and Opie 1978, Davidheiser et al. 1984, Lynch and Paul 1983, Paul et al. 1986). In neural tissue there is also evidence to suggest that there is a similar type of energy compartmentalization. Fast axonal transport appears to depend upon oxidative metabolism (Ochs and Hollingsworth 1971, Kirkpatrick et al. 1972, Ochs 1972 and Smith 1971) and ion pumps appear relatively refractory to hypoxic damage (Milito et al. 1988). Considering this body of evidence, it is reasonable to assume that the immediate post-traumatic increases in glycolysis reflect a specific energy demand caused by intense membrane pump activity needed to restore ionic homeostasis following traumatic depolarization.

As to why lactic acidosis appears during this period of high energy demand, a dissociation between glycolytic production and respiratory consumption of pyruvate must be proposed. Dissociation between the rates of oxygen and glucose uptake have been reported experimentally (Chapman et al. 1977, Sactor et al. 1966) in situations where neither cerebral blood flow (Howse and Duffey 1975) nor oxygen availability (Duckrow et al. 1981) have been shown to be limiting, implying that increased glycolytic flux is not necessarily due to substrate limitation of oxidative phosphorylation. It is suggested that generally increased oxidative and glycolytic metabolism is a physiologic response to situations of high energy demand (Sactor et al. 1966, Howse and Duffey 1975), however, the maximum rate of glycolysis is significantly higher than that of the TCA cycle, perhaps due to transport systems that link glycolysis to the citric acid cycle acting as rate limiting steps (Chapman et al. 1977). This disparity between oxidative and glycolytic flux during maximal stimulation results in the production of surplus pyruvate.

Excessive amounts of pyruvate can be converted to lactate in an effort to maintain glycolytic activity. In the normal state, glycolysis phosphorylates ADP to ATP, metabolizes glucose to pyruvate and reduces NAD^+ to NADH. During periods of high energy demand due to trauma, neither ADP (Sacktor et al. 1966) nor glucose availability are usually limiting (Unterberg et al. 1988, DeSalles et al. 1987). NAD^+ is normally produced by oxidative phosphorylation which resupplies glycolysis with this necessary electron carrier. However, if production of NAD^+ is inadequate, it could limit the rate of glycolysis if it were not for the fact that pyruvate can be converted to lactate by lactate dehydrogenase (E.C. 1.1.1.27) and in the process, convert NADH back to NAD^+. This situation allows glycolysis to continue but produces lactic acid as a by-product (Grootegoed et al. 1986).

We believe that the acidosis seen soon after trauma in our model results from glycolytic output exceeding citric acid cycle input rather than assuming a defect in oxidative phosphorylation. Our reasons for rejecting mitochondrial damage or ischemia as a cause for the uncoupling of the rates of glycolysis and oxidative phosphorylation are two-fold.

First of all, high energy phosphates (PCr/Pi ratio) did not decrease. As we reported in a previous work (Andersen et al. 1988), glycolytic pathways of energy production alone are not adequate to maintain the PCr/Pi ratio in the normal range. Thus, in order for the PCr/Pi ratio to remain constant (as reported), glycolytic production of high energy phosphates must be supplemented by other sources (i.e. oxidative phosphorylation), implying functional mitochondria.

Additionally, Duckrow (Duckrow et al. 1981) reported that following fluid percussion trauma there is a consistent increase in the ratio of oxidized to reduced cytochrome aa_3, demonstrating that this degree of fluid percussion trauma does not produce a period of cerebral hypoxia in the post-traumatic period, and suggesting that trauma of this type does not damage mitochondrial energy production.

To summarize, we observed increased glycolysis and consequent cerebral acidosis following trauma in non-ischemic, normoxic animals. We believe this is a result of stimulation of glycolysis without a commensurate increase in the rate of oxidative phosphorylation. This condition allows lactate, a glycolytic endproduct and citric acid cycle precursor, to accumulate in spite of adequate global cerebral blood flow, normal oxygenation, and non-damaged mitochondria. We believe the cause for this marked increase in glycolytic flux is an increased demand for high energy phosphate compounds by membrane pumps in order to re-establish cellular ionic homeostasis that is disturbed following trauma. Disparity between the rates of glycolytic and oxidative energy metabolism have not been previously reported following fluid percussion trauma and may complicate the interpretation of increased brain lactate levels in traumatic head injury.

Acknowledgements. Supported by the Richard Roland Reynolds Neurosurgical Research Fund and NIH Grants 5RO1NS19235 and 2RO1NS12587.

References

Andersen BJ, Unterberg AW, Clarke GD, Marmarou A (1988) Effect of post-traumatic hypoventilation on cerebral energy metabolism. J Neurosurg 68:601–607

Benjamin AM, Verjee ZH (1980) Control of aerobic glycolysis in the brain in vitro. Neurochem Res 5:921–934

Bricknell OL, Opie LH (1978) Effects of substrates on tissue metabolic changes in the isolated rat heart during underperfusion and on release of lactate dehydrogenase and arrythmias during reperfusion. Circ Res 43:102–115

Chapman AG, Meldrum BS, Siesjö BK (1977) Cerebral metabolic changes during prolonged epileptic seizures in rats. J Neurochem 28:1025–1035

Davidheiser S, Joseph H, Davies RE (1984) Separation of aerobic glycolysis from oxidative metabolism and contractility in rat anococcygeus muscle. Am J Physiol 247:C335–341

DeSalles AAF, Kontos HA, Becker DP, Yang MS, Ward JD, Moulton R, Gruemer HD, Lutz H, Maset AL, Jenkins L, Marmarou A, Muizelaar R (1986) Prognostic significance of ventricular CSF lactic acidosis in severe head injury. J Neurosug 65:615–624

DeSalles AAF, Muizelaar JP, Young HF (1987) Hyperglycemia, cerebrospinal fluid lactic acidosis, and cerebral blood flow in severely head injured patients. Neurosurg 21:45–50

DeWitt DS, Jenkins LW, Wei EP, Lutz H, Becker DP, Kontos HK (1986) Effects of fluid percussion brain injury on regional cerebral blood flow and pial arteriolar diameter. J Neurosurg 64:787–794

Duckrow RB, LaManna JC, Rosenthal M, Levasseur JE, Patterson JL (1981) Oxidative metabolic activity of cerebral cortex after fluid-percussion head injury in the cat. J Neurosurg 54:607–614

Grootegoed JA, Oonk RB, Jansen R, van der Molen HJ (1986) Metabolism of radiolabelled energy-yielding substrates by rat Sertoli cells. J Reprod Fertil 77:109–118

Hellstrand P, Jorup C, Lydrup ML (1984) O_2 consumption, aerobic glycolysis and tissue phosphagen content during activation of the Na^+/K^+ pump in rat portal vein. Pflugers Arch 401:119–124

Howse DC, Duffy TE (1975) Control of redox state of the pyridine nucleotides in the rat cerebral cortex. Effect of electroshock-induced seizures. J Neurochem 24:935–940

Howse DC, Caronna JJ, Duffey TE, Plum F (1974) Cerebral energy metabolism, pH, and blood flow during seizures in the cat. Am J Physiol 227(6):1444–1451

Hubschmann OR, Nathanson DC (1985) The role of calcium and cellular membrane dysfunction in experimental trauma and subarachnoid hemorrhage. J Neurosurg 62:698–703

Inao S, Marmarou A, Clarke GD, Andersen BJ, Fatouros PP, Young HF (1988) Production and clearance of lactate from brain tissue, cerebrospinal fluid, and serum following experimental brain injury. J Neurosurg (in press)

Julian FJ, Goldman DE (1962) The effects of mechanical stimulation on some electrical properties of axons. J Gen Physiol 46:297–313

Katayama Y, Cheung MK, Alves A, Becker DP (1988) Effects of experimental concussive brain injury on extracellular ion concentration on the hippocampus as monitored by microdialysis. AANS Scientific Program: 380 (abstract)

Kirkpatrick JB, Bray JJ, Palmer SM (1972) Visualization of axoplasmic flow in vitro by Nomarski microscopy. Comparison to rapid flow or radioactive proteins. Brain Res 43:1–10

Lewelt W, Jenkins LW, Miller JD et al. (1980) Autoregulation of cerebral blood flow after experimental fluid percussion injury of the brain. J Neurosurg 53:500–511

Lewis DV, Schuette WH (1975) Temperature dependence of potassium clearance in the central nervous system. Brain Res 99:175–178

Lothman E, LaManna J, Cordingley G, Rosenthal M, Somjen G (1975) Responses of electrical potential, potassium levels, and oxidative metabolic activity of the cerebral neocortex of cats. Brain Res 88:15–36

Lynch RM, Paul RJ (1983) Compartmentalization of glycolytic and glycogenolytic metabolism in vascular smooth muscle. Science 222:1344–1346

McDonald TF, Hunter EG, MacLeod DP (1971) Adenosinetriphosphate partition in cardiac muscle with respect to transmembrane electrical activity. Pflugers Arch 322:95–108

McIntosh TK, Faden AI, Bendall MR, Vink R (1987) Traumatic brain injury in the rat: Alterations in brain lactate and pH as characterized by ^1H and ^{31}P nuclear magnetic resonance. J Neurochem 49:1530–1540

Milito SJ, Raffin CN, Rosenthal M, Sick TJ (1988) Potassium ion homeostasis and mitochondrial redox activity in brain: Relative changes as indicators of hypoxia. J CBF and Metab 8:155–162

Ochs S (1972) Fast transport of materials in mammalian nerve fibers. Science 176:252–260

Ochs S, Hollingsworth D (1971) Dependence on fast axoplasmic transport in nerve on oxidative metabolism. J Neurochem 18:107–114

Ochs S, Smith CB (1971) Fast axoplasmic transport in mammalian nerve in vitro after block of glycolysis with iodoacetic acid. J Neurochem 18:833–843

Paul RJ, Wuytack F, Raeymaekers L, Casteels R (1986) Association of an integrated glycolytic enzyme cascade with a smooth muscle plasma membrane fraction. Fed Proc 45(4):766

Sacktor B, Wilson JE, Tiekert CG (1966) Regulation of glycolysis in brain, in situ, during convulsions. J Biol Chem 241(21):5071–5075

Sullivan HG, Martinez J, Becker DP, Miller JD, Griffith R, Wist AO (1976) Fluid percussion model of mechanical brain injury in the cat. J Neurosurg 45:520–534

Takahashi H, Manaka S, Sano K (1981) Changes in extracellular potassium concentration in cortex and brain stem during the acute phase of experimental closed head injury. J Neurosurg 55:708–717

Unterberg AW, Andersen BJ, Clarke GD, Marmarou A (1988) Cerebral energy metabolism following fluid percussion brain injury in cat. J Neurosurg 68:594–600

Weiss J, Hiltbrand B (1985) Functional compartmentation of glycolytic versus oxidative metabolism in isolated rabbit heart. J Clin Invest 75:436–447

Young W, Koreh I (1986) Potassium and calcium changes in injured spinal cords. Brain Res 365:42–53

N-Methyl-D-Aspartate (NMDA) Receptor Antagonists in the Treatment of Experimental Brain Injury: [31]P Magnetic Resonance Spectroscopy and Behavioral Studies

T.K. McIntosh [1], R. Vink [2], H. Soares [1], and R. Simon [3]

[1] Surgical Research Center, Department of Surgery, University of Connecticut Health Center, Farmington, Connecticut 06032 (USA); [2] Department of Chemistry and Biochemistry, James Cook University, Townsville (Australia); [3] Department of Neurology, University of California, San Francisco, California (USA)

Introduction

The excitatory amino acid neurotransmitters (EAA) glutamate and aspartate and their various analogs can produce cell swelling and cell death after direct application to neurons (Olney 1978). Recent data also exist to support the hypothesis that these "excitotoxins" participate in the tissue damage caused by brain hypoxia and/or ischemia since both in vivo and in vitro treatment with N-methyl-D-aspartate (NMDA) receptor antagonists appears to protect against cell death (Rothman and Olney 1986, Simon et al. 1984). Because it is possible that EAA receptor activation may contribute to delayed damage after brain trauma, we evaluated the therapeutic efficacy of MK-801, a centrally-active, antagonist of the NMDA receptor, on brain metabolism (as measured by phosphorus nuclear magnetic resonance spectroscopy (^{31}P MRS)) and neurological outcome after fluid-percussion (FP) brain injury in the rat.

Methods

Male rats (400–450 g) were anesthetized with a constant infusion of sodium pentobarbital (60 mg/kg i.p. plus 20 mg/kg/hr i.v.), intubated, artifically ventilated with room air, and a craniotomy was made over the left parietal cortex. FP brain injury (2.8 atmospheres) was induced by injecting a rapid epidural saline bolus through the craniotomy (trauma site) (McIntosh et al. 1987). At 15 min postinjury, animals were randomly assigned to treatment with either MK-801 (1 mg/kg i.v.) or equal volume saline. One group of animals ($n = 12$/treatment) was allowed to recover and scored for neurological outcome over a 2-week postinjury period using a previously described battery of motor function tests (McIntosh et al. 1987). A second group of animals ($n = 4$/treatment) was injured, placed in a specially designed Plexiglas holder and a two-turn 5×9 mm MRS surface coil was positioned centrally around the trauma site. ^{31}P MRS spectra were obtained at 34.6 MHz in 20-min blocks prior to and for 4 h following FP brain injury using a GE CS-1 2 Tesla spectrometer (Vink et al. 1987). Intracellular pH was determined from the chemical shift of inorganic phosphate (Pi) relative to phosphocreatine (PCr).

Results and Discussion

Animals treated with MK-801 15 min prior to injury appeared slower and more unresponsive than saline-treated controls at 24 h postinjury. However, MK-801-treated animals showed a slight but non-significant trend towards improved post-traumatic neurological recovery when tested at 1- and 2-weeks postinjury (Table 1). In the NMR spectrometer, the PCR/Pi ratio of saline treated animals declined from $3.9+0.4$ (mean$+$SEM) to $2.5+0.6$ at 2 h and remained suppressed. The intracellular pH of control animals decreased somewhat by 40 min posttrauma (from $7.25+0.07$ to $6.9+0.06$) but recovered to preinjury values by 90 min. The PCr/Pi ratio in MK-801-treated animals fell from $3.9+0.4$ preinjury to $2.7+0.3$ by 2 hours and then recovered to remain significantly higher than that of control animals during the remainder of the study (mean$=3.6+0.4$). The intracellular pH in MK-801-treated animals showed no significant changes with respect to those values obtained from saline-treated controls.

Our results demonstrate that post-traumatic treatment with MK-801 (1 mg/kg) can cause a slight but significant improvement in cerebral metabolic status (PCr/Pi ratio) and a slight but non-significant improvement in neurological recovery at 1 and 2 weeks following traumatic brain injury. Combined with our previous results that MK-801 can improve brain ion homeostasis and prevent tissue water accumulation in the injured hemisphere after FP brain injury (McIntosh et al. 1988), these results suggest that excitatory amino acid neurotransmitters may be involved in the pathophysiology of traumatic brain injury.

Table 1. Median composite neuroscore following traumatic brain injury with treatment with either saline or MK 801

Time	Saline	MK 801 (1 mg/kg I.V.)
24 hours	15	12
1 week	22	25
2 weeks	25	29

Animals were scored from 4 (normal) to 0 (severely impaired) for each of the following indices: (A) forelimb flexion upon suspension by tail; (B) Decreased resistance to lateral pulsion; (C) Ability to stand on an inclined angle board with the maximal angle at which the animal can stand for 5 seconds recorded (angle board); (D) Ambulatory and vertical activity monitored over a period of 5 minutes. Combination of the four neurobehavioral scores yielded a composite neuroscore of 36

References

McIntosh TK, Noble LJ, Andrews B, Faden AI (1987) Traumatic brain injury in the rat: Characterization of a midline fluid-percussion model. CNS Trauma 4:119–134

McIntosh TK, Soares H, Hayes R, Simon R (1988) NMDA receptor antagonists prevent edema and restore magnesium homeostasis after traumatic brain injury in rats. In: Lehman J (ed) Recent advances in excitatory amino acid research. Alan R. Liss, New York

Olney J (1978) Neurotoxicity of excitatory amino acids. In: McGeer EG, Olney JT, McGeer PL (eds) Kainic acid as a tool in neurobiology. Raven, New York, pp 95–121

Rothman S, Olney J (1986) Glutamate and the pathophysiology of hypoxic-ischemic brain damage. Ann Neurol 19:105–111

Simon R, Swan J, Griffith T, Meldrum B (1984) Blockade of N-methyl-D-aspartate receptors may protect against ischemic damage in the brain. Science 226:850–852

Vink R, McIntosh TK, Weiner MW, Faden AI (1987) Effects of traumatic brain injury on cerebral high energy phosphates and pH: A ^{31}P magnetic resonance spectroscopy study. J Cereb Blood Flow Metab 7:563–571

Ion Fluxes and Cell Swelling in Experimental Traumatic Brain Injury: The Role of Excitatory Amino Acids

Y. Katayama, M.K. Cheung, A. Alves, and D.P. Becker

Division of Neurosurgery, University of California at Los Angeles, School of Medicine, Los Angeles, California 90024 (USA)

Several earlier studies have demonstrated, using ion-sensitive electrodes, that massive ionic fluxes across the brain cell membrane occur in response to traumatic brain injury even when the cell membrane is not primarily damaged (Takahashi et al. 1981, Tsubokawa 1983, Hubschman and Kornhauser 1983, DeSalles et al. 1986). However, no data are currently available regarding the exact mechanism of such ionic events. Similar changes in ionic distribution in anoxic or ischemic brain injury have been shown to produce cellular swelling as a direct consequence (Van Harreveld and Ochs 1956, Hansen et al. 1980). While the occurrence of cellular swelling in traumatic brain injury is not well documented to date, the massive ionic fluxes are likely to result in changes in cell volume regardless of their cause. Therefore, understanding these phenomena would provide insight into the intraparenchymal pathology seen clinically in traumatic brain injury.

Recently, procedures for the determination of changes in substances in the extracellular space using brain microdialysis have been reported. The brain microdialysis technique not only enables us to monitor various neurochemical changes occurring in the extracellular space simultaneously but also provides a means of administering various agents in situ through the dialysis probe. Employing this technique, the present study demonstrated ionic fluxes and associated cellular swelling following traumatic brain injury, and yielded data indicating that these events result from the pathological opening of well defined ion channels rather than non-specific breakdown of the brain cell membrane.

Traumatic brain injury was induced in rats by epidural fluid-percussion described in detail elsewhere (Dixon et al. 1987), at the level of concussive injury which produced unconsciousness for 2–12 min without overt morphological damage. The dialysis probe (O.D. 300 μm) was positioned in the hippocampus or the midbrain. At the moment of injury, the probe was temporarily withdrawn and re-positioned at the same site immediately after the injury. Animals were anesthetized with gas mixture (66% N_2O, 33% O_2 and 1–2 ml/min enflurane). Delivery of anesthetic gases was terminated 1-min before injury induction and restarted on recovery from unconsciousness. Respiration was mechanically supported during the period of apnea. The concentration of extracellular ions ($[K^+]_e$ and $[Ca^{2+}]_e$) and various neurotransmitters were determined for sequential 1-min fraction of the dialysate in vitro.

Immediately after the injury, an increase in $[K^+]_e$ of varying magnitudes was observed. A transient, small increase (1.5–1.9 fold) was induced by relatively mild insult, whereas a longer-lasting, more pronounced increase (4.7–5.6 fold) resulted from more severe insult (Fig. 1). A transition between these two patterns occurred relatively abruptly when the severity of injury reached a certain threshold (4–6 min unconsciousness). Maximum $[K^+]_e$ was always observed in the initial 1-min fraction of post-injury dialysate. Since this increase represents the average $[K^+]_e$ increase during 1-min period for the collection of each dialysate fraction, the peak increase should be higher than these values. The $[K^+]_e$ increase taking place immediately after the injury could not be accounted for by failure of energy-dependent ion pumps due primarily to anoxia or ischemia since the ionic fluxes in these conditions occur more than a minute after their onset (Astrup et al. 1980, Hansen and Olsen 1980).

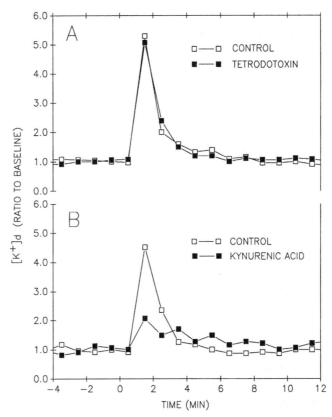

Fig. 1 A, B. Representative examples of changes in the concentration of potassium in the dialysate ($[K^+]_d$, ratio to 5-min preinjury baseline) following concussive brain injury. A pair of dialysis probes were positioned in the hippocampus (CA-1, *dentate area*) bilaterally. *Open square*, control probe; *solid square*, test probe perfused with tetrodotoxin (10^{-5} M, **A**) or kynurenic acid (10^{-2} M, **B**). Each square is located at a midpoint of 1-min period in which the fraction was collected. The injury is administered at time zero. The delay of the response from the time of injury is due to the dead space (5.0 μl) of the dialysis system (perfusion rate, 5.0 μl/min). Therefore, 2nd 1-min fraction following the injury contained initial postinjury dialysate

In order to test the hypothesis that the observed potassium fluxes are due to openings of voltage-gated ion channels associated with neuronal discharges, the effect of tetrodotoxin, a potent depressant of neuronal discharge, was examined. The tetrodotoxin (10^{-5} M), administered in situ through the dialysis probe, significantly attenuated the small increase in $[K^+]_e$ after mild insult but had no effect to the large increase in $[K^+]_e$ after severe insult (Fig. 1 A). Thus, while neuronal discharges resulting presumably from sudden deformation of neural tissue explain the small $[K^+]_e$ increase, the large $[K^+]_e$ increase must be mediated by other mechanism. An alternative possibility for the mechanism of the ionic fluxes is the opening of ligand-gated ion channels, which is consistent with the idea of massive neurotransmitter release.

Among the various neurotransmitters, excitatory amino acids appear to be the most likely substances which could mediate such a large potassium flux (Mayer and Westbrook 1987). Excitatory amino acid receptors exist throughout the brain and probably more than one-fifth of neurons within the brain utilize excitatory amino acids as a neurotransmitter. In fact, it was found that, concomitantly with the large $[K^+]_e$ increase, an elevation of excitatory amino acids, especially glutamate (4.1–5.0 fold), occurred in the dialysate. This increase is comparable to the change seen in transient ischemia (Benveniste et al. 1984). Although non-specific slight increase was observed also in other amino acides, such a large increase was noted only in excitatory amino acids. Furthermore, kynurenic acid (10^{-2} M), a broad spectrum antagonist of excitatory amino acids, administered in situ was found to attenuate effectively the large increase in $[K^+]_e$ following concussive brain injury (Fig. 1 B). This observation indicates that a major component of the large ionic flux has been caused by the opening of ligand-gated ion channels activated by excitatory amino acids. Evidence has accumulated indicating that, when $[K^+]_e$ is elevated beyond the level of physiological ceiling, synaptic terminals are depolarized and an indiscriminate release of neurotransmitter ensues. Thus, it appears that $[K^+]_e$ initially increases due to sudden intense neuronal discharge and then, when $[K^+]_e$ surpasses the physiological ceiling, extracellular excitatory amino acids are massively elevated resulting in much greater potassium flux.

Excitatory amino acids activate quisqualate- and kainate-preferring receptors which open channels permeable to both sodium and potassium. They also activate N-methyl-D-aspartate-preferring receptor which opens channels permeable to calcium in addition to sodium and potassium. The occurrence of potassium fluxes through excitatory amino acid-activated channels, therefore, indicates that large sodium and calcium fluxes must also occur through these same channels. This implies that neuronal swelling described in anoxic or ischemic brain injury (Van Harreveld and Ochs 1956, Hansen and Olsen, 1980) occurs in traumatic brain injury as well, since the osmotic pressure of the intracellular impermeable anions is no longer counteracted. In addition, the excessive neuronal release of neurotransmitters and potassium stimulate glial swelling. We, therefore, next examined changes in the volume of the extracellular space. The ^{14}C-sucrose (10^{-2} M) was perfused through the dialysis probe before the injury, as a marker of the extracellular space. It was found that the concentration of ^{14}C-sucrose in the extracellular space increases immediately following the injury (1.3–2.5 fold,

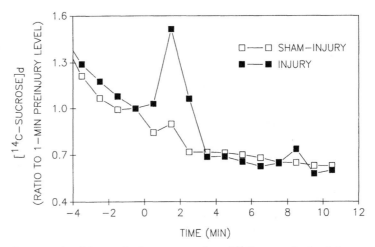

Fig. 2. A representative example of changes in the concentration of ^{14}C-sucrose in the dialysate ([^{14}C-sucrose]$_d$, ratio to 1-min preinjury level) following concussive brain injury. Thje dialysis probe was positioned in the hippocampus (CA-1, *dentate area*). The perfusion of ^{14}C-sucrose through the dialysis probe was continued for 20-min and terminated 18-min prior to the injury. Open square, sham-injury; solid square, actual injury. *See also* legend for Fig. 1

Fig. 2). This observation confirms a shrinkage of the extracellular space and cellular swelling resulting from a large flux of water into the cell.

When the large increase in $[K^+]_e$ was observed, a decrease in $[Ca^{2+}]_e$ (0.6–0.8 fold), preceded by transient increase (1.0–2.0 fold), was also demonstrated. The presence of initial increase suggests that the observed profile of $[Ca^{2+}]_e$ changes are a sum of a transient incrementing response and a longer-lasting decrementing response occurring simultaneously. While the incrementing response may partly be a result of the shrinkage of the extracellular space, the other possible source of the $[Ca^{2+}]_e$ increase is calcium fluxes from the capillary due to its permeability change. Thus, calcium fluxes into the brain cells may be much larger than what is expected simply from the change in $[Ca^{2+}]_e$. These events may also be the cause of the non-specific slight increase in other substances in the extracellular space, although a remarkable rise in $[K^+]_e$ and excitatory amino acids are apparently not accounted for by these mechanisms alone (see above).

The present study demonstrated that ionic fluxes following concussive brain injury are mediated by ligand-gated ion channels, especially those activated by excitatory amino acids, rather than a non-specific breakdown of the membrane. While the present study was concerned with concussive brain injury in order to separate pathological processes associated with primary brain cell damage, the ionic fluxes and cellular swelling described above must occur also in more severe forms of traumatic brain injury. These events are quite likely to trigger metabolic derangements at subcellular levels, which may be an important component of pathological processes contributing to secondary brain cell damage.

Acknowledgements. (This work is supported by Grants from Lind Lawrence Foundation and Sunny Von Bulow Coma and Head Trauma Research Foundation.)

References

Astrup J, Rehncrona S, Siesjo BK (1980) The increase in extracellular potassium concentration in the ischemic brain in relation to preischemic functional activity and cerebral metabolic rate. Brain Res 199:161–174

Benveniste H, Drejer J, Schousboe A, Diemer NH (1984) Elevation of the extracellular concentration of glutamate and aspartate in rat hippocampus during transient cerebral ischemia monitored by intracerebral microdialysis. J Neurochem 43:1369–1374

DeSalles AAF, Jenkins LW, Anderson RL, Opoku-Edusei T, Marmarou A, Hayes RL (1986) Extracellular potassium activity following concussion. Soc Neurosci Abstr 12:967

Dixon CE, Lyeth BG, Povlishock JT, Findling RL, Hamm RJ, Marmarou A, Young H, Hayes RL (1987) A fluid percussion model of experimental brain injury in the rat. J Neurosurg 67:110–119

Hansen AJ, Olsen CE (1980) Brain extracellular space during spreading depression and ischemia. Acta Physiol Scand 108:355–365

Hubschman OR, Kornhauser D (1983) Effects of intraparenchymal hemorrhage on extracellular cortical potassium in experimental head trauma. J Neurosurg 59:289–293

Mayer ML, Westbrook GL (1987) Cellular mechanisms underlying excitotoxicity. TINS 10: 59–61

Takahashi H, Manaka S, Sano K (1981) Changes in extracellular potassium concentration in cortex and brain stem during the acute phase of experimental closed head injury. J Neurosurg 55:708–718

Tsubokawa T (1983) Cerebral circulation and metabolism in concussion. Neurol Surg 11:563–573

Van Harreveld A, Ochs S (1956) Cerebral impedance changes after circulatory arrest. Am J Physiol 189:159–166

Neuron-Specific Enolase and S-100 Protein in CSF: Objective Markers of Structural Brain Damage

L. Persson, N. Eriksson, H.-G. Hårdemark, and Z. Kotwica

Department of Neurosurgery, University Hospital, S-751 85 Uppsala (Sweden)

Introduction

Despite the modern imaging techniques such as CT, PET, and MRI, it is often difficult to differentiate between reversible (e.g. edematous) and irreversible (e.g. infarction) brain damage during the acute phase of cerebral injury or disease. Biochemical CSF and serum markers specific for brain damage have therefore been sought as means of measuring the tissue destruction. Many substances, especially proteins, have been found in the CSF in conjunction with brain damage (Bakay et al. 1986). We have developed methods for quantifying neuron-specific enolase (NSE) and S-100 protein in CSF and serum (Påhlman et al. 1984, Persson et al. 1987). These cytoplasmic proteins are regarded as nervous-system specific, and are present in high concentrations in neurons and glial cells, respectively. They are currently under evaluation as brain damage markers at our institution. We have found a quantitative relationship between the CSF-NSE and S-100 concentrations and brain damage in patients with various types of stroke, subarachnoid hemorrhage, and head injury (Persson et al. 1987, Persson et al. 1988). However, the exact relationship between the concentrations of these markers in CSF and the degree of irreversible brain damage is difficult to study in patients.

The pattern of NSE and S-100 concentrations in CSF was therefore studied in two experimental rat models involving brain damage (middle cerebral artery (MCA) occlusion and cortical contusion). Further, the concentrations of NSE and S-100 in these experiments were compared with the CSF findings in 2 patients, 1 with subarachnoid hemorrhage (SAH) complicated by embolic infarction and 1 with severe head injury.

Materials and Methods

NSE and S-100 protein were measured by radioimmunoassay (Påhlman et al. 1984, Persson et al. 1987). In the rats $25-50$ µl and in the patients 100 µl samples were used.

Rat Experiments. Focal brain ischemia was induced by occlusion of the MCA (Tamura et al. 1981). Brain contusion was produced by dropping a weight on the exposed dura under controlled conditions (Feeney et al. 1981). CSF was sampled repeatedly before and after the production of the brain lesion via an indwelling catheter in the cisterna magna (Hårdemark et al. 1988).

Patients. CSF was aspirated via a ventricular catheter inserted primarily for ICP measurements.

Results

Rats (Fig. 1). Following MCA occlusion the NSE concentrations rose to a maximum after about 3 days. The concentrations then decreased, returning to normal after ca. 6 days. S-100 concentrations measured in one rat remained rather low for 3 days following occlusion, after which a significant increase was noted.

Following the experimental contusion injury the NSE concentrations reached a peak only ca. 7.5 h in all rats. The NSE concentrations then dropped and reached normal values within 3–4 days. S-100 protein has not yet been analysed in this model.

Patients. Case 1. This patient suffered a severe SAH; 24 h later he was Hunt and Hess Grade III. Angiography showed an anterior communicating artery aneurysm. The angiography caused an embolus in the left posterior cerebral artery. This was confirmed during the angiography. In spite of this complication the aneurysm was clipped the same day. The postoperative course was uneventful,

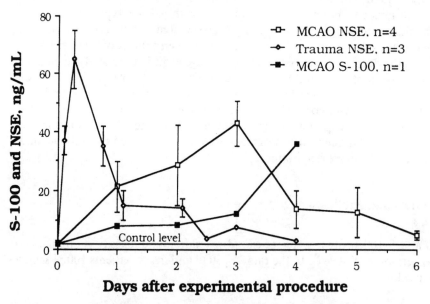

Fig. 1. Cerebrospinal fluid NSE and S-100 protein concentration curves (ng/ml) after middle cerebral artery occlusion or cortical contusion (NSE only) in the rat. The traumatic injury resulted in an earlier peak concentration than did the ischemic injury

590

apart from the development of an occipital infarction which caused hemianopsia. The S-100 concentration curve showed a maximum 24 h after ictus. However, the S-100 concentration remained raised for about 6 days. The NSE curve showed a somewhat different pattern, the peak concentration being noted about 6 days after ictus.

Case 2. This 16-year-old girl sustained severe head injury with multiple small contusions and progressive brain swelling. The resulting raised intracranial pressure was successfully controlled with artificial hyperventilation and barbiturates. Raised NSE and S-100 concentrations were recorded in the first CSF sample obtained about 24 h after the injury. Lower values were subsequently found, but the NSE concentration remained moderately raised for 2 weeks. The S-100 concentration returned to normal values within a few days.

Discussion

Studies on biochemical brain damage markers are based on the assumption that the quantity of markers found in the CSF reflects the number of injured brain cells. The concentration of such markers can be used clinically as an objective measure of the extent of brain damage. However the presence of markers in CSF in conjunction with brain damage is transient and CSF must be sampled within a critical period. The timing of this period depends on several factors including the distance between the lesion and the CSF pathways. The present study demonstrates that the CSF-NSE and S-100 concentration curve patterns were different after ischemic and traumatic injury, implying that the type of brain injury is also important. The reason for the difference is obscure, but a number of factors may be involved.

Cerebral trauma probably causes instant mechanical rupture of especially the cell membranes which could result in escape to the extracellular space from a large number of cells of cytoplasmic proteins such as NSE and S-100, producing a "wave" of proteins which reach the CSF shortly after the injury. The cellular injury following ischemia, on the other hand, is probably more gradual. Necrosis per se is a slow process, and some cells may die several days after ictus (e.g. delayed neuronal death). This may explain why the peak concentration of a marker in CSF occurs later than after trauma. The ischemic process also involves coagulation and degradation of tissue proteins, probably including also the marker proteins. The concentration of marker per volume of destroyed tissue may therefore be lower after ischemia than after trauma.

MCA occlusion and cortical contusion in the rat are useful models for studies on the relation between brain damage and biochemical markers in the CSF.

References

Bakay RA, Sweeney KM, Wood JH (1986) Pathophysiology of cerebrospinal fluid in head injury: Part 2. Neurosurgery 18:376–382

Feeney DM, Boyeson MG, Linn RT, Murray HM, Dail WG (1981) Responses to cortical injury: I. Methodology and local effects of contusions in the rat. Brain Res 211:67–77

Hårdemark H-G, Persson L, Bolander HG, Hillered L, Olsson Y, Påhlman S (1988) Neuron-specific enolase in rat cerebrospinal fluid: Marker of infarction development and size in a focal ischemia model. Stroke 19:1–5

Påhlman S, Esscher T, Bergvall P, Odelstad L (1984) Purification and characterization of human neuron specific enolase: Radioimmunoassay development. Tumour Biol 5:127–139

Persson L, Hårdemark H-G, Gustafsson J, Rundström G, Mendel-Hartvig I, Påhlman S (1987) S-100 protein and neuron-specific enolase in cerebrospinal fluid and serum: Markers of cell damage in human central nervous system. Stroke 18:911–918

Persson L, Hårdemark H-G, Edner G, Ronne E, Mendel-Hartvig I, Påhlman S (1988) S-100 protein in cerebrospinal fluid of patients with subarachnoid hemorrhage. Acta Neurochir (in press)

Time Course of Brain Tissue Pressure in Temporal Fluid Percussion Injury

N. Wako, K. Shima, and A. Marmarou

Richard Reynolds Neurological Research Laboratories, Division of Neurosurgery, Medical College of Virginia, Richmond, Virginia 23298 (USA)

Introduction

Fluid percussion injury is known to produce an immediate rise in systemic blood pressure (MABP) which gradually returns to near normal levels within a 30 minute period (Sullivan et al. 1976, Lewelt et al. 1980, 1982; Rosner et al. 1982, 1984). It is reasonable to suspect that the brain tissue experiences a similar surge. However, intracranial pressure (ICP) measures thus far have been restricted to fluid coupled devices which may not accurately reflect the brain tissue pressure (TP) changes during the percussion transient.

The purpose of this study was to determine to magnitude of change in TP produced by fluid percussion injury and determine if pressure gradients develop in an experimental model of mechanical trauma.

Materials and Methods

Eight adult cats (2.5–3.8 kg) were anesthetized with titrated 1% methohexal sodium and å-chlorolase (40 mg/kg). Animals were tracheotomized, paralyzed with gallamine triethiodine (4 mg/kg), and maintained normocapnic using a gas mixture containing 30% oxygen and room air by means of mechanical ventilatory support. An arterial cannula was inserted into the femoral artery for measurement of MABP and for withdrawal of blood samples to confirm normal levels of carbon dioxide, oxygen, and pH. The animals were fitted into a stereotaxic frame and two small burr holes were made over the frontoparietal region for measuring TP and ventricular fluid pressure (VFP). A stainless steel screw was secured at the vertex for "Far-Field Brainstem Auditory Evoked Response" (BAER), and a second reference electrode was inserted into the inner pinna of the ear. An additional electrode at the bough served as ground. A large burr hole 11 mm in diameter was made over the temporoparietal region and a hollow metal screw was tightly fitted into the burr hole without opening the underlying dura mater. The fluid percussion device described previously (Sullivan et al. 1976) was then attached and fixed with dental acrylic to the hollow injury screw. A miniaturized fiber optic device (Camino) for measuring the TP was inserted stereotactically in white matter (AP + 12, LAT + 6.5, DEP + 10) in the impacted hemisphere. After surgical preparation, measurements of MABP, TP, and BAER were performed to determine the resting control values. Brain trauma was produced by the release of a weighted pendulum which struck a fluid-filled plexiglass column attached to the injury screw. All animals were subjected to a percussion impact of 3.0 atmospheres. Ventricular and cisterna fluid pressure catheters were implanted within 1 hour after impact and the pressures were followed for a period of 8 hours post-trauma. BAERs were also measured. Cisterna magna pressure (CMP) was recorded continuously.

Results

Brainstem Auditory Evoked Response: Injured animals were divided into two groups according to the severity of brain stem damage as assessed by BAER. Low tissue pressure animals (LO-TP) were characterized by a preservation of BAER while in High tissue pressure animals (HI-TP), BAERs were absent due to the more extensive damage in the brain stem.

Arterial Blood Pressure: Control MABP values in LO-TP and HI-TP groups were not significantly different. Immediately following injury there was an average increase in MABP of 104 ± 11 mm Hg in the LO-TP group. MABP returned to control levels within 15 min and throughout the remainder of the experiment, MABP was not significantly different from control. In the HI-TP group, the MABP rose by 139 ± 16 mm Hg transiently, but one hr later was 23% below control and continued to fall without returning to baseline throughout the experiment.

Intracranial Pressure: Before injury, baseline TP values ranged from 8 to 10 mm Hg in all animals. Immediately following trauma, TP increased synchronously with blood pressure to levels in excess of 100 mm Hg in HI-TP group, while in LO-TP group, the TP rise was limited to 29 mm Hg. This peak TP rise occurred within 3 min post-injury, returning to near baseline values by 30 min and was closely related to the extent of brain stem injury. By one hr, TP in HI-TP group were still 6 mm Hg above baseline, subsequently elevating gradually to reach a level of 21 mm Hg by the end of experiment. Animals which developed high tissue pressure had high CSF pressures by 3 hours post-trauma, small tissue pressure gradients developed on the order of 5 mm Hg. The development of the small gradients was coincident with the point of dissociation between VFP and CMP indicating a gradual tissue impaction, which was significant at 7 hr post-trauma. At 7 hr, the TP fell between the boundaries set by VFP and CMP. In the LO-TP group, tissue and fluid pressures were within a very close range, with the exception of small tissue gradients, again on the order of 5 mm Hg, developing at 5 hr post-injury, which gradually dissipated and approached the range of the fluid pressures at 7 hours (Fig. 1).

Cerebral Perfusion Pressure: The cerebral perfusion pressure (CPP) was calculated by taking the difference of MABP and TP values for each animal. Because MABP rose more than TP immediately after the injury, there was a transient

594

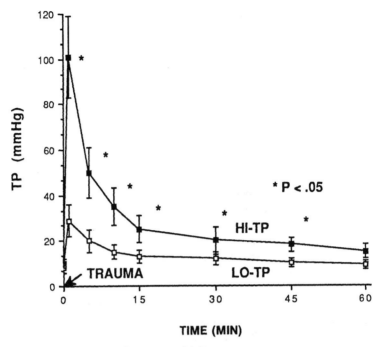

Fig. 1. Tissue pressure after temporal injury

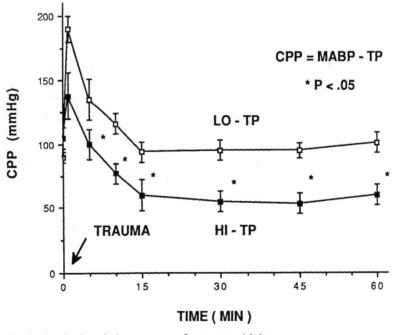

Fig. 2. Cerebral perfusion pressure after temporal injury

increase in CPP. CPP in the LO-TP group returned to baseline levels within 15 min after injury and maintained this level throughout the experiment. In the HI-TP group, CPP was 26% below baseline 15 min after injury and 43% one hr post-trauma. With the combined effects of a reduced MABP and a slight elevation of TP, the HI-TP group had a statistically lower mean CPP values than the LO-TP group over the eight hr period (Fig. 2).

Discussion

Summarizing these observations, we have observed that the MABP rises to levels greater than 200 mm Hg as previously reported (Sullivan et al. 1976, Lewelt et al. 1980, 1982; Rosner et al. 1982, 1984). We speculate that the differential response observed in TP is caused by the degree of impairment of autoregulation of the two groups of animals. We further speculate that vessel constriction was adequate and that those animals which maintain a greater degree of regulation, produced less rise in TP. These animals, despite the high CPP, developed less ICP over time. In animals in which vessel constriction was not as marked, a greater loss of regulation was exhibited allowing pressure to be transmitted downstream to the vascular bed to produce high TP levels, approaching 100 mm Hg. These animals developed higher ICP over time and a more immediate reduction in PVI.

We also observed that following mechanical injury, small tissue pressure gradients developed (on the order of 5 mm Hg), then gradually resolved to fall within the bounds set by VFP and CMP. The finding that animals which develop higher levels of ICP are associated with a greater degree of vascular impairment and volume disregulation, adds support to our concept that the rise of ICP in man is mediated primarily to our concept that the rise of ICP in man is mediated primarily by a vascular mechanism. This notion is further supported by the immediate reduction of brain compliance in these animals, measured 1 hr post-injury when there was not sufficient time for edema to develop.

To our knowledge, these are the highest pressures recorded in tissue in response to mechanical trauma. It is a matter of concern that neurons are subjected to extraordinarily high levels of pressure for a period of time. Obviously, transmission of this high tissue pressure wave to the brain stem resulted in permanent damage as assessed by auditory evoked responses. It is also clear, when compared to previous studies of ICP following impact (Sullivan et al. 1976, Lewelt et al. 1980, 1982, Rosner et al. 1982, 1984), that CSF coupled pressures underestimate the pressure seen by the brain tissue.

Acknowledgements. This research was supported in part by Grants NS-12587 and RO1-NS-19235 from the National Institutes of Health. Additional facilities and support were provided in part by the Richard Roland Reynolds Neurosurgical Research Laboratories.

References

Lewelt W, Jenkins LW, Miller JD (1980) Autoregulation of cerebral blood flow after experimental fluid-percussion injury of the brain. J Neurosurg 53:500–511

Lewelt W, Jenkins LW, Miller JD (1982) Effects of experimental fluid-percussion injury of the brain on cerebrovascular reactivity to hypoxia and to hypercapnia. J Neurosurg 56:332–338

Rosner MJ, Bennet MD, Becker DP (1982) The clinical relevance of labolatory head injury models: prerequisites of therapeutic testing. In: Grossman RG, Gildenberg PL (eds) Head injury: basic and clinical aspect. New York, Raven, pp 103–115

Rosner MJ, Newsome HH, Becker DP (1984) Mechanical brain injury: the sympathoadrenal response. J Neurosurg 61:76–86

Sullivan HG, Martinez J, Becker DP et al. (1976) Fluid percussion model of mechanical brain injury in the cat. J Neurosurg 45:520–534

Improved Outcome as a Result of Recognition of Absent and Compressed Cisterns on Initial CT Scans

T.G. Luerssen, K. Hults, M. Klauber, L.F. Marshall, and the TCDB Group

Pediatric Neurosurgery, James Whitcomb Riley Hospital for Children, 702 Barnhill Drive, Room 214, Indianapolis, Indiana 46321 (USA)

Introduction

The identification of absent or compressed basal cisterns on CT scans obtained after closed head injury has been shown to be related both to mortality and to the subequent development of elevated intracranial pressure (Murphy et al. 1983, van Dongen et al. 1983, Toutant et al. 1984). One of these studies (Toutant et al. 1984) was performed using data acquired from the pilot phase of the Traumatic Coma Data Bank. Recently, the main phase of this study has been completed and the data is undergoing initial analyses. We felt it would be of interest to compare the relationship of the findings of absent or compressed cisterns on initial CT scans to outcome in this larger group of patients and hypothesized that the information gained from the pilot study suggesting that recognition and aggressive management of patients with this radiographic finding would result in improved outcome.

Methods

In the pilot phase TCDB, which involved six participating medical centers, data was collected on 581 patients between January, 1980 and May, 1982. Information regarding the status of the basal cisterns was available in the last 218 patients studied. In this project, the CT appearance of the basal cisterns was classified as "absent", "compressed", "present" or "not visualized".

In the main phase study, data collection began in 1983 and was completed early in 1988. In this study of over 1000 head injuries, there were 746 patients who had closed head injuries and were not brain dead on admission, whereby knowledge of the basilar cisterns was available. In this study, however, the cisterns were categorized as "absent or compressed", "present", or "unknown".

For this report, the data from both of these studies was organized into comparable groups. Therefore, the "absent" and "compressed" groups from the pilot study were combined. Injury severity was categorized using the Glasgow Coma Scale score (GCS), and outcomes at last follow up were categorized using the Glasgow Outcome Scale score (GOS) (Teasdale and Jennett 1974, Jennett and Bond 1975).

Results

In the pilot study 118/218, or 54%, had "absent or compressed" cisterns compared to 379/746, or 51%, in the main phase. Similarly, 82/218, or 37.6%, versus 294/746, or 39%, had cisterns that were categorized as "present" on the initial CT scans. Those categorized as "not visible" in the pilot study represented 8.3% of the population, and those categorized as "unknown" in the main phase represented 9.7% of the population.

Table 1 shows the outcome for all GCS scores with outcomes grouped as either good (that is GOS scores of good or moderate) or poor (GOS scores of severe, vegetative, and dead). In the pilot study 27.1% of patients with "absent or compressed" cisterns had good outcomes compared to 31.9% of patients in the main phase. Of those with "present" cisterns in the pilot phase 57.3% had good outcomes compared to 61.6% of those in the main phase.

Table 1. Outcome for all Coma Scores

Cisterns	GOS	Pilot	Main
ABS/Comp	G+M	32/118 (27.1%)	121/379 (31.9%)
	S+V+D	86/118 (72.9%)	258/379 (68.1%)
Present	G+M	47/82 (57.3%)	181/294 (61.6%)
	S+V+D	35/82 (42.7%)	113/294 (38.4%)

Table 2 shows a comparison of the populations grouped by GCS and categorized by outcomes for both the pilot phase and the main phase. One can see that there was little improvement in outcome between the two studies for patients with admitting GCS of 3, 4, or 5. However, for the less severely injured, that is GCS scores of 6, 7, or 8, and 9–15, more patients achieved good outcomes in the main phase study than in the pilot phase study. The small numbers in each group, however, do not allow these differences to achieve statistical significance.

The groups in whom the status of the cisterns was known, absolutely, seemed to exhibit similar outcomes. However, clear differences in outcome were noted between the groups of patients in the pilot phase whose cisterns were "not visible" and those in the main phase whose cisterns were "unknown". In the pilot phase, patients with "not visible" cisterns exhibited outcomes almost identical to those whose cisterns were "absent or compressed". In the main phase, patients whose cisterns were categorized as "unknown" exhibited outcomes intermediate to those patients who had "absent or compressed" cisterns and those who had "present" cisterns. Furthermore, data from the main phase study allowed the extraction of those patients who were "treated" early, that is, those patients who arrived at the hospital pharmacologically paralyzed and mechanically ventilated. These patients, previously categorized as GCS of 3 were reassigned a GCS of 3.3, indicating that they were being treated. As shown in Table 2, this group of patients has much better outcomes than those categorized as GCS of 3–5.

Table 2

Pilot phase

Outcome	Cisterns	GCS				
		3–5	6–8	3–8	9–15	All
Good/ Moderate	ABS/Comp	9/60 (15%)	16/39 (41%)	25/99 (25%)	7/19 (37%)	32/118 (27%)
	Not visible	1/10 (10%)	2/5 (40%)	3/15 (20%)	1/3 (33%)	4/18 (22%)
	Present	11/33 (33%)	30/37 (81%)	41/70 (59%)	6/12 (50%)	47/82 (57%)
Severe/ Vegetative/ Dead	ABS/Comp	51/60 (85%)	23/39 (59%)	74/99 (75%)	12/19 (63%)	86/118 (73%)
	Not visible	9/10 (90%)	3/5 (60%)	12/15 (80%)	2/3 (67%)	14/18 (78%)
	Present	22/33 (67%)	7/37 (19%)	29/70 (41%)	6/12 (50%)	35/82 (43%)

Main phase

Outcome	Cisterns	GCS					
		3–5	6–8	3–8	9–15	3.3	All
Good/ Moderate	ABS/Comp	36/228 (16%)	67/117 (57%)	103/345 (30%)	18/34 (53%)	14/35 (40%)	121/379 (32%)
	Unknown	5/12 (42%)	11/18 (61%)	16/30 (53%)	1/4 (25%)	3/4 (75%)	17/34 (50%)
	Present	33/86 (38%)	129/184 (70%)	162/270 (60%)	19/24 (79%)	11/19 (58%)	181/294 (62%)
Severe/ Vegetative/ Dead	ABS/Comp	192/228 (84%)	50/117 (43%)	242/345 (70%)	16/34 (47%)	21/35 (60%)	258/379 (68%)
	Unknown	7/12 (58%)	7/18 (39%)	14/30 (47%)	3/4 (75%)	1/4 (25%)	17/34 (50%)
	Present	53/86 (62%)	55/184 (30%)	108/270 (40%)	5/24 (21%)	8/19 (42%)	113/294 (38%)

In the pilot study, of those patients in whom ICP was measured who had "absent or compressed" cisterns on the initial CT scan, 74% demonstrated intracranial pressures (ICPs) of greater than 30 mm Hg. This compares favorably to the finding in the main phase study whereby 63% of those with "absent or compressed" cisterns exhibited ICPs of greater than 30 mm Hg. Only 28% of patients with cisterns characterized as "present" on the initial CT scan demonstrated ICP elevations of this magnitude. Finally, the added effect of the presence of a shift or mass effect along with "absent or compressed" cisterns could be compared between the pilot and main phase. In the pilot study, those patients with "absent or compressed" cisterns who had a shift of greater than 15 mm on the initial CT scan, regardless of the cause, exhibited a mortality of 100 percent. However, in the main phase study, patients with a shift of greater than 15 mm and "absent or compressed" cisterns exhibited a mortality of 59%. Furthermore, the data from the main phase study indicated that 88% of patients with "absent or compressed" cisterns and a shift of 15 mm or more had surgical mass lesions.

Discussion

The finding of "absent or compressed" basal cisterns on admitting CT scans continues to be an ominous predictor of both ultimate outcome and the development of elevated ICP. The two studies allow some assessment of the effects of improved recognition and aggressive therapy. However, little improvement in outcome occurred between the pilot phase and the main phase studies for those patients with the most severe injuries, suggesting that the magnitude of the primary injury is the major factor determining outcome. In contrast, the outcome for all other groups improved, probably the effect of an overall improvement of care for head injured patients. The most dramatic improvement came from the group of patients who exhibited the most severe CT findings, that is "absent or compressed" cisterns, associated with large shifts of midline structures. For this group of patients there was a significant reduction in mortality between the two studies ($p = 0.004$, Fisher's exact test). This reduction in mortality is heartening, because this group of patients had a very high incidence of surgical mass lesions, suggesting that aggressive management of even very large lesions and shifts is rewarding.

In general, the two study populations are similar. The incidence of elevated ICP is similar, and the outcomes are similar. There are some differences between the two populations, however. In the pilot study, patients who had cisterns that were "not visible" presumably due to poor scan quality had outcomes essentially the same as those patients whose cisterns were "absent". This suggests that these cisterns were truly "not visible" and not the result of a poor quality scan. In contrast, during the main phase study, in an era where CT scans had improved significantly in quality, those patients whose cistern status was "unknown" had outcomes suggesting that this population was distributed in injury severity through a fairly large range. This suggests that there was an improved level of confidence regarding the characterization of the basilar cisterns in the main phase study.

601

The outcome of patients in the main phase study who were undergoing therapy for their injury at the time of arrival at a data bank hospital was much better than those with the severe head injuries, who were not being treated. Whether or not this is an effect of the early treatment, or simply due to the inability to carefully characterize the initial severity of the injury remains to be seen.

In conclusion, this study suggests that there has been some improvement in the ability of physicians to correctly identify the status of the basilar cisterns after trauma. There has been improved outcome for the patients except for those with GCS of 3–5. The most improvement in outcome occurred for patients with large shifts due to surgical mass lesions.

Acknowledgements. This work was supported by the Pilot Traumatic Coma Data Bank under Contracts NO1-NS-9-2306, 2307, 2308, 2309, 2313, 2340 and the Traumatic Coma Data Bank (TCDB) under Contracts NO1-NS-3-2339, NO1-NS-3-2340, NO1-NS-3-2341, NO1-NS-3-2342, NO1-NS-6-2305 from the National Institute of Neurological and Communicative Disorders and Stroke (NINCDS). The TCDB Manual of Operations which includes the TCDB data forms is available from the National Technical Information Service (NTIS), U.S. Department of Commerce, 5285 Port Royal Road, Springfield, VA 22161 (NTIS Accession No. PB87 228060/AS).

References

Jennett B, Bond M (1975) Assessment of outcome after severe brain damage. A practical scale. Lancet I:480–484

Murphy A, Teasdale E, Matheson M et al. (1983) Relationship between CT indices of brain swelling and intracranial pressure after head injury. In: Ishii S, Nagai H, Brock M (eds) Intracranial pressure V. Springer, Berlin Heidelberg New York, pp 562–565

Teasdale GM, Jennett B (1974) Assessment of coma and impaired consciousness. A practical scale. Lancet II:81–84

Toutant SM, Klauber MR, Marshall LF et al. (1984) Absent or compressed basal cisterns on first CT scan: Ominous predictors of outcome in severe head injury. J Neurosurg 61:691–694

van Dongen KJ, Braakman R, Gelpke JG (1983) The prognostic value of computerized tomography in comatose head injured patients. J Neurosurg 59:951–957

An Effacement Score for Basal Cisterns to Predict ICP Level and Outcome After Severe Closed Head Injury

F. Artru, Ch. Jourdan, J. Convert, J. Duquesnel, and R. Deleuze

Neurological Hospital, "Pierre Wertheimer", F-69394 Lyon (France)

Introduction

In severe head injury, obliteration of basal cisterns on the initial CT-scan is associated with intracranial hypertension and poor outcome (Van Dongen et al. 1983, Teasdale et al. 1984, Toutant et al. 1984). In this study, we proposed a practical scale to evaluate the degree of cistern effacement. The cistern effacement score (CRS) was then correlated in a series of patients to the level of ICP. In addition, the relationship of the CES score with outcome, in particular with the risk of brain death, was examined.

Methods

The initial CT-scan of 149 patients in coma from closed, non-surgical head injury was reviewed. CT-scans were all performed with 24 hrs of the trauma, most of them between the 5th and the 8th hour and 12% within the first two hours.

Evaluation of cisterns focused on two scanning slices, lying parallel to the cantho-meatal line, one running through the perimesencephalic cistern at the level of the dorsum sellae, the second running 10 mm above and showing the quadrigeminal cistern. Both cisterns were decomposed in segments, the former, grossly rhombic in four segments, the latter, semicircular in three segments. Each segment was assigned a score: 0 = normal, 1 = compressed, 2 = absent. The total cistern effacement score ranged therefore from 0 (no effacement) to 14 (absent cisterns).

ICP was monitored from the epidural space in 55/149 patients. In each patient, mean ICP and maximal ICP (highest level reached for at least 15 min) were determined for the 24 hrs period following the initial CT-scan.

The level of coma at admission was scored with the Glasgow Coma Score. Outcome was classified in the following categories: 1 = good recovery, 2 = moderate outcome, 3 = severely disabled or vegetative, 4 = dead from complications, 5 = brain dead.

Results

Relationship of CES Score with ICP (Fig. 1)

The CES score correlated linearly with maximal ICP ($p < 0.01$) and mean ICP ($p < 0.01$) recorded during the post CT-scan day.

All patients whose CES score was <6 had a mean ICP level remaining below 30 mm Hg, except for one whose CT-scan was performed within two hours of the trauma.

In the group of patients with a CES score of >6, 82% had a mean ICP above 30 mm Hg. Patients with maximal ICP exceeding 40 mm Hg had a CES score of >6 except for one.

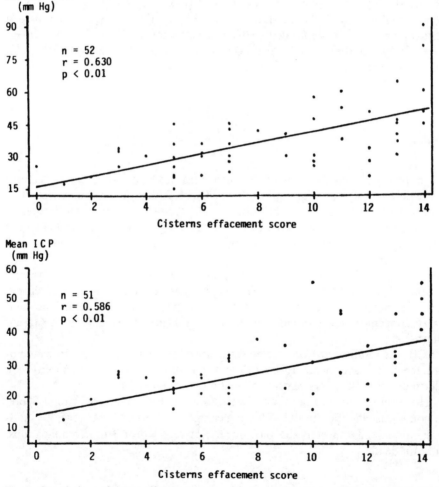

Fig. 1. Correlations of cistern effacement score with maximal and mean ICP recorded during the 24 hrs following the initial CT-scan

In this series, the incidence of brain death was clearly related to the CES score. In patients with a CES score of >10 ($n = 39$), the rate of brain death was 92% whereas in the group with a CES score of >3 ($n = 55$) only three patients progressed to brain death. One of them developed a secondary hematoma. In the two others, the CT-scan was misleading due to preexistent post-traumatic brainstem atrophy in one case, and to an excessively short time interval from injury to scanning in the other case. The rate of good recovery was inversely related to the CES score. Pataient outcome was generally more closely related to CES score than to GCS score.

Discussion

The progressive obliteration of basal cisterns may be regarded as one of the buffer mechanisms against the development of intracranial hypertension. In each patient, at a given time from the injury, the size of cisternal spaces is likely to be reduced in proportion to the severity of traumatic brain lesions. A linear relationship of CES score with ICP is therefore not too surprising. In each patient the CES score may help to decide wether ICP is to be monitored and allows us to predict rather precisely the level of its mean and maximal values.

Since the risk of brain death is very low in patients with a CES score of <3 the monitoring of ICP, in this category representing 37% of our population, does not appear of immediate necessity.

References

Teasdale E, Cardoso E, Galbraith S, Teasdale G (1984) CT-scan in severe diffuse head injury: physiological and clinical correlations. J Neurol Neurosurg Psychiatry 47:600–603

Toutant SM, Klauber MR, Marshall LF, Toole BM, Bowers SA, Seeling JM, Varnell JB (1984) Absent or compressed basal cisterns on first CT-scan: ominous predictors of outcome in severe head injury. J Neurosurg 61:691–694

van Dongen KJ, Braakman R, Gelpke GJ (1983) The prognostic value of computerized tomography in comatose head-injured patients. J Neurosurg 59:951–957

The Relation Between Glasgow Coma Scale (GCS) and a Regional Lesion Index Based on CT-Scans in Patients with Extradural Hematomas

J.O. Espersen and O.F. Petersen

Departments of Neurosurgery and Neuroradiology, University Hospital, Aarhus (Denmark)

The purpose of our work has been to try to make a lesion grading based on CT-scans and to compare this scaling to the GCS.

59 patients with extradural hematomas – admitted consecutively from Dec. 1st 1977 to Nov. 30th 1981 – had CT-scan performed just prior to surgery and the GCS was recorded at this time. All intracranial lesions and findings on the CT-scan were recorded without knowledge of the patient's condition.

The most simple approach of CT-scaling is to use the size of the basal cisterns. We found that a relation between GCS and the conditions of the cisterns exist.

The lesion number i.e. the sum of all different types of lesions seen at the CT-scans – irrespective of the extent and number in different regions, gives a fair correlation to the GCS based on the mean values.

The Regional Lesion Index is defined by the sum of lesions (as indicated above) in 13 brain regions. (Frontal, Parietal, Temporal, Occipital, Central (Striate corpus and Diencephalon), Cerebellar – and the unpaired brainstem.)

The average values of this index have nearly linear correlation to the clinical stage, but the index cannot be used to replace the GCS in the individual patient (Fig. 1).

It is concluded that despite the fact that the CT-scan gives a rather precise picture of the lesions, a CT-scaling of patients with head injuries faces the following problems:

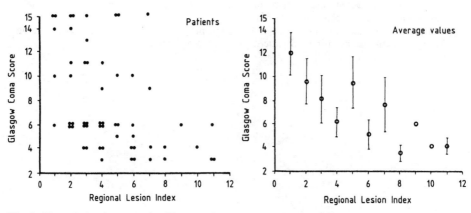

Fig. 1. The relation between the Glasgow Coma Scale and the Regional Lesion Index

Eds.: J.T. Hoff and A.L. Betz
© Springer-Verlag Berlin Heidelberg 1989

1) Different pathological lesions have different prognostic values.
2) Identical lesions have different prognostic values, dependig on their regional placement.
3) Identical lesions of varying extent have probably no linear relation to prognosis, due to the intracranial pressure/volume relationship.
4) The CT-scan underestimates contusions in the acute phase.

These reasons, and the fact that Glasgow Coma Scale mostly measures the brainstem function, will make it impossible to devise a similar simple scaling based on CT-scans which could replace the GCS in the individual patient.

Volume/Pressure Rebound with Mannitol in Head Injured Patients with Raised ICP

A. Marmarou and A. Wachi

Richard Reynolds Neurological Research Laboratories, Division of Neurosurgery, Medical College of Virginia, Richmond, Virginia 23298 (USA)

Mannitol has been shown to improve the pressure/volume status in head injured patients. This improvement in compliance has been considered to be the basis for ICP reduction (Miller et al. 1975). We posed the question that if compliance is improved with Mannitol, why does ICP gradually return and in some cases continue to rise? One view is that, in the presence of a compromised blood brain barrier, the osmolarity gradient between blood and brain produced by Mannitol is gradually dissipated as the Mannitol eventually leaks into damaged tissue. An alternative view, offered by many investigators, is that the rate of brain swelling caused by continued extravasation of edema or vascular engorgement following traumatic injury exceeds the volume that can be accommodated by hyperosmolar therapy. The objective of this study was to examine the time course of PVI and ICP following mannitol administration to determine the duration of improvement of the pressure/volume status in severely head injured patient and relate these changes to serial measurements of ICP, osmolarity and blood viscosity.

Methods

All patients studied were severely injured (GCS < 8) mechanically ventilated and under routine intensive care monitoring at the time of study. ICP was monitored by intraventricular catheters which allowed bolus manipulation of CSF for the determination of the Pressure Volume Index (PVI). The pressure transducer was referenced to a position equivalent to the foramen of Monro and PVI was calculated according to the standard equation with no constant term. Serial measurements of blood viscosity were obtained using a coneplate digital viscometer. When possible, blood samples were obtained at 0, 15, 30, 60, and 90 minutes after Mannitol administration for determination of blood viscosity, arterial blood gases and serum osmolarity. PVI measurements were obtained at the same time intervals and at 120, 150, and 180 minutes after Mannitol use. All studies were conducted when Mannitol was required for control of elevated ICP.

Eds.: J. T. Hoff and A. L. Betz
© Springer-Verlag Berlin Heidelberg 1989

Results

We observed that PVI gradually increased (189% of control) in all patients and reached a maximum at 40 minutes following bolus Mannitol. Thereafter PVI gradually declined and reached pre-Mannitol levels by 3 hours after treatment (Table 1). The maximal ICP reduction (15.9 mm Hg) was coincident with maximal PVI increase and return of ICP tracked the gradual return of PVI to pre-Mannitol levels. The maximum change in blood viscosity occurred at 30 minutes and was close to the time interval of maximum PVI increase. Interestingly, higher PVI levels in response to Mannitol were reached in patients in whom the osmolarity gradient was not significantly changed relative to control at 90 minutes.

Table 1. Response of PVI, ICP, CPP, osmolarity, and blood viscosity in head injured patients

	0	15	30	45	60	90	120	180 (min)
PVI (ml)	10.8	17.2**	20.5**	21.0**	15.9*	16.5**	12.9	11.9
	(4.0)	(8.4)	(7.1)	(6.5)	(7.0)	(5.7)	(4.0)	(4.2)
ICP (mm Hg)	31.7	22.7**	20.8**	16.4**	16.3**	19.1**	21.2**	24.7**
	(4.6)	(6.5)	(6.0)	(6.9)	(7.3)	(7.8)	(8.3)	(7.1)
CPP (mm Hg)	69.2	80.5*	81.3**	86.5**	78.8*	82.3**	78.0	74.6
	(14.5)	(17.1)	(15.2)	(11.7)	(9.7)	(10.6)	(9.3)	(10.3)
Osm (mm Osm)	299					308*		305
	(11)					(14)		(15)
Visc (%)	100	89.6	80.9**		85.2*	89.9	93.9	
	(control)							

*$p < 0.05$, **$p < 0.01$, mean (S.D.).

Discussion

This study shows that the improvement in pressure/volume status with Mannitol is not sustained, but rebounds within a 3 hr period coincident with the gradual return of ICP to pre-Mannitol levels. The increase in PVI, with no significant rise in osmolarity measured at 90 minutes, supports the contention that the improvement in PVI occurs as a result of a vascular effect rather than reduction of excess water in the acute phase of Mannitol action (Muizelaar et al. 1983). The time course of viscosity change was also synchronous with the PVI course and was altered in the direction to favor an autoregulatory response. We have shown in laboratory studies (Inao et al. 1988) that ICP was significantly reduced in the absence of water reduction measured 30 minutes following bolus Mannitol. Taking these studies in concert, it is clear that a vascular mechanism for improvement of the pressure/volume status following Mannitol therapy cannot be excluded. We speculate that the gradual return of PVI which occurs coincident with the return of ICP is related to dissipation of the vascular response to Mannitol.

Acknowledgements. This research was supported in part by Grants NS-12587 and RO1-NS-19235 from the National Institutes of Health. Additional facilities and support were provided in part by the Richard Roland Reynolds Neurosurgical Research Laboratories.

References

Inao S, Fatouros P, Marmarou A (This Volume) Effect of mannitol on experimental infusion edema.

Miller JD, Leech P (1975) Effects of mannitol and steroid therapy in intracranial volume pressure relationships in patients. J Neurosurg 42:274–281

Muizelaar JP, Wei EP, Kontos H (1983) Mannitol causes compensatory cerebral vasoconstriction and vasodilation in response to blood viscosity changes. J Neurosurg 59:822–828

Prospective, Randomized Trial of THAM Therapy in Severe Brain Injury: Preliminary Results

M.J. Rosner, K.G. Elias, and I. Coley

University of Alabama at Birmingham, Division of Neurosurgery, University Station, Birmingham, Alabama 35294 (USA)

We have previously reported a salutary effect of tromethamine (THAM) in a laboratory model of head injury using cats. Tromethamine therapy resulted in improved survival and reduced intracranial pressure (ICP) when compared to control animals. The putative mechanism for this action was neutralization of intracellular hydrogen ion. Multiple studies of traumatic brain injury have demonstrated an associated CSF lactic acidosis. Presumably this lactic acid had originated in the neural parenchyma and "percolated" into the ventricular system via the cerebral extracellular space. The CSF lactate then becomes a "marker" for certain intracellular events. By neutralizing excess hydrogen ion within tissue, the "internal millieu" of the parenchyma would be more effective at self repair and resistant to progressive edema. Other mechanisms are possible such as a shift in ionized calcium changes in other cellular enzymatic processes, change in vascular reactivity related to change in intracellular pH at the level of the cerebral smooth muscle wall and/or neutralization of other compounds which may be produced but unmeasured.

Based upon these findings and rationale, we undertook a randomized prospective trial of THAM therapy in head injured patients testing the hypotheses that:

1) THAM therapy would be associated with reduced ICP when compared to controls,
2) THAM therapy would be associated with reduced CSF lactate levels when compared with controls,
3) THAM therapy would be associated with improved survival and/or reduced morbidity when compared with controls.

Methods

37 severely brain injured patients were admitted to this study. Decision about admission to the study was made by the clinician and then the clinical coordinator was contacted for the code relating to treat vs. no treat. Informed consent was obtained from patients' families and this was approved and monitored by the IRB committee. Patients with severe traumatic brain injury of GCS less than 8 were candidates for this study.

Once entered, all patients underwent placement of a frontal ventriculostomy using standard techniques. ICP was continuously monitored as was systemic arterial blood pressure (SABP). All patients were intubated and ventilated. All patients underwent active management of cerebral perfusion pressure (CPP) in an effort to maintain this value at 70 mm Hg or greater. All patients were nursed in the flat position. CPP was actively maintained using Dopamine and/or phenylephrine infusions. Mannitol was used when CPP declined below 70 mm Hg for a significant period of time and did not respond to ventricular drainage. Mannitol was usually administered in 0.5 gm – 1.0 gm/kg doses.

Initial attempts to maintain the ET-CO_2 at 35 mm Hg for both groups were used. If intracranial pressure and/or if perfusion pressure was difficult to maintain at CPP ≥ 70 mm Hg and this was due to an ICP increase then the pCO_2 was gradually lowered by 2 to 3 mm Hg decrements as required for ICP management. If the patient randomized to THAM therapy, this was begun at 2 cc/kg/hr for one hour and then reduced to 1 cc/kg/hr. All patients underwent daily sampling of CSF for lactate and pyruvate as well as pH. Daily and often more frequent electrolyte, CBC, blood gas analysis and at least q3d determinations of bilirubin, SGOT, SGPT, alkaline phosphatase and LDH were obtained.

THAM was stopped only if renal failure supervened and hyperkalemia was a potential or actual problem. When ICP required only CSF drainage for control of CPP then THAM was tapered by reducing the dose by 20% of the initial dose each day. Tapering was accomplished within 3 to 4 days.

Results

There was no difference between the two groups with regard to the initial ICP which was measured at the time of ventricular tap. However, by the end of day 1 when average ICP's from each hour were added for all patients in both groups, the effect of THAM had already become apparent with a tendency for the treated patients to have lower ICP. This trend continued throughout the hospital course. The greatest effect of THAM seemed to be related to prevention of the increase in intracranial pressure which occurred in many of the patients in the control group. This was much less prominent than in the THAM treated patients. All of these group differences between treated and untreated patients in ICP were significant at the $P < 0.05$ level or better (Fig. 1).

Table 1 gives the SABP, CPP and $PaCO_2$ values between the control and THAM treated patients for the first 10 days of observation. As can be seen, THAM patients demonstrated lower SABP which was significant from day 1. However, the initial SABP for each group was not different. This was reflected in the slightly lower CPP in the THAM patients. This difference remained statistically reliable only for the first three days of observations. It was clear that there was a 3 to 4 mm Hg difference in pCO_2 during the first week with THAM treated patients being consistently higher. Toward the end of 10 days there was no difference between the groups.

There were no group differences detected between age, GCS (median = 5), mass lesion the amount of mannitol, furosemide, albumin, dopamine, serum

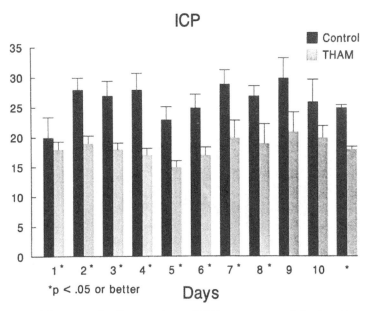

Fig. 1. Course of intracranial pressure for first ten days of ICU management. It is clear that intracranial pressure is characterized by a slight reduction from day 1 onward. The effect is more prominent when one realizes that the increase in ICP that seems to occur from day 2 and 3 onward in the control patients does not occur in the THAM patients. There was no difference between *initial* intracranial pressures between the two groups though after the first full 24 hours of therapy there was a reliable difference

Table 1. SABP, CPP and PaCO$_2$ values

Day	MAP		CPP		pCO$_2$	
	CONT	THAM	CONT	THAM	CONT	THAM
1	107±4.1	86±2.2*	87±4.4	68±2.1*	29±0.8	33±1.1*
2	108±3.0	87±1.6*	81±3.2	68±1.9*	32±1.4	37±1.2*
3	110±3.0	89±1.6*	83±3.2	71±1.3*	31±0.9	36±1.0*
4	106±2.5	90±2.1*	78±3.3	73±1.6	30±1.1	35±0.9*
5	104±2.1	93±1.8*	81±3.5	78±1.7	29±1.0	36±0.8*
6	106±3.2	92±1.6*	81±4.2	76±1.5	29±1.2	35±0.8*
7	109±3.4	91±2.6*	80±4.4	71±3.1	29±1.5	33±1.0*
8	104±2.8	92±3.6*	77±3.2	74±2.0	32±1.5	36±1.7
9	105±3.1	95±4.6	75±3.0	75±2.8	33±1.3	33±1.7
10	107±3.3	99±3.1	81±3.0	81±2.3	34±2.2	33±1.3

* $p<0.05$ or better.

osmolarity, serum potassium, PaO$_2$. Intake, output, respirations and heart rate did not vary between the groups and there was no difference in bilirubin or serum enzymes which might be related to liver function. There were significant differences between the THAM and control patients with regard to creatinine (1.05 ± 0.10 vs 1.96 ± 0.12 mg%) and BUN (17 ± 2.1 vs 49 ± 4.9). In essence, the

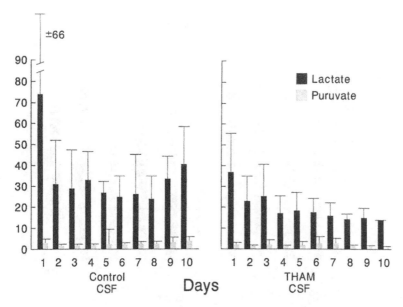

Fig. 2. CSF lactate and pyruvate levels in THAM and control patients: From day 3 onward the difference in CSF lactate levels was significant ($p < 0.05$ level or better). From day 3 onward, THAM treated patients had reduced CSF lactate levels when compared to controls ($p < 0.05$ or better)

treated patients had a creatinine almost 50% that of the control patients and this was significant at the $P = 0.03$ level.

There were 20 patients in the control group of which 9 survived. There were 17 patients treated with THAM of whom 12 survived (Fisher Exact Test, $P < 0.1$, one-tail test).

Discussion

While our survival results may have occurred by chance the apparent improvement in survival is encouraging. These groups were small and the difference of only a couple of patients in either category could have accounted for these differences. However, ICP was reliably and significantly improved in the patients on THAM therapy. This difference in intracranial pressure occurred from the first 24 hour period of monitoring onward. It was clearly not the result of either greater amounts of mannitol, lower pCO_2, etc. In fact, the pCO_2 in the THAM treated patients was slightly higher and would have tended to increase ICP in this group. The difference in SABP between the two groups is intriguing. While this may have been a pharmacologic action of tromethamine on the general cardiovascular system we can speculate that a salutory effect of the drug on neural tissue may actually have reduced the sympthoadrenal drive to hypertension seen in most severely brain injured patients. The results with regard to CSF lactate concentrations are extremely interesting and suggest that lactate metabolism, probably within the neural parenchyma, has been improved in some way. Whether this actually is due to buffering of intracellular hydrogen which might allow enzyme systems an improved milieu in which to metabolize lactate and pyruvate or whether this is due to some other effect of the drug is not clear from these data. However, the effect seems to be real and is consistent with a beneficial effect of THAM therapy in the context of severe brain injury. Differences in survival ICP, and CSF lactate cannot be attributed to a difference in age, Glasgow Coma Score (median = 5) between the groups, difference in initial intracranial pressure, nor in any other measured variable (Fig. 2).

We conclude that THAM therapy is associated with improved intracranial pressure levels and ease of control, improved CSF lactate levels and pattern of response and probably improved survival.

These results are preliminary and require further study. However, the drug can be administered safely for long periods of time with no evidence of nephrotoxicity or hepatotoxicity.

THAM (Tromethamine, "Tris-Buffer"): Effective Therapy of Traumatic Brain Swelling?

M.R. Gaab, K. Seegers, and C. Goetz

Neurosurgical Department, Hanover Medical School, Konstanty-Gutschow-Str. 8, D-3000 Hannover 61 (FRG)

Introduction

The rapid development in diagnostic technology (CT, MRI) for acute brain damage is not accompanied by comparable improvement in therapy and prognosis (Mendelow 1988). In spite of easy detection of operable space occupying lesions like intracranial hematomas after trauma, the outcome of severely head injured patients with a fatality of 40–60% (Mendelow 1988) is far from satisfying. The main problem after severe brain trauma remains the delayed development of "*secondary brain damage*", which causes brain swelling leading to *intracranial hypertension*.

Therapy of secondary brain damage and intracranial hypertension has been based on osmotherapy and general intensive care for decades. The pathophysiological significance of "engorgement" and acidotic tissue dysmetabolism after trauma (Mendelow 1988), however, suggests new therapeutic concepts. While barbiturates were disappointing due to severe side effects, *Tris buffer* (THAM, trometamol) has been reported to be effective in lowering ICP after head injury (Akioka et al. 1976, Gaab et al. 1980, Knoblich et al. 1978). In addition, THAM was found to be more effective in animal trauma models than osmotherapy (Gaab et al. 1980, Knoblich et al. 1978). We therefore investigated the effects of THAM on acute brain trauma in *experimental and clinical conditions*.

Materials and Methods

Animal Experiments

In a first series of experiments *cold brain injury* edema was produced in groups of 5 *cats* each. After trephination, the cold stamp with a constant tip temperature of $-73°C$ was positioned on the dura for 3.5 min. The trephination was closed with an integrated pressure transducer in a cast. In addition, the ICP over the opposite hemisphere (Gaeltec microtransducer), the systemic arterial pressure (SAP) and the central venous pressure (cvP) were registered. The EEG was evaluated over both hemispheres (bipolar lead) by computer (FFT, Dr. Weiss Neuromonitor). Each group of animals was treated either with osmotherapy (sorbit 40% 8 ml/kg for 30 min) or with THAM (isoosm., 5 mmol/kg for 1 hr).

Eds.: J.T. Hoff and A.L. Betz
© Springer-Verlag Berlin Heidelberg 1989

In a second series of experiments, cold injury edema was produced in *rats*. The animals were anesthetized with ketamine, relaxed by pancuronium and ventilated after tracheostomy (Kesting 1984). The cold stamp was placed over the right skull for 4 min after removal of the skin. With continued ventilation, the animals were treated either with placebo ("controls", Ringers solution), with pentobarbital (1 mg bolus, 1 mg/6 h), with dexamethasone (1 mg bolus, 2 mg/6 hr) or with THAM (0.66 mmol bolus, 3.3 mmol/5 hr) i.v. in groups of 12 animals. After 6 h, the rats were decapitated, and water, sodium and potassium contents were measured in both hemispheres.

Clinical Investigations

In patients with severe head injury, the ICP is routinely measured by epidural transducer (Gaeltec, Hellige). By recording the SAP in addition, the CPP is continuously evaluated on-line by the Dr. Weiss Neuromonitor®. This computer provides histogram statistics of ICP, SAP and CPP over any desired period (Gaab et al. 1986). All patients were ventilated (CMV). Any increase in ICP exceeding 30 mm Hg was treated by using either osmotherapy (mannitol or sorbitol, 0.5 g/kg b.wt i.v. over 20 min) or THAM (50–100 mmol i.v. for 60–120 min resp) in a randomized manner. The effects of ICP, SAP, CPP, and EEG were compared statistically.

Results

Animal Experiments

In the *cat* experiments, a rapid increase in ICP develops 2–3 h after injury. THAM reliably produces a steep *drop in ICP* followed by a slow increase within 1 h. As the SAP rises, in addition, the CPP is increased overproportionally (Gaab et al. 1980, Knoblich et al. 1978, Knoblich et al. 1978). The *survival time* is *significantly longer* than with osmotherapy (Table 1 A) and is only exceeded by that after trephination and edema resection. In the experiments with *rats,* the tissue edema parameters water content and sodium are significantly decreased by THAM therapy. The *effect is better* than with any other drug investigates (Table 1 B). The K^+ loss (a sign of tissue necrosis) is diminished by THAM.

Clinical Investigations

The infusion of THAM (diluted with Ringers solution, isoosmolar) results in a *rapid decrease of the ICP* especially in pts with "isodense" brain swelling and large pulse amplitudes/tendency towards plateau waves. Not only the individual record, but also the statistical evaluation shows that the effect on ICP and CPP is at least as pronounced as with osmotherapy. In patients with severe intracranial

Table 1 A, B. THAM in experimental brain edema

A Survival time in cats significantly prolonged by THAM

Survival times of cats after 4-min-cold brain injury

Treatment	n	$\bar{x}$ (min)	s_x (min)	Signif. therapy group against controls
Controls (without therapy)	15	160	57	
Osmotherapy (40%, 8 ml/kg b.w.)	13	205	33	$p < 0.05 > 0.02$
Tris-buffer-Th. (Trometamol 5 mmol/kg)	5	234	49	$p < 0.01$
Operative Ther. (Resection of edematous brain tissue)	5	354[a]	(33)[a]	$p < 0.0005$

[a] 4 of the 5 animals were still alive and spontaneous respirating at 6 h after the injury (end of experiment with KCl i. v.).

B Tissue edema parameters in rats with controlled respiration

Therapy groups	n	Water content (rel. %)		Na^+ (mval/kg d.wt.)		K^+ (mval/kg d. wt.)	
		Right	Hemisphere left	Right	Left	Right	Left
Normals (no ed.)	20	76.97 ± 0.92	77.01 ± 0.82	158 ± 13	156 ± 12	355 ± 20	359 ± 15
Controls (no th.)	21	79.56 ± 1.00	77.92 ± 0.42	292 ± 46	239 ± 24	320 ± 29	370 ± 24
Tris-buffer (THAM)[3]	20	78.18 ± 0.74	77.27 ± 0.70	201 ± 35	164 ± 20	345 ± 31	353 ± 18
Na-bicarbonate[4]	20	79.14 ± 1.04	77.66 ± 1.14	258 ± 52	173 ± 40	331 ± 28	357 ± 28
Dexamethasone[5]	20	78.99 ± 0.82	77.53 ± 0.86	252 ± 43	184 ± 42	330 ± 56	352 ± 40
Barbiturate[6]	20	78.57 ± 0.88	77.45 ± 0.88	198 ± 34	166 ± 15	343 ± 22	349 ± 15

hypertension after trauma, therapy with alternation osmotherapy and THAM is therefore our routine procedure today provided that Tris buffer can be given according to blood gas analysis. Regarding the *EEG*, the effect of THAM is clearly *better* than that of osmotherapy. No side effects were seen in 53 patients up to now.

Conclusions

In *animal experiments* THAM is at least as effective in reducing the ICP as are osmotherapy or barbiturates. The effect on tissue edema parameters and on animal survival is even better. In *clinical investigations,* too, the ICP is decreased as reliably as with osmotherapy and the effect on the EEG as a parameter of tissue metabolism is more pronounced than with any other drug therapy. No side effects were seen with a dosage of $1-1.5$ mmol THAM/kg b.wt over $60-120$ min under conditions of controlled respiration provided that the base excess (BE) was $\leqq 3$ when starting Tris infusion.

Further investigations on THAM in acute brain damage seem to be justified and a *double blind clinical trial* is suggested.

References

Akioka T, Ota K et al. (1976) The effect of THAM on acute intracranial hypertension. An experimental and clinical study. In: Beks JWF, Broch DA, Brock M (eds) Intracranial pressure III. Springer, Berlin Heidelberg New York, pp 219–223

Gaab MR, Knoblich OE, Fuhrmeister U (1980) Effect of THAM on ICP, EEG and tissue edema parameters in experimental and clinical brain edema. In: Shulman K et al. (eds) Intracranial pressure IV. Springer, Berlin Heidelberg New York, pp 664–668

Gaab MR et al. (1986) Routine computerized neuromonitoring. In: Miller MD, Teasdale GM, Rowan JO, Galbraith SL, Mendelow AD (eds) Intracranial pressure VI. Springer, Berlin Heidelberg New York Tokyo, pp 240–247

Kesting U (1984) Medikamentöse Therapie beim experimentellen Hirnödem mit Natriumbikarbonat und THAM. Ph. D. Thesis, Julius-Maximilian-Universität, Würzburg (FRG)

Knoblich OE, Gaab MR et al. (1978) Comparison of the effects of osmotherapy, hyperventilation and THAM on brain pressure and EEG in experimental and clinical brain edema. In: Frowein RA et al. (eds) Advances in neurosurgery, vol 5. Springer, Berlin Heidelberg New York, pp 336–345

Knoblich OE, Gaab MR et al. (1978) Wirkung von Hyperventilation und THAM-Behandlung auf Hirndruck und elektrische Hirnaktivität im experimentellen Hirnödem. Neurochirurgia (Stuttg) 21:109–119

Mendelow AD (1988) Head injuries. Curr Opinion Neurol Neurosurg 1:37–45

rCBF Following an Experimental Missile Wound to the Brain

H.C. McKowen, J.B. Farrell, M.E. Carey, and J.S. Soblosky

Department of Neurosurgery, Louisiana State University Medical Center, 1542 Tulane Avenue, New Orleans, Louisiana 70112 (USA)

Introduction

The purpose of this experiment was to study the effect of a missile wound to the brain (MWB) on global and regional cerebral blood flow (rCBF).

Materials and Methods

CBF was measured by radioactive microspheres in 28 cats (23 test; 5 controls). Animals were anesthetized with i.v. or i.p. pentobarbital (30 mg/kg), intubated, and placed in a stereotaxic head frame. After paralysis with gallamine (5 mg/kg), they were placed on a respirator for control of respirations. Arterial blood gases were maintained at normal feline values. A left parietal epidural pressure transducer was placed and sealed with methylmethacrylate to reform a closed cranial vault.

Animals were wounded by a 2 mm, 31 mg steel sphere shot through the intact cranium. Brain entrance was through the right upper frontal pole (cruciate gyrus). The trajectory angled 20° away from the sagittal plane so that the missile exited the brain but not the skull in the right parietal-occipital area. Three different missile velocities were used: 225 meters/sec (m/s), 300 m/s and 380 m/s which provided missile energies of 0.9 Joules (J), 1.4 J and 2.4 J. Prior experiments had shown that 2.4 J wounds caused fatal apnea in about two thirds of cats. CBF determinations were made prior to injury and again 1 min, 30 min, 60 min and 90 min following MWB.

After the final blood flow measurement brains were fixed-perfused with 10% formalin, removed, and sectioned into 32 regions. Following initial gamma counting for rCBFs, each wounded hemisphere was reassembled. Hollow circular cylinders of tissue were then cored out in successive shells surrounding the entire length of the missile track and recounted to determine the radial distribution of blood flow changes adjacent to the missile track after wounding.

All data were analyzed by ANOVA, and individual CBF comparisons were made by Tukey's test. Significance was taken at $p < 0.05$.

Results

Nine cats developed intracranial hematoma after MWB (subdural or intracerebral hematoma expanding the missile track) while 14 exhibited no significant post wounding intracranial hematoma. Animals *with* post wounding intracranial hematomas had a progressive and severe diminution in global CBF attributable to a progressive rise in ICP and concomitant fall in CPP. All brain regions in this group showed diminished rCBFS paralleling drops in global CBF. Animals *without* intracranial hematomas showed no significant changes in global CBF over the 90 in post wounding period despite an ICP plateau of ~40 mm Hg and a drop in CPP to ~75 mm Hg. Post wounding rCBF changes consequent to missile wounding alone were most clearly delineated in those cats which did not develop intracranial hematoma after injury.

rCBF in Cats Without Post Wounding Intracranial Hematomas

Brain-wounded cats without hematomas showed distinct rCBF elevations early (1 minute) and late (30 minutes) following wounding (Fig. 1).

Early (1 Min) rCBF Changes. Following MWB significant, early rCBF elevations occurred about the area of entry in the right upper frontal pole as well as in the left upper frontal pole (*coup* regions). rCBF was also significantly increased in the left upper occipital pole (*contrecoup* region) in the same horizontal plane as the entry site. Gross structural lesions, other than the wound track itself, were generally not seen in these areas of rCBF increases. Mean arterial blood pressure (MABP) was elevated at this time.

Late (30 Min) rCBF Elevation. Late rCBF elevations were confined to the cores of tissue immediately surrounding the missile track. These areas alone showed a significant correlation between missile energy and the magnitude of the periwound track rCBF elevations. Increases in rCBF adjacent to the wound track

Early CBF Elevations   Late CBF Elevations

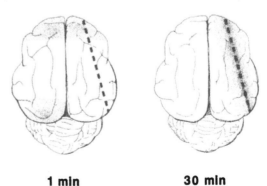

Fig. 1. Distribution of *early* (*1 min*) and *late* (*30 min*) rCBF elevations following missile wounding (*n* = 14, no intracranial hematoma)

1 min　　　　　　**30 min**

varied inversely with the distance from the missile track itself: higher flows were observed closer to the wound track; lower blood flows were seen at greater distances from the missile track. In all cases the late increased rCBF around the wound track returned to prewounding levels by 60 min. CPPs had returned to base line when these late rCBF elevations occurred indicating a significant, graded drop in cerebrovascular resistance (CVR) in tissues surrounding the missile track.

Discussion

The chronologic and anatomic separation of observed rCBF elevations following MWB suggests two different causative mechanisms: one due to concussion (early) and one due to penetration of brain tissue (late). Early rCBF elevations occurred in coup and contrecoup regions, and possibly represent a focal injury to cerebral blood flow autoregulatory mechanisms caused by pressure waves emanating from the impact site. MABP was invariably elevated at this time point and no significant CVR changes were demonstrable. The timing of these focal CBF elevations was identical to global CBF elevations seen in percussion hammer experiments of brain injury (DeWitt 1986). Late rCBF elevations about the wound track occurred after MABP had returned to normal control values. This indicated a graded loss of CVR in damaged brain tissue surrounding the missile track. Focal injury around the missile track appears to be related to the radial displacement of tissue outward from the path of the missile which occurs with temporary cavity formation in ballistic wounding. The late decrease in periwound track CVR following this early energy transfer suggests a mediator within damaged tissue the nature of which is under investigation.

In this model significant brain ischemia did not occur except in the face of intracranial hematoma, which caused a high ICP and low CPP.

References

DeWitt DS et al. (1986) Effects of fluid-percussion brain injury on regional cerebral blood flow and pial arteriolar diameter. J Neurosurg 64:787–794
Marcus ML et al. (1976) Total and regional cerebral blood flow measurements with 7–10, 15-, 25- and 50 μm microspheres. J Appl Physiol 40:501–507

Transtentorial Brain Herniation in the Monkey: Predictive Value of Brain-Stem Auditory and Somatosensory Evoked Responses

J.L. Stone, R.F. Ghaly, K.S. Subramanian, and P. Roccaforte

Division of Neurosurgery, Department of Surgery and Anesthesiology, Cook County and University of Illinois Hospitals, Chicago, Illinois 60612 (USA)

The monitoring of short-latency auditory (BAER) and somatosensory (SSER) evoked responses were studied extensively in head injury and states of increased intracranial pressure (ICP) (Stone et al. 1988). However, this study is a monkey model of transtentorial brain herniation (TBH) over a four hour period which was developed from our experience with traumatic intracranial hematomas.

Methods

Twelve cynomolgus monkeys were given pancuronium and placed on a ventilator with equal mixture of nitrous oxide and oxygen. Systemic arterial and intracranial pressure (subdural bolt) monitors were placed. An auditory click stimulus (85 dB pe SPL, 10/sec, 0.1 msec) was delivered to one ear. Electrodes were placed to stimulate each median nerve independently and to record EKG, EEG, BAER and SSER. A latex balloon was inserted into the temporal region extradurally. The balloon inflation rate was 1 ml followed by 0.5 ml every 30 minutes. At about 3 ml balloon inflation, systemic hypertension, bradycardia, and rise in ICP temporally followed each instillation. Mean ICP values were obtained 1 hour before (4 ml), 30 minutes before (4.5 ml), and at TBH (5 ml) were 16, 23, and 44 mm Hg respectively. TBH was documented as bilaterally dilated fixed pupils and generally came at about 4 hours, at a balloon volume representing 10% of the animal's brain volume. Following balloon deflation, the ICP dropped to control levels, and the pupils returned to normal size. Each animal was considered its own control and an analysis of variance performed for ICP, BAER, and SSER.

Results

Seven animals survived neurologically intact, five were either vegetative or died. This latter group showed central brainstem hemorrhages. Whole head pathologic preparations with the balloon inflated documented medial temporal TBH with marked midbrain shift. The ICP was increased from baseline 1 hour before ($p < .05$), 30 minutes before ($p < .01$), and at TBH ($p < .001$). The crebral perfusion pressure remained above 45 mm Hg in all but one animal. Wave V of the

BAER showed depressed amplitude 1 hour before ($p < .05$), 1/2 hour before ($p < .001$), and at TBH ($p < .001$). Wave IV of the BAER had depressed amplitude at TBH ($p < .01$). The later (P3N3) components of the SSER were lost 1/2 hour before ($p < .01$) or at TBH ($p < .001$). P2N2 of the SSER was also depressed at TBH ($p < .01$). By 30 minutes after deflation BAER and SSER were not significantly different from baseline. Immediate post-deflation ICP level was not significant from the baseline value. These findings in a primate model confirm observations made with similar experiments performed in our laboratory in cats (Nagao et al. 1979). These findings suggest that BAER and SSER in addition to ICP may be used to predict TBH.

References

Nagao S, Roccaforte P, Moody RA (1979) Acute intracranial hypertension and auditory brain-stem responses. Part 1: Changes in the auditory brain-stem and somatosensory evoked responses in intracranial hypertension in cats. J Neurosurg 51:669–676

Stone JL, Ghaly RF, Hughes JR (1988) Evoked potentials in head injury and states of increased intracranial pressure. J Clin Neurophysiol 5:135–160

Relationship Between Clinical Course, CT Scan and ICP in Post-Traumatic Diffuse Lesions

G. Tomei, E. Sganzerla, D. Spagnoli, P. Guerra, S. Gaini, and R. Villani

Institute of Neurosurgery, University of Milan, I-20122 Milan (Italy)

Introduction

There is strong anatomicopathological and experimental evidence that widespread axonal damage in the white matter (Diffuse Axonal Injury = DAI) is the primary brain lesion in posttraumatic diffuse injuries (Adams et al. 1982, Langfitt et al. 1982). Focal hemorrhages in the corpus callosum, basal ganglia and brain stem (shearing injury) are the distinctive macroscopic features of DAI (Strich 1961). DAI patients are comatose immediately after trauma and the CT scan shows deep hemorrhages that are indicative of the lesion. Patients in coma with a normal CT may belong to the same clinicopathological syndrome as the hemorrhagic components of DAI, demonstrated in these patients by Magnetic Resonance Imaging (Wilberger et al. 1987). DAI may be associated with diffuse brain swelling (Langfitt et al. 1982), hyperemia and increased cerebral blood volume playing the main role in its pathogenesis. The typical CT picture of diffuse brain swelling shows reduction in size of lateral ventricles (slit like ventricles) and absence of the 3rd ventricle and basal cisterns.

Patients and Methods

Our series includes 150 patients selected from 2100 cases of head injuries admitted to the Neurosurgical Institute of the University of Milan over the period 1981–87. The criteria of selection were immediate coma lasting more than 24 hrs and the CT appearance of diffuse lesions that were classified as follows: (1) *Diffuse axonal injury (DAI):* (a) normal CT (50 cases); (b) Shearing injury (20 cases) and (2) *Diffuse brain swelling (DBS)* (80 cases). Among these, a subgroup of 44 pts (55%) presented with either subarachnoid hemorrhage (SAH) or, in a limited number of cases, minimal subdural blood effusion which never evolved in a true hematoma. All patients were admitted to our Intensive Care Unit. Intracranial pressure (ICP) was continuously monitored during the acute phase by means of both intraventricular catheter or subarachnoid bolt in 31% of the cases. The jugular vein was cannulated in a group of patients and arteriojugular venous oxygen difference (AVDO$_2$) along with arterial and jugular venous lactate levels were measured twice a day during the first 3 days after admission. In a limited number of cases ventricular CSF lactate was determined. Injury severity was evaluated according to the Glasgow Coma Scale (GCS) score. The age of the patients ranged from 16 to 73 yrs (mean 25.5 ± 17).

Results

Clinical course, ICP trend and overall mortality rate were substantially different in the 2 groups of diffuse lesions.

1) Clinical Picture. Evaluation of the clinical picture showed that GCS on admission was lower (3–5) in patients with shearing injuries (60%) and in those with diffuse brain swelling and SAH (95%) (Table 1). In contrast, 65% of patients with a normal CT and 55% of those with diffuse brain swelling without SAH had a GCS=6 on admission (Table 1). Patients with no CT abnormalities usually showed rapid neurological improvement, on average obeying commands after 3 days from trauma. The latter patients showed no fluctuations in clinical condition over the following 2 weeks and their GCS was always higher than 12. Patients who died (7 cases=14%) had the lowest GCS on admission and all of them were older than 60. Patients with shearing injury needed more time to recover from coma (i.e. eyes opening, 10 days on average) and executed simple commands after 18 days on average. The mortality rate in this group was 25% (5 cases).

The different clinical course in patients with Diffuse Axonal Injury (normal CT and shearing injury patients) was characterized by a diverse incidence of persistent vegetative state. This complication, in fact, accounted for 8% (4 cases) in patients with normal CT and 25% (5 cases) in those with shearing injury. Surprisingly, the fate of patients with persistent vegetative state was better than expected. In fact, only 3 patients died and 2 are severely disabled after one year followup.

Table 1

	DAI			Diffuse brain swelling		
	Normal CT	Shearing injury	Total	DBS	DBS +SAH	Total
GCS on admission:						
3	–	–		10%	30%	20%
4–5	35%	60%		35%	65%	50%
6	65%	40%		55%	5%	30%
Duration of coma days (mean *)	3 *	10 *		3 *	3–7	
Persistent vegetative state	8%	25%		–	–	
Mortality rate	14%	25%	17%	42%	80.5%	63%
ICP (mm Hg):						
Normal	100%	85%				23%
20–60 (changeable)	–	15%		–		32%
> 60 (monotonous)	–	–	–	–		45%

In patients with diffuse brain swelling a clearcut distinction was noted between patients who died and those who survived. Those with fatal outcome had a mean GCS on admission of 4.5 ± 1.2. Patients with associated SAH had the highest rate (95%) of the lowest GCS ($= 3.5$). During the following days no significant neurological changes were apparent and death occurred shortly after injury (3–7 days). The mortality rate was 42% in patients with diffuse swelling and it reached its highest value (80.5%) in patients who had brain swelling associated with SAH or minimal subdural effusion. Patients who survived had a mean GCS on admission of 5.8 ± 1.4 and rapidly regained consciousness (3 days on average) when the therapy was effective in reducing intracranial hypertension. Moreover, a tendency to clinical deterioration was observed between the 5th and the 10th day from admission, often due to the appearance of respiratory disturbances, fever and other complications. These patients eventually awakened by the 15th day.

2) ICP Study. Forty per cent of patients with DAI were continuously monitored. Values exceeding 15 mm Hg were never recorded in patients with a normal CT. In patients with shearing injury ICP was usually within normal ranges except for 3 cases (15%) in which the presence of blood in the third ventricle caused a mild dilatation of the lateral and 3rd ventricles and an ICP increase. Intracranial hypertension was controlled by continuous CSF external drainage that never exceeded 100 ml/day.

Intracranial hypertension was the hallmark of patients with diffuse brain swelling and it was noticed in 77% of the cases (62 pts). In general, a strict relationship exists in these patients between GCS on admission, ICP trend and outcome. No survival occurred in those patients (36 cases $= 45\%$) whose recording was characterized by monotonous high pulse wave (45–90 mm Hg) over a baseline of 20–30 mm Hg and ICP was never normalized with hyperventilation, barbiturates, or CSF external drainage. When ICP was changeable with recurrent elevations no higher than 60 mm Hg (32%) and when all resources aimed at reducing intracranial hyperemia were effective in producing a moderate increase of ventricular size, intermittent CSF drainage resulted in a definite decrease and eventual normalization of ICP. The amount of CSF withdrawn was 2–3 ml/hr and it was never followed by a flattening of the recording. During such maneuvers, hyperventilation, barbiturate and mannitol infusion were not discontinued. In 23% of patients, ICP was normal despite the presence of CT findings strongly suggestive of diffuse brain swelling. These patients were always mechanically ventilated, keeping the pCO_2 above 32 mm Hg.

$AVDO_2$, obtained in 11 pts, resulted in a wide arteriovenous difference approaching ischemic levels ($AVDO_2 = 8.2 \pm 0.7$ and 7.9 ± 0.9) during the first 24 hours after admission (Fig. 1). In the same group of patients venous jugular and CSF lactate (the latter obtained in 5 patients) had a peculiar trend (Fig. 1). On admission, lactate levels were markedly abnormal with an AV difference approaching 30% of jugular increase. During the following 12 hours, lactate production remained below normal, yet in a limited number of patients (2 cases) a renewed elevation was noticed during the following 2 days (Fig. 1). These patients, whose $AVDO_2$ on admission was high, died.

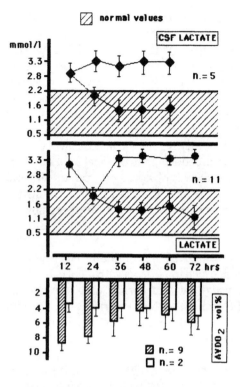

Fig. 1. Arteriovenous jugular oxygen difference ($AVDO_2$), venous jugular lactate levels (*LACTATE*) and CSF lactate levels (*CSF LACTATE*) trends during the first 3 days after trauma in patients with CT indicative of diffuse brain swelling and normal ICP

Discussion

Analysis of the clinical course of our patients clearly shows that the severity of diffuse injury depends on the brain lesion itself. The good results obtained in deeply comatose patients with no CT abnormalities are due to the fact that a diffuse lesion – namely, diffuse axonal injury – involves brain parenchyma to a less severe degree. Appearance of deep hemorrhages on CT scan is indicative of a wider extension of axonal damage from the cerebral hemispheres to the corpus callosum and brain stem. This leads to more serious neurological impairment (60% of patients with GCS = 4–5 on admission), a greater incidence of persistent vegetative state (25%) and a higher mortality rate (25% vs 14% in patients with normal CT).

Diffuse axonal injury can be considered as the primary posttraumatic lesion (Adams et al. 1982; Langfitt et al. 1982) and it usually does not cause an increase of ICP.

Appearance of secondary vascular involvement brings about a series of secondary intracranial lesions (Fig. 2), in which diffuse brain swelling plays an important role due to its frequency (45%) and its mortality rate (63%). Hypoxemia, anemia and other unknown causes seem to be the basis factors in the pathogenesis of diffuse brain swelling. The degree of severity of this lesion rises with the presence of subarachnoid hemorrhage or subdural effusion. The main causes of progressive elevation of ICP in these patients are vasoparesis and

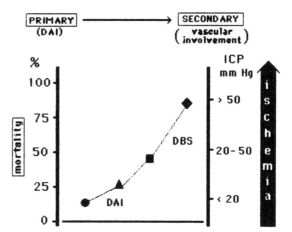

Fig. 2. Mortality rate and lesion categories of diffuse lesions. *DAI:* Diffuse Axonal injury (● *normal CT;* ▲ *shearing injury*); *DBS:* Diffuse Brain Swelling (■ *diffuse brain swelling;* ◆ *diffuse brain swelling and subarachnoid hemorrhage*)

increase of cerebral blood volume and brain water content (Langfitt et al. 1982; Teasdale et al. 1986). Intracranial hypertension is responsible for rapid neurological deterioration (70% of patients had a GCS = 3–5). The possibility to treat ICP effectively is related to the degree of intracranial hypertension and to the promptness of therapy, mainly aimed at the prevention of ischemia. Continuous ICP monitoring and $AVDO_2$ lactate measurements seem useful in the early detection of ischemia, particularly in those patients in whom CT indicates diffuse swelling and ICP is normal. In these cases, such determinations prevent excessive hyperventilation and worsening of brain ischemia.

References

Adams HJ, Gennarelli TA, Graham DI (1982) Brain damage in non missile head injury: observations in man and subhuman primates. In: Smith TW, Cavanagh JB (eds) Recent advances in neuropathology. Churchill Livingstone, Edinburgh London Melbourne New York, pp 165–190

Langfitt TW, Gennarelli TA, Obrist WD, Bruce DA, Zimmermann RA (1982) Prospects for the future in the diagnosis and management of head injury: pathophysiology, brain imaging and population based study. Clin Neurosurg 29:353–376

Strich SJ (1961) Shearing of nerve fibers as a cause of brain damage due to head injury. Lancet II:443–448

Teasdale GM, Mendelow AD, Galbraith S (1986) Causes and consequences of raised intracranial pressure in head injuries. In: Miller JD, Teasdale GM et al. (eds) Intracranial pressure VI. Springer, Berlin Heidelberg New York Tokyo, pp 3–8

Wilberger JE, Deeb Z, Rothfus W (1987) Magnetic resonance imaging in cases of severe head injury. Neurosurgery 4:571–576

Effect of Prophylactic Hyperventilation on Outcome in Patients with Severe Head Injury

J.D. Ward, S. Choi, A. Marmarou, R. Moulton, J.P. Muizelaar, A. DeSalles, D.P. Becker, H.A. Kontos, and H.F. Young

Division of Neurosurgery, Medical College of Virginia, MCV Station Box 508, Richmond, Virginia 23298 (USA)

Introduction

Severe head injury remains a major problem despite advances in recent years. The mortality of patients with a coma score of eight or less is still between 45–55% (Miller et al. 1981). In an attempt to improve outcome in a significant number of these patients, we have directed our efforts toward therapeutically influencing the brain and its environment after a severe head injury. Severe mechanical brain injury initiates a series of complex events in the brain which are thought to secondarily influence the ultimate outcome of the patient. One of these proposed secondary events is cerebral acidosis. The presence of cerebral acidosis has been inferred by the presence of lactate in the CSF of patients sustaining a severe mechanical brain injury (Cold et al. 1975, Enevoldsen et al. 1977, Sood et al. 1980). In addition, prognostic significance has been attached to high levels of lactate in the CSF after a severe brain injury (Crockard et al. 1972; Seitz and Ocker 1977). Furthermore, it has been shown that acidosis itself, when present as the result of any pathologic process, is harmful to the brain (Pulsinelli and Petito 1983). It was felt therefore that outcome from severe head injury might be improved if cerebral acidosis present after a head injury was treated.

Several investigators have used a variety of agents to buffer acidosis. Sietz and coworkers used intrathecal sodium bicarbonate in patients in coma from severe head injury (Seitz and Ocker 1977). Gaab used THAM both clinically and experimentally in the treatment of brain edema (Gaab et al. 1980). Others have also used THAM or similar agents to buffer suspected acidosis (Akiota et al. 1976). Based on our experience from laboratory investigation, we decided to use THAM to treat our severely head injured patients in a prospective controlled trial (Rosner and Becker 1984).

Since the aim of the trial was to treat brain tissue acidosis, it was reasoned that hyperventilation might be sufficient to raise systemic pH and buffer the brain tissue acidosis. Hyperventilation is in widespread use as an adjunct in the treatment of patients with severe head injury. In fact, it has been suggested that hyperventilation might attain its beneficial effect as a result of compensation of CSF acidosis and improve outcome in head injured patients (Gordon and Rossanda 1970, Rossanda et al. 1973). Although hyperventilation is in common use, there has never been a randomized trial of its use in severe head injury. Therefore, a randomized controlled trial was conducted with the following objectives: to improve outcome in patients with a severe head injury by treating cerebral acidosis with hyperventilation and THAM. This paper is a report on the results of the first part of the study, that is, the use of prophylactic hyperventilation in the treatment of patients with a severe head injury.

Methods

The present study consists of all patients over the age of three years who arrived at the Medical College of Virginia from January 1983 until December 1987, with a severe nonpenetrating head injury and a Glasgow Coma Score (GCS) of eight or less after six hours. Patients were randomized into one of the three groups using a baseline motor score as a stratifying factor: 1) control (C), 2) hyperventilation (HV), and 3) THAM plus hyperventilation (TH-HV). In the control group P_aCO_2 was maintained at 35 ± 2 mm Hg while the other two groups had their P_aCO_2 maintained at 24 ± 2 mm Hg. P_aCO_2 was checked every 4–6 hours. All patients underwent aggressive resuscitation, diagnosis, and treatment of mass lesions. All patients were treated in the neuroscience intensive care unit and had intracranial pressure monitoring either with a ventricular catheter if possible, a subarachnoid bolt, or Camino device. All patients had hemodynamic monitoring with appropriate arterial and central venous or pulmonary artery lines. All patients had a catheter inserted into the jugular bulb for determination of A-VdO$_2$ every 4–6 hours. A baseline battery of multimodality evoked potentials and again at 12, 24, and 36 hours were obtained on a routine basis. CBF, CMRO$_2$, and autoregulation was measured at similar intervals using the intravenous xenon technique. Blood and CSF lactate (in patients with ventricular catheter) was drawn every 12 hours for 5 days. THAM levels were drawn daily in the treated group.

Upon completion of all baseline tests, the control group P_aCO_2 was adjusted to 35 mm Hg, the hyperventilation group P_aCO_2 set to 24 mm Hg, and a THAM dose was calculated for the THAM group (TH-HV). The THAM dose is calculated by determining the bicarbonate at a P_aCO_2 of 35, then extrapolating the bicarbonate level at a pH of 7.6. The difference gives the base deficit, which was then multiplied by the patient's body weight. The calculated THAM amount was then given in bolus over the next two hours. A maintenance dose was then given at a rate of 1 cc per kilogram per hour for five days. The ventilator was adjusted to maintain the P_aCO_2 at 24 ± 2 mm Hg. Glucose and electrolytes were watched carefully and fluid administration determined and adjusted in all groups to maintain normal central pressures, i.e.: a pulmonary capillary wedge pressure of 10–15 mm Hg.

All patients had their outcome assessed at three, six, and twelve months using the Glasgow outcome categories of good, moderately disabled, severely disabled, vegetative and dead.

Results

A total of 114 patients were studied: 36 in the THAM group, 36 in the hyperventilation group, and 42 in the control group. Table 1 lists the number of cases, their age and sex, neurological deficits, GCS on admission, ICP of admission and the number of mass lesions. There was a statistical difference among results in these three groups. In addition, a comparison was made between the admission multimodality evoked potentials of all three groups and there was no statistical difference. The randomization process was therefore adequate. There was no difference between the baseline P_aCO_2 values of the other two groups on the corresponding days. Table 1 shows the three and six month outcome of the three groups respectively. There was a statistical difference between the control and the hyperventilation groups in the good and moderately disabled categories at three and six months. The hyperventilation group did less well at these intervals than the control group. There was no difference between the control group and THAM plus hyperventilation group as far as outcome was concerned. An analysis of expected outcome based on our past 350 patients using the entry data of each of the three groups was also performed. This showed that the control groups did as was predicted while the hyperventilation group did worse than predicted. CBF, $CMRO_2$, and A-VdO$_2$ were analyzed for both groups. Although there was a difference between the amount of change from day one to day three between the control and the hyperventilation groups, none of the values in the hyperventilation group reached values that would be considered ischemic. In addition, A-VdO$_2$ in the hyperventilation groups did not reflect any persistent failure to meet metabolic demands.

The hyperventilation group had pH measurements in the CSF and blood that were alkalotic when compared to control.

The findings of this study are that hyperventilation, if used prophylactically and not just in the course of ICP control, results in a poorer outcome for patients at three and six months. That is, recovery is retarded by the prophylactic use of hyperventilation.

The implication of these findings are clear. In the treatment of elevated ICP, hyperventilation is utilized only after drainage, sedation, paralysis, and mannitol have been used and are no longer effective.

Table 1. 3 and 6 month outcome of control and hyperventilation groups

	G	MD	SD	V	D
Three month outcome					
Hyperventilation	2	2	15	8	9
Control	1	11	9	9	12
Six month outcome					
Hyperventilation	3	5	15	5	8
Control	4	12	11	2	13

G = good, MD = moderately disabled, SD = severely disabled, V = vegetative, D = dead

Acknowledgements. This research was supported in part by the Grants NS-12587 and RO1-NS 19235 from the National Institutes of Health. Additional facilities and support were provided in part by the Richard Roland Reynolds Neurosurgical Research Laboratories.

References

Akioka T, Ota K, Matsumoto A, et al. (1976) The effect of THAM on acute intracranial hypertension. An experimental and clinical study. In: Beks JWF, Bosch DA, Brock M (eds): Intracranial pressure III. Springer, Berlin Heidelberg New York, pp 219–233

Cold G, Enevoldsen E, Malmros R (1975) Ventricular fluid lactate, pyruvate, bicarbonate, and pH in unconscious brain-injured patients subjected to controlled ventilation. Acta Neurol Scand 52:187–195

Crockard HA, Taylor AR (1972) Serial CSF lactate-pyruvate values as a guide with acute severe head injury coma. Europ Neurol 8:151–157

Enevoldsen EM, Jensen FT (1977) Cerebrospinal fluid lactate and pH in patients with acute severe head injury. Neurol Neurosurg 80:213–225

Gaab M, Knoblich OE, Spohr A, Bourke H, Fuhrmeister U (1980) Effect of THAM on ICP, EEG, and tissue edema parameters in experimental and clinical brain edema. In: Shulman K, Marmarou A, Miller JD, Becker DP, Hochwald GM, Brock M (eds) Intracranial pressure IV. Springer, Berlin Heidelberg New York, pp 664–709

Gordon E, Rossanda M (1970) Further studies in cerebrospinal fluid acid-base status in patients with brain lesions. Acta Anaesthesiol Scand 14:79–109

Miller JD, Butterworth JF, Gudeman SK, et al. (1981) Further experience in the management of severe head injury. Neurosurgery 54:289–299

Pulsinelli WA, Petito CK (1981) The neurotoxicity of hydrogen ion. Stroke 14:13

Rosner MJ, Becker DP (1984) Experimental brain injury: Successful therapy with a weak base tromethamine with an overview of CNS acidosis. J Neurosurg 60:961–971

Rossanda M, Selenati, Villa L, et al. (1973) Role of automatic ventilation in treatment of severe head injuries. J Neurosurg Sci 17:265–270

Seitz HD, Ocker H (1977) The prognostic and therapeutic importance of changes in the CSF during the acute stage of brain injury. Acta Neurologica 38:211–231

Sood SC, Gulati SC, Kumar M, Kak VK (1980) Cerebral metabolism following brain injury. II. Lactic acid changes. Acta Neurochir (Wien) 53:47–51

The PA/ICP-Relation in Head-injured Patients: is There only one Relationship?

A. Brawanski, J. Meixensberger, R. Zöphel, and W. Ullrich

Department of Neurosurgery, University of Würzburg, Josef-Schneider-Str. 11, D-8700 Würzburg (FRG)

Introduction

Many remarkable results have been published which show a correlation of the pulse amplitude (PA)–mean ICP (PM) relationship to the intracranial reserve capacity. However, many of the results were accomplished by animal experiments and the clinical studies were performed during relatively short time intervals. Our study investigates whether the PA/PM relationship remains stable in a single patient during a prolonged period of time.

Patients and Methods

Epidural ICP, the arterial blood pressure and the respiratory pattern of 8 head injured patients was recorded continuously for the first 5 days after admission. All patients had diffuse brain edema on CT scan, all were treated conservatively with barbiturate coma and hyperventilation. Any changes of ventilation, barbiturate dosage or fluid imbalance were recorded separately. The clinical status was examined according to the Glasgow Coma Scale several times a day.

The data were stored on tape at eight hour intervals and transferred to a computer at 4 hour or 2 hour intervals. In order to eliminate respiratory induced ICP and PA undulations, we calculated the mean PM and the mean PA at 15 sec intervals. Using these data the PM and PA were plotted against each other. The variance of each single mean point was calculated in order to have a criterion which would indicate whether other PA/PM data of the sampling interval belonged to the same mathematical distribution. With this mathematical approach, 8 hour intervals and 2 hour intervals were checked for the distribution of the PA/PM relationship.

Results

The 8 hour intervals revealed multiple PA/PM curves in 67 of the 89 patients (Fig. 1). Similarly, we found multiple PA/PM relations in 15% of the two hour intervals corresponding to our "variance criteria". Some of these multiple curves

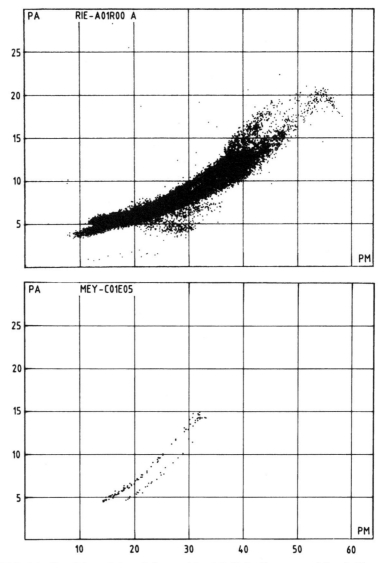

Fig. 1. The PA/PM plot of an 8 hour interval shows at least 2 distinctive curves (*above*). The same phenomenon was found during a plateau wave (*below*)

were clearly caused by external stimuli, like changes in respiration or arterial blood pressure. However, in many instances we did not find any obvious reason. All of the multiple curves occurred during marked ICP changes, including plateau waves or other major ICP undulations (Fig. 1).

Discussion

Our data indicates that, in one patient, several PA/PM relationships may occur. Some of them are caused by changes of blood pressure and pCO_2. These results correspond to findings by Eijndhoven et al. (1983). On the other hand, significant changes of the ICP itself showed a similar effect. These findings are in agreement with the concept of Sullivan et al. (1977) (increasing edema, formation of brain contusions, etc.). These issues are under further investigation.

Consequently, our results have one major implication for the clinical use of the PA/PM relationship as an indirect measure of intracranial reserve capacity: The existence of several PA/PM curves in one patient renders the intracranial system unstable during prolonged periods. A different PA may occur at the same ICP levels. Furthermore, volume pressure tests (Szewczykowski et al. 1977) seem to be unreliable, an issue which already has been investigated by Kosteljanetz (1986). Thus, it seems likely that PA/PM relationship cannot simply be used as an indicator for intracranial reserve capacity.

References

Eijndhoven JH, Avezaat CJ (1983) Cerebrospinal Fluid Pulse Pressure as Parameter of Intracranial Elastance. In: Wood J (ed) Neurobiology of cerebrospinal fluid 2. Plenum Publishing Corporation, pp 643–660
Kosteljanetz M (1986) Acute Head Injury: Pressure-Volume Relations and Cerebrospinal Fluid Dynamics. Neurosurgery 18:17–24
Sullivan HG, Miller JD, Becker DP, Flora RE, Allen GA (1977) The physiological basis of intracranial pressure change with progressive epidural brain compression. Neurosurgery 47:532–550
Szewczykowski J, Sliwka S, Kunicki A et al. (1977) A fast method of estimating the elastance of the intracranial system. Neurosurgery 47:19–26

Tomographic Mapping of CBF, CBV and Blood Brain Barrier Changes in Humans After Focal Head Injury Using SPECT-Mechanisms for Late Deterioration

R. Bullock, P. Statham, J. Patterson, G.M. Teasdale, E. Teasdale, and D. Wyper

Departments of Neurosurgery and Clinical Physics, Institute of Neurological Sciences, Southern General Hospital, Glasgow G51 4TF (UK)

Introduction

Ischemic brain damage due to reduced global cerebral perfusion pressure is a major determinant of outcome after head injury, and its recognition has led to major changes in management over the last few years (Graham et al. 1978). However, the effects of focal injury upon the local cerebral microcirculation has received little attention despite experimental evidence that progressive abnormalities can occur and may account for the delayed deterioration which often occurs in patients with cerebral contusions, intracerebral or subdural hematomas (Bullock et al. 1984). Serial CT scanning in patients with focal injury have shown hematoma enlargement in under 10% of patients while progression of surrounding brain edema occurs in one third of cases, and may cause raised intracranial pressure (Kobayashi et al. 1983). Hyperaemia has also been cited as a cause of raised ICP after diffuse injury and has been demonstrated after focal injury, but its role in causing later deterioration is not known (Kuhl et al. 1980).

We have used SPECT to explore the following questions:

1. How is regional CBF influenced by focal brain injury?
2. How do changes in regional CBF and CBV vary with time after focal injury?
3. Which forms of focal injury induce a blood brain barrier lesion?
4. What are the effects of surgical evacuation of a focal lesion on the blood brain barrier?

Patients and Methods

Twenty patients with focal cerebral contusion, two with intracerebral hematomas and four with acute subdural hematoma were studied. CT, MRI and serial SPECT imaging (NOVO 810 scanner) were carried out at various time intervals 1–30 days after head injury. RCBF was mapped using 90 mTc HMPAO (Ceretec), RCBV was mapped using 99 mTc labelled red cells and blood brain barrier changes were mapped using 99 Technicium pertechnetate. Eight SPECT slices 10 mm apart were made and abnormalities were graded visually with reference to the contralateral hemisphere and normal volunteers. Both the extent and intensity of the abnormality on SPECT were considered in grading the lesion as mild, moderate or marked for each parameter.

Results

In 9 patients, *serial CBF* maps were made, 10–20 days apart, 1–25 days after injury, and these showed varied patterns of evolution (Table 1).

- Zones of hypoperfusion
  - – ENLARGED in 3 (contusions)
  - – REDUCED in 3 (SDH, 2 contusions)
  - – UNCHANGED in 3 (ICH, 2 contusions)

- Zones of hyperperfusion
  - – Absent in 6 (ICH, SDH, 4 contusions)
  - – Present in 3 (contusions) disappeared within 5 days of injury

Table 1. SPECT; Abnormalities in 26 focal head injury patients

	HMPAO CBF		CBV ^{99}mTc red cells	BBB lesion ^{99}mTc per-technetate
	Hypoperfusion	Hyperperfusion	Engorgement	
Contusion n = 20	Nil 0	Nil 5	Nil 0	Nil 0
	Mild 4		Mild 1	Mild 1
	Moderate 1	Moderate 1		Moderate 2
	Marked 3	Marked 2	Marked 1	Marked 4
ICH n = 2	Nil 0	Nil 2		Nil 0
	Moderate 1			Mild 1
	Marked 1			Marked 1
ASDH n = 4	Nil 2	Nil 4	Nil 0	Nil 0
	Mild 1		Mild 1	Mild 1
	Moderate 1		Moderate 1	Moderate 1
				Marked 2
26				

Blood-brain barrier maps were made in 13 patients. Zones of barrier breakdown were most marked with contusion.

RCBF and BBB Lesions

RCBF and Blood-brain barrier maps were made at similar times in 7 patients. In 5 cases with a zone of blood-brain barrier disturbance, a corresponding zone of hypoperfusion was present. In the remaining 2 patients, neither rCBF nor blood brain barrier changes were present.

BBB Lesions

BBB lesions were most marked surrounding contusions. After surgical removal of a focal lesion, the size of the barrier lesion was reduced in four of five patients studied pre- and post-operatively.

In three of four acute SDHs in whom blood brain barrier maps were made, a zone of barrier opening was seen under the SDH.

Conclusions

1. Zones of reduced CBF are common around ICH and contusions, and occur under some ASDHs.
2. Hypoperfusion may co-exist with hyperperfusion, but the latter disappears a few days after injury.
3. Focal peri-lesional hypoperfusion coexists with regions of breakdown of the blood-brain barrier, and may worsen with time, after injury.
4. Surgical removal of contusions is associated with a reduction in the size of the blood-brain barrier lesion, on SPECT.

Acknowledgements. This study was funded by the Institute of Neurological Sciences Research Trust, Glasgow, The SPECT imager was funded by the Wellcome Trust.

References

Bullock R, Mendelow AD, Teasdale GM, et al. (1984) Intracranial hemorrhage induced at arterial pressure in the rat. Part 1. Neurol Res 6:184–188
Graham DI, Adams JH, Doyle D (1978) Ischemic brain damage in fatal nonmissile head injuries. J Neurol Sci 39:213–234
Kobayashi S, Nakazawa S, Otsuk T (1983) Clinical value of serial computer tomography with severe head injury. Surg Neurol 20:25–29
Kuhl DE, Alavi A, Hoffmann EJ, et al. (1980) Local cerebral blood volume in head injured patients. J Neurosurg 52:309–320

Optimal Cerebral Perfusion Pressure in Head Injury

D.G. Changaris[1], C.P. McGraw[1], and R.A. Greenberg[1]

[1] Division of Neurological Surgery, Department of Surgery, [2] Department of Community Health, The School of Medicine, The University of Louisville, Health Sciences Center, Louisville, Kentucky 40292 (USA)

Introduction

The lowest Cerebral Perfusion Pressure (CPP) sustainable for days is unknown. An acute reduction in CPP below 45 alters sensorium (Stone et al. 1965, Williams 1968). Cerebral ischemia is reported to occur when CPP falls below 25–30 mm Hg (Tyson and Jane 1982). It seems likely that the brain should be more sensitive to prolonged reductions in CPP. Previously published works by the authors show that all severely head injured patients who had a 48-hour CPP below 60 mm Hg died (of 136 patients with severe head injury, 24 fell into this category; Changaris et al. 1988). We sought to determine if early clinical improvement was more frequent when the 48-hr CPP was greater than 80 mm Hg.

Materials and Methods

Patient Population

The 88 chosen from 562 patients monitored with either subarachnoid or intraventricular devices during the years 1981 to 1988, had a Highest Glasgow Coma Score (HGCS) equal to 5 or 6 on day 1. Clinical improvement was defined as improvement in the day 2–3 HGCS. This study excluded patients with operated epidural, subdural, and intracranial hematomas. Continuous and hourly measurements of intracranial pressure guided the therapy. This included fluid restriction, selective colloid administration, hyperventilation, mannitol, and furosemide. The hourly CPP consisted of the hourly difference between the Mean Arterial Pressure (MAP) and Intracranial Pressure (ICP). The averages of the individual hourly readings over the entire 48 hr period (days 2 and 3) were done for day 2–3 MAP, ICP, and CPP.

Of the 88 patients with an HGCS equal to 5 or 6 recorded for day 1, 74% were male and 26% were female. Their ages ranged between 15 and 84 with a mean of 26 years of age. Slightly fewer than half had multiple system injury requiring orthopedic or general surgical intervention.

Eds.: J.T. Hoff and A.L. Betz
© Springer-Verlag Berlin Heidelberg 1989

Statistical Analysis

The ridit transformation (Fleiss 1981) of the three clinical groups [improved, unchanged, and worsened] generated numerical scores [ridits: 0.83, 0.46, 0.13, respectively]. Ridits above 0.5 indicate above average clinical improvements: conversely, a ridit below 0.5 indicates a greater tendency to clinical deterioration.

Because the initial hypothesis was whether the patients with a day 2–3 CPP greater than 80 mm Hg show more clinical improvement, patients with the day 2–3 CPP ≥ 80 mm Hg were used as the reference group (mean ridit normalized to 0.500).

Results

Ridit Analysis

Table 1 shows the frequency distributions from the reference (≥ 80 mm Hg) and comparison groups (< 80 mm Hg). The 95% confidence interval for the ridit of the comparison group is 0.187 to 0.440 with a mean $r = 0.321$ and standard error s.e. $(r) = 0.,0608$. The z score (-2.944) is significant ($P = 0.0032$). This estimates that the odds of showing clinical improvement is more than doubled ([$1.000 - 0.321$]/$0.321 = 2.11$) for an CPP above 80 mm Hg during the first three days after head injury as compared with a CPP below 80 mm Hg.

70 mm Hg Cerebral Perfusion Pressure

Plotting the population showing clinical improvement (Fig. 1; MAP vs. ICP) and the line corresponding to the CPP = MAP – ICP = 70 mm Hg shows that all the patients who show clinical improvement lie above this line.

Table 1. Frequency distributions from reference (≥ 80 mm Hg) and comparison ($\leq$) groups

	≥ 80 mm Hg Reference group (N_j)	≤ 80 mm Hg Comparison group (n_j)	Total ($N_j + n_j$)
Status			
Worsened	8	15	23
Unchanged	26	9	35
Improved	23	7	30
Total	57	31	88

Mean ridit $= \bar{r} = 0.321$; S.E. $(\bar{r}) = 0.0608$; Z $= 2.944$; $P = 0.0032$
(For computational details see Fleiss, 1981, p. 154)

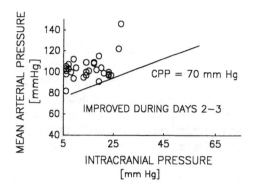

Fig. 1. The patients showing clinical improvement during days 2–3 ($n=30$) are shown. All the patients fall above the line $CPP=70$ mm Hg. This provides an estimate of lowest day 2–3 CPP tolerated

Discussion

Statistical (ridit) analysis of the *a priori* hypothesis shows that an ACPP above 80 mm Hg doubles the chance of clinical improvement. However, the visual inspection of the data shows that some patients improve when the day 2–3 CPP is close to 70 mm Hg. This suggests that the CPP should be maintained above 70 mm Hg and preferably above 80 mm Hg.

References

Changaris DG, McGraw CP, Richardson JD, Garretson HD, Arpin EJ, Shields CB (1988) Correlation of cerebral perfusion pressure and Glasgow coma scale to outcome. J Trauma 27:1007–1013

Fleiss JL (1981) Statistical methods for rates and proportions. John Wiley and Sons, New York, pp 151–156

Stone HH, Donnelly CC, MacKrell TN, Brandstater BJ, Nemir P Jr (1965) The effect of acute hemorrhagic shock on cerebral circulation and metabolism of man. In: Mills LC, Moyer JH (eds) Shock and hypotension: Pathogenesis and treatment. Grune and Stratton, New York, pp 257–264

Tyson GW, Jane JA (1982) Pathophysiology of head injury. In: Cowley RA, Trump BF (eds) Pathophysiology of shock, anoxia, and ischemia. Williams and Wilkins, Baltimore, pp 570–600

Williams LF (1968) Hemorrhagic shock as a source of unconsciousness. Surg Clin North Am 48:263–272

Effect of Stable Xenon Inhalation on ICP in Head Injury

J.M. Darby, H. Yonas, J.J. Moossy, J.R. Boston, and D.W. Marion

University of Pittsburgh, School of Medicine, Pittsburgh, Pennsylvania (USA)

Introduction

Stable xenon enhanced CT (Xe/CT) allows for the measurement of local cerebral blood flow (LCB F) with high resolution and anatomic specificity. Its application in head injury victims may ultimately provide important prognostic and clinical information as well as insight into basic pathophysiology (Harrington et al. 1986; Latchaw et al. 1986). Animal and human studies have suggested that stable xenon inhalation may cause cerebral blood flow to increase (Gur et al. 1985; Junck et al. 1985; Obrist et al. 1985). In the head injured population, this effect might result in an increase in intracranial pressure (ICP). We evaluated changes in ICP in patients with head injury while undergoing clinical cerebral blood flow studies using Xe/CT.

Methods

Ten patients with severe head injury (GCS ≤ 8), four with intracranial mass lesions, underwent a total of 22 CBF evaluations with the GE 9800 CT scanner adapted for blood flow imaging. All patients were intubated at the time of the study and were receiving controlled ventilation with a volume cycled ventilator modified to deliver a 33% xenon, 67% oxygen gas mixture during CBF imaging. ICP was monitored through a closed ventriculostomy or via direct brain tissue pressure monitoring with a transducer tipped fiberoptic system. Arterial blood pressure was monitored continuously. Exhaled xenon and CO_2 were monitored continuously in end-tidal air during gas delivery.

Following baseline CT scans, sequential enhanced CT scans were obtained during 4½ minutes of inhalation of the gas mixture. Arterial pCO_2 was measured directly at the end of the examination in 19 observations and indirectly by capnography in the remainder of the observations. For the purposes of analysis, blood pressure and ICP data were evaluated immediately before xenon inhalation and at peak end-tidal xenon concentration at the end of the inhalation period (Peak xenon $= 30-31\%$). Data were analyzed with a two-tailed t-test.

Intracranial Pressure VII   643
Eds.: J. T. Hoff and A. L. Betz
© Springer-Verlag Berlin Heidelberg 1989

Results

The ICP and blood pressure data of ten patients with severe head injury undergoing CBF imaging are presented in Table 1. Baseline ICP was ≥ 20 mm Hg in 54% of the observations. At a mean arterial pCO_2 of 24 mm Hg, there were no significant differences from baseline in mean arterial pressure or ICP with xenon inhalation. ICP rose to ≥ 5 mm Hg in two patients during xenon inhalation. One of the patients had unstable ICP before CBF study requiring CSF venting and the other patient developed secretions in the tracheobronchial tree resulting in coughing and an increase in peak airway pressures during delivery of the gas mixture. The maximum rise in ICP observed in this study during xenon inhalation did not exceed 6 mm Hg.

Table 1. Intracranial pressure and blood pressure in patients with severe head injury undergoing CBF imaging [a]

	Baseline (mean $\pm$ SD)	Peak xenon (mean $\pm$ SD)	P
ICP	19.4$\pm$ 4.9	19.6$\pm$ 5.4	NS
MAP	96.0$\pm$16.4	94.8$\pm$17.2	NS

[a] $n=22$; CBF evaluations in 10 patients.

Discussion

If stable xenon increases CBF, patients with head injury undergoing CBF imaging with XE/CT might be at risk for increases in ICP during the procedure. Harrington et al. (1986) reported variable increases in ICP in 28 patients undergoing CBF imaging with a 7 minute xenon inhalation period. However, they did not report absolute changes in ICP nor did they report the arterial pCO_2 at which their patients were ventilated. With a 4½ minute xenon inhalation period, under hypocapnic conditions, we observed no consistent increase in ICP during xenon inhalation. Potentially important rises in ICP that were observed in two patients were related to factors other than xenon inhalation itself.

Our observations suggest that under hypocapnic conditions, inhalation of a 33% Xe/67% O_2 gas mixture for CBF imaging does not cause ICP to increase in head injured patients.

References

Gur D, Yonas H et al. (1985) Measurement of cerebral blood flow during xenon inhalation as measured by the microspheres method. Stroke 16(5):871–874

Harrington TR, Manwaring K et al. (1986) Local basal ganglion and brain stem blood flow in the head injured patient using stable xenon enhanced CT scanning. In: Miller JD, Teasdale

GM, Rowan JO (eds) Intracranial Pressure VI. Springer, Heidelberg New York Tokyo, pp 680–686

Junck L, Dhawan V et al. (1985) Effects of xenon and krypton on regional cerebral blood flow in the rat. J CBF Metab 5:126–132

Latchaw RE, Yonas H et al. (1986) Xenon/CT cerebral blood flow determination following cranial trauma. Acta Radiologica (Suppl) 369:370–373

Obrist WD, Jaggi J et al. (1985) Effect of stable xenon inhalation on human CBF. J CBF Metab 5 (Suppl 1): 557–558

Experimental Epidural Bleeding in Swine: ICP Course, Mass Displacement, Changes in Brain Tissue Water and the Effects of INFIT

J. Ganz, N.N. Zwetnow, U. Ponten, P. Nilsson, K.A. Thuomas, and K. Bergstroem

Section of Experimental Neurosurgery, Institute for Surgical Research, The National Hospital, Oslo (Norway) and Departments of Neurosurgery and Neuroradiology, Academic Hospital, Uppsala (Sweden)

Introduction

Loefgren and Zwetnow (1972), in 1972 found that intracranial arterial bleeding is an essentially self-limiting process. Haematoma volume is determined by the interplay of 5 factors. Three of these factors, counterpressure, haemostasis and possibly vasospasm act to reduce bleeding. The remaining two factors, CSF outflow and cerebral homeostasis, consisting of autoregulation and increased O_2 extraction, compensate for the presence of an intracranial haematoma.

Epidural bleeds have been shown to differ from other intracranial bleeds in two respects (Habash et al. 1983). These are the effects of dura adherence to the skull and an arteriovenous shunt, which develops during the stripping of dura from the skull. In earlier work (Ganz and Zwetnow 1988) it has been shown that the greater the degree of dura detachment the faster the volume increase of the haematoma. Thus dura attachment represents an extra element of counter-pressure to bleeding. On the other hand the arteriovenous shunt reduces the epidural pressure and thereby increases the bleeding pressure, since this is the difference between arterial pressure and epidural pressure. The higher bleeding pressure is associated with a greater bleeding rate and tends to prolong bleeding. Moreover while the shunt reduces the epidural pressure this is associated with a reduction in intradural pressure so that a pressure gradient is maintained. The force acting on the dura to detach it from the bone may be reduced in this situation but never enough to preclude further dura detachment and thus haema-toma volume growth. Thus in epidural bleeding dural attachment and the arterio-venous shunt alter the course of bleeding without affecting the basic principles governing haematoma volume, as stated above.

Aims

It is known that the volume increase of an intracranial haematoma is rapid from the start and decreases exponentially (Loefgren and Zwetnow 1972), and that this also applies to epidural bleeding (Habash et al. 1983). Thus this study compares the sequence of mass shifts during epidural bleeding compared with those seen with expansion of an epidural balloon from an infusion pump, which gives a linear volume input. MRI was used for this examination and at the same time brain tissue water, in association with epidural bleeding was measured. Moreover the effect of artificial counterpressure on the course of epidural bleeding was studied using the technique of Intracranial Fluid Infusion Tamponade or INFIT.

Materials and Methods

Bleeding was induced in anesthetized swine, imitating the natural bleeding course by leading blood from the femoral artery, via an electronic drop recorder into a collapsed epidural balloon. An epidural balloon was used since the arteriovenous shunt that develops during epidural bleeding prevents the continuous measurement of haematoma volume using the drop recorder. This is because leakage of blood out of the epidural space through the shunt makes the bleeding volume different from the haematoma volume. The use of a balloon together with a drop recorder obviates this problem. In infusion experiments the epidural balloon was expanded with saline from a Braun-Melsinger infusion pump. Intraventricular pressure, cisterna magna pressure, epidural pressure, arterial pressure, central venous pressure, respiration, EEG and ECG were monitored continuously. INFIT was applied through an additional cisterna magna catheter (Fig. 1).

Magnetic Resonance Imaging. Superconductive 0.5 T equipment (Magnetom, Siemens) was used. SE sequences with TR 2000 ms and TE 35, 120 ms were applied in the frontal and sagittal planes. The time-interval between each registration was 8 mins. Slice thickness was 10 mm.

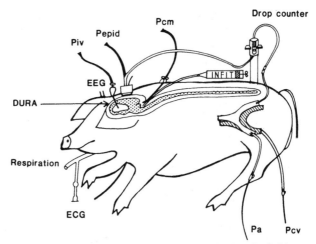

Fig. 1. The model used in the INFIT experiments is shown here diagrammatically. The fluid was injected into the cisterna magna to ensure even distribution of pressure throughout the CSF spaces. A separate needle was used from that used for Pcm measurement so as not to distort that measurement

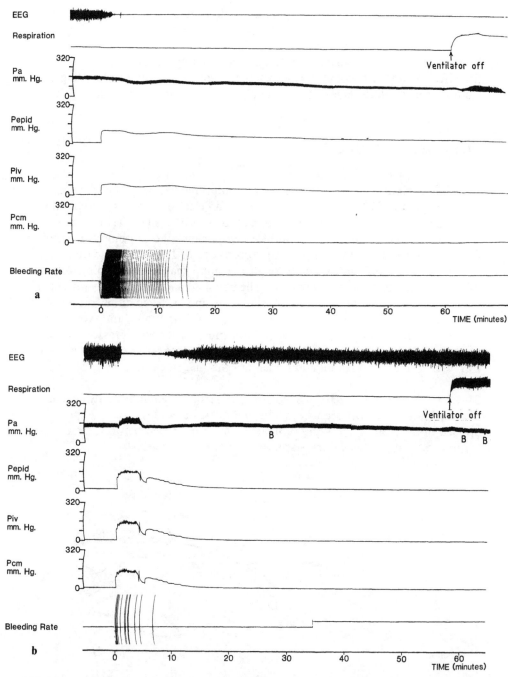

Fig. 2. a Epidural bleeding in a ventilated pig following detachment of the dura over the entire hemisphere. The course of pressures is typical and the lethal outcome inevitable. **b** Epidural bleeding in a model identical with that depicted in **a** but with the application of INFIT. Note the rise in all intracranial pressures and the concomitant rise in Pa. (*B*) under the Pa trace indicates i.v. injection of barbiturate anaesthetic. The animal survived and breathed adequately. For further details see text

648

Results

There was an orderly sequence of compressions and shifts of the ventricular system with infusion experiments. There was a similar orderly sequence of herniations from above downwards. In the case of epidural bleeding the same mass shifts occurred but they occurred earlier and almost together. Moreover herniation occurred virtually simultaneously. It was also found that tissue water, expressed as normalized T2 weighted signal intensity increased following the development of a haematoma, indicating the development of cerebral oedema.

Figure 1 shows the model used in the INFIT experiments. Fig. 2 shows the characteristic pressure changes during an epidural bleed in a ventilated animal with dura detached over the entire hemisphere. In seven experiments this bleeding model was invariably lethal. There was a rapid initial bleeding rate which decreased exponentially and stopped. The intracranial pressures rose rapidly and a transtentorial pressure gradient developed early. There was a fall in arterial pressure at the beginning of the bleeding. The haematoma volume increased so rapidly that the EEG became isoelectric within 2–3 minutes. After 1 hour, following disconnection of the ventilator, the animal could not breath spontaneously. After an attenuated Cushing Response cardiovascular collapse occurred. In the experiment depicted in Fig. 2b INFIT was applied by injecting cooled, mock CSF into the cisterna magna. This produced a rise in all intracranial pressures and at the same time a rise in arterial pressure. The cerebral perfusion pressure fell below 30 mm Hg and the EEG became isoelectric. The INFIT was regulated by watching the pulsating drop in the drop counter and allowing 1–2 drops through every minute by reducing the INFIT pressure and thus temporarily increasing the cerebral perfusion pressure. After 5 minutes the INFIT pressure was decreased stepwise and finally stopped. The intracranial pressures returned to near control levels. No herniations developed. The EEG began to recover before the intracranial pressures had normalized and reached normal amplitude after about 15 minutes. After one hour the animal was able to breathe spontaneously. Blood gas measurements indicated that this respiration was adequate. This outcome was consistent in the seven experiments performed which were identical with the lethal preparation illustrated in Fig. 2a except for the application of INFIT.

Discussion

MRI Study

This study showed two major findings of interest. Firstly the difference in sequence of mass shifts and compressions between epidural bleeding and epidural infusion mirror the different patterns of volume expansion in the two situations. Infusion gives a linear volume input while bleeding gives a rapid early volume input, the rate of which decreases exponentially. The linear volume growth is probably more like the clinical expansion seen in non-haemorrhagic space occupying lesions. Compressions and shifts and herniations occurred in sequence, with herniations occurring late in the course of the expansion. The early herniations following epidural bleeding are clearly clinically relevant. The finding that water accumulated in the hemisphere in association with an epidural bleed suggests that cerebral oedema can develop in the presence of epidural bleeding in the absence of direct brain trauma, and would thus exacerbate the clinical condition.

INFIT Study

The earlier finding that counterpressure, developing during intracranial bleeding reduces the rate of increase of haematoma volume has been applied in the present study by using the artificial counterpressure in INFIT. This technique converted a lethal epidural bleeding model into a survival model. The probable explanation is related to the different effects of epidural bleeding and INFIT on outflow resistance. A bleed left a haematoma mass in the cranial cavity which increased outflow resistance of producing herniations and by compression of cerebral veins. INFIT produced a temporary rise in pressure, which dissipated as the infused fluid drained out of the cranium. The haematoma volume remaining in the epidural balloon was insufficient to produce herniation or to produce significant compression of cerebral veins. Thus the ICP could return to normal or near normal levels and the cerebral perfusion pressure could return to adequate levels.

Conclusions

1. Brain shifts and herniations occur early in epidural bleeding.
2. Cerebral oedema can develop in association with epidural bleeding in the absence of direct brain trauma.
3. INFIT can prevent the lethal outcome of an aggressive epidural bleed.

References

Ganz JC, Zwetnow NN (1988) Analysis of the dynamics of experimental epidural bleeding in swine. Acta Neurochir (Wien) (In Press)
Habash AH, Zwetnow NN, Ericson H, Loefgren J (1983) Arteriovenous epidural shunting in epidural bleedings – radiological and physiological characteristics. An experimental study in dogs. Acta Neurochir (Wien) 63:291–313
Loefgren J, Zwetnow NN (1972) Kinetics of arterial and venous hemorrhage in the skull cavity. In: Lundberg N, Ponten U, Brock M (eds) Intracranial pressure II. Springer, Berlin Heidelberg New York, pp 155–159

Cerebral Concussion Suppresses Hippocampal Long-term Potentiation (LTP) in Rats

S. Miyazaki, P.G. Newlon, S.J. Goldberg, L.W. Jenkins, B.G. Lyeth, Y. Katayama, and R.L. Hayes

Division of Neurosurgery, Medical College of Virginia, Richmond, Virginia 23298 (USA)

Introduction

Patients suffering even mild head injury commonly have residual memory deficits (Rimel et al. 1981), the mechanisms of which are unknown. Recent experimental studies have shown that prolonged memory deficits exist following moderate head injury without any gross pathological change (Lyeth et al. 1987). It is our hypothesis that such enduring behavioral deficits may result following even mild trauma due to membran depolarization and excitatory transmitter release (Katayama et al. 1988; Hayes et al. 1988). It has been proposed that such events maladaptively alter synaptic efficacy (Hayes et al. 1988). In contrast, hippocampal long-term potentiation (LTP) provides a model of adaptive synaptic modification possibly involved in the formation of memory (Teyler et al. 1984). The present study examined for the first time the effects of cerebral concussion on hippocampal LTP in rats.

Material and Methods

Male Sprague-Dawley rats were subjected to cerebral concussion at 1.5 atm of fluid percussion brain injury. Animals were surgically prepared under Nembutal anesthesia 24 hours prior to injury. The transient behavioral effects of injury were evaluated by measuring the duration of righting response suppression. LTP was evaluated in the Schaffer collateral/CA1 pathway under urethane anesthesia (1.1 g/5 ml/kg i.p.) 2 to 3 hours following injury. The population EPSP and the population spike were recorded in response to 0.2 Hz stimulation before and 15 min after tetanic stimulation. To avoid contamination by the population spike, the measurements of the population EPSP were taken as the initial slope. The amplitude of the population spike was measured from the onset of the spike on the population EPSP to the negative peak of the spike. LTP of the population spike was expressed as the ratio of the post to pre tetanus spike amplitude in each animal. LTP of the population EPSP was also expressed as a ratio of the post to pre tetanus EPSP slope. LTP was evaluated at the stimulus intensity that would cause 15% of the maximum amplitude of the population spike before the tetanus. All animals were examined histologically after the experiments to confirm electrode placement and any possible pathological lesion or hemorrage.

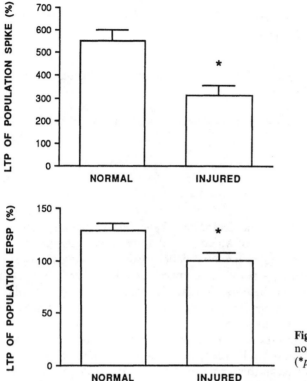

Fig. 1. Comparison of LTP in normal and injured animal (*$p < 0.02$)

Results

Righting response of all the injured animals was restored within 9 min following injury. Injured animals also did not exhibit convulsion and prolonged apnea. The threshold for eliciting the population spike decreased significantly in the injured animals. The input-output curve of the population spike showed a significantly decreased amplitude before the tetanus in the injured animals at the higher stimulation current. This was in contrast to the increase observed at the lower current intensity. Although a similar finding was shown on the curve of the population EPSP, the difference were not significant. LTP of population EPSP and population spike were significantly suppressed in the injured animals. There was no significant difference between the control animals and the injured animals in the latency of population EPSP. There was not any gross pathological change in the injured animals except for mild subarachnoid hemorrage overlying the traumatized convexities. Proper electrode placement was verified histologically in all animals (Fig. 1).

Conclusion

1. Cerebral concussion alters synaptic efficacy and excitability in the Schaffer collateral/CA1 system of the rat hippocampus.
2. LTP in the Schaffer collateral/CA1 system of the rat hippocampus is suppressed following cerebral concussion in the rat.
3. According to the putative role of LTP in memory function, similar mechanisms that produce alteration in LTP following cerebral concussion may also produce memory deficits following injury.

Acknowledgements. This work was supported by NS 21458 and NS19550.

References

Hayes RL, Lyeth BG, Jenkins LW (1988) Neurochemical mechanisms of mild and moderate head injury: implications for treatment. In: Levin HS, Eisenberg H, Bention AL (eds) Mild head injury. Oxford University Press, London (in Press)

Katayama Y, Cheung MK, Madsen P, Becker DP (1988) Excitatory amino acids mediate an increase in extracellular potassium following concussive brain injury in the rat hippocampus. J Neurotrauma (in Press)

Lyeth BG, Jenkins LW, Hamm RJ, Robinson SE, Dixon CE, Geibel ML et al. (1987) Enduring short term memory deficits in the absence of hippocampal cell death following moderate head injury in the rat. Soc Neurosci Abstr 13:1253

Rimel RW, Giordani B, Barth JT, Boll TJ, Jane JA (1981) Disability caused by minor head injury. Neurosurgery 9:221–228

Teyler TJ, DiScenna P (1984) Long-term potentiation as a candidate mnemonic device. Brain Res Rev 7:15–28

Histological Changes of the Brain by Experimental Extradural Compression

O. Sakuta, J. Mukawa, E. Takara, M. Nakata, T. Kinjo and H. Kuda

Department of Neurosurgery, University of the Ryukyus, 207 Uehara, Nishihara-cho Okinawa 903-01 (Japan)

Introduction

This experimental study was designed to clarify the effects of long-standing brain compression.

Materials and Methods

26 adult cats, 2.4–3.2 kg in body weight, were anesthetized with halothane in a 70:30 mixture of nitrous oxide and oxygen delivered through an intubated tube, and ventilated artificially. The brain was compressed by inserting 10–15 steel balls (5 mm in diameter every 10 minutes) into the extradural space through a small burr hole at the left parietal bone. Systemic arterial pressure (SAP) was monitored from an aortic catheter via the femoral artery, and intracranial pressure (ICP) was measured by a plate-type pressure transducer placed in the right parietal epidural space.

The animals were divided into six groups depending on the duration of compression (1 hour, 6 hours, 2 days, 7 days, 1 month and 6 months).

After the period, the animals were anesthetized again and maintained normocapnia ($PaCO_2$ 35–43 mm Hg). The brains were perfused via both carotids with 10% buffered formalin, and additional fixation was followed for 2–3 weeks. The brains were sectioned coronally, (5 mm in thickness) perpendicular to the orbit-meatal line with a reference point in the interauricular line.

From these slices, the cross-sectional areas of affected and contralateral brains were measured using a microcomputer.

The cross-sectional area-ratio (CAR) of affected brain was calculated from the following equation.

$$CAR(Lt/Rt) = S(Lt)/S(Rt)$$

S: Cross-sectional Area; Lt: Affected Brain; Rt: Contralateral Brain

These slices were cut into 10 μm thick sections and stained with hematoxylin-eosin or with a combination of Nissl and Luxolfast blue. Histological examination was made under conventional light microscope to identify sequential changes caused by longstanding brain compression.

Eds.: J. T. Hoff and A. L. Betz

Results

Systemic Parameters

ICP was progressively increased up to 35 mm Hg during ball insertion, and gradually decreased down to 20 mm Hg within 2 hours after it. It had a tendency to regain normal level within 6 hours. SAP and ECG did not alter significantly during these periods.

Cross-Sectional Area-Ratio (CAR)

The CAR remained unchanged in 1 hour group. There was significant reduction in CAR in the 1 and 6 month groups. ($p < 0.05$ Student-t-test and Wilcoxon rank sum test.)

Histological Changes (Table 1)

The focal shrinkage of neurons with dark-staining nuclei was seen in the 1 hour to 7 day groups. Chromatolysis and rupture of neurons appeared predominantly at the deeper cortex in the 2 day group, and remained in the 1 month group. Infiltration of microglia was found with chromatolysis. Dense gliosis, calcification around vessels and disappearance of cortical architecture were found in the 6 month group.

Table 1. Histological changes of compressed brain

	1 hr	6 hrs	2 days	7 days	1 month	6 months
Shrinkage of neurons	+	+	+	+	−	−
Chromatolysis	−	±	+	+ +	+	±
Infiltration of microglia	−	−	+	+ +	+	−
Gliosis	−	−	−	−	+	+
Calcification	−	−	−	−	−	+
Destruction of cortex	−	−	−	±	+	+ +

Discussions

This study has confirmed that intracranial mass makes brain tissue progressively atrophic. The histological changes of the compressed brain divide into two phases from this study, the first is focal shrinkage of neurons as an acute reaction, the second is chromatolysis as a chronic reaction. Chromatolysis seems to be a major finding of long-standing compressed brain and it causes rupture of neurons and destruction of cortical architecture. It is suggested that brain compression by intracranial mass should be relieved within two days in order to avoid the chronic reaction.

Conclusions

The following conclusions were drawn concerning the effects of long-standing brain compression in the cat:

1. One of the effects of long-standing compression on the brain is a progressive atrophic process; chromatolysis → rupture of neuron → infiltration of microglia → gliosis → destruction of cortical architecture.
2. This process begins after two days of compression and is completed within six months.

Effect of Hemorrhagic Hypotension on CBF and ICP After Brain Missile Wounding in Anesthetized Paralyzed Cats

D. Torbati, B.J. Farrell, J.F. Davidson, and M.E. Carey

Louisiana State University Medical Center, Department of Neurosurgery, 1542 Tulane Avenue, New Orleans, Louisiana 70112 (USA)

Introduction

The intracranial pressure (ICP) may increase following brain missile wounding (BMW), leading to a corresponding decrease in cerebral perfusion pressure (CPP). Extreme reductions in CPP (i.e. <40 mm Hg), can affect both CBF auto-regulation (Zwetnow 1968) and reduce brain energy metabolism (Zwetnow 1970). BMW-induced pathology may also impair CBF autoregulation, while hemor-rhagic hypotension (associated with multiple wounds) could further aggravate the breakdown of CBF autoregulation. In the present study alterations in ICP and CPP in relation to CBF autoregulation by means of hemorrhagic hypoten-sion were investigated in unwounded and brain wounded anesthetized paralyzed cats.

Method

The complete description of our experimental BMW model using anesthetized cats is presented elsewhere (Carey et al. 1988). Briefly however, pentobarbital anesthetized cats were cannulated in femoral and brachial arteries for CBF mea-surements by radioactive microspheres (Gd, Sn, Ru, Nb, and Sc; 10 µc/kg ran-domly injected through an intraventricular cannula inserted via a femoral artery), recording of MABP and bleeding to induce hypotension. An epidural ICP probe was placed over the left parietal cortex and 3 EEG electrodes were implanted, 2 over the right parietal and one over the left parietal cortex. After completion of surgery, cats were paralyzed with 10 mg/kg gallamine and were artificially respi-rated. BMW was inflicted by a 2 mm, 31 mg steel sphere penetrating the intact cranium into the right cerebral hemisphere at 280 m/s corresponding to 1.4 J. Experimental groups included:

A – Normotensive Unwounded ($n=8$; control)
B – Hypotensive Unwounded ($n=10$; control)
C – Normotensive Wounded ($n=8$)
D – Hypotensive Wounded ($n=10$)

In cats that were not subjected to bleeding (groups A and C), CBF was measured 10 min before BMW or a sham-injury (time zero) and at 5, 20, 45 and 90 min thereafter. In cats that were subjected to hemorrhagic hypotension (group B and D), after a control CBF measurement (10 min before time zero), the CBF was measured at 3 steady-state levels of hypotension corresponding to time points 5, 20 and 45 min after BMW or sham-injury. The last CBF measurement was made at 90 min time point, after all collected blood was reinfused and a normotensive MABP was achieved.

In all groups, MABP, ICP, EEG and ECG were continuously recorded throughout the experiments, while blood samples were taken for gas analysis during each CBF measurement.

Results

Changes in total CBF, MABP, ICP and CPP in all groups are illustrated in Fig. 1.

Among unwounded, normotensive controls MABP slightly increased during the course of the experiment (Fig. 1 A), while CBF remained constant. CBF autoregulated in unwounded cats made hypotensive by bleeding. After reinfusion of shed blood MABP returned to normal levels (Fig. 1 C). Among normotensive wounded cats, CBF decreased after BMW, but on the average remained above 20 ml/100 g/min (Fig. 1 B), which is above critical level required for metabolic demands (Zwetnow 1970).

Brain wounded cats made simultaneously hypotensive did not autoregulate CBF and the brain became ischemic at relatively high levels of MABP. Reinfusion of shed blood did not completely restore MABP and further decreased CBF (Fig. 1 D). Both hemorrhage and BMW produced severe metabolic acidosis. However, the CVR was significantly reduced only during hemorrhagic hypotension without BMW, while it was significantly increased during hemorrhagic hypotension followed by BMW or BMW without hemorrhage. Brain functional activity was reduced after BMW or BMW and hemorrhagic hypotension as judged by severe reductions in frequency and amplitude of the EEG. Cardiac arrythmias developed immediately after BMW in both normotensive and hypotensive cats.

Discussion

The ICP may increase following BMW because of intracranial hemorrhage, increased rate of CSF formation or decrease rate of CSF absorption, as well as, due to an increase in the intracerebral vascular volume and vasogenic brain edema. The expected rise in ICP, lowering the CPP could compromise CBF autoregulation. These data indicate that the CBF autoregulation was impaired following BMW. Lack of CBF autoregulation after BMW led to brain ischemia even after mild degrees of hemorrhagic hypotension. Reinfusion of blood after BMW and hemorrhagic hypotension further increased ICP (absence of CBF autoregulation) and did not restore CBF to levels known to maintain brain functional activity.

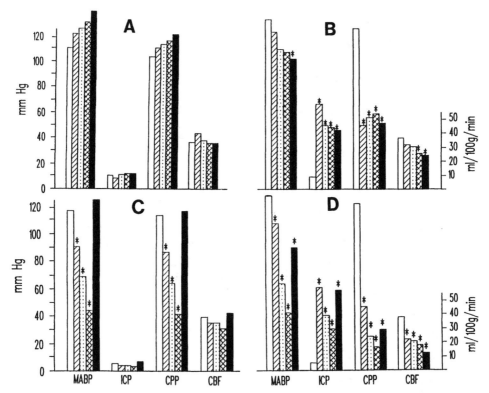

Fig. 1. Alterations in CBF in relation to systemic and cranial pressure changes in anesthetized paralyzed cats during 5 consecutive measurements in normotensive unwounded (**A**), normotensive wounded (**B**), hypotensive unwounded (**C**) and hypotensive wounded groups (**D**)

☐ Control measurement during which all cats were normotensive and unwounded corresponding to 10 min before time zero for BMW, bleeding, both or none.

▨ 5 min after time zero; 5 min post-BMW in B and D and 5 min post-bleeding in C and D.

⊡ 20 min after time zero.

▧ 45 min after time zero; before blood reinfusion started in C and D

■ 90 min after time zero after reinfusion in C and D completed.

* significant; p<0.05; analysis of variance

This may have significant clinical importance concerning treatment of BMW which is accompanied by hemorrhagic hypotension. The underlying mechanisms of the above phenomena are currently investigated.

References

Carey ME, Sarna GS, Farrell JB, Happel LT (1988) Experimental missile wound to the brain. A new model in the anesthetized cat. Submitted for publication

Zwetnow N (1968) CBF autoregulation to blood pressure and intracranial pressure variations. Scand J Lab Clin Invest [Suppl] 102V:A

Zwetnow N (1970) The influence of an increased ICP on the lactate, pyruvate, bicarbonate, phosphocreatine, ATP, ADP and AMP concentrations of the cerebral cortex of dog. Acta Physiol Scand 79:158–166

The Relation Between Mass Effect of Extradural Hematomas and Glasgow Coma Scale (GCS)

J.O. Espersen and O.F. Petersen

Departments of Neurosurgery and Neuroradiology, The University Hospital, Aarhus (Denmark)

Fifty-nine consecutive patients with extradural hematoma – admitted from Dec. 1st. 1977 to Nov. 30th 1981 – had a CT-scan performed prior to surgery. The GCS was recorded at the time of CT-scanning, and the "best GCS" recorded for the time period from the injury to the CT-scanning.

The volume of 54 measurable extradural hematomas were measured by the volume summation method, i.e. $V = T \times (A_1 + A_2 + \ldots A_n)$, where T = slice thick-

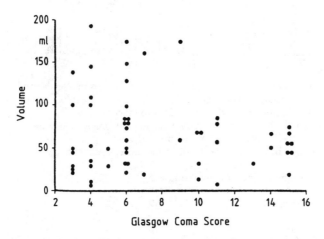

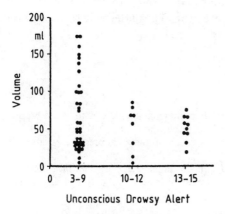

Fig. 1. All patients with measurable hematomas (54 patients)

ness and A = area of the single slice. The reliability was tested using silicone "hematomas" in a skull. The "hematomas" were measured by volume summation on a CT-scan and replacement by water.

The material as a whole showed no clearcut relationship between the size of the hematoma and the clinical condition – apparently due to the fact that many patients had other severe brain lesions. In unconscious patients (GCS between 3 and 9) the range of the hematoma was 5 to 192 ml (Fig. 1).

In patients with a "best GCS" of 11 or more and no other hematomas at the time of the CT-scan – indicating only slight primary brain injury – a good correlation between the GCS and the volume was found. No patients with a hematoma exceeding 75 ml were conscious at the time of the CT-scan, indicating the critical extradural volume, above which unconsciousness always appears (Fig. 2).

It is concluded that man can compensate for up to 75 ml extradural hematoma. If this limit is exceeded, the patient's condition rapidly worsens. The critical volume is, of course, dependent on other lesions, hydrocephalus and brain atrophy. More than half of the patients with extradural hematomas had severe additional lesions affecting the level of consciousness.

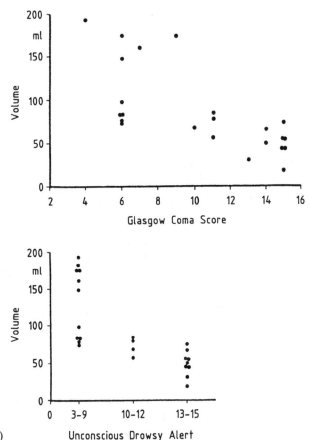

Fig. 2. Patients having a best GCS of 11 or more and no other hematomas (25 patients)

Predicting Neuropsychological Outcome by Physiological Parameters of Severe Head Injured Patients

C.P. McGraw, M.J. Ball, and N.A. Davis

Department of Surgery, University of Louisville, School of Medicine, Louisville, Kentucky 40292 (USA)

Introduction

This study was conducted to determine if there is a significant relationship between the severity of brain injury (as indicated by the first 72 hours of intensive care unit monitoring in severe head injury patients) and the degree of cognitive recovery.

Methods

Thirty patients who had survived severe closed head injury were administered a battery of neuropsychological tests. These patients were comatose upon admission, were unable to perform appropriate motor response to painful stimuli and had a Glasgow Coma Scale (GCS) of less than 8. These patients, who were in the intensive care unit, received hourly evaluation and the hourly GCS, ICP and blood pressure were recorded in a computer data bank. All patients had intracranial pressure (ICP) monitors for at least 72 consecutive hours. Readings of elevated ICP were combared with hyperventilation, mannitol, furosemide, intermittent ventricular drainage, or a combination. Subjects were screened to insure that no other prior history of head injury, pretraumatic psychological problems and no history of alcohol or drug abuse existed. Patients were followed at least 1 year following the injury. The patients used in this study had Glasgow outcome scores of 4 (unable to return to work or school but can provide domestic self maintenance) or 5 (return to full function with residual deficits). All were given a battery of neuropsychological tests: Logical Memory Section of the Wechsler Memory Scale Form I, Selective Reminding Test, Trail Making Test A and B, Wisconsin Card Sort, Benton Visual Retention Test, Milner Facial Memory Test, Seashore Rhythm Test, and the Object Assembly Section of the Wechsler Adult Intelligence Scale Revised. Total test time per patient ranged from 75 minutes to 105 minutes.

The resulting data were examined by Pearson Correlation Coefficients, scatter plots and "t" testing using the BMDP* Statistical Software package. The following for each consecutive 24 hour period of monitoring was statistically analyzed with each test score: highest ICP (HICP), highest GCS (HGCS), average ICP (AICP), lowest GCS (LGCS), average GCS (AGCS), lowest CPP (LCPP), aver-

Eds.: J. T. Hoff and A. L. Betz
© Springer-Verlag Berlin Heidelberg 1989

Table 1. Pearson correlations

Test	Day 1			Day 2			Day 3		
	W 0	W 30	SEL	W0	W 30	SEL	W 0	W 30	SEL
% ICP > 30	<0.01	<0.01	<0.01						
HICP	<0.04	<0.01			<0.01		<0.03	<0.02	<0.01
AICP	<0.01	<0.01	<0.04						<0.01
% CPP < 60	<0.02	<0.05	<0.02				<0.04		

Test	WIS	TRB	BEN	WIS	TRB	BEN	WIS	TRB	BEN
AMABP						<0.03	<0.01	<0.01	<0.01
LMABP								<0.01	<0.03
HMABP	<0.02			<0.01		<0.05	<0.01	<0.04	<0.04
ASBP								<0.01	<0.04
LSBP								<0.01	<0.02
HSBP				<0.03				<0.03	
ADBP	<0.03			<0.05		<0.05	<0.01		<0.02
HDBP	<0.01			<0.01			<0.01		<0.04
LCPP								<0.01	<0.04
ACPP					<0.05		<0.01	<0.01	

age CPP (ACPP), percent time the CPP was below 60 mm Hg, average Mean Arterial Blood Pressure (AMABP), lowest MABP (LMABP), highest MABP (HMABP), average Systolic Blood Pressure (ASBP), lowest SBP (LSBP), highest SBP (HSBP), average Diastolic Blood Pressure (ADBP), lowest DBP (LDBP), and the highest DBP (HDBP).

Results

Poor test scores for Wechsler at zero time (W0), Wechsler 30 minutes later (W30), and the Selective Reminding Test (SEL) were associated (Pearson correlations) with higher ICP readings and the percent time the CPP was low (Table 1). Poor test scores for the Wisconsin card sort (WIS), Trail Making Test B (TRB), and the Benton Visual Retention Test (BEN) were associated with higher blood pressure readings and higher CPP readings (Table 1).

Discussion

Verbal memory was significantly affected by elevations of ICP and reductions of Cerebral Perfusion Pressure. Since ICP is not localized to a specific area of the brain, this finding supports such studies demonstrating memory deficiencies associated with head injury. It was also noted that the first 24 hour period was the most critical for predicting verbal memory damage.

The poor test scores associated with high CPP and blood pressure levels were observed most frequently on the third day. This finding suggests that higher CPP and blood pressure levels are associated with increasing edema. There was not an explicit increase in ICP or a corresponding decrease in CPP on the third day. However, local edema may be compromising tissue perfusion to the extent that higher blood pressures are required in order to adequately perfuse the tissue.

In conclusion, deficiencies in verbal memory were associated with elevated ICP and the percent time CPP was below 60 mm Hg. Deficiencies were also associated with higher levels of blood pressure and average CPP on the third day suggesting that this may be an association secondary to the peak of edema. Thus, the upper limits of blood pressure and CPP were associated with poor test scores measuring reaction time, concentration, mental tracking, and higher level complex reasoning.

Acknowledgement to Dennis Buchholz, Ph. D., Neuropsychologist for his aid in testing these patients and preliminary efforts with respect to the project.

Neuronal Dysfunction and Intracranial Pressure: Multimodal Monitoring of Severely Brain-Damaged Patients

T. Shiogai, T. Sakuma, M. Nakamura, E. Maemura, C. Kadowaki, M. Hara, M. Ogashiwa, and K. Takeuchi

Department of Neurosurgery, Kyorin University School of Medicine, 6-20-2, Shinkawa, Miataka, Tokyo 181 (Japan)

Introduction

Neuromonitoring of brainstem auditory evoked potentials (BAEP), short-latency somatosensory evoked potentials (SSEP), compressed spectral arrays (CSA) and/ or conventional EEG can provide useful information on neuronal dysfunction within the brainstem and cerebrum in severely brain-damaged patients with elevated intracranial pressure (ICP). This study was undertaken to delineate the evolution of neuronal dysfunction in terms of the relationships among neuromonitoring and neurological findings, ICP and cerebral perfusion pressure (CPP).

Patients and Methods

Forty-nine patients with severe brain damage (Glasgow Coma Scale score of 7 or less) whose ICP had been continuously monitored (epidural pressure in 40 patients and intraventricular pressure in 9) were selected. They were divided into two groups: group D comprised 34 patients who died (27 were brain-dead), and the 15 survivors composed group S. Their mean age was 46 years (range, 11–79). Nineteen were treated with pentobarbital. Brain damage resulted from cerebrovascular accident in 27 patients and head injury in 22. All but 6 patients (3 with diffuse brain swelling, 2 with subarachnoid hemorrhage, and 1 with brainstem hemorrhage) had CT-confirmed supratentorial mass lesions. All but 10 patients continuously underwent neuromonitoring every 10 to 30 minutes (BAEP in 44 patients, SSEP in 18, and CSA in 23). Electrodes were placed at Cz and on the earlobes for BAEP and CSA and, for median nerve-stimulated SSEP, at Cv2 and C3'(C4') referred to Fz in 8 patients and to the earlobes in 10. Systemic blood pressure and body temperature were also monitored.

Neuronal dysfunction was defined as loss of components in I to V of BAEP and SSEP after N14, electrocerebral silence on CSA and/or EEG, and neuological criteria of brain death (deep coma, absent brainstem reflexes, and apnea). Mean ICP and CPP data were analysed at the first appearance of each dysfunction.

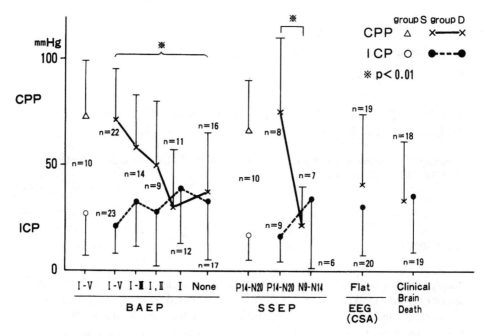

Fig. 1. Relationship of neuronal dysfunction to ICP and CPP in survivors (*group S*) and non-survivors (*group D*). The graph illustrates changes in *ICP* (mean − S.D.) and *CPP* (mean + S.D.) at the initial appearance of each finding of neuronal dysfunction. The preserved *BAEP* and *SSEP* components are shown in the *abscissa*

Results

1) Relationship of BAEP to ICP and CPP

In group D, rostral-caudal deterioration of BAEP components was correlated with decreased CPP (I−V, 71 ± 24 mm Hg; I−III, 59 ± 25; I and II, 50 ± 30; I, 30 ± 28; flat, 36 ± 28: $F = 5.82, p < 0.01$). However, there was no apparent correlation between ICP and deterioration of BAEP (I−V, 21 ± 13 mm Hg; I−III, 33 ± 21; I and II, 28 ± 26; I, 39 ± 26; flat, 33 ± 28: $F = 1.48$, ns).

In group S, BAEP waves I−V were preserved in all 10 patients monitored, and mean ICP and CPP were 27 ± 20 mm Hg and 73 ± 26, respectively.

2) Relationship of SSEP to ICP and CPP

In group D, the difference in CPP values in the presence (75 ± 35 mm Hg) and absence (21 ± 19) of SSEP components after N14 was significant ($t = 3.4$, $p < 0.01$). However, ICP did not differ significantly in the presence (16 ± 12 mm Hg) and absence (34 ± 33) of SSEP after N14.

In group S, P14 or P15, and/or N18–N20 components were preserved in all 10 patients examined. Their mean ICP and CPP were 17 ± 12 mm Hg and 66 ± 24, respectively.

3) Relationship of Loss of Neuronal Function to ICP and CPP (Fig. 1)

Mean ICP and CPP were 30 ± 23 mm Hg and 41 ± 33, respectively, when the EEG (CSA) was flat, and were 35 ± 26 and 33 ± 28 when the neurological criteria for brain death were met. Decreased CPP became more apparent than increased ICP upon loss of neuronal function.

Discussion

Neuronal dysfunction caused by severe brain damage is not always associated with increased ICP. Also, mechanical factors associated with transtentorial herniation may affect BAEP (Garcia-Larrea et al. 1987). However, loss of neuronal function as a consequence of brain ischemia is thought to be closely related to decreased CPP. In fact, regardless of the ICP, rostral-caudal deterioration of BAEP is correlated with decreased CPP. It has been noted that CPP plays an important role in the depression of BAEP in experimental animals (Sohmer et al. 1986) and in pediatric patients (Goitein et al. 1983).

The relationship between SSEP and CPP has not been clarified because the SSEP brainstem components are not easily identified with scalp references (Desmedt 1985). Loss of SSEP, including the P14 brainstem component, was related to decreased CPP in this study.

Therefore, we consider ischemia of the posterior fossa associated with decreased CPP to be the most important factor in the loss of BAEP and SSEP after N14.

In conclusion, it is difficult to determine irreversible loss of neuronal function by only one monitoring modality because false-positive and false-negative results may be obtained. Therefore, CPP measurement together with neuromonitoring is necessary in evaluating severely brain-damaged patients.

References

Desmedt JE (1985) Critical neuromonitoring at spinal and brainstem levels by somatosensory evoked potentials. CNS Trauma 2:169–186

Garcia-Larrea L, Bertrand O, Artru F, Pernier J, Mauguière F (1987) Brain-stem monitoring. II. Preterminal BAEP changes observed until brain death in deeply comatose patients. Electroencephalogr Clin Neurophysiol 68:446–457

Goitein KJ, Fainmesser P, Sohmer H (1983) Cerebral perfusion pressure and auditory brainstem responses in childhood CNS diseases. Am J Dis Child 137:777–781

Sohmer H, Freeman S, Gafni M, Goitein K (1986) The depression of the auditory nerve-brainstem evoked response in hypoxaemia – mechanism and site of effect. Electroencephalogr Clin Neurophysiol 64:334–338

Methodology of Spectral Analysis of the Intracranial Pressure Waveform in a Head Injury Intensive Care Unit

I.R. Piper, N.M. Dearden, J.R.S. Leggate, I. Robertson, and J.D. Miller

Department of Clinical Neurosciences, University of Edinburgh, Western General Hospital, Crewe Road, Edinburgh, EH4 2XU (UK)

Introduction

Chopp and Portnoy (1980) were the first to apply spectral analysis of the intracranial pressure (ICP) waveform, in experimental models of intracranial hypertension, as the basis of a systems analysis approach whereby the amplitude and phase of the arterial pressure (BP) waveform and the ICP waveform were studied as measures of input and output functions respectively to the cerebrovascular bed (CVB). We are applying, in an observational study, spectral analysis of the ICP and BP waveforms as a systems analysis approach towards determining the range of values in head injured patients of the pressure pulse transfer characteristics of the CVB. This paper describes our methods.

Pressure Monitoring

ICP is monitored subdurally and BP via the radial artery using two methods. One method uses a fluid filled catheter-transducer system while the other method uses a Camino fibre-optic catheter-tip transducer system. Transient response analysis of the fluid filled catheter-transducer system currently in use in our head injury intensive care unit (ICU) showed it to be underdamped (damping factor 0.310 ± 0.021) with a damped resonant frequency of 21 Hz. Resonant frequency and damping were determined by the pop test method (Gabe 1972). Underdamped systems can produce significant amplitude distortion in the waveform component harmonic frequencies greater than 9 Hz, while producing less marked amplitude distortion at the harmonic frequencies less than 9 Hz. Acudynamic adjustable damping devices were used to correct underdamping in the fluid filled catheter-transducer systems ensuring an optimally damped (damping factor 0.622 ± 0.04) flat frequency response with minimal amplitude distortion of the higher harmonics up to 14 Hz (Allan 1988). In a group of patients with overdamped fluid filled catheter-transducer systems, Camino fibre-optic catheter-tip ICP transducers could discriminate ICP waveform harmonics up to 9 Hz compared with only 6 Hz for the overdamped fluid filled systems.

Data Collection

Five minute samples of ICP and BP waveform data, timed to coincide with half-hourly clinical recordings by the nursing staff, are stored to magnetic tape. Data collection is under automatic microcomputer control. Manual starting and stopping of waveform data collection can be carried out at any time. With each waveform segment stored to tape, a computer file is created storing the starting tape count and the time and date the sample was collected. Comments can be entered and stored to the current active computer file at any time. ICP and BP waveform data are collected every half hour during the entire patient monitoring period in the head injury ICU. A 32-bit microcomputer system forms the basis of the waveform analysis system. All software is written in the C programming language. Waveform data were filtered prior to digitizing by analogue 5th order low pass filters with a corner frequency of 70 Hz rolling off at 30 db per octave. The entire waveform analysis system, including pressure transducers, preamplifier, patient monitor, FM tape recorder and anti-aliasing low-pass filter, has a flat amplitude frequency response from DC to 70 Hz ± 2 db (DC to 20 Hz ± 2 db with the optimally damped fluid filled catheter-transducer system) and a linear phase shift of 0.09 radians/Hz. Phase shifts are corrected in the software for the linear phase shifts inherent in the waveform analysis system. Each waveform segment (4096 points) is digitized at a sampling rate of 400 Hz. Sampling rates slower than 400 Hz (200 Hz and 100 Hz) produced spectral artifacts due to aliasing as a result of high energy input signals still having sufficient energy outwith the pass band of our low pass filters to alias with the sampling frequency.

Data Analysis

In systems analysis an attempt is made to define the physical characteristics of a system using only the system input and output signals. The assumption is made that the BP waveform is the chief input signal to the cerebrovascular system and the ICP waveform is the output signal emanating from the CVB. The system transfer function is defined as the relationship that describes how the stimulus signals are transformed by the system into response signals. A 4096 point fast fourier transform (FFT) is calculated on each waveform segment. The modulus of the transformed data is plotted against frequency as the amplitude spectrum. The frequency resolution of the amplitude spectrum is 0.098 Hz. The transfer function consists of amplitude and phase components. Both the amplitude and phase components of the transfer function are calculated from the amplitude spectrum and raw fourier transformed data by standard methods (Marmareliz 1978).

Methodological Considerations

Use of the radial artery waveform site as a measure of the input signal to the CVB requires special justification. The abdominal and thoracic aorta, subclavian,

The effect of two different B.P. measuring sites (Carotid vs Radial artery) on the amplitude transfer fuction, phase transfer function and coherence function

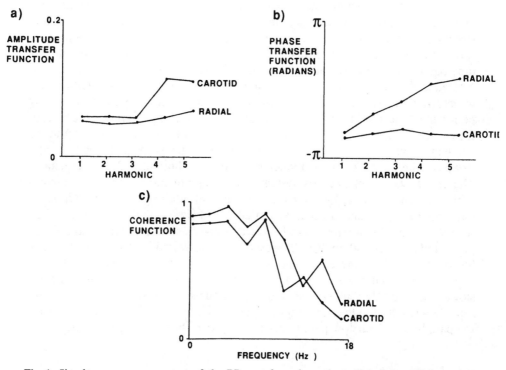

Fig. 1. Simultaneous measurement of the BP waveform from the radial and carotid arteries allow comparison of the amplitude transfer function (**a**) and phase transfer function (**b**) between both BP waveform measurement sites and the ICP waveform. The coherence function (**c**) is a measure of the correlation between two signals. The coherence function calculated between ICP/Radial and ICP/Carotid pressure waveforms were compared and found to show a similar configuration. In this patient the ICP/Radial coherence function showed the better coherence particularly at higher frequencies

lingual and brachial arterial pressure waveforms have each been used by previous workers in this field, in experimental studies, as the input signal to the CVB. During a change of arterial pressure monitoring from the carotid to the radial sites, we were able to monitor and compare simultaneously the carotid with the radial artery pressure waveform and the transfer functions between both sites and the ICP waveform (Fig. 1a, b). The amplitude transfer functions (ICP/Carotid, ICP/Radial) showed a marked similarity in configuration. The ICP/Carotid amplitude transfer function was slightly greater at all frequencies, although the ICP/Radial phase transfer function remained greater at all frequencies. The coherence function has been used as a measure of the correlation between two signals. If a system is linear and free of contaminating noise, or if there is only one input signal, then the output signal will show a high cross correlation with the

670

input signal. The coherence functions between ICP/Radial and ICP/Carotid waveforms in this patient were of similar configuration (figure 1 c). The ICP/Radial correlation showed higher coherence than the ICP/Carotid correlation, particularly at the higher frequencies. Furthermore, a factor derived from the amplitude spectrum (distortion factor – k) is calculated as an index that represents the extent to which a given waveform is distorted or different from a pure sine wave. The value of the distortion factor is zero if it is a pure sine wave. The distortion factor (k) is calculated as a check on a divergence between the amplitude transfer function and the ICP spectrum. If the amplitude transfer function is increasing as a result of a true frequency dependent change in the cerebrovascular system, then one would expect this to be detectable in both the amplitude transfer function and the output waveform amplitude spectrum. If, however, frequency-selective changes in the BP waveform at the radial artery are being produced independently of the true input signal to the CVB, then the amplitude transfer function produced will be artifactual. If the BP waveform distortion factor alters significantly between measurement events and in an opposite direction to the ICP distortion factor, then one might suspect that the amplitude transfer function is invalidated because a true measure of the input signal to the CVB has not been used. While there are differences in the amplitude and phase transfer functions between carotid and radial artery measurement sites, the overall frequency relationship appears similar and, provided measures are taken to detect when the BP waveform at the radial site is changing independently of the BP waveform input to the CVB, then the choice of the radial artery site does not invalidate our method.

Acknowledgements. This work has been supported by Action Research for the Crippled Child (Grant number A/8/1671).

References

Allan MWB et al. (1988) Measurement of arterial pressure using catheter-transducer systems. Br J Anaesth 60:413–418

Chopp M, Portnoy H (1980) Systems analysis of intracranial pressure. J Neurosurg 53:516–527

Gabe IT (1972) Cardiovascular fluid dynamics. Academic Press, London. General Part. Acta Physiol Scand 19:306–332

Marmareliz PZ, Marmareliz VZ (1978) Analysis of physiological systems: The whitenoise approach. Plenum, New York

Effects of Intracranial Hypertension on Evolution of Post-Traumatic Acute Subdural Hematoma

G. Tomei, D. Spagnoli, P. Guerra, L. Ceretti, M. Giovanelli, and R. Villani

Institute of Neurosurgery, University of Milan, 35, F. Sforza Str., I-20122 Milan (Italy)

Introduction

Acute subdural hematoma (SDH) is a posttraumatic lesion that results in a severe neurological impairment and a high mortality rate due to the effects of the mass expanding lesion, the resulting intracranial hypertension and the presence of injury to brain parenchyma (Becker 1986; Cooper 1982).

The aim of this paper is to point out the relevance of the association of diffuse brain lesions to SDH, the role of ICP in its evolution and the incidence of postoperative intracranial complications.

Patients and Methods

The present series includes 60 patients with SDH, admitted to our Department within 24 hours of injury and operated on shortly after. CT examination allowed distinction of 2 main groups of SDH: (a) *SDH associated with brain swelling (BS)* (19 cases = 32%). Associated findings in this group were: hematoma of small size; 3rd ventricle and basal cisterns absent (100%); compressed or absent unilateral ventricle (54%); partially enlarged contralateral ventricle (30%); and deep hemorrhages (shearing injury) (15%). The mean age of these patients was 36 ± 16. In 90% of the cases head injury was due to a traffic accident; (b) *SDH not associated to brain swelling (BS)* (29 cases = 48%): Associated findings were: hematoma of large size; compressed or absent unilateral ventricle (28%); 3rd ventricle and basal cisterns always present. The mean age of these patients was 60.7 ± 18. In 81% head injury was due to a domestic accident (fall). In the remaining 12 patients a clear distinction between the two groups was not evident.

Results

In the first group surgery was never effective in improving clinical status. In fact, during the first postoperative week, persistence of motor posturing and pupillary abnormalities was observed in patients who died (mean GCS = 4.8 ± 1.2). Surviv-

Eds.: J. T. Hoff and A. L. Betz

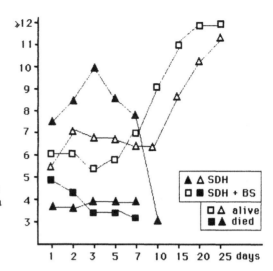

Fig. 1. Post-operative clinical course in patients with acute subdural hematoma (SDH) associated with brain swelling (□ = survived, ■ died) and in SDH patients without brain swelling (△ = survived; ▲ died)

ing patients (mean GCS = 5.9 ± 1.3) remained comatose for more than 7 days, then progressively regained consciousness (Fig. 1). The mortality rate was 74%.

The poor outlook for patients with SDH and BS could be ascribed to the appearance of major intracranial complications documented on CT scan: including brain ischemia (10%), brain stem hemorrhage (10%), hemispheric edema (31%), and multiple intracerebral hematomas (37%). A normal CT was present in only 10% of the cases. A marked difference was marked in the second group of patients with SDH not associated with BS. In fact, normalization of the CT scan after operation was demonstrated in 55% of the cases (16 pts), whereas in the remaining 45% brain ischemia (10%), brain stem hemorrhage (10%) and hemispheric edema (25%) were evident.

As shown in Fig. 1, the postoperative clinical course had different trends. In spite of dramatic clinical improvement and CT normalization, 62% of the patients (10 cases) eventually died due to the occurrence of respiratory disturbances, pneumonia and heart attack (Fig. 1). All these patients were older than 70. Persistence of severe coma lasting a week on average was marked the second group of patients who died (12 cases) (Fig. 1). In patients who survived (7 cases), no remarkable clinical amelioration was noticed before the 10th day after surgery. Then, they progressively regained consciousness, often after a phase of persistent vegetative state.

Hemispheric edema and multilocated intracerebral hematomas resulted in severe intracranial hypertension. ICP tracings were often similar to those recorded in patients with diffuse brain swelling (Tomei et al., this volume). The increase of cerebral blood volume (hyperemia), brain water content and CSF (due to sudden obstruction of CSF pathways) should be considered as relevant mechanisms for the ICP increase. As a consequence, hyperventilation, mannitol and CSF withdrawal were commonly used, depending upon the ICP course and AVDO$_2$, attempting to keep values as normal as possible to avoid brain ischemia. In patients with documented brain stem hemorrhage and brain ischemia, ICP basal values were always below 15 mm Hg. During routine nursing maneuvers, long lasting ($\sim$20 min) elevations of ICP up to 25–30 mm Hg were often recorded and they were usually controlled by means of 2–3 ml/hr, CSF drainage or patient sedation.

Discussion

The unfavorable clinical course observed in the present series and reported in other studies (Becker 1986) was mainly influenced by 2 factors: (1) the associated injury to brain parenchyma (Cooper 1982; Stone et al. 1983) and (2) the presence of a mass lesion. In our experience co-existing brain swelling or shearing injury was demonstrated in 32% of patients with SDH. This association was common in young patients involved in vehicle accidents. In older patients SDH was often the consequence of domestic accidents and such association was not evident, but outcome was deeply influenced by the appearance of extracranial complications. Postoperative intracranial complications have to be considered the third factor influencing outcome.

The appearance of hemispheric edema and multilocated intracerebral hematomas had the highest incidence (68%) in patients with SDH and brain swelling on admission, resulting in severe intracranial hypertension. Successful treatment of ICP was seldom obtained in these patients. Moreover, normal ICP did not necessarily indicate a good prognosis. In fact, in patients who died with brain ischemia and brain stem hemorrhage, elevated ICP was never recorded.

References

Becker DP (1986) Acute subdural hematoma. In: Vigouroux RP (ed) Advances in neurotrauma-tology, vol 1 – Extracerebral collections In: McLaurin RL (ed). Springer, Wien New York, pp 51–100

Cooper PR (1982) – Post-traumatic intracranial mass lesions. In: Cooper PR (ed) Head injury. Williams and Wilkins, Baltimore London, pp 185–232

Stone JL, Rifai MHS, Sugar D, Lang RGR, Oldershaw JB, Moody RA (1983) Subdural hema-toma. I. Acute subdural hematoma: progress in definition, clinical pathology and therapy. Surg Neurol 19:216–231

Experimental Arterial Subdural Bleeding

J. Orlin and N.N. Zwetnow

Section of Experimental Neurosurgery, Rikshospitalet, The National Hospital,
University of Oslo, Oslo (Norway)

Introduction

Acute subdural hematoma is perhaps the intracranial bleed considered to carry
the highest rate of mortality. Most authors regard subdural bleeding to arise from
ruptured veins. In recent literature, however, arteries are increasingly indicated as
the bleeding source (Drake 1961; Hoff and Gauger 1975; Rengachary and Szymanski 1981; Shenkin 1982). A quantitative analysis of the pathophysiological
characteristics and the lethal mechanism of this condition has hitherto been
lacking.

In this paper induced acute experimental subdural bleeding has been studied
with emphasis on the dynamic course of intracranial pressures, changes in vital
physiological parameters and their correlation to volume and rate of bleeding and
to concomitant intracranial anatomical changes as displayed with Magnetic Resonance Imaging (MRI). Attempts were also done to stop a lethal subdural bleeding by means of the Intracranial Fluid Infusion Tamponade (Zwetnow 1988)
(INFIT) technique.

Material and Methods

The study was done on dogs and swine anesthetized with pentobarbital, intubated
and either ventilated mechanically or allowed to breathe spontaneously. Subdural
bleeding was induced by leading blood from the abdominal aorta through an
electronic drop recorder and a craniotomy into the subdural space over the left
cerebral hemisphere. Thus the bleeding was propagated by the systemic arterial
pressure. The diameter of the subdural catheter was the major determinant of the
bleeding intensity, and led to lethal outcome when exceeding 1.6 mm. Intracranial
pressures, measured at three to five sites within the craniospinal system, systemic
arterial and central venous pressures, respiration, EEG, ECG and rate and volume of bleeding were monitored continuously and registered on a Grass Polygraph model 7D. In 12 animals regional cerebral blood flow was measured with
radioactive microspheres in the early and in the late bleeding phase. In 8 animals
Magnetic Resonance Images were repeatedly taken in frontal and sagittal planes
of the cranium to study shifts of intracranial structures during bleeding. Each
animal was observed for 1–2 hours after bleeding stop, and then sacrificed with

an overdose of Nembutal and a saturated solution of potassium chloride. Thereafter brain and spinal cord were meticulously removed for microscopy. Details of the experimental procedure are given elsewhere (Steiner et al. 1975).

Results

Pressure Course

In experiments with spontaneously respiring animals start of bleeding led to rapid rise in all intracranial pressures and to a transtentorial pressure gradient within 1–2 min. (Fig. 1). Bleeding intensity decreased exponentially during the same time period, parallel with the decrease in heart rate, respiration rate and EEG amplitude. Small bleeds, produced through a catheter with a diameter less than 0.8 mm, stopped within 3–5 minutes, and subsequently resulted in normalization of intracranial pressures, recovery of EEG and other vital parameters, and to acute survival. Large bleedings led to progressive intracranial hypertension with marked transtentorial pressure gradients, to a marked rise in arterial pressure (Cushing effect) and ultimately to cardiovascular collapse within about 5 min. EEG always turned isoelectric at an early stage. ECG exhibited cardiac rhythm disturbances during the period of arterial hypertension.

In experiments with mechanical ventilation the hemorrhage volumes were usually smaller, but their duration somewhat longer. The rises in ICP and SAP were quantitatively less dramatic. Moderate, early transtentorial pressure gradients were the rule, likewise an early isoelectric EEG and a final cardiovascular collapse leading to death in 12/17 animals. Thus, of 17 animals 5 animals survived a lethal subdural hemorrhage when mechanically ventilated.

Regional Blood Flow

Regional blood flow measured in 20 cerebral regions with radioactive microspheres was on the average unchanged in the early phase of the bleeding. However, rCBF decreased in all regions in the late bleeding phase to less than 5 ml/100 g/min. This decrease was grossly proportional to the decrease in cerebral perfusion pressure suggesting that CBF autoregulation was largely abolished.

Magnetic Resonance Imaging (MRI)

In collaboration with Ponten, Bergstroem and Thuomas at the Academic Hospital of Uppsala, MR images were taken in frontal and in sagittal planes at 1–8 min intervals throughout the bleeding course. Compression and shift of the homolateral side ventricle and the third ventricle occurred within a few minutes concomitant to the initial rapid rise of bleeding. Local tissue water, as evaluated from T_2-weighted images, increased linearly after the start of bleeding. The rise was grossly uniform in the 8 regions measured.

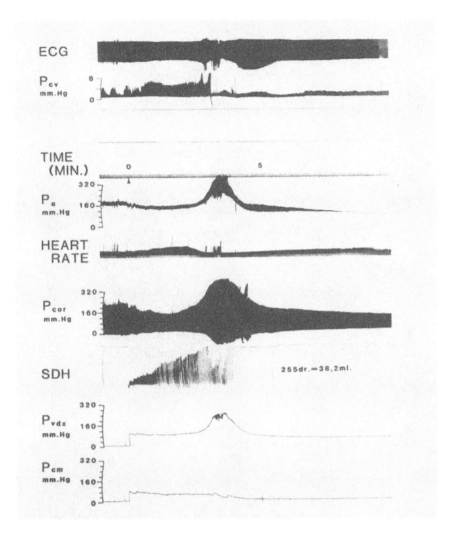

Fig. 1. Lethal subdural bleed in a swine. Bleeding starts at time 0 and leads to cardiovascular collapse within 5 min. Note rapid rise in intracranial pressures, a progressive decrease in subdural bleeding rate, bradycardia and disturbances in ECG during the marked Cushing effect

Application of INFIT

The last objective of this study was to test the therapeutic effect of INFIT upon the mortality rate in lethal bleeding models in 7 mechanically ventilated swine. The bleeding was produced through catheters with a subdural orifice of 16 mm in diameter.

INFIT was applied shortly after the start of bleeding. The intracranial pressure then rose simultaneously in all leads while the bleeding intensity rapidly and

677

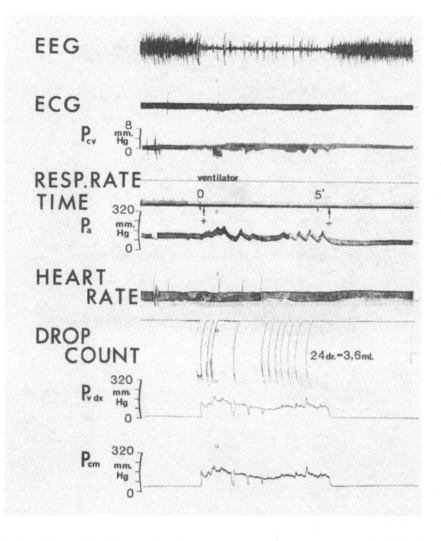

Fig. 2. Lethal, subdural haemorrhage in swine treated with mechanical ventilation and INFIT. Note the decrease in bleeding rate at onset of INFIT. Note also that the total bleeding volume is about $\frac{1}{10}$ of the total bleeding volume in the lethal control experiments in Fig. 1. Observe also normalization of intracranial pressures and recovery of EEG after cessation of INFIT

Table 1

Animal group	Group size (n)	Volume of bleeding $\bar{x} \pm$ SD ml.	Bleeding time $\bar{x} \pm$ SD min.	Number of acute survivors
Spontaneous respiration	8	47.1 ± 10.1	10.8 ± 2.7	0/0
Mechanical ventilation	17	35.0 ± 7.7	13.6 ± 6.0	5/17
Mechanical ventilation + INFIT	8	10.3 ± 7.1	7.9 ± 3.0	8/8

markedly decreased. The EEG amplitude became rapidly reduced, but was not always isoelectric. After 4–5 minutes INFIT was discontinued. Intracranial pressures then rapidly fell to near-normal values while the EEG amplitude recovered gradually. After 60 min the animals were taken off the respirator and then had spontaneous, regular respiration. A typical course is illustrated in Fig. 2.

Table 1 shows the total material. While the mortality was 100% in the spontaneously breathing animals and 71% in the ventilated ones, it was 0% in the group treated with INFIT.

Discussion

Very few quantitative studies of acute subdural bleeds are reported in the literature. This seems surprising in view of the clinical importance of the clinical importance of the condition, but may partly be explained by technical difficulties in producing arterial bleeding within the subdural space. The subdural positioning of the catheter tip is crucial. In our experiments its location was scrupulously checked by means of subarachnoid infusion of saline before the experiment and by ascertaining the position of the catheter tip in microscopic sections after the experiment. Additional data were obtained from studies with horseradish peroxidase to delineate the functional anatomy and the bulk flow properties of the subdural space.

The bleeding volumes from subdural bleedings in this study are comparable to the volumes from intracranial subarachnoid bleeds described earlier (Loefgren and Zwetnow 1972; Steiner et al. 1975; Zwetnow et al. 1983). This similarity is probably due to the subdural hematomas extending into the spinal subdural space. Like the subarachnoid bleeding, the arterial subdural bleeding appears to parallel intracranial bleeding rather closely (Loefgren and Zwetnow 1972). However, unlike subarachnoid hemorrhage, the regular occurrence of an early transtentorial pressure gradient, which increases as bleeding continues, contrasts with the uniform pressure increase found in progressive tissue herniation (Steiner et al. 1975). In fact, both transtentorial and transforaminal herniation were observed on MRI.

The measurements of CBF were done in situations where cerebral perfusion pressure diminished progressively and slowly and where transient hyperemia thus was avoided. Under these circumstances the flow figures provided by the microsphere method should be valid. The intact autoregulation found in the initial part of each subdural bleeding accords with what has been observed in epidural and subarachnoid bleeds and obviously contributes to survival in moderate bleeds.

Recovery of vital parameters, leading to acute survival in almost one fourth of the lethal bleeding experiments with mechanical ventilation accentuates the importance of adequate oxygenation in treating intracranial expanding lesions. Furthermore, acute survival in 100% of the animals treated with INFIT, is promising and warrants further experimental work. Clinical data and the present experimental results make a possible use of INFIT in hyperacute clinical situations feasible. However, more experimental data are needed concerning the therapeutic range of the method, its optimal application, and its possible side effects before steps are taken to introduce it in clinical practice.

Acknowledgements. This study has been supported by The University of Oslo, The Anders Jahre Foundation for Advancement of Science and by The Norwegian Society for Fighting Cancer. Mrs. Solveig Hassfjell has typed the manuscript and Chief Veterinarian Leif Schjerven has been in charge of the animal care.

References

Drake GG (1961) Subdural hematoma from arterial rupture. J Neurosurg 18:591–601
Hoff J, Gauger G (1975) Arterial subdural hematomas of unusual origin. J Trauma 15:528–531
Loefgren J, Zwetnow NN (1972) Kinetics of arterial and venous hemorrhage in the skull cavity. In: Brock M, Dietz E (eds) Intracranial pressure. Springer, Berlin Heidelberg New York, pp 155–159
Rengachary SS, Szymanski DC (1981) Subdural hematomas of arterial origin. Neurosurgery 8:166–172
Shenkin HA (1982) Acute subdural hematoma. Review of 39 consecutive cases with a high incidence of cortical artery rupture. J Neurosurg 57:254–257
Steiner L, Loefgren J, Zwetnow NN (1975) Characteristics and limits of tolerance in repeated subarachnoid hemorrhage in dogs. Acta Neurol Scand 52:241–267
Steiner L, Loefgren J, Zwetnow NN (1975) Lethal mechanism in repeated SAH in dogs. Acta Neurol Scand 52:268–293
Zwetnow NN (1989) Hyperacute arrest of intracranial bleeding with intracranial fluid infusion tamponade treatment (INFIT). This volume, pp 681–687
Zwetnow NN, Habash AH, Loefgren J, Håkansson S (1983) Comparative analysis of experimental epidural and subarachnoid bleedings in dogs. Acta Neurochir (Wien) 67:67–101

Hyperacute Arrest of Intracranial Bleeding with Intracranial Fluid Infusion Tamponade Treatment (INFIT)

N.N. Zwetnow

Section of Experimental Neurosurgery, Rikshospitalet, The National Hospital,
University of Oslo, Oslo (Norway)

Introduction

While evacuation of craniospinal space-occupying hematomas has long been a routine procedure in neurosurgical practice no efficient method has hitherto been available for treatment of craniospinal bleeding in the hyperacute stage. Two evident reasons for this lack are the short survival time of brain tissue during ischemia and the necessity of anatomic localization of the bleeding source. As a consequence the clinical attitude towards subarachnoid bleeds in the hyperacute stage has largely been nihilistic. Decompressing maneuvers like hyperventilation, ventricular drainage and hyperosmolar agents have been rather discouraging.

In this paper the opposite principle, i.e. intracranial *compression,* has been tested to arrest intracranial bleeds in the hyperacute stage. The intracranial compression has been effected manually by infusing mock cerebrospinal fluid under pressure into the cerebrospinal fluid space. This therapeutic principle has accordingly been termed Intracranial Fluid Infusion Tamponade (INFIT). The theoretical basis of the method, the experimental results and its possible therapeutic application in clinical situations are discussed below.

Theoretical Background

At the first ICP symposium in 1971 in Hanover, and at later ICP meetings it has been experimentally shown how various types of craniospinal bleeds tend to follow a general maxim in being shortlasting, self restricting and in leading to survival provided an efficacious temporal interplay of five survival factors (Loefgren and Zwetnow 1972). The most important survival factor was the build-up of intracranial counterpressure leading to immediate decrease in bleeding pressure and bleeding intensity and eventually to intracranial hemostasis. It has further been shown (Steiner, Loefgren and Zwetnow 1975a and b, 1976) that survival depends on intracranial hemostasis occurring before the volume of the bleed reaches a certain threshold value ("the lethal bleeding volume"). This threshold value usually varies with the anatomical location, being smallest in intracerebral bleeds (about 10% of the intracranial volume).

Our previous animal experiments and some recent in vitro experiments prompted us to test whether INFIT could arrest intracranial bleeding before the bleeding had reached its lethal volume.

Material and Methods

INFIT was tested both in acute and chronic dog experiments. In the acute experiments 2 lethal bleeding models were used. The animals were anesthetized with intravenous pentobarbital and intubated with an inflatable tracheal tube. They were either breathing spontaneously or mechanically ventilated. Systemic arterial pressure, central venous pressure, CSF pressures in the lateral ventricle and cisterna magna, heart rate, respiration, EEG and ECG were continuously monitored and registered on a 16 channel Grass Polygraph model 7 D. A polyethylene catheter was introduced into the cisterna magna for manual infusion of mock CSF.

Model 1: Intracranial Section of Major Arteries. Through a craniotomy the internal carotid artery or the middle cerebral artery (immediately at the offshoot from the carotid artery) was transected with rapid restoration of the closed-box integrity of the skull. INFIT was applied immediately after sectioning by manual infusion of mock CSF into the cisterna magna at a rate which maintained an intracranial pressure of 100–120 mm Hg and which led to marked rise in systemic arterial pressure (Cushing effect). Infusion was discontinued at 2–3 minute's intervals to check maintenance of high ICP as a sign of ongoing bleeding.

Model 2: Extracorporeal Bleeding Shunt. Through a polyethylene catheter in the femoral artery blood was led from the abdominal aorta into the cisterna magna via a electronic drop recorder. The experimental lay-out was essentially the same as has been described in earlier papers (Loefgren and Zwetnow 1972; Steiner, Loefgren and Zwetnow 1975 a, b). INFIT was applied as in Model 1 a few seconds after start of bleeding. However, the infusion rate was manually checked to be just adequate to prevent blood from passing the drop recorder. Discontinuation of infusion at intervals served to check whether bleeding was still going on. The chronic experiments were only performed on Model 2, using a sterile set-up. In case of survival each dog received regular neurosurgical postoperative treatment, including antibiotics and parental nutrition, and were meticulously observed for prolonged periods.

The material was grouped as follows:

Model 1:

Transection of the internal carotid artery (1 spontaneously ventilated, 4 mechanically ventilated)	5 dogs
Partial section of the internal carotid artery (mechanical ventilation only)	2 dogs
Transection of the middle cerebral artery (2 spontaneously ventilated, 3 mechanically ventilated)	5 dogs

Model 2:

Extracorporal shunt bleeding into the cisterna magna (4 spontaneously ventilated, 6 mechanically ventilated)	10 dogs
Extracorporeal shunt bleeding into one lateral ventricle (only mechanically ventilated)	4 dogs

Survival experiments

Extracorporeal shunt bleeding into the cisterna magna (only mechanically ventilated)	4 dogs
Total	30 dogs

Controls

Extracorporeal shunt bleeding into the cisterna magna (spontaneous respiration 9+4, mechanical ventilation 3)	16 dogs
Intracranial transection of the internal carotid artery (1 mechanically ventilated, 1 spontaneously breathing)	2 dogs
Transection of the middle cerebral artery (spontaneous respiration 3, mechanical ventilation 4)	7 dogs
Extracorporeal shunt bleeding into one lateral ventricle (all dogs spontaneously breathing)	5 dogs
Total	30 dogs

Results

I. Acute Experiments

a) Controls. The general course of all control experiments was characterized by rapid rise in intracranial pressures at the start of bleeding, decrease in cerebral perfusion pressure, flattening of EEG, terminal rise in arterial pressure and cardiovascular collapse. Respiratory arrest occurred in the spontaneously respiring animals. Ultimately all control animals succumbed.

b) Experiments with INFIT. Intracranial sectioning of the internal carotid artery always led to a fatal bleed despite treatment. However, after *partial* sectioning of the carotid artery INFIT always led to recovery of an isoelectric EEG, to falling of all CSF pressures towards normal, to spontaneous respiration and usually also to occasional spontaneous body movements appearing within 1 hour after bleeding. Likewise, application of INFIT in animals with transected middle cerebral artery and mechanical ventilation always led to recovery (Fig. 1), while the spontaneously respiring animals in this group succumbed. In the extracorporeal bleeding shunt experiments, application of INFIT led to a drastic reduction of the registered bleeding rate and to arrest of bleeding within a few minutes (Fig. 2). In

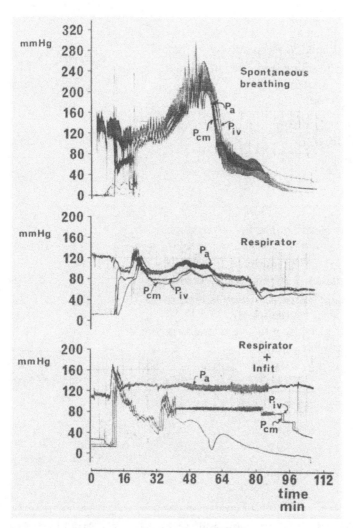

Fig. 1. Pressure course in three different dog experiments after transection of the middle cerebral artery (Model 1). *Upper curves:* Dog with spontaneous respiration. Note marked reduction in perfusion pressure despite the extreme rise in arterial pressure (Cushing Effect), followed by cardiovascular collapse. *Middle curves:* Dog with mechanical ventilation. Pressure course is similar to the one with spontaneous respiration, but blood pressure falls slower and the Cushing Effect is very moderate. *Lower curves:* Dog with mechanical ventilation. INFIT is applied twice. After initial hemostasis at 16 min a rebleeding occurred at 32 minutes. INFIT was re-applied with new hemostasis at 40 min, and was then maintained for 50 minutes to avoid rebleeding. Note better maintenance of arterial pressure and decrease in intracranial pressures secondary to bleeding arrest

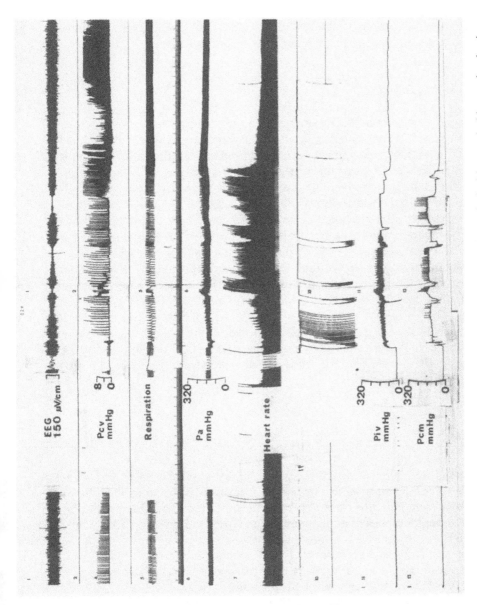

Fig. 2. INFIT applied in an extracorporeal shunt bleed. Bleeding start is marked with a vertical bar under the time scale. Note decrease in bleeding drop rate (*curve 10*) EEG amplitude (*curve 1*) and heart rate (*curve 7*) during intermittent application of INFIT during 15 minutes. Note also decrease in *ICP* and recovery of *EEG* upon bleeding arrest after *INFIT*

685

the mechanically ventilated dogs INFIT always led to survival, but it did not prevent a fatal outcome in the spontaneously respiring animals.

II. Chronic Experiments

Permission to perform survival experiments was granted by The Norwegian State Board of Animal Experimentation. In 4 pilot experiments (type Bleeding Model II) INFIT treatment was applied with prolonged observation. All 4 animals survived and recovered during the respective observation periods 18 hrs, 7 days, 19 days and 23 days after which they were sacrificed by order from the Board's inspector. One dog (19 days observation) had a severely impaired neurologic status immediately after bleeding reacting only to pain stimuli, exhibiting a transient left hemiparesis and becoming probably cortically blind. After a few days it reacted to human voice and regained purposeful movements and natural functions. Two animals woke up without neurological defects already a few hours after the bleed, and remained alert during 7 and 23 days, respectively. The fourth dog had, after bleeding and INFIT, continuous registration of EEG on the operating table for about 18 hours. During this period EEG continuously improved in frequency and amplitude. Initial normalization of the CSF pressure in this dog after INFIT was followed by a secondary rise in CSF pressure during the next 3–6 hours. Thereafter ICP fell again and remained steady on the pre-bleeding level.

Discussion

The results of this animal study demonstrate that lethal subarachnoid and intraventricular bleedings may be arrested with survival if INFIT is applied in the hyperacute phase. This effect has also been demonstrated in acute experimental subdural and epidural bleeds at this symposium (Orlin and Zwetnow 1988; Ganz et al. 1988).

The main therapeutic objective of INFIT administration is to avoid a prolonged elevation of static CSF pressure by extravasated blood by induction of a transient controlled rise in *dynamic* CSF pressure.

Obviously, this transient rise in CSF pressure implies a risk of morbidity caused by ischemic damage to the brain. Accordingly, careful evaluation must be done of the relation of morbidity degree to INFIT duration and to volume of bleeding, further of the optimal mode of INFIT application and of its therapeutic range before INFIT can be adopted for clinical purposes.

Acknowledgements. This study has been supported by The University of Oslo, The Anders Jahre Foundation for Advancement of Science and by The Norwegian Society for Fighting Cancer. Mrs. Solveig Hassfjell has typed the manuscript and Chief Veterinarian Leif Schjerven has assisted with animal care.

References

Loefgren J, Zwetnow NN (1972) Kinetics of arterial and venous hemorrhage in the skull cavity. In: Brock M, Dietz E (eds) Intracranial pressure I. Springer, Berlin Heidelberg New York, pp 155–159

Loefgren J, Steiner L, Zwetnow NN (1976) Intracranial pressure course in repeated SAH. In: Beks et al. (eds) Intracranial pressure III. Springer, Berlin Heidelberg New York, pp 113–117

Steiner L, Loefgren J, Zwetnow NN (1975) Characteristics and limits of tolerance in repeated subarachnoid hemorrhage in dogs. Acta Neurol Scand 52:268–293

Steiner L, Loefgren J, Zwetnow NN (1975) Lethal mechanism in repeated SAH in dogs. Acta Neurol Scand 52:268–293

Blood Volume Responsivity to ICP Change in Head Injured Patients

A. Marmarou and A. Wachi

Richard Reynolds Neurological Research Laboratories, Division of Neurosurgery,
Medical College of Virginia, MCV Station, Box 508, Richmond, Virginia 23298 (USA)

Our studies of severely head injured patients have shown that CSF parameters play a relatively minor role in the sequence of events leading to intracranial hypertension. We hypothesized that the major factor leading to raised ICP is mediated by a vascular mechanism (Marmarou et al. 1987). These findings prompted us to examine means by which the cerebrovascular system could be challenged to permit a quantitative assessment of the blood volume – intracranial pressure relationship. In this study, we tested the vessel responsivity in head injured patients by quantifying the change in ICP for a known change in PCO_2 introduced by varying ventilatory rate.

Methods

We defined four indices for assessment of the pressure responsivity of the vessels in response to changes in PCO_2. The pressure Reactivity Coefficient to Hyperventilation (PRCR) was defined as the change in steady state ICP per torr change in arterial PCO_2. It was determined by measuring the average ICP and arterial PCO_2 and then modifying the ventilator setting to lower PCO_2 by 2 or 3 torr. When ICP stabilized at a new level (12–15 min), the change in steady state pressure (P1–P0) divided by the measured change in PCO_2 was defined as the PRCR. A similar procedure was used for determining PRCO with mild hypoventilation. The change in Estimated Blood Volume (EBV) in response to PCO_2 change was estimated by calculating the change in volume as the ICP traverses along the exponential Pressure/Volume curve from an initial steady state pressure of Pa to a new steady state pressure Pb. Having determined the PVI prior to altering PCO_2, the EBV was calculated according to the equation: $EBV = (PVI) * \log (Pb/Pa)$. The estimation is based on the assumption that the PVI remains constant during manipulation of the PCO_2. This also permitted calculation of the Blood Volume Reactivity (BVR) according to the equation: $BVR = EBV/\text{delta } PCO_2$.

Results

These indices were measured in 41 severely head injured patients (GCS < 8) upon stabilization in the ICU and at 24 hr intervals. Vessel responsivity as assessed by

PRCR was markedly impaired during the first 24 hr, averaging 0.7 mm Hg ICP per mm Hg delta PCO_2. The PRCR increased nearly two fold (1.3) over the next 48 hr and remained stable thereafter. The vessel responsivity to increased PCO_2 (PRCO) was also impaired, averaging 0.6 ± 1.9 on day 1 and increased by three fold on day 2 to a level of 1.9 ± 1.8. The impairment of vessel responsivity as assessed by PRCR and PRCO 24 hr post trauma was statistically significant (Table 1), ($p < 0.05$). Responsivity parameters were grouped for those patients who were hyperventilated and maintained at PCO_2 less than 30 and had PVI measures of less than 13. We reasoned that vessels would be maximally constricted under these conditions. We found that the amount of blood (EBV) expelled under these conditions per torr PCO_2 was quite small and equaled 0.22 ± 0.06 ml/mm Hg PCO_2 for non-survivors.

Table 1.

Day	mm Hg/mm HgP$_{CO_2}$	Number of studies
PRCR		
1	0.7 ± 0.7 ($p < 0.05$)	41
2	1.3 ± 1.1	35
PRCO		
1	0.6 ± 1.6 ($p < 0.05$)	21
2	1.9 ± 1.8	16

Discussion

We have found that cerebral vessel reactivity is markedly impaired during 24 hr post trauma. We view this impairment as a contributing factor toward the early development of raised ICP. As time progresses, the vessel responsivity as assessed by these methods tends toward recovery. The blood volume responsivity averaged 0.56 ml for each mm Hg delta PCO_2 for survivors of severe head injury. We were concerned that these estimates of blood volume change were low. However, Grubb et al. (1974) measured the relationship between cerebral blood volume and PCO_2 in Rhesus monkeys by determining the change in transit time using Oxygen-15 labeled carboxyhemoglobin and a diffusible tracer, oxygen labeled water. Based on values obtained from 28 primates, the change in CBV extrapolated to a 1500 gm human brain equals 0.615 cc per torr change in PCO_2 which is close to our values obtained 2 and 3 days post injury. We believe that these new indices, which are easily obtained by evaluating the PVI and observing the ICP response to known changes in PCO_2, provide an additional tool which can be used to assess vascular impairment following traumatic injury and efficacy of therapeutic measures directed toward ICP management.

Acknowledgements. This research was supported in part by Grants NS-12587 and RO1-NS-19235 from the National Institutes of Health. Additional facilities and support were provided in part by the Richard Roland Reynolds Neurosurgical Research Laboratories.

References

Grubb RL, Raichle ME, Eichling JO, Ter-Pogossian MM (1974) The effects of changes in PCO_2 on cerebral blood volume, blood flow, and mean transit time. Stroke 5:630–639

Marmarou A, Maset A, Ward JD et al. (1987) Contribution of CSF and vascular factors to elevation of ICP in severely head injured patients. J Neurosurg 66:883–890

Relation Between CBF, ICP and PVI in Severely Head Injured Children

J.P. Muizelaar, A. Marmarou, and J.D. Ward

Division of Neurosurgery, Medical College of Virginia, Virginia Commonwealth University, Richmond, Virginia 23298-0631 (USA)

Bruce et al. (1979; 1981) and Obrist et al. (1979; 1984) have drawn attention to the correlation between elevated ICP and hyperemia, occurring more often in children. According to these authors, the increased cerebral blood volume (CBV) which, they propose accompanies the increased CBF, is the chief cause of high ICP. The exceptional results obtained by Bruce et al. (1979; 1981) were ascribed specifically to the generous use of hyperventilation to decrease CBF and CBV, resulting in control of ICP. On the other hand, the use of mannitol to control ICP in children was discouraged, as this agent had been found to increase CBF in a number of head injured patients in the past.

It has been noted, however, that hyperemia cannot be defined by CBF criteria alone, but that the $AVDO_2$ and cerebral metabolic rate of O_2 ($CMRO_2$) must be taken into account as well (Obrist et al., 1984). Obrist et al., have also suggested some measure of brain compliance be considered, such as the pressure-volume index (PVI) of Marmarou et al. (1978). We, therefore, present in this paper a series of 32 children in whom measurements of CBF, $AVDO_2$ and $CMRO_2$ could be correlated with measurements of ICP and PVI.

Materials and Methods

The sample consists of 32 children admitted within 12 hours from their injury, aged from 3 to 18 years (mean 13.6 ± 4.8 years), and with a GCS of 7 or lower following resuscitation in the first 6 hours post-injury (mean GCS 5.4 ± 1.2). ICP was continuously recorded in all patients, in 28 with an intraventricular catheter and in 4 with a subarachnoid bolt. PVI measurements were performed with injections and withdrawals of $0.5-1.5$ ml bolus of CSF. Normal PVI in children between 3 and 14 years of age varies between 18 and 30 ml, depending on head circumference and spinal length of the child (Shapiro et al. 1980). In this paper, PVI is considered moderately depressed down to levels of 18 ml and considered markedly depressed below this value, with danger of ICP elevation.

CBF measurements were performed by the ^{133}Xe i.v. injection technique with $10-16$ detectors over both hemisphere. Normal CBF in awake, young adults at $PaCO_2$ 34 mm Hg is 44.1 ± 5.6 ml/100 g/min. Obrist et al. (1984) have defined CBF during coma below normal minus 2 SD (32.9 ml/100 g/min) as "reduced flow," between normal minus or plus 2 SD (between 32.9 and 55.3 ml/100 g/min) as "relative hyperemia," and above normal plus 2 SD (55.3 ml/100 g/min) as "absolute hyperemia". The same definitions are used in this paper.

Results

Table 1 shows ICP and PVI values taken at the same time as the CBF measurements were performed. Obviously, ICP was not different whether CBF was reduced, normal or high. There was possibly a trend for PVI to be lower (=stiffer brain) with higher CBF, but this was not statistically significant.

In Table 2, the temporal relationship between the ICP and PVI measurements and the CBF measurements is not maintained. However, also with this method of grouping the data, no correlation could be established between CBF and ICP or PVI. It is noteworthy that there were seven patients who were hyperemic at some time in their acute course in whom PVI remained above 18 ml all the time. On the other hand, three children with the lowest PVI values (around 6 ml) and most consistently below normal (total $19 \times <18$ ml, $2 \times >18$ ml) also had the highest flows consistently (absolute hypermia $8 \times$, normal $+2$ SD $1 \times$, average flow 74 ± 36 ml/100 g/min, $n=9$). Interestingly, all these three children had a favorable outcome.

$AVDO_2$ varied between 0.6 and 9.5 vol%, mean 4.5 ± 1.9 ($n=60$) which is markedly lower than normal (around 7 vol%), indicating luxury perfusion in the great majority of cases.

Table 1. ICP and PVI at the time of CBF measurements

	Reduced flow		Relative hyperemia		Absolute hyperemia
	(n=16)	(n=8)	(n=16)	(n=8)	(n=20)
CBF (34)	<32.9	32.9–38.3	38.4–49.7	49.8–55.3	>55.3
Average ICP	15.3±7.5	12.8±7.1	16.2±4.0	16.9±8.9	15.5±8.2
% ICP > 20 mm Hg	29	20	13	25	25
PVI above 18 ml (n)	0	0	2	1	2
PVI below 18 ml (n)	1	0	2	2	6

Table 2. CBF findings in two groups of head-injured children, classified according to ICP and PVI

Acute CBF findings	Total cases	ICP > 20 mm Hg no.	ICP < 20 mm Hg no.	PVI < 18 ml no.	PVI > 18 ml no.
Hyperemia	28	19	9	10	7
Reduced flow	4	4	0	1	0
Totals	32	23	9	11	7

Discussion

We have been unable to establish a correlation between "hyperemia" and high ICP or low PVI in head injured children. First, real hyperemia is uncommon. We measured CBF in 4 normal children aged 11–16 (mean 12.8) years and found an average of 68 ± 4 ml/100 g/min. Values above 76 (normal + 2 SD) were found in only 8 instances, of 73 measurements (11%). Second, there is no linear relation between CBF and CBV. Thus, increased CBV may still play an important role in high ICP in pediatric head injury, but this cannot be shown with CBF measurements. For the same reason mannitol can freely be used in children; even if it would increase CBF, it would not increase CBV and still may be effective because of its dehydrating effect.

References

Bruce DA, Raphaely RC, Goldberg AL et al. (1979) Pathophysiology, treatment and outcome following severe head injury in children. Childs Brain 5:174–191

Bruce DA, Alavi A, Bilaniuk L et al. (1981) Diffuse cerebral swelling following head injury in children: The syndrome of "malignant brain edema." J Neurosurg 54:170–178

Marmarou A, Shulman K, Rosenda RM (1978) A nonlinear analysis of the cerebrospinal fluid system and intracranial pressure dynamics. J Neurosurg 48:332–344

Obrist WD, Gennarelli TA, Segawa H et al. (1979) Relation of cerebral blood flow to neurological status and outcome in head injured patients. J Neurosurg 51:292–300

Obrist WD, Langfitt TW, Jaggi JL et al. (1984) Cerebral blood flow and metabolism in comatose patients with acute head injury. Relationship to intracranial hypertension. J Neurosurg 61:241–253

Shapiro K, Marmarou A, Shulman K (1980) Characterization of clinical CSF dynamics and neural axis compliance using the pressure-volume index: I. The normal pressure-volume index. Ann Neurol 7:508–514

Biochemical and Biophysical Parameters Under Thiopental Infusion in Severe Head Injured Patients

F. Della Corte, P. Carducci, A. Clemente, M. Sciarra, R.S. Brada, C. Anile, and R. Proietti

Istituto Di Anestesiologia E Rianimazione, Istituto Di Neuochirurgia, Universitá Cattolica S. Cuore, Largo A, Gemelli 1, 00167 Rome (Italy)

The rationale for the use of long term high dose barbiturates depends still on two debated considerations:

a) their efficacy in long term control of intracranial hypertension (IH) refractory to conventional treatment (Rockoff et al. 1979); b) their role in improvement of prognosis through control of ICP (Nordby et al. 1984).

The aim of the study was to evaluate the effects of continuous thiopental (TPS) infusion on intracranial biophysical and biochemical parameters in severe head injured patients.

Materials and Methods

Eight severe head injured patients (5 males and 3 females, from 24 to 42 years, GCS < 5 on admission) were studied. All patients developed, between 24 to 72 hours after admission, a persistent IH (ICP > 20 mm Hg) not amenable to a surgical procedure and refractory to conventional medical therapy. ICP (by means of an intraventricular catheter), systemic arterial pressure, central venous pressure, EtCO$_2$ and body temperature were continuously monitored. A loading dose of TPS (5 mg/kg) was followed by a continuous infusion of 3–5 mg/kg/h for at least 36 hrs; the infusion rate was then gradually reduced and adjusted to maintain a CPP > 50 mm Hg. CSF and blood samples were simultaneously collected before infusion was started and thereafter twice a day. Blood gas analysis, electrolytes, lactate, CK-BB, conjugate dienes, and TPS (by HPLC) were determined. The data obtained have been used for statistical analysis through the multiple linear regression method and subjected to a step-wise regression.

Results

A statistically significant correlation between the CSF TPS concentration (considered as the dependent variable) and serum TPS concentration and the CSF pH (viewed as independent variables) was ascertained. The stepwise regression analysis proved TPS serum concentration to be the main factor for the explanation of the dependent variable (F = 7455, DF = 1,28, $p < 0.01$).

Eds.: J. T. Hoff and A. L. Betz
© Springer-Verlag Berlin Heidelberg 1989

The linear regression between CSF lactate concentration and time, infusion rate, serum and CSF TPS concentrations was statistically significant. The most important factor was time ($F = 11.207$, $DF = 1,28$ $P < 0.002$). Conversely, no regression equation significantly linked the CSF pH and CSF lactate, CSF and serum lactate, and CSF lactate and ICP.

The regression analysis of CK-BB with time ($F = 12,950$, $DF = 1,28$, $p < 0.001$) and with lactate concentrations ($F = 17,063$, $DF = 1,28$, $p < 0.0005$) was significant. Considering only the infusion phase, the analysis of the multiple regression of ICP with time, with infusion rate and with serum and CSF TPS concentrations appeared to be significant. In this regression analysis the major contribution was rate of infusion. Finally, referring to the first 36 hrs of infusion, a linear correlation linked CSF lactate to CSF TPS concentration, and the serum barbiturate concentrations was capable of influencing the CSF lactate significantly. Regarding CSF conjugate dienes, higher concentrations than the control group were found; during TPS infusion a significant reduction in CSF dienes concentration was observed.

Discussion

Our preliminary data emphasizes a positive linear correlation between CSF and serum concentrations of TPS. This is probably due to simple diffusion of its free, non ionized form through the BBB. pH may be a less important and not significant factor in determining CSF TPS concentrations. Moreover, a linear relationship could not be found between TPS infusion rate and serum and CSF concentrations, which might have explained the complex pharmacokinetics of TPS, chiefly determined by the redistribution phenomenon.

No relationship was found between CSF lactate concentration (an index of cerebral metabolic conditions) and pH, as reported by DeSalles and Kontos (1986); the correlation between serum lactate on CSF lactate, although existing to some extent, did not appear to be significant.

In all patients high lactate concentrations were found prior to barbiturate infusion, whilst a significative reduction was recorded during the continuous TPS infusion (depending upon TPS CSF concentrations and not on plasma concentrations or upon the administered dose). A local effect on the cerebral oxidative metabolism may be involved that may help to remove the suspicion that barbiturate therapy is only used to delay inevitable death.

Finally, we also intended to show the presence of metabolic products of polyunsaturated fatty acids (conjugate dienes) in the CSF to prove the production of free radicals. Even if, at present, it appears impossible to advance the physiopathological hypothesis about their increase in head injury a "protective" effect of TPS on the oxidative process at the cerebral level may be assumed.

References

Rockoff MA et al. (1979) High dose barbiturate therapy in humans: A clinical review of 60 patients. Ann Neurol 6:194–199

Nordby HK et al. (1984) The effect of high dose barbiturate after severe head injury – a controlled clinical trial. Acta Neurochir (Wien) 72:157–166

DeSalles AA, Kontos HA (1986) Prognostic significance of ventricular CSF lactic acidosis in severe head injuries. J Neurosurg 65:615–624

ICP-Course After Weaning from Artificial Ventilation in Patients with Severe Brain Trauma

R. Schedl, G. Ittner, R. Jaskulka, F. Kiss, N. Mutz, and W. Thurner

II. Universitätsklinik für Unfallchirurgie, Spitalgasse 23, A-1090 Wien (Austria)

Introduction

The impact of different modes of artificial ventilation on intracranial pressure (ICP) curves has been reported by several groups in patients as well as in animal experiments (Richard and Karimi-Nejad 1977; Shapiro and Marshall 1978; Babinsky et al. 1981; Mutz et al. 1984; Schedl et al. 1984; Schedl et al. 1986). In this retrospective study we analyzed changes of ICP-course in severely brain injured patients, that were weaned from controlled mechanical ventilation (CMV).

Patients and Methods

Our experience includes 191 patients, the survival rate is 46.1%. In 29 patients ICP was continuously monitored when the ventilatory mode was changed from CMV continuous positive airway pressure (CPAP). In this group we investigated:

1. Immediate alterations of ICP.
2. Mean ICP-values from ICP recordings 6 hours before and up to 6 hours after changing the ventilary mode (if weaning was successful).
3. Highest and lowest ICP-levels in the observation periods.
4. Mean blood pressure (BP) and blood gases.

Results (Table 1)

At the moment of changing the ventilatory mode a short, transient peak in ICP was observed in almost all patients. During the 6 hour period – in 22 patients no remarkable changes were found. In 7 patients (24.1%) however, increases of mean-ICP-levels from $4-15$ mm Hg were observed. In 4 patients these elevations of ICP correlated with increased $paCO_2$, but in 3 patients blood gases remained unaffected.

The individual highest and lowest ICP-levels showed the same tendency as the mean-ICP; mean BP was not markedly influenced. In all patients except one, the ventilatory mode had to be changed to CMV due to elevation of ICP. All were successfully weaned later.

Table 1. Patients with elevation of ICP after changing ventilatory mode from CMV to CPAP

Initials	H. M.	Z. J.	E. G.	S. J.	O. R.	H. P.	T. A.
Sex	f	m	m	m	m	m	m
Age (years)	28	48	23	17	17	42	24
Diagnosis	br. cont.	depr. fr.	br. cont.	g. s.	depr. fr.	br. cont.	br. cont.
m. b. s	II	I	II	III	III	II	I
Weaning	4	4	2	6	2	9	3
MBP	100/95	90/90	93/94	80/80	93/92	96/105	94/95
ICPh	38/48	36/40	25/42	9/15	21/29	31/36	26/35
ICPl	31/43	30/32	19/33	6/13	19/27	24/33	24/30
ICPm	35/46	33/37	22/37	8/14	21/28	28/34	25/32
PaCO$_2$	33/33	32/32	34/33	32/38	29/34	32/37	33/39

br. cont. = brain contusion; *depr. fr.* = depression fracture; *g. s.* = *gun shot; m. b. s.* = mid brain syndrome on admission; *weaning* = weaning after *n* days from trauma; *MBP* = mean blood pressure; *ICPh* = highest ICP-level; *ICPl* = lowest ICP-level; *ICPm* = mean ICP-level

Discussion and Conclusion

Our experience shows that increases of ICP are observed frequently in brain injured patients that are weaned from artificial ventilation. Surprisingly these elevations are not dependent on simultaneous increases of PaCO$_2$ in every patient. The reason for this phenomenon might be due to alterations of thoracic pressure or in some unnoticed difficulty breathing. Further prospective investigations will be necessary to elucidate this problem. We propose to continue ICP-monitoring in mechanically ventilated patients until the critical period of weaning from CMV has passed.

References

Babinsky MF, Albin M, Smith RB (1981) Effect of high frequency ventilation in ICP. Crit Care Med 9:159

Mutz N, Baum M, Benzer H, Goldschmied W, Schedl R, Koller W (1984) Beatmung mit hohen Frequenzen in der Intensivmedizin, In: Lawin P, Peter K, Scherer R (Hrsg) Maschinelle Beatmung gestern – heute – morgen. Thieme, Stuttgart New York, pp 340–354

Richard KE, Karimi-Nejad A (1977) Intrakranielle Druckänderung unter Atemtherapie. Unfallheilk 132:208–214

Schedl R, Mutz N, Benzer H, Fasol P (1984) Conventional mechanical ventilation versus high-frequency ventilation – Influence on elevated intracranial pressure. Crit Care Med 12:262

Schedl R, Baum M, Benzer H, Fasol P, Ittner G, Mutz N, Spängler H (1986) Elimination of ventilator-related ICP-fluctuations by special techniques of artificial ventilation. In: Miller JD, Teasdale GM, Rowan JO, Galbraith SL, Mendelow AD (eds) Intracranial pressure VI. Springer, Berlin Heidelberg New York Tokyo, pp 740–746

Shapiro HM, Marshall LF (1978) Intracranial pressure response to PEEP in head-injured patients. J Trauma 18:254–256

Evaluation of Medical Management for Severe Head Injury

M. Shigemori, T. Moriyama, T. Tokutomi, K. Harada, N. Nishio,
and S. Kuramoto

Department of Neurosurgery, Kurume University School of Medicine, 67 Asahi-machi,
Kurume City, Fukuoka 830 (Japan)

Introduction

Barbiturates, hyperosmotic agents, hyperventilation and head elevation have
been widely used for the control of ICP in patients with severe head injury. But
controversies still exist on the efficacy and limitation of these managements. In
the present study, these medical managements were evaluated by analyzing their
effects on ICP, cerebral perfusion pressure (CPP), and blood flow velocity in the
middle cerebral artery (MCAFV).

Clinical Materials and Methods

We studied 50 patients with severe head injury including 40 with acute intracranial hematomas who had GCS scores of 8 or less on admission. The mean age
of the patients was 39 years. The extradural ICP monitoring was performed by
use of ICT/b catheter tip transducer (Gaeltec) and systemic arterial blood pressure (SABP) was also recorded simultaneously and therefrom CPP was calculated. MCAFV was recorded using transcranial Doppler ultrasonography (TCT
2064, EME) (Aaslid et al. 1982) under end-tidal CO_2 monitoring. The mean
velocity on the side of ICP monitoring was measured.

30 patients with GCS scores of 7 or less had barbiturate therapy consisting of
an initial dose of 5 mg/kg of thiopental and a loading dose of 2–3 mg/kg/hr. The
therapy was continued for 3–4 days after the operation (Shigemori et al. 1986).
As a hyperosmotic agent, Sendai Cocktail (Suzuki et al. 1985) was infused as a
bolus in 6 patients. To evaluate the effect of hyperventilation, the cerebrovascular
CO_2 reactivity was investigated in 9 patients by obtaining the K value in the
modified Olesen's formula of cerebral blood flow calculation according to Markwalder's report (In % $MCAFV = K \cdot PCO_2 + A$) (Markwalder et al. 1984), in
which mean velocity at 40 mm Hg of PCO_2 was determined as 100%. The control
of K value was 0.033 ± 0.007 (n: 50). The effect of head elevation was studied in
10 patients by elevating their heads from 0° (horizontal), 15°, 30° and 45°. SABP
was measured with reference to that measured at the level of the foramen of
Monro.

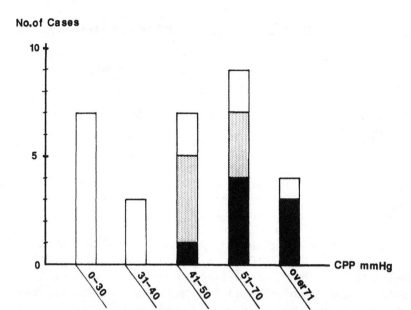

No. of Cases

Fig. 1. The mean CPP (cerebral perfusion pressure) during barbiturate therapy is closely related to outcome

Results

The outcomes of the patients with barbiturate therapy were good in 8 patients (26.7%), poor in 7 (23.3%), and dead in 15 (50%). There were no survivors in those with GCS score of 3 and those older than 60 years. Out of 30 patients, 17 (56.7%) responded to the therapy, but all 8 patients with initial ICP over 41 mm Hg also died irrespective of the response to barbiturate (Fig. 1). The Sendai Cocktail beneficially affected ICP and MCAFV in patients with normal mean MCAFV before the administration. The K value, examined twice in each patient, was low in the patients with GCS score of 5 or less. In the patients whose GCS score improved, the K values returned to nearly normal values. As the degree of head elevation was increased, there was a gradual decrement in CPP in association with a decrease of mean MCAFV in patients with low GCS scores. The reduction of CPP was induced either by reduction of SABP at the head level or by an increase of ICP. The average decreases of CPP and mean MCAFV were not remarkable in less severe patients (Fig. 2 A, B).

Discussion

Despite the widespread uses of barbiturate, hyperosmotic agents, hyperventilation, and head elevation there is no absolute evidence that they can effectively control

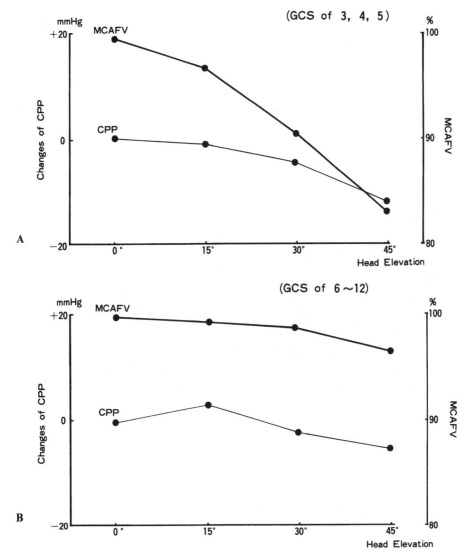

Fig. 2 A, B. The changes of CPP and mean MCAFV in head elevation in the patients. **A** Low GCS scores. **B** Less severe GCS scores

ICP and maintain adequate CPP and cerebral circulation. The present study on barbiturate therapy indicates that the best candidates for the treatment are the patients with GCS score of 4 or more, younger than 60 years, and with the initial ICP not exceeding 40 mm Hg. It is also found that CPP should be maintained at least higher than 40 mm Hg throughout the course of the treatment.

It is well known that hyperventilation effectively controls ICP by reducing cerebral blood flow. But, cerebrovascular CO_2 reactivity was apparently impaired in patients with low GCS scores so that the beneficial effect of hyperventilation are limited to patients with less severe brain injury. Hyperosmotic agents used as the Sendai Cocktail also failed to improve mean MCAFV and to reduce ICP when significant brain ischemia already existed. Since the severities of brain injury and brain ischemia were the main determinant of the efficacy of these managements, inappropriate employment of them should be avoided. The horizontal position is the optimal one to keep adequate CPP and mean MCAFV since the maximum CPP and mean MCAFV was always present with the head in the horizontal position. This finding is inconsistent with the report by Rosner and Coley (1986). MABP at the head level was reduced frequently in patients with dehydration. Therefore adequate hydration and the horizontal head position are recommended in patients with severe head injury.

References

Aaslid R, Markwalder TM, Nornes H (1982) Noninvasive transcranial Doppler ultrasound recording of flow velocity in basal cerebral arteries. J Neurosurg 57:769–774

Markwalder TM, Grolimund P, Seiler RW, Roth F, Aaslid R (1984) Dependency of blood flow velocity in the middle cerebral artery on end-tidal carbon dioxide partial pressure – a transcranial ultrasound Doppler study. J Cereb Blood Flow Metab 3:368–372

Rosner MJ, Coley IC (1986) Cerebral perfusion pressure, intracranial pressure, and head elevation. J Neurosurg 65:636–641

Shigemori M, Kawaba T, Yamamoto F, Kawasaki K, Yuge T, Tokutomi T, Nakashima H, Kuramoto S (1986) Efficacy and limitation of postoperative barbiturate therapy for severe head injury. Neurol Surg 14:637–642

Suzuki J, Imaizumi S, Kayama T, Yoshimoto T (1985) Chemiluminescence in hypoxic brain – The second report: cerebral protective effect of mannitol, vitamin E and glucocorticoid. Stroke 16:695–700

Intracranial Pressure Changes in Response to Deep Brain Stimulation in Traumatic Prolonged Coma Patients

T. Tsubokawa, Y. Katayama, and S. Miyazaki

Nihon University School of Medicine, Department of Neurological Surgery, Ohyaguchi Kamimachi 30, Itabashi-ku, Tokyo (Japan)

In an attempt to facilitate recovery from traumatic prolonged coma, chronic intermittent deep brain stimulation was applied on 8 cases (Hassler et al. 1969; Hassler et al. 1969; McLardy et al. 1968; Strum et al. 1979). These cases were selected by the following criteria; (1) coma prolonged more than 4 months, (2) no localized gross brain damage on CT, and (3) low amplitude of early components of the somatosensory evoked potentials, but not prolonged central conduction time more than three times standard deviation.

Stimulation targets were the ventral anterior thalamic nucleus (VA), thalamic reticular nucleus (R), thalamic intralaminal nucleus (CM) and the midbrain reticular formation (MRF: nucleus cuneiformis).

In this presentation, the differences of change of intracranial pressure and EEG alteration with behavioral expression were studied during chronic stimulation of the thalamic nuclei group and the midbrain reticular formation.

Method

A stimulating electrode was inserted into the target by stereotaxic surgery and a pressure sensor was placed to measure ICP from the epidural space. In some cases, two electrodes were inserted into both the thalamic nucleus and the midbrain reticular formation.

Results

EEG showed an arousal pattern during stimulation of either the thalamic nucleus or the midbrain reticular formation. After stimulation, the EEG changed from a slow wave pattern to α waves predominantly. Four-five weeks after chronic stimulation, this alteration was more marked with arousal behavior expression. Alteration of arousal behavior expression during MRF stimulation was typically of the sympathetic excitation type; the eyes opened with dilated pupils; the mouth also opened widely with vocalization. In contrast, the eyes opened without dilated pupils and the mouth opened slightly without vocalization during stimulation of the thalamic nucleus (VA, R and CE).

Intracranial Pressure VII
Eds.: J. T. Hoff and A. L. Betz
© Springer-Verlag Berlin Heidelberg 1989

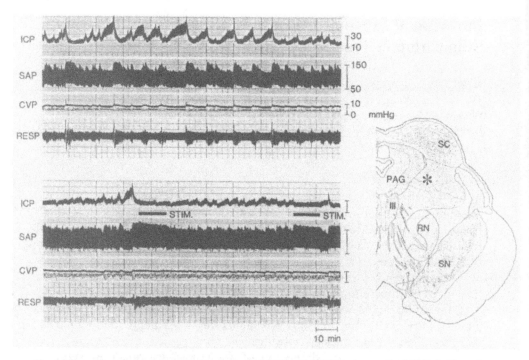

Fig. 1. Spontaneous pressure waves suppressed by chronic stimulation at the MRF (indicated by *star* on the right side anatomical diagram). *ICP:* intracranial pressure, *SAP:* systemic arterial pressure, *CVP:* central venous pressure, *RESP:* respiration, *STIM:* MRF stimulation

Baseline intracranial pressure did not change during or after stimulation of either the thalamic nucleus or the midbrain reticular formation, in spite of behavioral sympathetic excitation which appeared during stimulation of the midbrain reticular formation. Spontaneously occurring pressure waves (A and/or B waves) ceased immediately after the onset of MRF stimulation. The pressure waves did not continue as stimulation continued. After stimulation, pressure waves reappeared. Whenever such inhibitory effects on pressure waves were observed, the EEG showed an arousal pattern with sympathetic excitation behavioral expression (Fig. 1).

Such inhibitory effects on pressure waves were not observed during stimulation of VA, CE or the thalamic reticular nucleus.

Conclusion

These observations suggest that unstable activity from certain reticular formation cell groups within the brain stem are involved in the production of pressure waves.

References

Hassler R et al. (1969) Behavioural and EEG arousal induced by stimulation of unspecific projection systems in a patient with post-traumatic apallic syndrome. Electroencephalogr Clin Neurophysiol 27:306–310

Hassler R et al. (1969) EEG and clinical arousal induced by bilateral long-term stimulation of pallidal systems in traumatic vigil coma. Electroencephalogr Clin Neurophysiol 27:689–690

McLardy T, Ervin F, Sweet W (1968) Attempted inset-electrodes -arousal from traumatic coma: Neuropathological Findings. Trans Am Neural Ass 93:25–30

Strum V et al. (1979) Chronic electrical stimulation of the thalamic unspecific activating system in a patient with coma due to midbrain and upper brain stem infarction. Acta Neurochir (Wien) 47:235–244

The Use of Narcotics and Hyperventilation for the Treatment of Posttraumatic Brain Swelling: Theoretical Basis and Clinical Experience

A. Yabuki, M. Maeda, and S. Ishii

Department of Neurosurgery, Juntendo University, 2-1-1 Hongo, Bunkyo-ku, Tokyo (Japan)

Introduction

Mortality and morbidity rate of the severe head injury remains unacceptably high (Alberico et al. 1987; Langfitt 1978). Treatments for post-traumatic brain swelling such as hyperventilation, osmotic diuretics, and barbiturates, if used simply to reduce ICP without consideration of various types of imbalance in CBF and $CMRO_2$ known to be present in severe head injury (Obrist et al. 1984, Overgaard and Tweed 1983), may worsen ischemia or hyperemia in some cases, thus influencing outcome adversely. Furthermore, barbiturates may sometimes be harmful because of potent cardiovascular suppression (Traeger et al. 1983). We have been using serial measurement of arterial-jugular venous oxygen difference ($AVDO_2$), equivalent to cerebral oxygen extraction, as a guideline for various treatments. Morphine has also been used in large doses as an adjunct to barbiturates in an attempt to reduce the dose of the latter. The results are discussed here.

Material and Method

Thirty patients with GCS of 3 to 8, aged 5 to 76 years (mean 39), male 25 and female 5, were included in the study. Their intracranial lesion consisted of 9 diffuse injuries and 21 focal injuries. All patients were placed in 30 degrees head-up positions, ICP was measured by either Gaeltec or Camino Transducer, and systemic blood pressure and central venous pressure were monitored continuously. $AVDO_2$ was measured at 3 to 6 hour intervals, and auditory brain stem responses were also studied as required. If ICP exceeded 20 mm Hg for more than 5 minutes whilst $PaCO_2$ remained around 30 mm Hg by controlled hyperventilation, our next treatment was chosen on the basis of $AVDO_2$. If the $AVDO_2$ was below 5 vol%, hyperventilation was increased; if $AVDO_2$ was 5–9 vol% dehydrating agents (either glycerol or mannitol), were given; and, if $AVDO_2$ was over 9 vol% cerebral metabolic depressants (such as barbiturate or morphine) were given.

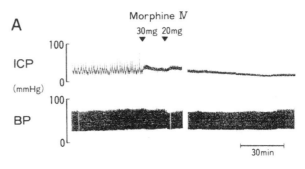

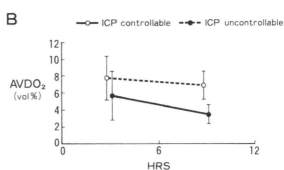

Fig. 1. A Rapid decrease of ICP (intracranial pressure) and disappearance of pressure waves following bolus injection of morphine hydrochloride. **B** Time course of mean AVDO$_2$ of first and 6 hrs in group of patients with controllable ($n=13$) and uncontrollable ICP ($n=9$)

Results

Our overall mortality was 47%. Patients who had G/R or M/D (Glasgow Outcome Scale) comprised 46% of all cases. All patients whose initial ICP exceeded 40 mm Hg died; all patients whose maximum ICP throughout the course remained below 30 mm Hg survived. Fig. 1 A shows the rapid reduction of ICP and disappearance of pressure waves as a result of the bolus injection of Morphine Hydrochloride. Morphine (0.5–1 mg/kg) was given in 10 patients; amongst 20 trials, 12 caused reduction of ICP. As demonstrated in Fig. 1 B, mean AVDO$_2$ of the first and next six hours were compared between the group of patients whose ICP was controllable ($n=13$), and patients whose ICP was uncontrollable and died ($n=9$). Although there was no statistical difference in the first 6 hours ($p=0.05$), the mean AVDO$_2$ was significantly lower in the next 6 hours in patients with uncontrollable intracranial hypertension ($p=0.001$), (Wilcoxon's test).

Discussion

Buchwitz et al. (1984) demonstrated the cerebral metabolic depressant effect of morphine. Morphine also reduced ICP in more than half of our cases, while cardiovascular suppression was minimal. Taking these observations into consideration, it may be reasonable to say that morphine can be a useful adjunct to barbiturates in the treatment of head injury. The sharp decrease of AVDO$_2$ in cases who died from uncontrollable intracranial hypertension is interpreted to be relative cerebral ischemia followed by rapid metabolic failure of cells. We believe, therefore, that monitoring the time course of $AVDO_2$ during the first 12 hours may be useful in predicting reversibility of brain dysfunction. There were also some of our patients with a favorable outcome who had high $AVDO_2$ value initially, decreasing within the first 12 hours. This may indicate the presence of an initial ischemic state, followed by relative hyperemia probably accompanying hypometabolism. If this is true, it is reasonable to speculate that hyperventilation, in the early course of the disease, might exaggerate relative ischemia and worsen outcome in some cases, and that treatment protocols using $AVDO_2$ may be useful in these situations. The number of cases demonstrated here is small. Further experience is required before drawing final conclusions.

References

Alberico AM, Ward JD, Choi SC, Marmarou A, Young H (1987) Outcome after severe head injury. J Neurosurg 67:648–656

Buchwitz E, Grandison L, Weiss HR (1984) Effect of morphine on regional cerebral oxygen consumption and supply. Brain Res 291:303–308

Langfitt TW (1978) Measuring the outcome from head injuries. J Neurosurg 48:673–678

Obrist WD, Langfitt TW, Jaggi JL, Cruz J, Genarrelli TA (1984) Cerebral blood flow and metabolism in comatose patients with acute head injury. J Neurosurg 61:241–253

Overgaard J, Tweed WA (1983) Cerebral circulation after head injury, Part 4: Functional anatomy and boundary zone flow deprivation in the first week of traumatic coma. J Neurosurg 59:439–446

Traeger SM, Henning RJ, Dobkin W, Giannotta S, Weil MH, Weiss M (1983) Hemodynamic effects of pentobarbital therapy for intracranial hypertension. Crit Care Med 11:697–701

Relationship Between Attenuation Changes on CT and Posttraumatic CSF-CKBB-Activity in Severely Head-Injured Patients

L. Rabow, D. Cook, A. DeSalles, M.H. Lipper, H. Gruemer, A. Marmarou, and D.P. Becker

From the Department of Neurosurgery, University of Umeå, Sweden, the Division of Neurological Surgery, Department of Surgery, and the Department of Radiology, Medical College of Virginia, Commonwealth University, Richmond, Virginia

CT-scanning has made it possible to separate the high attenuation of a hematoma from the low attenuation of localized edema. A contusion is usually recognized as scattered areas of high attenuation (blood) within areas of normal or even low attenuation, i.e. so-called mixed density areas, it is difficult, however, to delineate a contusion exactly.

Previous work from this institution (Lipper et al. 1985) has shown a correlation between the volume of an intracranial expanding mass on CT with outcome in head injured patients. Van Dongen et al. (1983) have also shown correlations between CT-scans and outcome, although they were looking not only at intracerebral contusions, but also at the type and site of intra- and extracerebral pathology.

CKBB, the so-called brain type isoenzyme of creatine kinase, has been shown by Bakay et al. (1983), Hedman and Rabow (1979), Nordby and Urdal (1982), and Rabow et al. (1987) to increase in the CSF after a brain contusion. Determination of CSF-CKBB-activity thus affords a method to estimate the amount of cell damage, i.e. the volume of a cerebral contusion in a head-injured patient.

The purpose of this study was to evaluate volume of a brain contusion from CT-images, assuming that maximal CSF-CKBB activity reflects the amount of damaged parenchyma. Since CSF cannot be obtained easily at standardized intervals after the trauma, a clearance curve for CSF-CKBB must be constructed. Such a curve allows us to estimate CKBB-activity at 6 hours after trauma, when the CSF-activity seems to peak (Nordby and Urdal 1982).

Material and Methods

CSF-CKBB-activity was analyzed in a consecutive series of patients with severe head injury, defined as not reacting to verbal stimuli, and with eyes continuously closed. There were 29 patients, 21 males and 8 females, aged 9–61 (median age, 25 years). Creatine kinase isoenzymes were separated on agarose film at pH 7.8. CKBB-activity was measured by a fluorescence technique involving NADPH (Wilkinson and Steciw, 1970). A CSF-CKBB-clearance curve was constructed from a series of selected patients with head injury (Rabow et al. 1987).

CSF-CKBB-activity at 6 hours after trauma was estimated from the clearance curve, and compared with the CT-scan. The initial admission CT-scans, usually carried out less than 6 hours after trauma, were examined. There were 8–10 images (1.0 cm thick) for each patient.

The number of images showing intracerebral pathology, i.e. hyperdense, hypodense, or mixed density lesions, was determined and compared with the CSF-CKBB-activity. For higher accuracy, each half of the brain was examined separately, giving a possible number of pathological images of 0–20.

As only areas of mixed density can be considered pathognomonic for brain contusion, the number of images on the CT-scan showing this feature was also counted and compared separately with CSF-CKBB-activity.

Results

With one exception, the maximum CSF-CKBB-activity developed within 24 hours after trauma. It was invariably increased in the first sample, even when this was obtained within 6 hours (5 cases). There was a significant correlation between the number of contusion locations and outcome. The relation between CSF-CKBB as estimated after 6 hours and outcome was even more significant (Table 1 A). There was, however, no correlation between the number of contusion images and CKBB (Table 1 B). This correlation was not improved if the highest measured CSF-CKBB-activities instead of the estimated 6 hour values, or/and those CT-images with mixed density areas only, were used for comparison.

Table 1. Outcome after severe head injury related to acute CT-scan and $CSF-CK_{BB}$

A	Good recovery or moderate disability $n=13$	Severe disability, vegetative or dead $n=16$	
CK_{BB} (6 h)	65 ±31	532±586	$p \leq 0,01$
Pathological CT-images (number of)	2.0± 2.0	5.7±3.6	$p < 0,05$

B		
Number of pathological (contusion) images on CT	Mean CK_{BB}-activity 6 h after trauma	n
0–2 (small contusion)	216 (34– 890)	9
3–5 (moderate contusion)	279 (38–1600)	12
6–15 (large contusion)	316 (34– 888)	6

Discussion

If CSF-CKBB-activity is accepted as an index of the extent of brain damage after a head injury, the first question is: At what time after trauma should the CSF be collected and CKBB-activity analyzed? Nordby and Urdal (1982), studying

15 patients with brain contusion, found significantly increased CKBB-activity in the CSF within four hours and a maximum within six hours in most of their patients.

The enzyme is supposed to leak from the cells through injured membranes to the extracellular space and from there to the CSF, where it presumably reaches the ventricular CSF almost as fast as the subarachnoid space. Based upon the studies mentioned above and our own findings, we have chosen to consider six hours after trauma as a point where the enzyme activity is most probably at its maximum level.

The process of denaturation does not seem to be very important for our clearance of CKBB from the CSF in vivo (Kjekshus et al. 1980). Our finding of a monoexponential clearance curve confirms that a simple production/absorption of CSF is the most probable mechanism involved. The unexpected lack of correlation between the CT-findings, as described above, and the CSK-CKBB-activity makes it necessary to consider what we are looking at on CT-images. The attenuation of damaged brain is probably not different from that of normal tissue until after some time, and then what we see on CT initially may be mainly extravasated blood and edema. Although the blood and edema are most often related to the severity of injury and therefore to prognosis, they are not correlated with the volume of damaged parenchyma, as reflected by the CSF-CKBB-activity. If the intracranial pressure is high, then the bleeding will often stop, and the local CT-changes may be limited, even if the enzyme leak may be substantial. Furthermore, traumatic intracerebral bleeds are sometimes better seen after evaluation of an extracerebral hematoma.

Localized expanding lesions on CT do not, per se, reflect the actual volume of a brain contusion, defined as the number of destroyed cells, but the combined effect of the primary parenchymal destruction, bleeding from the injured tissue, and secondary edema. Prognosis is not, however, dependent on the number of injured brain cells only, but also on the location of the lesions, intracranial pressure, the degree of ischemia, and, hopefully, also on the efficacy of treatment.

References

Bakay RAE, Ward AA Jr (1983) Enzymatic changes in serum and cerebrospinal fluid in neurological injury. J Neurosurg 58:27–37

Hedman G, Rabow L (1979) CKBB-isoenzymes as a sign of cerebral injury. Acta Neurochir (Wien) [Suppl] 28:108–112

Kjekshus JK, Vaagenes P, Hetland V (1980) Assessment of cerebral injury with spinal fluid CSF-CK in patients after cardiac resuscitation. Scand J Clin Lab Invest 40:437–444

Lipper M, Koshore PRS, Enas GG et al. (1985) Computed tomography in the prediction of outcome in head injury. Am J Neurol Rad 6:7–10

Nordby HK, Urdal P (1982) The diagnostic value of measuring creatine kinase BB activity in cerebrospinal fluid following acute head injury. Acta Neurochir (Wien) 65:93–101

Rabow L, DeSalles AAF, Becker DP et al. (1987) CSF brain creatine kinase levels and lactic acidosis in severe head injury. J Neurosurg 65:625–629

Van Dongen KJ, Braakman R, Gelpke GJ (1983) The prognostic value of computerized tomography in comatose head-injured patients. J Neurosurg 59:951–957

Wilkinson JH, Steciw B (1970) Evaluation of a new procedure for measuring creatine kinase activity. Clin Chem 16:370–374

ICP and Biomechanical Responses After Closed Impact Injury to the Spinal Cord

M. Albin and L. Bunegin

Department of Anesthesiology, University of Texas, Health Science Center, San Antonio, Texas 78284-7838 (USA)

Impact injury to the spine carries with it a tremendous release of energy, a portion of which is absorbed and transmitted by the cerebrospinal fluid. In a previous study (Hung et al. 1975) using an *open* impact injury model (anesthesia, laminectomy, impact at T_9 vertebral level and $F = 5.85 \times 10^5$ dynes), the CSF pressure wave generated immediately after impact 2.0 cm cephalad to the impact site reached a maximal of 50 mm Hg.

In this study we used a closed impact injury technique (lower thoracic column) to study the propagation of the CSF pressure wave from the point of impact to brain.

Methods

This experimental protocol received the prior approval of the Institutional Animal Care Committee, University of Texas Health Science Center at San Antonio. Seven (7), cats were anesthetized with 25 mg/kg of pentobarbital, intubated, and ventilated to normoxia and normocarbia. Closed impact injury was carried out at the T_9-T_{10} interspace using an air-cannon missile impacting upon an impounder resting within an optic-electronic module on the dorsum of the cat (Bunegin et al. 1986). A twist drill burr-hole was made in the temporal-parietal junction of the skull and the dura incised. A subarachnoid bolt was inserted into the burr-hole and a watertight seal obtained. A fast rise-time semiconductor transducer was connected to the subarachnoid bolt with a lead connected to an oscilloscope. Thus, intracranial pressure (ICP) and impact force could be simultaneously recorded. We delivered an impact force of 1.0×10^7 dynes/kg, which we demonstrated in an earlier study was capable of producing paraplegia in all the animals subjected to this closed impact injury (Bunegin et al. 1986). CSF waves were then digitized and averaged after subtraction of impact artifact.

Results

As can be noted in the Figure 1, the CSF pressure wave in the cranium following impact was noted to have an amplitude of 30 mm Hg over a period of approximately 8.0 msec, with the peak pressure occurring approximately 3.8 msec after impact.

Eds.: J. T. Hoff and A. L. Betz

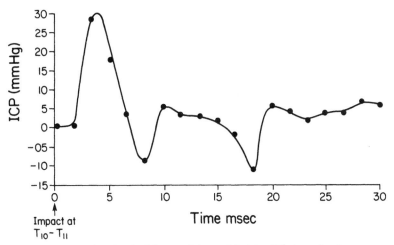

Fig. 1. ICP following $T_{10}-T_{11}$ closed spinal impact injury with 1.0×10^7 dynes/kg force

Discussion

In a previous study (Hung et al. 1975) using the Allen-Albin weight drop open impact injury method (Allen 1911; Albin et al. 1968), we determined that as much as 97% of the energy delivered during spinal cord impact is absorbed at and immediately adjacent to the impact site. This is one of the many limitations of the Allen-Albin *open* model, since the laminectomy removes the anatomical energy-attenuating structures so that a relatively small amount of force can produce major damage.

We used a force directed at the lower thoracic vertebra that was shown to produce severe histological damage which was directly correlated with a neurobehavioral recovery score. In this *closed* impact injury model study, it is noted that the unabsorbed energy can be propagated by the CSF to the brain via a pressure wave. Based on our findings, it is logical to hypothesize that the peak pressure recorded at the cranial level would be of a higher order of magnitude were impact performed higher up on the spine. It has also been noted in a recent animal study that cervical transection at the C_4 vertebral level produces early marked transitory physiopathological responses. These changes include a decrease in CBF, increase in brain water, increase in ICP, increase in blood-brain barrier permeability, an increase in mean arterial blood pressure and an increase in extravascular lung water (Albin et al. 1985).

If we put our experimental data within the framework of cervical cord injuries where intracranial lesions occur concomitantly (falls, motor vehicle and diving accidents), then this information may have clinical relevance. Thus, the impact associated ICP rise may further place the brain at risk.

References

Albin MS, White RJ, Acosta-Rua G, Yashon D (1968) Study of functional recovery produced by delayed localized cooling after spinal cord injury in primates. J Neurosurg 29:113–120

Albin MS, Bunegin BS, Wolf S (1985) Brain and lungs at risk after cervical spinal cord transection: Intracranial pressure, brain water, blood-brain barrier permeability, cerebral blood flow, and extravascular lung water changes. Surg Neurol 24:191–205

Allen AR (1911) Surgery of experimental lesion of spinal cord equivalent to crush injury of fracture dislocation of spinal column. A preliminary report. JAMA 57:878–881

Bunegin L, Albin MS, Martinez J, Bernal K, Rauschhuber R (1986) A new closed impact injury model for experimental spinal cord trauma. Soc Neuroscience Abstract 12:388

Hung TK, Albin MS, Brown TD, Bunegin L, Albin R, Jannetta PJ (1975) Biomechanical responses to open experimental spinal cord injury. Surg Neurol 4:271–276

Intracranial Pressure in Experimental Subarachnoid Haemorrhage

N. Dorsch[1,2], N. Branston[1], L. Symon[1], and J. Jakubowsky[3]

[1] Department of Neurological Surgery, Institute of Neurology, London WC1N 3BG (UK)
[2] Department of Surgery, Westmead Hospital, Westmead, N.S.W. 2145 (Australia)
[3] Department of Neurosurgery, Royal Hallamshire Hospital, Sheffield S10 2JF (UK)

Subarachnoid haemorrhage (SAH) has profound effects on cerebral circulation and intracranial pressure (Nornes 1975). Previous studies have analysed experimental subarachnoid haemorrhage in baboons (Kamiya et al. 1983, Jakubowsky et al. 1984, Kuyama et al. 1984). We review data from these and other experiments, in particular the effects on intracranial pressure (ICP) and cerebral blood flow (CBF).

Methods

From the above series and from a fourth (Dorsch et al. in preparation), sufficient data were available for inclusion of 29 animals. Six were treated with nimodipine and eight with its vehicle, without significant effects on the parameters discussed below.

SAH was produced via a transorbital approach (Kamiya et al. 1983), by avulsion usually of a posterior communicating artery, with the skull closed and data obtained for one half to two hours afterwards.

Results

Intracranial Pressure. In one animal there was no significant haemorrhage, as ICP never rose above 20 mm Hg; its data have not been used further. In the other 28, ICP increased sharply from resting levels of 0–20 mm Hg, peaking within half a minute at 50–210 mm Hg (mean 121, SD 48). ICP fell rapidly after reaching its peak in many cases, and after a further six minutes was already back to normal (< 20 mm Hg) in four animals. Sixteen minutes after the peak, mean ICP was 42 mm Hg (SD 44), and by 31 minutes the mean was 30 mm Hg (SD 22).

Cerebral Perfusion Pressure (CPP). Perfusion pressure fell drastically immediately after the haemorrhage, and by the time peak ICP was reached, was between 0 and 90 mm Hg. It reached zero in nine of the 28 experiments, and was 50 mm Hg or less in 25. Mean CPP at this time was 26.3 mm Hg, SD 25.7.

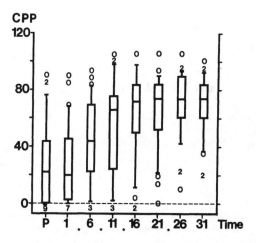

Fig. 1. Box Graph of CPP (mm Hg) changes, showing median and 10th, 25th, 75th and 90th percentile values. *Abscissa* – time intervals in minutes from peak ICP immediately after SAH (*P*); number of cases of zero CPP shown underneath. * – intervals with significant rise in perfusion pressure (Wilcoxon rank sum test); from *left to right P* < 0.0001, < 0.01, < 0.001, < 0.025

The time course of perfusion pressure is shown in Fig. 1. As with ICP the recovery of CPP was reasonably rapid; it was zero for longer than five minutes in only three cases. However, it took over ten minutes for the mean CPP to reach above 50 mm Hg. Significant rises occurred during several of the five-minute measurement intervals.

Differential ICP. Although the site of haemorrhage was always near the midline, and no intracerebral haematomas or large localised clots were found at post mortem, some animals showed differential pressures after SAH. In 19 cases, satisfactory bilateral measurement of ICP was possible; at the peak of ICP, nine showed a differential between the two sides of at least 5 mm Hg, with the higher pressure always on the side of the avulsed artery. The mean difference was 17.8 mm Hg (SD 11.2), and the highest 35 mm Hg. Two more animals showed delayed pressure differentials, 1 and 6 minutes later. Even half an hour later diffential pressures were still present in five cases, ranging from 10 to 30 mm; the mean differential at this time was 19 mm (SD 8.9).

Systemic Circulation. Many animals showed a considerable rise in systemic blood pressure. Some increase occurred in all but four, but 18 showed a significant pressor response (defined arbitrarily as a rise of at least 30 mm Hg), with an increase in blood pressure of up to 125 mm Hg. The mean rise in these 18 was 63 mm, SD 27. The rise in pressure persisted for the whole study period in two cases; in the other 16 it lasted for an average of 8 minutes.

Seven of these 18 had a zero perfusion pressure at the time (out of a total of 9 with zero CPP). However the mean CPP (23.9 mm, SD 25.8) was similar to that of the other 10 (mean 30.5, SD 26.3, $T = 0.65$, $P > 0.5$). If the pressor response had not occurred, then their calculated mean CPP of 1.4 mm (SD 5.9) would have been much lower than in the remainder ($T = 4.56$, $P < 0.001$). Mean CPP over the whole series would have been 10.9 instead of the measured 26.3 mm Hg. CPP would have been zero in 19 instead of 9.

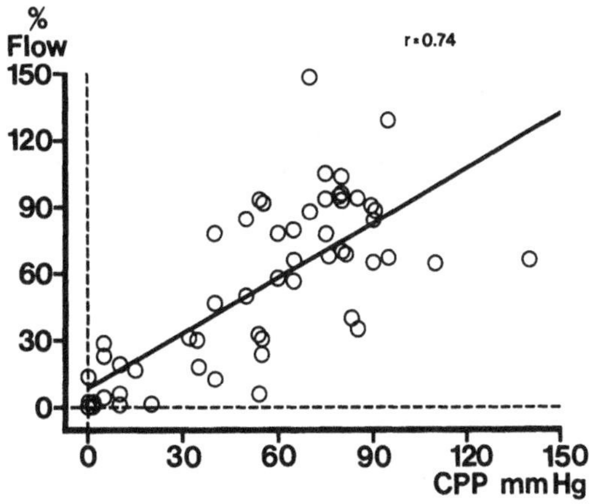

Fig. 2. Plot of post-haemorrhage CBF (expressed as percentage of resting pre-haemorrhage flow for each animal) against cerebral perfusion pressure, showing a more or less linear relationship.
Flow % = 9.315 + 0.828 CPP.
T = 7.94, DF = 53, $P < 0.0005$

Cerebral Blood Flow. CBF was measured by hydrogen clearance, and results are available for 16 animals. Prior to haemorrhage, mean flow was 69.4 ml/100 G/min (SD 29.3), falling immediately after by nearly 80%, to 14.3, SD 22.1. It reached zero in four (persisting in one for over 90 minutes), and was less than 10 ml/100 G/min, the threshold for loss of ionic homeostasis (Astrup et al., 1977) in 8 cases.

CBF then improved fairly rapidly, recovering to over 80% of pre-haemorrhage levels within 15 minutes in half (8 cases), and within 30 minutes in 12. Autoregulation of flow was, as would be expected, lost. There was a more or less linear, significant relationship between perfusion pressure and flow expressed as a percentage of the pre-SAH flow (Fig. 2).

Discussion

The changes seen here parallel those of human SAH (Nornes 1975), with considerable variation in the levels of ICP and CPP reached. In some cases where perfusion pressure was zero or very low, this presumably allowed cessation of the haemorrhage. In others where a reasonable perfusion pressure was maintained, it was presumably another factor, most likely an immediate local arterial spasm, that stopped the haemorrhage.

The duration of dangerously low CPP was usually brief. By one minute after the peak of pressure, it was already starting to recover, and significant further increases took place in subsequent time intervals. By 11 minutes over half the cases had an adequate perfusion pressure (50 mm Hg or greater).

Much of the credit for the maintenance of a reasonable perfusion pressure must be due to the pressor response seen in the systemic blood pressure in nearly two-thirds of cases. As noted above, if it had not occurred then the overall fall in CPP would have been much greater; it is suggested that the Cushing response can

717

be a useful one, at least under these conditions. The maintenance of perfusion pressure is of obvious importance for maintaining a continued satisfactory CBF. This applies even more when cerebral autoregulation has been lost, as was the case in all of this series (Fig. 2).

The occurrence of differential intracranial pressures is interesting in this model, where although the pathological process is severe, it is almost in the midline. It is probably due to the accumulation of increased water in the involved hemisphere (Kuyama et al. 1984), and illustrates how rapidly this can develop.

References

Astrup J, Symon L, Branston NM, Lassen NA (1977) Cortical evoked potential and extracellular K^+ and H^+ and critical levels of brain ischemia. Stroke 8:51–57

Jakubowski J, Bell BA, Symon L, Zawirski MB, Francis BM (1982) A primate model of subarachnoid hemorrhage: change in regional cerebral blood flow, autoregulation, carbon dioxide reactivity, and central conduction time. Stroke 13:601–611

Kamiya K, Kuyama H, Symon L (1983) An experimental study of the acute stage of subarachnoid hemorrhage. J Neurosurg 59:917–924

Kuyama H, Ladds A, Branston NM, Nitta M, Symon L (1984) An experimental study of acute subarachnoid haemorrhage in baboons; changes in cerebral blood volume, blood flow, electrical activity and water content. J Neurol Neurosurg Psychiatry 47:354–364

Nornes H (1975) Monitoring of patients with intracranial aneurysms. Clin Neurosurg 22:321–331

Cortical Tissue Pressure in Injured Brain After Subarachnoid Hemorrhage

J. Chen, S. Hatashita, and J.T. Hoff

Section of Neurosurgery, University of Michigan Hospitals, 1500 E. Medical Center Dr., Ann Arbor, Michigan 48109-0338 (USA)

Introduction

Alterations in blood-brain barrier, impaired cerebral circulation, toxic effects of extravasated blood, edema, and sudden increase in intracranial pressure are important early factors causing cerebral dysfunction after subarachnoid hemorrhage. This study examines the effects of experimental subarachnoid hemorrhage on intracranial CSF and tissue pressure, cerebral blood flow, and brain water content in order to determine how cerebrovascular homeostasis is influenced by cortical tissue pressure.

Materials and Methods

Adult cats were anesthetized with intravenous sodium pentobarbital (20 mg/kg). Mechanical ventilation was utilized and blood gases and blood pressure were maintained in the physiologic range. Left orbital exenteration allowed placement of a small catheter into the perichiasmatic cistern.

Subarachnoid hemorrhage (SAH) was simulated in eight cats by injection of 3 cc of autologous blood over a two minute period.

Intracranial pressure (ICP) was measured at the cisterna magna and cerebral blood flow (rCBF) and tissue pressure (TP) were measured in the left sylvian and suprasylvian gyrus according to methods described by Pasztor et al. (1973) and Iannotti et al. (1984). Grey matter water content was determined after sacrifice 6 hrs after SAH by the gravimetric method (Nelson et al. 1971).

A control group of four cats underwent injection of mock CSF by the same method. The statistical significance of all results was determined by the students t-test with $P < 0.01$ considered significant.

Results

Tissue pressure in the sylvian gyrus increased from 6.2 ± 0.6 (M + SE) to 12.5 ± 0.8 mm Hg ($n = 8$, $P < 0.01$) one hour after SAH, with a similar rise in the suprasylvian gyrus. Six hours after SAH tissue pressure had risen further to 18.8 ± 1.7 mm Hg ($n = 8$, $P < 0.01$).

Intracranial Pressure VII
Eds.: J.T. Hoff and A.L. Betz
© Springer-Verlag Berlin Heidelberg 1989

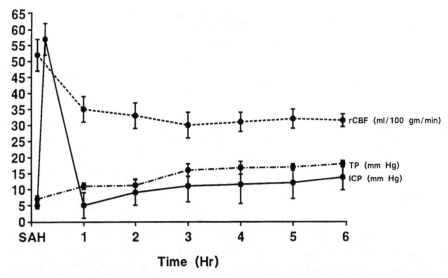

Fig. 1. Effects of SAH on blood flow, intracranial CSF and tissue pressure. There is a significant decline in rCBF and a significant increase in TP ($p < 0.01$)

Experimental SAH caused an immediate rise in ICP to values approaching diastolic blood pressure with rapid decline and subsequent slow rise. The overall rise in ICP was less than the rise in TP with a difference between TP and ICP of about 4.5 mm Hg 6 hr after SAH.

Cerebral blood flow fell from 51.12 ± 6.03 ml/100 g/min in the sylvian gyrus to 34.40 ± 3.38 ($n = 8$, $P < 0.01$) one hour after SAH and to 30.91 ± 1.89 ml/100 g/min at 6 hrs. The TP increase correlated with the decrease in rCBF at 6 hrs ($r = 0.97$) (Fig. 1).

Brain water content did not change significantly compared to controls by 6 hrs.

Discussion

Alterations in blood-brain barrier (BBB) may occur in both large and microvessels after SAH. While no increased brain water content was evident at 6 hrs, other studies suggest that a longer time period may be required for this to occur (Doczi et al. 1986). Cerebral blood flow studies in animals and humans after SAH generally reveal diminished flows with increased blood volume. This experiment also demonstrates a significant decline in rCBF correlated with a rise in tissue pressure. Indeed, some studies have shown dilatation of arterioles and venules acutely after SAH (Grubb et al. 1977) which could cause increased tissue pressure.

In addition to electrolyte and neurotransmitter alterations, cerebrovascular homeostasis may be affected at the autonomic level. Alterations in hypothalamic function have been shown to alter cerebral blood flow in the acute stage of SAH

720

(Delgado et al. 1986). The overall fall in cerebral blood flow seen in this study may be a major factor in the pathophysiology of delayed ischemic deficits.

We conclude that acute SAH causes reduced blood flow and increased tissue pressure which may be critical in the genesis of clinical vasospasm.

References

Delgado TJ, Diemer NH, Svendgaard NA (1986) Subarachnoid hemorrhage in the rat: cerebral blood flow and glucose metabolism after selective lesions of the catecholamine systems in the brainstem. J Cereb Blood Flow Metab 6:600–606

Doczi T, Joo F, Adam G et al. (1986) Blood-brain barrier damage during acute stage of subarachnoid hemorrhage, as exemplified by a new animal model. Neurosurgery 18:733–739

Grubb RL, Raichle ME, Eichling JO et al. (1977) Effects of subarachnoid hemorrhage on cerebral blood volume, blood flow and oxygen utilization in humans. J Neurosurg 46:446–453

Iannotti F, Hoff JT, Schielke GP (1984) Brain tissue pressure: physiological observations in anesthetized cats. J Neurosurg 60:1219–1225

Nelson SR, Mantz ML, Maxwell JA (1971) Use of specific gravity in the measurement of cerebral edema. J Appl Physiol 30:268–271

Pasztor E, Symon L, Dorsch NWC et al. (1973) The hydrogen clearance method in assessment of blood flow in cortex, white matter and deep nuclei of baboons. Stroke 4:556–567

Experimental Hypertensive Putaminal Hemorrhage

Part 1. Physiological Study

S. Waga, Y. Morooka, A. Morikawa, M. Sakakura, and T. Kojima

Department of Neurosurgery, Mie University Hospital, 2-174 Edobashi, TSU, Mie 514 (Japan)

Putaminal hemorrhage is the most common among the hypertensive intracerebral hemorrhages. The optimal form of treatment still remains controversial. Some neurosurgeons, especially in Japan, believe surgical treatment is superior, while others hold that hypertensive putaminal hemorrhage should be treated conservatively. Our clinical results have shown that the surgical treatment is not superior to the conservative one and that the results depend upon the size and extent of the hemorrhage (Waga and Xamamoto 1983; Waga et al. 1986).

This paper describes experimental hypertensive putaminal hemorrhage induced in dogs, and resultant changes in intracranial pressure, the electroencephalogram, somatosensory evoked potentials, auditory brain stem evoked responses and thalamic blood flow, compared between groups treated with and without surgery.

Clinical observations, intracranial pressure, electroencephalograms, somatosensory evoked potentials, thalamic blood flow, and brain stem evoked responses did not show any difference between the surgical and non-surgical treatment groups.

Results of this study do not support the view that surgical treatment is superior to the conservative one in the management of hypertensive putaminal hemorrhage.

References

Waga S, Yamamoto Y (1983) Hypertensive putaminal hemorrhage: Treatment and results. Is surgical treatment superior to conservative one? Stroke 14:480–485

Waga S, Miyazaki M, Okada M et al. (1986) Hypertensive putaminal hemorrhage: Analysis of 182 patients. Surg Neurol 26:159–166

Experimental Hypertensive Putaminal Hemorrhage

Part 2. Pathological Study

S. Waga, H. Tochio, Y. Morooka, A. Morikawa, K. Knamaru, and T. Kojima

Department of Neurosurgery, Mie University Hospital, 2-174 Edobashi, Tsu, Mie 514 (Japan)

Hypertensive putaminal hemorrhage was stereotactically produced in the dogs who had been hypertensive for more than 4 weeks by means of the Goldblatt procedure. In the surgical group the hemorrhage was aspirated stereotactically 3 hours after bleeding. The comparative pathological study included perifocal edema, number of neutrophils and macrophages, glial reaction, neovascularity, volume of hemorrhage, and degree of hemolysis and absorption.

This study did not demonstrate any difference between the surgical group and the non-surgical group.

Thus, the study supports our clinical results in humans (Waga and Yamamoto 1983; Waga et al. 1986) that the surgical treatment for hypertensive putaminal hemorrhage did not give better results than the conservative one.

References

Waga S, Yamamoto Y (1983) Hypertensive putaminal hemorrhage: Treatment and results. Is surgical treatment superior to conservative one? Stroke 14:480–485
Waga S, Miyazaki M, Okada M et al. (1986) Hypertensive putaminal hemorrhage: Analysis of 182 patients. Surg Neurol 26:159–166

Estimation of Intracranial Pressure in Acute Subarachnoid Hemorrhage Based on CT

C. Kadowaki, M. Hara, M. Numoto, and K. Takeuchi

Department of Neurosurgery, Kyorin University School of Medicine, 6-20-2 Shinkawa, Mitaka, Tokyo 181 (Japan)

Introduction

The predictive values of certain features of computed tomography (CT) scans in estimating intracranial pressure (ICP) were investigated during the acute stage of subarachnoid hemorrhage (SAH) to determine if noninvasive CT can be useful for the identification of patients not requiring ICP monitoring.

Materials and Methods

Thirteen patients with acute SAH are included in the present study, included 9 females and 4 males with a mean age of 57 years (range 40–77 years). All were admitted within 24 hours of SAH onset. There were four Hunt and Kosnik clinical grade II patients, five grade III, two grade IV, and two grade V. All were treated without early surgery for various reasons.

ICP (intraventricular pressure or epidural pressure) was continuously monitored for a mean of 6 days (range: 6 hours – 17 days) after the initial hemorrhage.

Various features of CT scans selected for the present study included: (1) blood in the basal cisterns, (2) blood in the Sylvian fissure, (3) presence in the cortical sulci and on the cortical surface, (4) ventricular dilation in the acute stage, (5) blood in the ventricles, (6) associated intra- and/or extra-axial hemorrhagic lesion, and midline shift.

Results

CT. Eleven cases showed SAH into the basal cisterns and/or intraventricular hemorrhage on admission CT scans, ten with blood into the Sylvian fissures and six with blood onto the cortical surface, and four with disappearance of the interspaces of the cortical sulci. One case showed a large subdural hematoma without SAH and one case showed SAH associated with an intracerebral hematoma. Both showed marked ventricular compression and midline shift greater than 5 mm. Three patients had blood in both lateral ventricles, two in the lateral third and fourth ventricles with moderate ventricular dilation including an Evans'

Eds.: J. T. Hoff and A. L. Betz
© Springer-Verlag Berlin Heidelberg 1989

ratio of more than 35 resulting from acute obstruction of the cerebrospinal fluid (CSF) pathway, and three in the fourth ventricle only.

ICP. Eight patients had moderately increased ICP of 15–40 mm Hg during the monitoring period, and four had severe increased ICP (> 40 mm Hg). There were plateau waves in 3 cases and B waves in 10 cases.

Correlation Between Features in CT and ICP. No correlation could be found between the amounts and distribution of blood in the basal cisterns and Sylvian fissures, and rises in ICP. Cases with diffuse SAH extending to the cortical surface showed ICP rises of more than 30 mm Hg. There was no significant correlation between the degree of ventricular dilation on admission CT scan and rise in ICP, but cases with acute blockage of CSF pathway, showing rapid progressive enlargement of the ventricles in repeated CT scans, showed moderate elevation of ICP greater than 30 mm Hg. Cases with intraventricular blood in the lateral ventricles exhibited moderate elevations in ICP of more than 30 mm Hg, while cases with blood in the third and fourth ventricles as well showed severe ICP elevation (more than 40 mm Hg). Patients with a midline shift greater than 5 mm on CT due to mass lesions such as an intracerebral hematoma (4 cm in diameter) or acute subdural hematoma (thickness of 2 cm) showed severe rise of ICP.

Discussion

Several reports have attempted to correlate ICP with the CT scan features in head injuries because of the potential risk and limitations of ICP monitoring (Kishore et al. 1981; Miller et al. 1979; Sadhu et al. 1979; Tabaddor et al. 1982). However, we have found it difficult to estimate ICP with a CT scan in the acute stage of SAH. Our results suggest a poor correlation between various features in CT and ICP in the acute stage of SAH. Our findings suggest that rises in ICP are dependent on a variety of factors, such as metabolism vasodilation resulting from stimulated neurogenic pathways and adrenergic activity (Hayashi 1976). Good correlation, however, was obtained between diffuse bleeding into the ventricles and onto the cortical surface, progressive hydrocephalus and rises in ICP.

Conclusion

The predictive features of CT scans in estimating ICP were as follows: intraventricular bleeding into the lateral ventricles, and lateral, third and fourth ventricles, diffuse SAH onto the cortical surface and acute enlargement of the ventricles.

References

Hayashi M, Maruyama S, Fujii H, Kitano T, Furubayashi H, Yamamoto S (1976) Effects of norepinephrine and phentolamine on acute intracranial hypertension. Brain Nerve 28:143–149

Kishore PRS, Lipper MH, Becker DP, Domingues das Siilva AA, Narayan RK (1981) Significance of CT in head injury: Correlation with intracranial pressure. AJNR 2:307–311

Miller JD, Gudeman SK, Kishore PRS, Becker DP (1979) CT scan, ICP and early neurological evaluation in the prognosis of severe head injury. Acta Neurochir (Wien) [Suppl] 28:86–88

Sadhu VK, Sampson J, Haar FL, Pinto RS, Handel SF (1979) Correlation between computed tomography and intracranial pressure monitoring in acute head trauma patients. Radiology 133:507–509

Tabaddor K, Danziger A, Wisoff HS (1982) Estimation of intracranial pressure by CT scan in closed head trauma. Surg Neurol 18:212–215

Intracranial Pressure (ICP) and Cerebral Blood Flow Velocity (BFV) in Patients with Subarachnoid Hemorrhage Under Treatment with Nimodipine

K.E. Richard, P. Sanker, and M. Alcantara

Neurosurgical University Hospital, Joseph-Stelzmann-Str., 5000 Cologne (FRG)

Introduction

Cerebral vasospasm and critical increases of intracranial pressure (ICP) are considered to be unfavorable prognostic factors, as well after an acute subarachnoid hemorrhage (SAH), as after the clipping of a cerebral aneurysm.

In recent years calcium-antagonists have been employed for prevention and treatment of vasospasm. But, several authors have called attention to the possibility that the treatment may provoke critical ICP increases, if the intracranial compliance is restricted (Bedford et al. 1983; Brinker and Spring 1987).

In patients with an acute SAH or in patients after clipping of a cerebral aneurysm we therefore investigated, in relation to the outcome, the behaviour of ICP and cerebral blood flow velocity (BFV) under treatment with the calcium-antagonist nimodipine.

Patients and Methods

Our study is based upon 26 patients, who were treated with continuous nimodipine infusions in a dosage of 15–36 µg/kg/h. Ten of these were treated after the acute SAH and 16 of these after clipping of the aneurysm. During a period of 1 to 3 weeks ICP, BFV, blood pressure and neurologic state (Brussels Coma Scale) were registered. ICP was monitored epidurally with a Gaeltec transducer, cerebral BFV by transcranial Doppler ultrasound measurements.

Results

ICP and BFV after acute subarachnoid hemorrhage (Table 1 A).
The ICP reached peak values from 30 to 9 mm Hg between the first and the ninth day after SAH. An effective lowering of high ICP values was accomplished by hyperosmotic bolus therapy. In two patients (pats. 5, 9) a temporary interruption of nimodipine infusion became necessary. Intracranial pulse pressure decreased immediately in both.

Table 1 A, B

A Intracranial pressure (ICP) and cerebral blood flow velocity (BFV) after subarachnoid hemorrhage (SAH) (n: 10). Outcome: ↑ fully recovered; (↑) slightly disabled; ↓ severely disabled; † deceased

No.	Pat.	Age	Sex	Location of aneurysm	Duration of Meas. after SAH	Peak values				Day of normalisation			Nimodipine continuously dosage			Outcome
						ICP (mmHg)	Day	BFV (cm/s)	Day	ICP	BFV	Neurol. state	Yes	No	(µg/kg/h)	
1	J., C.	46	f	SAH u. O.	0–14	40	8	170	7	13	no	no	yes		30	†
2	T., H.	44	m	MCA	1–24	46	9	212	10	?	24	24	yes		15–30	↑
3	G., F.	59	m	A A	1–24	27	5	105	14	?	23	no	yes		15–30	↓ Hydr.
4	S., M.	42	f	ICA	1–16	50	5	180	5/6	16	10	11	yes		15–36	↑
5	H., H.	33	m	A A	1–11	90	4	50	2	7	2	5		no	15–30	↑
6	S., L.	54	f	MCA	1–11	38	3	228	7	8	12	4	yes		15–30	↑
7	B., S.	22	f	MCA	1–6	40	1	180	4	6	11	27	yes		15–30	↑
8	D., B.	40	m	ICA	2–8	38	3	156	6	4	?	6	yes		10–15	(↑) Aph.
9	B., S.	66	f	SAH u. O.	4–17	80	7	94	4	14	6	21		no	15–30	(↑) Paresis
10	R., G.	49	f	ACA	13–24	38	17	140	16	21	21	21	yes		15–30	↑

B Intracranial pressure (ICP) and cerebral blood flow velocity (BFV) after clipping of cerebral aneurysms (*n*: 16)

No.	Pat.	Age	Sex	Location of aneurysm	OP after SAH	Peak values ICP (mmHg)	Day	BFV (cm/s)	Day	Day of normalisation ICP (mmHg)	BFV (cm/s)	Neurol. state	Nimodipine continuously dosage Yes	No	(µg/kg/h)	Outcome ↑ (↑)↓ †
1	S., M.	42	f	ICA	0	50	4	180	5/6	16	10	22	yes		15–36	↑
2	T., H.	44	m	MCA	1	47	8	212	9	?	24	24	yes		15–30	↑
3	J., K.	38	f	ACA	7	14	5	65	3	6	4	14	yes		15–30	↑
4	H., G.	51	f	ICA	7	28	1	186	7	2	>25	25	yes		30	↑
5	H., H.	58	m	MCA	11	36	0	100	0	4	4	30	yes		30	↑
6	S., L.	54	f	MCA	12	16	2	90	1	4	2	7	yes		30–36	↑
7	Z., S.	28	m	ACA	14	30	1	90	0–2	3	3	4	yes		15–30	↑
8	N., M.	62	f	MCA	17	13	1	90	0–2	3	3	17	yes		30–36	↑
9	E., U.	51	f	MCA	30	15	1	75	2	2	2	2	yes		15–30	(↑) Aph.
10	T., H.	48	m	ICA	30	26	7	140	2	8	8	16	yes		36–45	(↑) Hydr. †
11	S., M.	67	f	ICA	30	74	5	200	1	–	4	3	yes		15–30	↑
12	T., U.	38	f	ACA	42	50	2	90	0/2	3	4	3	yes		15–30	
13	R., G.	49	f	ACA	49	80	7	90	1	16	5	54		no	15–30	(↑) Hydr.
14	L., A.	33	f	MCA	78	16	1	90	4	3	?	5	yes		30	↑
15	B., S.	22	f	MCA	85	6	1	80	1	2	2	2	yes		15	↑
16	S., W.	50	f	MCA	155	18	2	64	4	3	6	3	yes		15–36	↑

BFV and neurologic state did not normalize simultaneously with the ICP. Peak values of BFV mostly appeared around the 5th day after SAH. Normalization of BFV occurred between day 10 and day 24. ICP and BFV did not correlate. We found high ICP values in connection with high BFV values (pat. 4), increasing BFV values in connection with decreasing ICP values (pat. 6), and critical ICP increases together with normal BFV values (pat. 5). Even in patients with temporary elevation of ICP and BFV increases the course of the treatment was favorable.

ICP and cerebral BFV after clipping of cerebral aneurysm (Table 1 B).

After an early clipping of the aneurysm (pats. 1–4), the outcome was generally favorable, even in patients with an ICP increase up to 50 mm Hg or with an BFV increase up to 212 cm/s. In patients operated on within 2nd to 4th week after SAH (pats. 5–10), ICP and BFV levels were significantly lower. A 67-year-old female, operated on day 30 after SAH (pat. 11), died after an extreme BFV increase of 100 cm/s and development of a severe postischemic brain edema with a final ICP increase up to the level of the diastolic blood pressure.

In patients operated on after the 4th week (pats. 12–16) BFV values did not rise above the normal range. Early ICP peaks were temporary (pat. 12). The reason for later ICP increases was the development of posthemorrhagic hydrocephalus (pats. 10, 13).

Conclusion

After an acute SAH as well as after clipping of the cerebral aneurysm, various but typical patterns of ICP and BFV behavior were observed. A significant correlation between these two parameters was not recognizable. We have not seen a general decrease of ICP with nimodipine treatment as observed in a primate model by Hadley et al. (1987). Temporary ICP increases occurred frequently. Only in 3 incidents were we forced to discontinue the infusion for several hours. After subarachnoid hemorrhage BFV values in 90% of the patients increased above the normal range and reached peak values above 180 cm/s in 40% of the patients. After clipping the aneurysm the BFV in 75% of the patients increased above the normal range, reaching peak values above 180 cm/s in 25% of the patients. But, these extreme rises of BFV did not essentially impair the outcome.

Our results correspond with those of other authors (Allen et al. 1983; Seiler et al. 1987), who also found a significant reduction of neurological deficits and an improvement of the final outcome.

References

Allen GS, Ahn HS, Preziosi TJ, Battye R (1983) Cerebral arterial spasm – a controlled trial of nimodipine in patients with subarachnoid hemorrhage. N Engl J Med 308:619–624
Bedford T, Dacey R, Winn HR, Lynch C (1983) Adverse impact of a calcium entry blocker (verapamil) on intracranial pressure in patients with brain tumors. J Neurosurg 59:800–802

Brinker T, Spring A (1987) Risiken der Nimodipin-Therapie bei erhöhtem Hirndruck. Anasth Intensivther Notfallmed 28:221–224

Hadley MN, Spetzler RF, Fifield MS, Bichard WD, Hodack JA (1987) The effect of nimodipine on intracranial pressure. Volume-pressure studies in a primate model. J Neurosurg 67:387–393

Seiler RW, Grolimund P, Zurbruegg HR (1987) Evaluation of the calcium-antagonist nimodipine for the prevention of vasospasm after aneurysmal subarachnoid haemorrhage. A prospective transcranial Doppler ultrasound study. Acta Neurochir (Wien) 85:7–16

ICP in the Diagnosis of Acute Hydrocephalus After Aneurysmal Subarachnoid Hemorrhage

H.-P. Stoiber, J.-P. Castel, P. Dabadie, and H. Loiseau

Université Bordeaux II, Groupe Hospitalier Pellegrin, Neurochirurgie A,
Place Amélie-Raba-Léon, 33076 Bordeaux Cedex (France)

Acute hydrocephalus is an early and dramatic complication occurring after sub-arachnoid hemorrhage (SAH) from ruptured intracranial aneurysm. Hydro-cephalus is well detected by a CT scan, but ventricular dilatation may be absent or doubtful in the early stage of this complication. The aim of this study is to demonstrate that, in this situation, an Intraventricular Fluid Pressure measure-ment is recommended, as it is highly effective to achieve the diagnosis and to guide ventricular drainage.

Material and Methods

Forty-seven patients out of 345 consecutive cases (14%) of aneurysmal subarach-noid hemorrhage (SAH) confirmed by CT scan and early four-vessel angiography were admitted to the neurosurgical unit from January, 1980, to December, 1986. Initial clinical condition and severity of SAH on the first CT scan were respective-ly graded on the Hunt and Hess Scale and Fisher's classification (Fisher et al. 1980). Ventricular size was measured by the Bicaudate Index, whenever it was possible, and by the Cella Media Index for the others. These values were com-pared to the normal values reported in the literature (Vassilouthis and Richardson 1979; Meese et al. 1980). Intracranial pressure (ICP) was measured with an intra-ventricular cannula, connected to an external transducer. Ventricular drainage was used in all patients within the first week after bleeding for management of acute hydrocephalus, diagnosed either on CT scan or ICP measurement, or both.

Results

Clinical Findings. There were 22 men (47%) and 25 women (53%), with a mean age of 55 years (SD ± 13.6). On admission no patient was grade 1. There were 10 patients grade II, 23 grade III, 13 grade IV and one grade V (Fig. 1). Evidence of clinical deterioration (at least 1 grade on Hunt and Hess Scale) was found in 62% of the patients (27/47). Sixty-six percent of patients (31/47) improved within 2 days after treatment (Fig. 1). The overall mortality rate was 49% (23/47). For survivors, the Glasgow Outcome Scale was scored 1 year after bleeding: 13 pa-

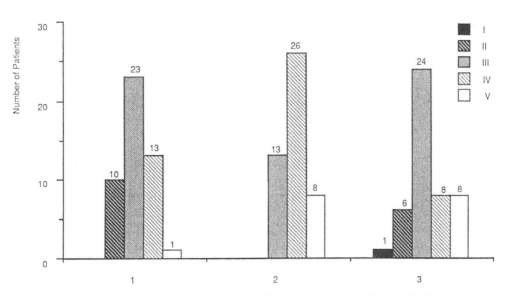

Fig. 1. Clinical grade, scored on the Hunt and Hess Scale: *1* on admission; *2* before treatment (ventricular drainage); *3* after treatment

Table 1. Computerized tomography findings

Classification of Fisher	Number of patients	Group A "Non dilated"	Group B "Dilated"
1	–	–	–
2	7	2	5
3	7	4	3
4	33	13	20
Total	47	19	28

tients had good recovery (28%), 6 had moderate disability (13%), one had severe disability (2%), and 4 were in a permanent vegetative state (8%).

Computerized Tomography Findings. As shown in Table 1, 70% of the patients were classified on the first CT scan in Fisher's group 4 (i.e., presence of intraventricular or intracerebral hemorrhage). After measurement of the ventricular dilatation two groups were compared. In group A, "non-dilated" patients (19/47), there was no ventricular enlargement or only minimal dilatation (Bicaudate Index ≤ 0.2 of Cella Media Index ≥ 4). In group B, "dilated" patients (28/47), the ventricular enlargement was moderate or marked (Bicaudate Index > 0.2 or Cella Media Index < 4).

Intracranial Pressure Findings. Intraventricular Fluid Pressure was measured in 81% of the patients (38/47). The difference between group A ("non-dilated") and group B ("dilated") is not significant (T-test: $0.1 < p \leq 0.375$).

733

Discussion

The incidence of acute hydrocephalus occurring after SAH is reported to range from 15 to 21% (Kassell et al. 1985; Milhorat 1987; Van Gijn et al. 1985). 14% of the patients affected by this complication in this study can be compared to other series reported in terms of initial clinical grading (79% of grade III–IV patients), clinical signs of progressive deterioration leading to the diagnosis (62% of the patients), CT scan findings of intraventricular hemorrhage occurring in 70% of the patients, and mortality rate of 49% (Mohr et al. 1983; Van Gijn et al. 1985).

Computerized tomography has proved to be highly reliable in detecting hydrocephalus. After SAH, ventricular enlargement may be absent or underestimated when there is only a minimal degree of dilatation (Kosteljanetz 1984; Van Gijn et al. 1985). In this study 40% of the patients ("non-dilated" group-A) and "dilated" group-B patients were comparable according to initial clinical grading and the presence of intraventricular blood. Similarly, when intraventricular fluid pressure was assessed, an intracranial hypertension was always present, with comparable mean values. Immediate clinical improvement after ventricular drainage was observed in 59% of the cases in group A, and in 71% of group-B patients, but this difference was not significant (Chi-square test; $p > 0.3$).

Acute hydrocephalus after SAH is due to mechanical obstruction of the cerebrospinal fluid (CSF) pathways by blood clots, especially in the basilar cisterns (Wenig et al. 1979; Black et al. 1985). This leads to elevation of CSF outflow resistance and a consecutive increase in intracranial pressure with ventricular dilatation. However, high ICP and increased resistance to CSF outflow do not necessarily cause ventricular dilatation. Changes in biomechanical properties of the surrounding brain may be responsible for this non-uniform behavior of the ventricular system (Kosteljanetz 1984; Hansen et al. 1987). Presumably high intraventricular fluid pressure precedes ventricular dilatation for hours or maybe even days after CSF blockade. In that way ICP measurement may be as important as CT scan for an early and accurate diagnosis.

In conclusion, secondary clinical deterioration or lack of clinical improvement in the first week following SAH is always an indication for CT scanning. In the absence of rebleeding or vasospasm or evidence of ventricular dilatation, intracranial pressure should be monitored, as intracranial hypertension from CSF blockade might be present and can be successfully treated by ventricular drainage.

References

Black PMcL, Tzouras A, Foley L (1985) Cerebrospinal fluid dynamics and hydrocephalus after experimental subarachnoid hemorrhage. Neurosurgery 17:57–62
Fisher CM, Kistler JP, Davis JM (1980) Relation of cerebral vasospasm to subarachnoid hemorrhage visualized by computerized tomography scanning. Neurosurgery 6:1–9
Hansen K, Gjerris F, Sorensen PS (1987) Absence of hydrocephalus in spite of impaired cerebrospinal fluid absorption and severe intracranial hypertension. Acta Neurochir (Wien) 86:93–97

Kassel NF, Torner JC, Jane JA (1985) The international cooperative study on the timing of aneurysm surgery. In: Auer LM (ed) Timing of aneurysm surgery. de Gruyter, Berlin New York, pp 277–278

Kosteljanetz M (1984) CSF dynamics in patients with subarachnoid and/or intraventricular hemorrhage. J Neurosurg 60:940–946

Meese W, Kluge W, Grumme T, Hopfenmüller W (1980) CT evaluation of the CSF spaces of healthy persons. Neuroradiology 19:131–136

Milhorat TH (1987) Acute hydrocephalus after aneurysmal subarachnoid hemorrhage. Neurosurgery 20:15–20

Mohr G, Ferguson G, Khan M, Malloy D, Watts R, Benoit B, Weir B (1983) Intraventricular hemorrhage from ruptured aneurysm. J Neurosurg 58:482–487

Van Gijn J, Hijdra A, Wijdicks EFM, Vermeulen M, Van Crevel H (1985) Acute hydrocephalus after aneurysmal subarachnoid hemorrhage. J Neurosurg 63:355–362

Vassilouthis J, Richardson AE (1979) Ventricular dilatation and communicating hydrocephalus following spontaneous subarachnoid hemorrhage. J Neurosurg 51:341–351

Wenig C, Huber G, Emde H (1979) Hydrocephalus after subarachnoid bleeding. Eur Neurol 18:1–7

Resistance to Cerebrospinal Fluid Outflow Following Subarachnoid Haemorrhage

F. Gjerris[1], S.E. Børgesen[1], J.F. Schmidt[1], O. Fedders[1], A. Gjerris[2], and P. Soelberg-Sørensen[3]

University Clinics of Neurosurgery[1], Psychiatry[2] and Neurology[3], Rigshospitalet, DK-2100 Copenhagen (Denmark)

Subarachnoid haemorrhage (SAH) often causes an increase in intracranial pressure (ICP) either by inpairment of the cerebrospinal fluid (CSF) resorption or by brain oedema (Kosteljanetz 1984, Voldby 1985). Fifteen to 20% of the patients sufferin from SAH develop hydrocephalus (Vassilouthis 1984).

Only a few investigations of CSF-dynamics in the acute phase of SAH have been done. Gjerris et al. (1982) reported that resistance to CSF outflow (R_{out}) in actue hydrocephalus after SAH, determined by a perfusion test, was very high, and by bolus-injection Kosteljanetz (1984) found that R_{out} was linearly correlated to ICP. A similar linear relationship between ICP and R_{out} was found by Gjerris et al. (1982), who also showed that patients with high pressure hydrocephalus (HPH) often had a bad outcome. In normal pressure hydrocephalus (NPH) after SAH the prognosis is usually good after shunting (Børgesen and Gjerris 1982).

The purpose of the present study was to measure R_{out} in patients with SAH and with early or late developed hydrocephalus after SAH and to correlate R_{out} with the ICP variables and the clinical outcome.

Clinical Material and Methods

58 adult patients with verified spontaneous SAH were studied. In most of the patients SAH was caused by a saccular aneurysm, in the others by a vascular malformation or by an unknown cause, possibly arterial hypertension. 39 were females with a mean age 52 years (range 23–71), 19 were males with a mean age 39 years (range 29–72). The clinical grade was in the acute phase estimated after Hunt and Hess and in the hydrocephalic stage by functional grades according to Børgesen and Gjerris (1982).

All patients but two had serial computerized tomography (CT) for assessment of SAH. In all the size of the ventricular system was estimated by Evans ratio on CT before and after treatment of hydrocephalus.

ICP was monitored for at least 24 hours in all patients at the time of measurement of R_{out} via an intraventricular catheter. All pressure curves were evaluated for plateau waves and B-waves given in per cent of the monitored time. The steady-state ICP was estimated as the mean ICP of the monitored time.

R_{out} was measured by a lumbo-ventricular (Børgesen et al. 1978) or by a ventriculo-ventricular perfusion method (Gjerris et al. 1982). The CSF-formation

Eds.: J. T. Hoff and A. L. Betz

rate (V_{fr}) was assumed to be 0.4 ml per min. The absorbed CSF-volume per min (V_{abs}) could then the calculated from the following formula:

$$V_{abs} = V_{in} + V_{fr} - V_{out}$$

V_{abs} was then related to the different steady-state levels of ICP, and the regression coefficient expresses the resistance to CSF outflow; normal value is $<12.5 \text{ mm Hg} \times \text{ml}^{-1} \times \text{min}$ (Børgesen and Gjerris 1982, Ekstedt 1977). The statistics were computed on the SPSS/PC+ (SPSS inc. 444 N. Michigan Avenue, Chicago, Illinois, USA).

Results

All patients but one with *acute SAH* had increased intracranial pressure with plateau waves and B-waves in more than 10% of the monitored time.

After monitoring of ICP *in the hydrocephalic state* the patients could be divided into two groups: 21 with HPH and 37 with NPH. HPH patients had a mean ICP of 37.5 mm Hg, and a median R_{out} of 61 mm Hg $\times$ ml^{-1} $\times$ min (range 23–142). NPH-patients had a mean ICP of 7.7 mm Hg, the median R_{out} was 27 mm Hg $\times$ ml^{-1} $\times$ min (range 5–57), and nearly all had more than 10% B-waves. Four had normal values below 12.5 mm Hg; three were investigated 5–8 years after the SAH.

Of the 33 NPH-patients with high R_{out} 32 were shunted (Gjerris et al. 1989). Fig. 1 shows the relationship between R_{out} and mean ICP. A trend of the higher ICP the higher R_{out} is seen. Fig. 2 shows the relation between B-waves and R_{out}. An increasing number of B-waves is correlated to an increased R_{out}. R_{out} correlated to the size of the ventricular system (Evans ratio) showed a decreasing R_{out} value with increasing Evans ratio.

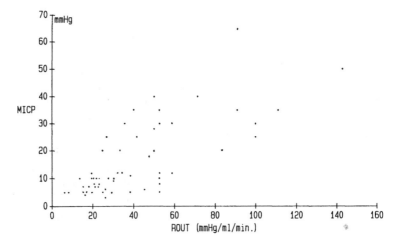

Fig. 1. Correlation between mean ICP and R_{out} in 58 patients with SAH or hydrocephalus after SAH ($n = 58$)

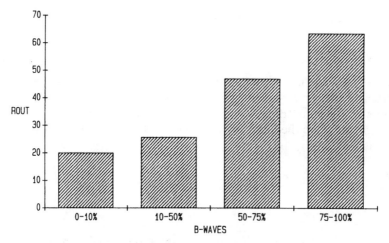

Fig. 2. Distribution of frequency of B-waves and R_{out} in 58 patients with SAH or hydrocephalus after SAH ($n = 58$)

All patients were followed at least one year after the episode of SAH or to their death. HPH-patients had a bad outcome and most of them died or were disabled. Of the NPH-patients all shunted patients improved, i.e. increased in the functional grade. All five non-shunted patients had an unchanged functional grading.

Discussion

The present study supports the contention that patients with SAH and hydrocephalus after SAH have a high R_{out}, and that patients with NPH after SAH can be treated successfully by shunt operation. It also confirms the findings of abnormal CSF-dynamics and increased ICP in SAH or hydrocephalus after SAH (Brock et al. 1975, Børgesen 1984, Kosteljanetz 1984, Hildebrandt et al. 1985; Voldby 1986). For the development of hydrocephalus an initial high intraventricular pressure is necessary (Hakum et al. 1976, Børgesen and Gjerris 1987). In patients with NPH no plateau waves were seen, but many patients had a high percentage of B-waves and a high R_{out}. Three patients investigated 5–8 years after SAH had a normal CSF-circulation.

Even up to 3 months after SAH we found xanthochromic CSF and a very high R_{out}. These patients had a very good prognosis after shunting. This suggests, that the decreased CSF-circulation is not only caused by subarachnoid adherences and inflammation secondary to the SAH (Ishii et al. 1979; Fuhrmeister et al. 1980), but that increased viscosity of the CSF also may be an important pathogenetic factor. An increased viscosity of CSF in the acute state of SAH is explained by the red cells and proteins in CSF. Studies have shown that increased viscosity of CSF causes increased R_{out}, both experimentally (Brock et al. 1975;

738

Blasberg et al. 1981) or in patients with protein producing spinal tumours and meningeal carcinomatosis (Hansen et al. 1987).

In conclusion patients with SAH or with hydrocephalus after SAH have an increased resistance to CSF-outflow. The patients with plateau waves or high R_{out} should be shunted preferably within the first 3 months after SAH.

Summary

R_{out} and ICP were measured in 58 patients suffering from SAH or hydrocephalus after SAH. Twenty-one had increased ICP (mean 37.5 mm Hg) and 37 had normal ICP below 15 mm Hg. The mean R_{out} in the patients with high ICP was 61 mm Hg $\times$ ml^{-1} $\times$ min (range 23–142). Mean R_{out} for patients with normal ICP was 27 mm Hg $\times$ ml^{-1} $\times$ min (range 5–57). Patients with acute SAH have a very high R_{out} and should be observed and treated for clinically significant HPH or NPH. Patients with a long interval from SAH to hydrocephalus often have normal ICP, normal CSF-dynamics and need no shunting.

Acknowledgements. The study has received financial support from the Research Foundation of Lundbeck, Eskofot A/S and DANICA, Medical Division, Denmark.

References

Blasberg R, Johnson D, Fenstermacher J (1981) Absorption resistance of cerebrospinal fluid after subarachnoid hemorrhage in the monkey; effect of heparin. Neurosurgery 9:686–691

Brock M, Furuse M, Hasuo M, Dietz H (1975) Influence of CSF-resorption pathways on intracranial capacitance. Adv Neurosurg 3:109–113

Børgesen SE (1984) Conductance to outflow of CSF in normal pressure hydrocephalus. Acta Neurochir (Wien) 71:1–41

Børgesen SE, Gjerris F (1982) The predictive value of conductance to outflow of CSF in normal pressure hydrocephalus. Brain 105:65–86

Børgesen SE, Gjerris F (1987) The relationships between intracranial pressure, ventricular size and resistance to CSF outflow. J Neurosurg (in press)

Børgesen SE, Gjerris F, Sørensen SC (1978) The resistance to cerebrospinal fluid absorption in humans. Acta Neurol Scand 56:88–96

Ekstedt J (1977) CSF hydrodynamic studies in man. I. Method of constant pressure CSF infusion. J Neurol Neurosurg Psychiatry 40:105–119

Fuhrmeister U, Ruether P, Dommasch D, Gaab M (1980) Alterations of CSF hydrodynamics following meningitis and SAH. In: Shulman K et al. (eds) Intracranial pressure IV. Springer, Berlin Heidelberg New York, pp 241–244

Gjerris F, Børgesen SE, Hoppe E, Boesen F, Nordenbo AM (1982) The conductance to outflow of CSF in adults with high-pressure hydrocephalus. Acta Neurochir (Wien) 64:59–67

Gjerris F, Børgesen SE, Schmidt J, Sørensen PS (1989) Resistance to outflow of cerebrospinal fluid in normal pressure hydrocephalus. In: Gjerris F et al. (eds) Outflow of the cerebrospinal fluid. Copenhagen, Munksgaard (in press)

Hakim S, Venegas JG, Burton JD (1976) The physics of the cranial cavity, hydrocephalus and normal pressure hydrocephalus: Mechanical interpretation and mathematical model. Surg Neurol 5:187–210

Hansen K, Gjerris F, Sørensen PS (1987) Absence of hydrocephalus in spite of impaired cerebrospinal fluid absorption and severe intracranial hypertension. Acta Neurochir (Wien) 86:93–97

Hildebrandt G, Werner M, Kaps M, Busse O (1985) Acute non-communicating hydrocephalus after spontaneous subarachnoid haemorrhage. Acta Neurochir (Wien) 76:58–61

Ishii M, Suzuki S, Julow J (1979) Subarachnoid haemorrhage and communication hydrocephalus. Scanning electron microscopic observations. Acta Neurochir (Wien) 50:265–272

Kosteljanetz M (1984) CSF dynamics in patients with subarachnoid and/or intraventricular hemorrhage. J Neurosurg 60:940–946

Vassilouthis J (1984) The syndrome of normal-pressure hydrocephalus. J Neurosurg 61:501–509

Voldby B (1986) Ruptured intracranial aneurysm. A clinical and pathophysiological study. Dan Med Bull 33:53–64

External Ventricular Drainage in the Management of Hypertensive Intracerebral Hemorrhage with Rupture Into the Ventricles

A. Taheri and M. Brock

Department of Neurosurgery, Steglitz Medical Center, Free University of Berlin, Hindenburgdamm 30, 1000 Berlin 45 (FRG)

Summary

The mortality of hypertensive intracerebral hemorrhage (HICH) with rupture into the ventricles (VR) is said to range between 60 and 85%. We report on 33 consecutive cases treated by external ventricular drainage (EVD). Only 12 patients (36.5%) died, and 12 of the survivors had no or only minor neurological deficit. The extension of intraventricular hemorrhage correlated with neurological deficit on admission in 29 (87%) and with outcome in 26 (78%) of the patients. A modification of the existing system of grading of the severity of intraventricular hemorrhages (IVH) in the posterior fossa is suggested. The pathophysiology is discussed on the basis of a review of the literature.

Key Words. Intracerebral Hemorrhage, Intraventricular Hemorrhage, Increased Intracranial Pressure, External Ventricular Drainage.

Hypertension is the main etiology of intraventricular bleeding (Little et al. 1977). The mortality of HICH with VR is reported to be about 60–85% (Graeb et al. 1982, Little et al. 1977, Sganzerla et al. 1984). Loew et al. (1980) and Miyagami et al. (1981) reported a few cases treated with EVD with a clearly higher survival rate, but the number of cases was too small to draw any definite conclusions. Sganzerla et al., on the other hand, did not observe any positive effect of EVD on the mortality of IVH (1984). In order to reevaluate the significance of the amount of blood in the ventricles for prognosis and to answer the question as to whether EVD has an influence on mortality and morbidity of HICH with VR, we carried out a retrospective study of 33 consecutive unselected patients.

Material and Methods

All patients had a history of hypertension or a diastolic BP above 100 mm Hg. Neurological findings were graded according to Hunt and Hess. The amount of blood in the ventricles was evaluated according to the criteria given in Table 1. Morbidity was assessed using the Glasgow Outcome Scale (Table 2). ICP was monitored continuously, and EVD was continued as long as CSF was bloody and whenever closure of the drainage caused a pathological increase in ICP.

Table 1. Scoring of severity of IVH[a] according to Graeb et al.

Lateral ventricles

    Score: 1 = trace of blood or mild bleeding
           2 = less than half of the ventricle filled with blood
           3 = more than half of the ventricle filled with blood
           4 = ventricle filled with blood and expanded

    (Each lateral ventricle is scored separately)

Third and fourth ventricles

    Score: 1 = blood present, ventricle size normal
           2 = ventricle filled with blood and expanded
    Total Score (maximum = 12)

Grading of IVH according to Ruscalleda et al.

    Score 1–3 = Grade I   = mild
    Score 4–6 = Grade II = moderate
    Score 7–9 = Grade III = severe
    Score 10–12 = Grade IV = very severe

Our modification for posterior fossa hemorrhage

    Score 1   = Grade 1 = mild
    Score 2   = Grade 2 = moderate
    Score 3–6 = Grade 3 = severe
    Score 7–12 = Grade 4 = very severe

[a] IVH: intraventricular hemorrhage.

Table 2. Relation of extention of ventricular occupation with blood to the neurological deficit on admission and to the outcome in 33 patients

Extention of ventricular occupation with blood, see Table 1		I	II	III	IV
Total no. of patients		1	14	12	6
Neurological deficit on admission, graded according to Hunt and Hess	I	0	0	0	0
	II	1	3	0	0
	III	0	8	[1]	0
	IV	0	[2]	8	3
	V	0	[1]	3	3
Morbidity and mortality, graded according to Glasgow Outcome Scale[a]	I	1	8	3	0
	II	0	2	[1]	[1]
	III	0	2	[2]	0
	IV	0	0	1	0
	V	0	[2]	5	5

[a] Glasgow Outcome Scale according to Jenett et al.
Grade I = normal or mild disability
Grade II = moderate disability
Grade III = major disability
Grade IV = vegetative state
Grade V = dead
□ Patients with uncorrelating features.

Results

The patients' mean age was 63 years (range: 37 to 81 y). Men predominated (63.6%). 16 hemorrhages (49%) occurred in the capsulolenticulostriate area and 6 (18%) in the posterior fossa. The positive relation between the amount of blood in the ventricles and the neurological deficit on admission in 29 (87%) and outcome in 26 (78%) patients is demonstrated in Table 2.

With the drainage system open, ICP was usually less than 15 Torr. 7 of the deceased patients but none of the survivors had a mean ICP of 15 Torr or more during the period preceding death. B-waves and Ramp-waves were observed in 19 cases, but an increase in their frequency, indicating the development of malresorptive hydrocephalus, was observed in only 3 cases.

Discussion

We had to modify the existing system of grading the severity of ventricular bleeding since our experience showed that the mere filling and expanding of the fourth and third ventricles with blood in posterior fossa hemorrhage has to be considered a severe hemorrhage (Table 1).

Primary damage of affected brain tissue in HICH was proved to be no longer reversible within a few hours after onset (Suzuki et al. 1980). Continuous pressure-regulated EVD appears to counteract the decrease in regional and global CBF, which depends upon both volume and speed of bleeding (Miyagami et al. 1981), and contributes towards restricting the extension of ischemic and compressive secondary lesions, thus providing better premises for the functional recovery of perilesional tissue.

Evacuation of intraventricular and central intracerebral hematoma did not reduce the total mortality of HICH with VR below 60% (Pia 1968). In conformity with this observation, an intracerebral hematoma was evacuated in only 1 patient.

The favorable outcome of our survivors (see Table 2) and the low mortality rate of 37.5% illustrates the positive influence of EVD on morbidity and mortality of HICH with VR.

References

Graeb DA, Robertson WD, La Pointe JS, Nugent RA, Harrison PhD (1982) Computed tomographic diagnosis of intraventricular hemorrhages. Etiology and prognosis. Neuroradiology 143:91–96
Jenett B, Bond H (1975) Assessment of outcome after severe brain damage. Lancet I:480–484
Little JR, Blomquist GA, Ethier R (1977) Intraventricular hemorrhage in adults. Surg Neurol 8:143–149
Loew F, Jaksche H (1980) Surgical treatment of intraventricular hemorrhage. In: Pia HW, Langmaid C, Zierski J (eds) Spontaneous intracerebral hematomas. Springer, Berlin Heidelberg New York, pp 326–329
Miyagami M, Murakami J, Wakamatsu K, Kondo T, Takeuchi T, Tsubokawa T, Mariyasu N

(1981) Experimental and clinical studies on prognosis-deteriorating factors in the acute stage of intraventricular hemorrhage. Neurol Med Chir (Tokyo) 21:73–75

Pia HW (1968) The prognosis and treatment of intraventricular hemorrhages. Prog Brain Res 30:463–470

Ruscalleda J, Peivo A (1986) Prognosis in parenchymatous hematoma with ventricular hemorrhage. Neuroradiology 28:34–37

Sganzerla EP, Rampini PM, Gaini SM, Granat G, Tomei G, Zavanone M, Villani RM (1984) Intraventricular hemorrhage: Role of early ventricular drainage. J Neurosurg Sci 28:61–65

Suzuki J, Ebina T (1980) Sequential changes in tissue surrounding ICH. In: Pia HW, Langmaid C, Zierski J (eds) Spontaneous intracerebral hematomas. Springer, Berlin Heidelberg New York, pp 121–128

Effects of Glycerol Infusion on Cerebral Blood Flow in Hypertensive Intracerebral Hematoma with Ventricular Hemorrhage

T. Yamada, T. Shima, S. Matsumura, Y. Okada, M. Nishida, K. Yamane, and S. Okita

Department of Neurosurgery, Chugoku Rousal Hospital, 1-5-1, Hiro-tagaya, Kure, Hiroshima, 737-01 (Japan)

Introduction

Glycerol has been known to be a cerebral dehydrating agent altering the dynamics of cerebrospinal fluid (CSF) (Guisado et al. 1976). The effect of glycerol on cerebral blood flow (CBF) has been studied mainly in cerebral infarction. In hypertensive intracerebral hematoma few reports on CBF can be found (Sasaki et al. 1983). Therefore, we studied glycerol effects on CBF in hypertensive intracerebral hematoma. Additionally, the effects on CBF in the presence of ventricular hemorrhage also has been considered.

Material and Method

We studied 13 cases, nine with putaminal hematomas and four with thalamic hematomas. Ventricular hemorrhage was found in six of the cases (three putaminal and three thalamic hematoma). The size of the hematoma ranged from 7 to 46 ml on CT scan. Five hundred ml of a 10% glycerol was infused intravenously for 60 min within four days of the hemorrhage. CBF was measured before and after glycerol infusion by single photon ECT with Xe-133 inhalation to obtain a CBF map 5 cm above the OM-line. Mean CBF was calculated in the affected and non-affected hemisphere. Epidural pressure was concomitantly recorded as intracranial pressure (ICP) during glycerol infusion in two of our cases, while measuring systemic arterial pressure (SAP).

Results

Reproducibility of the CBF measurements was considered to evaluate quantitative CBF changes. The ratio of mean CBF in the hemispheres between two measurements in the same person was 0.98 ± 0.05 (mean $\pm$ SD). We determined mean CBF change of more than 2 SD (10%) by glycerol infusion to be significant.

Table 1. Summary of the presented cases

No.	Age	Sex	Location of hematoma	Size of hematoma (ml)	CBF Before Aff	CBF Before Non	CBF After Aff	CBF After Non	Patterns of CBF increase
					(ml/100 g/min)				
Cases with ventricular hemorrhage									
1	66	F	Putamen	34	23	31	34*	38*	Homogeneous
2	48	M	Putamen	46	26	34	31*	37	Homogeneous
3	54	M	Putamen	35	17	21	26*	33*	Homogeneous
4	63	M	Thalamus	10	23	26	29*	28	Heterogeneous
5	53	M	Thalamus	27	21	22	29*	32*	Homogeneous
6	74	F	Thalamus	7	21	26	30*	35*	Heterogeneous
Cases without ventricular hemorrhage									
7	52	F	Putamen	10	33	36	41*	41*	Homogeneous
8	54	F	Putamen	20	28	34	32*	39*	Homogeneous
9	60	M	Putamen	40	17	22	18	21	Homogeneous
10	68	M	Putamen	10	31	34	30	31	Homogeneous
11	52	M	Putamen	25	23	31	23	29	Homogeneous
12	63	F	Putamen	24	31	32	32	39*	Homogeneous
13	65	F	Thalamus	9	38	39	38	38	Homogeneous

Aff: affected hemisphere; Non: non affected hemisphere; *: significant increase in CBF.

Mean CBF of the affected hemisphere increased significantly in all cases with ventricular hemorrhage (Table 1). In seven cases without ventricular hemorrhage, two showed a significant increase in mean CBF and five revealed no change. The size of the hematoma (26 ± 15 ml) in cases with ventricular hemorrhage was not significantly larger (20 ± 11 ml) without it.

CBF maps showed two patterns of CBF increase in cases with a significant increase in mean CBF. The first pattern was a homogeneous increase (seven cases). The second pattern was a heterogeneous increase (two cases). In the second pattern, CBF increased in the area around the hematoma and in the cerebral cortex close to hematoma. CBF was unchanged in the cerebral cortex distant from the hematoma.

In two cases in which ICP and SAP were recorded during the CBF study, mean CBF increased in both hemispheres with ICP reduction. Additionally, the mean CBF increase was proportional to a rise in perfusion pressure (SAP-ICP).

Discussion

The present study shows that mean CBF increased in nine cases and did not increase in the remaining four. In cases with ICP recording, CBF increased in proportion to a rise in perfusion pressure, indicating disturbed autoregulation. A previous study also showed that CBF increases in some cases with hypertensive intracerebral hematoma, but is unchanged in the others (Sasaki et al. 1983). Disturbed autoregulation was found in earlier cases with hypertensive intracerebral hematoma (Fieschi et al. 1968). From Fieschi et al. (1968) data, autoregulation should be disturbed in some cases with hypertensive intracerebral hematoma, in which case glycerol should increase CBF because of a rise in perfusion pressure. Additionally, a heterogeneous increase in a CBF map might indicate that autoregulation was heterogeneously disturbed in the hemisphere.

The present study shows that mean CBF increased more frequently in cases with ventricular hemorrhage. A previous study showed that CSF clearance is increased by glycerol to reduce ICP and edema (Guisado et al. 1976). From our current data, ventricular hemorrhage seriously disturbs cerebral circulation with edema and elevated ICP due to reduced CSF clearance, which is improved by glycerol infusion.

References

Fieschi C, Agnoli A, Battistini N et al. (1968) Derangement of regional cerebral blood flow and of its regulatory mechanisms in acute cerebrovascular lesions. Neurology 18:1166–1179
Guisado R, Arieff AL, Massry SG (1976) Effects of glycerol administration on experimental brain edema. Neurology 26:67–75
Sasaki T, Matsuzaki T, Nakagawara J et al. (1983) Improvement of CBF by glycerol administration in hypertensive intracerebral hemorrhage. Brain Nerve 35:505–510

Pressure Waves and Brain Stem Microcirculatory Disturbance Following Experimental Subarachnoid Hemorrhage

M. Hashimoto, S. Higashi, Y. Kogure, H. Fujii, T. Yamashima, K. Tokuda, H. Ito, and S. Yamamoto

Department of Neurosurgery, School of Medicine, University of Kanazawa, Takaramachi 13-1, Kanazawa City 920 (Japan)

Introduction

In a study of the intraventricular fluid pressure of patients with intracranial hypertension, Lundberg (1960) was able to distinguish three main forms of pressure waves. These waves that were seen generally in the process of secondary intracranial hypertension may be regarded as a pathophysiological basis of acute disorders of brain stem in patients with increased intracranial pressure (ICP). We have developed an experimental subarachnoid hemorrhage (SAH) model in which the pressure waves resemble those seen in clinical patients. The present study was performed to examine the relationship between acute intracranial hypertension and the topography of impaired microvascular perfusion of brain stem with special attention to the pathogenesis of pressure waves.

Materials and Methods

Twenty-four adult mongrel dogs, each weighting 8–12 kg, were anesthetized with intravenous thiopental sodium (10 mg/kg), intubated endotracheally, and immobilized with panchuronium bromide (1 mg/hour). The animal's head was fixed into a stereotaxic frame in the sphinx position. ICP was monitored using an epidural pressure transducer (Koningsberg P-3.5) placed in the parietal epidural space. To monitor systemic blood pressure (SBP) a catheter was introduced into the abdominal aorta via the femoral artery. Cerebral perfusion pressure (CPP) was expressed as the difference between SBP and ICP. A 21 gage needle was inserted into the chiasmatic cistern via the optic canal. Experimental SAH was induced by hand injection of hemolysed red blood cells (RBCs; 0.15–0.25 ml/kg) in twenty dogs.

In various stages of increased ICP, carbon black (CB; Kaimei, 200 ml) was injected with a pressure of mean SBP from the left vertebral artery. The brain was embedded in celloidin and the microvascular perfusion was examined serially from anterior commissure to medulla with sections of 100 μ thick.

Eds.: J. T. Hoff and A. L. Betz

Results

Intracranial hypertension and pressure waves after SAH. Secondary intracranial hypertension following intracisternal infusion of hemolized RBCs was observed over 3 to 15 hours with the occurrence of pressure waves (Fig. 1). In 17 of 20 animals, pressure waves were observed in a basal ICP range from 15 to 70 mm Hg. The pressure waves were classified into three types according to the wave form and the pattern of changes in SBP. First, plateau waves (10 dogs), ranged from 3 to 10 minutes in duration. These were accompanied by a simultaneous decrease in SBP (Fig. 2A). Second, pre-plateau waves (13 dogs), ranged from 30 seconds to 3 minutes in duration, accompanied by either some simultaneous decrease or by no changes in SBP (Fig. 2 A, B). Third, B-like waves (6 dogs), ranged from 10 to 30 seconds in duration. They were accompanied by a marked simultaneous rise in SBP (Fig. 2C). Pre-plateau waves often developed to plateau waves. Rhythmic sequence of B-like waves were seen for a while over 60 mm Hg of ICP in which pre-plateau and plateau waves had already disappeared.

Microcirculatory disturbance of brain stem in various ICP stages. In 4 control dogs, the brain stem was perfused fully with CB. In 4 dogs of group II (ICP; 15–40 mm Hg), in which pressure waves appeared and then showed rhythmic sequence, fine and coarse capillary networks were observed in the rostral hypothalamus. In 10 dogs of group III (ICP; 40–70 mm Hg), in which basal ICP increased progressively with the sequence of many pressure waves, macro-

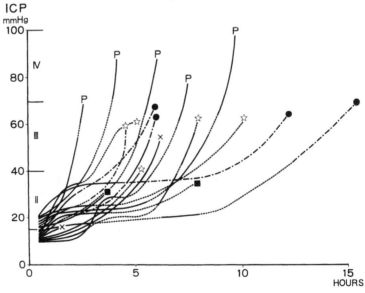

Fig. 1. Experimental time course of secondary increase in ICP and pressure wave types from the time of subarachnoid infusion of hemolysed RBCs to CB perfusion. The following symbols represent: ———×, no pressure waves; - - - - ■, pre-plateau waves; - - - - ☆, pre-plateau and plateau waves; —·—·—●, B-like waves; *P*, vasoparalysis respectively

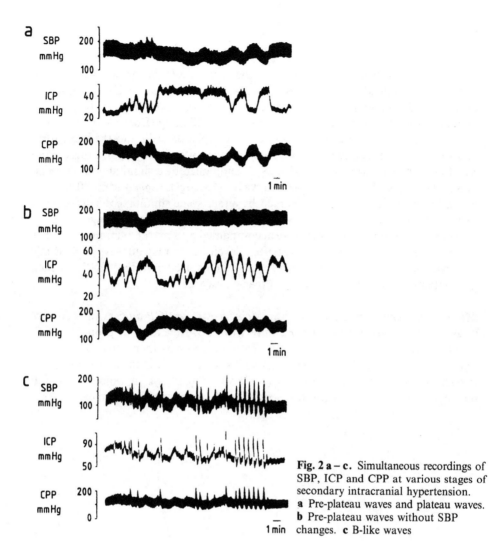

Fig. 2 a – c. Simultaneous recordings of SBP, ICP and CPP at various stages of secondary intracranial hypertension. **a** Pre-plateau waves and plateau waves. **b** Pre-plateau waves without SBP changes. **c** B-like waves

scopically scattered non-perfusion areas were found in the thalamus, rostral hypothalamus, periaqueductal gray, and tegmentum of the midbrain and upper pons (Fig. 3). In 4 dogs of group IV (70–100 mm Hg) these non perfusion areas extended downward to the pons and medulla along the floor of the IV ventricle and tegmentum. Two typical lesions were observed in the 7 dogs with pressure waves of group II and III (Fig. 4). The first lesions were in the basal forebrain area and rostra 1 hypothalamus. The second were columunar lesions in the central thalamus, midbrain and floor of the IV ventricle of the upper pons.

Discussion

In patients, concerning ICP changes immediately after SAH, some cases show a slow increase in ICP over the course of the next few hours. These subsequent slow

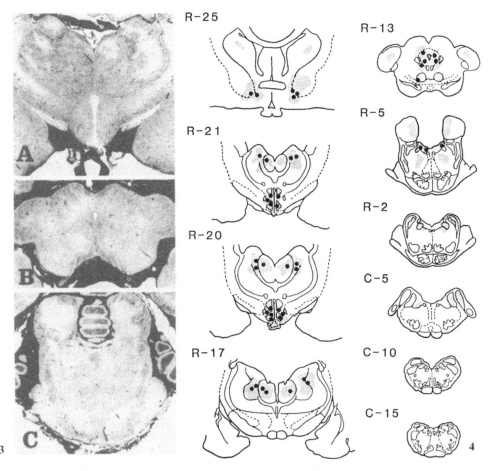

Fig. 3. Photomicrographs of coronal sections (100 μ thick). CB are perfused at the level of 60 mm Hg when rhythmic sequence of pressure waves are observed

Fig. 4. Topographic representation of microvascular impairments in brain stem. The following symbols represent: small dots shadow, microcirculatory disturbance of 7 dogs with pressure waves at the time of CB perfusion in group II and III; large dots, selectively vulnerable non perfusion areas in 3 dogs with pressure waves

elevations of ICP are thought to be dependent on cerebral ischemia and edema (Nornes et al. 1972). Likewise, secondary intracranial hypertension with pressure waves have been shown in our model. These facts suggest that the progressive rise in basal ICP in our study is due to the ischemic lesions.

Pressure waves have been possible to distinguish three main forms of variation (Lundberg 1960). Two are of a rhythmic nature and are related to periodic breathing of the Cheyne-Stokes respiration and Traube-Hering-Mayer waves of the SBP. The third type of pressure waves is called plateau waves. In this study, pressure waves were observed in group II and III dogs (ICP; 15–70 mm Hg). Pre-plateau waves often developed to plateau waves. Furthermore these two waves were associated with a decrease of CPP. These phenomena are thought to

751

be derived from active cerebral vasodilatation. B-like waves were accompanied by a marked simultaneous rise in SBP and were often observed for a while in later stages when pre-plateau and plateau waves disappeared. These facts suggest that the origin of B-like waves are different from the other two waves.

In our experiment, microcirculatory disturbance in the brain stem began to appear in group II dogs, and pressure waves were seen in group II and III dogs. Then vasomotor paralysis was observed in group IV dogs (ICP: over 70 mm Hg) and the pressure waves were never seen in these dogs. Langfitt et al. (1965) stated that the acute cerebral vasodilatation and the vasopressor mechanisms fail in terminal stage. These facts suggest that microcirculatory disturbance in the brain stem contributes to the occurrence of pressure waves.

Asano (1977) reported the symmetrical distribution of the no-reflow phenomenon in their SAH model, with a predeliction for locations in the thalamus, basal ganglia and arterial boundary zones. Crompton (1963) demonstrated numerous hypothalamic lesions in patients who had died after SAH. These lesions showed hemorrhagic or ischemic areas in the rostral hypothalamus. In our study, microcirculatory disturbances were observed predominantly in the basal forebrain, especially the rostral hypothalamus in group II and III. Those lesions extended to the mid brain and upper pons especially the periaqueductal gray and the floor of the IV ventricle with an increase in ICP. These facts suggest that pressure waves are induced by ischemia of the rostral hypothalamus and upper brain stem.

Hypothalamus and upper pons are considered as the upper center of vasomotor activity. Ueda et al. (1968) reported that electrical stimulations of the basal forebrain, especially the prechiasmatic area, induced hypotension with a decrease of sympathetic discharge. Langfitt et al. (1968) reported that stimulation of the upper pons and the floor of the IV ventricle produced both dilatation of the cerebral vessels and a rise of SBP. These facts suggest that microcirculatory disturbance in the rostral hypothalamus and upper pons plays an important role in the genesis of plateau and pre-plateau waves with a depressor response. In the present study, B-like waves were observed not only in group II and III, but also for a while over 60 mm Hg of ICP after disappearance of plateau and pre-plateau waves. Electrical vasopressor points are seen broadly in the brain stem. Therefore B-like waves may be governed by a wider region.

We conclude that microcirculatory disturbance in the brain stem, especially the rostral hypothalamus, periaqueductal gray and the floor of the IV ventricle, causes dysfunction of the vasomotor center in the brain stem which results in pressure waves.

References

Asano T, Sano K (1977) Pathogenetic role of no-reflow phenomenon in experimental subarachnoid hemorrhage in dogs. J Neurosurg 46:454–466

Crompton MR (1963) Hypothalamic lesions following the rupture of cerebral berry aneurysm. Brain 86:301–314

Nornes H, Maches B (1972) Intracranial pressure in patients with ruptured saccular aneurysm. J Neurosurg 36:537–547

Langfitt TW, Weinstein JD, Kassell NF (1965) Cerebral vasomotor paralysis produced by intracranial hypertension. Neurology 15:622–641

Langfitt TW, Kassel NF (1968) Cerebral vasodilation produced by brain stem stimulation: neurogenic control vs autoregulation. Am J Physiol 215:90–97

Lundberg N (1960) Continuous recording and control of ventricular fluid pressure in neurosurgical practice. Acta Psychiatr Scand [Suppl] 149:1–193

Ueda H, Katayama S (1968) Central nervous control of the blood pressure. Respir Circ 16:113–120

Raised Intracranial Pressure (RICP) and Cerebral Blood Flow (CBF): A Comparison of Xenon Clearance and Single Photon Emission Tomography (SPET)

M.S. Choksey, F. Iannotti, D. Campos Costa, P.J. Ell, and H.A. Crockard

Departments of Neurosurgery and Nuclear Medicine, Middlesex Hospital,
London W1N 8AA (UK)

The management of acute traumatic intracerebral hematomas is controversial. Some patients tolerate large clots with no deterioration, whereas others do not. There is a dilemma – whether to remove these clots, or undertake a trial period of conservative management. Given time, these clots either resolve or evolve into areas of low attenuation. However, many patients deteriorate – often days after injury. To date, our ability to predict this deterioration is limited.

We investigated the role of cerebral blood flow (CBF) measurement using Xenon-133 clearance, and Single Photon Emission Tomography (SPET) using Tc99m-Hexamethylene propylene amineoxime (Tc99m HM-PAO) as possible discriminators in the investigation of these patients.

Patients

Eight patients were studied. All were male, aged 14 to 75. They had all been admitted within 24 hr of sustaining their head injury. The Computerized Tomographic (CT) scans on admission showed intracerebral hematomas; 5 frontal, 1 temporal and 2 temporoparietal. 5 patients deteriorated neurologically, and required removal of their clots. None of the conservatively-managed group required any therapy other than fluid restriction for 72 hr.

All the patients survived. The two with temporo-parietal clots were left with a residual contralateral hemiparesis. The others made good recoveries.

Methods

All the patients were investigated within 48 hr of admission. The CT scans were all performed on a Siemens Somatom DR2 scanner, the CBF studies using a Novo Cerebrograph 10a system, and the SPET studies on a Starcam IGE400 computer system.

Analysis

The CT scan images were analyzed by measuring the largest mutually perpendicular diameters (Da, Db) on transverse slices, and multiplying these by the number of slices on which the hematoma was visible (N). The product (Da × Db × N) gave an indication of the relative size of the hematoma. These ranged from 18 to 120 (Fig. 1).

The Xenon clearance studies were expressed as both absolute values and as percentage ratios of the affected to the unaffected side.

The SPET data were analyzed on the STARCAM IGE400 system. We obtained transverse slices parallel to the orbito-meatal line. On each slice, we defined the perfusion defect as the area in which the activity in counts/pixel was less than 50% of the maximum on that slice. We summed the areas on all the slices in which the perfusion defect was visible, and obtained the percentage area that represented the clot (A%). The product of this and the number of slices was taken as an index of size (S).

$$\text{Severity} = \frac{\text{Percentage Area of Clot} \times \text{No. Slices}}{\text{Uptake Ratio (aff/non-aff)}}$$

We then calculated the ratio of the uptake on the affected and unaffected sides (R); dividing S by R gave us a figure which we have used as an index of severity of the perfusion defect. The most severe clots were seen as large perfusion defects associated with low uptake in the entire hemisphere.

Results

The CT scan appearances showed that the patients with larger clots were more likely to require surgery. However, there was some overlap of the two groups (Fig. 1).

There was no correlation between the Xenon CBF results and the likelihood of the patients needing surgery.

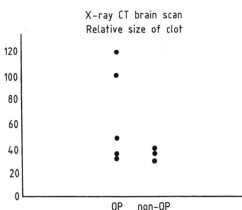

Fig. 1. The distribution of clot size in the two groups of patients, showing considerable overlap

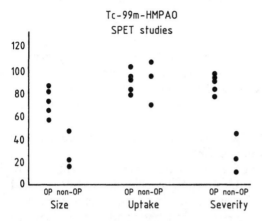

Fig. 2. The results of the SPET studies, showing marked differences between the two groups of patients

In contrast, the HMPAO studies fell into two distinct groups. Patients with large perfusion defects, particularly when associated with a marked hemisphere disturbance, were more likely to deteriorate. The index of severity in this group ranged from 76 to 93, whereas in those that did not deteriorate it ranged from 11 to 44 (Fig. 2).

Discussion

The management of intracranial hematomas is difficult. There is no means of predicting which patients will deteriorate, and therefore possibly benefit from more aggressive and anticipatory management. The CT scanner can be used to define the volume of intracranial hematomas very accurately, but this is of limited value as the volume of a clot is not the sole determinant of subsequent deterioration.

Likewise, we have found that the measurement of CBF is a poor guide to management, there being no significant difference between the two groups of patients.

Tc99m HMPAO is widely held to be a marker of regional perfusion in the brain (Ell et al. 1985; Holmes et al. 1985; Sharp et al. 1986). This gives rise to a possible explanation of our findings – that there are two separate phenomena being visualized here. The first is the perfusion defect associated with the clot itself, and the second is a concomitant lack of perfusion in the rest of the hemisphere. So, a large defect in uptake in the region of the clot, combined with diffuse low uptake in the whole hemisphere, may indicate a widespread disturbance in the brain, with a greater likelihood of subsequent swelling and deterioration.

In a series of this size we can not state definitely that the two phenomena are truly independent variables – it is possible that the size of defect and the hemisphere disturbance are both manifestations of the original traumatic insult. Alternatively, it may be that the presence of a clot provokes a widespread hemisphere disturbance. In this context, it is worth noting that one of our patients had a sizeable perfusion defect (44 units) but had unimpaired uptake in the rest of the hemisphere, suggesting that the two do occur separately. This patient did not require surgery.

Conclusion

We believe that SPET images of the uptake of Tc99m-HMPAO are complementary to conventional CT scan images, and may be useful in predicting late deterioration in patients with raised intracranial pressure due to intracerebral hematomas.

References

Ell PJ, Hocknell JML, Jarritt PH, Cullum I, Lui D, Costa DC, Nowotnik DP, Pickett RD, Canning LR, Neirinckx RD (1985) A ^{99m}Tc labelled radiotracer for the investigation of cerebrovascular disease. Nucl Med Commun 6:437–441

Holmes RA, Chaplin SB, Royston KG, Hoffman TJ, Volkert WA, Nowotnik DP, Canning LR, Cumming SA, Harrison RC, Higley B, Nechvatal G, Picket RD, Piper IM, Neirinckx RD (1985) Cerebral uptake and retention of ^{99m}Tc hexamethyleneamine (^{99m}Tc HM-PAO). Nucl Med Commun 6:443–447

Sharp PF, Smith RW, Gemmell HG, Lyall D, Evans NTS, Gvozdanovic D, Davidson J, Tyrell DA, Pickett RD, Neirinckx RD (1986) Technetium ^{99m}Tc HM-PAO stereoisomers as potential agents for imaging regional cerebral blood flow: human volunteer studies. J Nucl Med 27:171–177

Cerebral Energy Metabolism During Post-Traumatic Hypoventilation *

A.W. Unterberg [1], B.J. Andersen [2], G.D. Clarke [2], and A. Marmarou [2]

[1] Department of Neurosurgery, University of Munich, 8000 Munich 70 (FRG)
[2] Division of Neurosurgery and Department of Radiology, Medical College of Virginia, Richmond, Virginia (USA)

Introduction

There is evidence to suggest that severe head injury can cause disturbances of cerebral energy metabolism which can result in tissue acidosis and decreased energy production [2]. One objective of this study was to determine if fluid percussion brain injury affects cerebral energy metabolism. Additionally, since post-traumatic respiratory distress is a major complicating factor in head injury [5], another goal was to analyze the effect of hypoventilation immediately following trauma on cerebral energy metabolism.

Methods

Cats (2.5–3.5 kg) anesthetized with chloralose and ventilated under controlled conditions were used for the study. A first group ($n=8$) was subjected to a 3.2 atm. fluid percussion injury to the brain while being normoventilated [7]. A second group ($n=6$) was hypoventilated to a pO_2 of 35–40 mm Hg for 30 minutes, then normoventilated again. This group did not receive a fluid percussion injury. A third group ($n=11$) was subjected to fluid percussion brain injury immediately followed by 30 min of hypoventilation.

Before and after trauma (30 min, 1, 2, 4 and 8 hours) cerebral blood flow (CBF) was measured by injection of radioactive microspheres into the left atrium [3]. In addition, oxygen- and glucose-consumption ($CMRO_2$, CMR_{Gl}) were determined. Continuous acquisition of 31-P-MR-spectra enabled to non-invasively monitor tissue-pH, as well as the phosphocreatine/inorganic phosphate-ratio [6]. Detailed information is given elsewhere [1, 8].

Results and Discussion

Some pertinent parameters of cerebral energy metabolism of the experimental groups is given in Table 1.

---

* This work was supported by NIH-Grant Nos. 5R01NS 19235-03 and 2R01NS 12587-12 as well as by Deutsche Forschungsgemeinschaft: Un 56-1/1.

Table 1. Parameters of cerebral energy metabolism[a]

	Control	30 min postinsult	60 min postinsult
Trauma			
CBF	34.80 ± 3.80	33.60 ± 4.40	27.50 ± 4.60
$CMRO_2$	1.09 ± 0.19	0.91 ± 0.13	0.90 ± 0.17
CMR_{GI}	0.30 ± 0.06	0.32 ± 0.07	0.31 ± 0.03
pH	7.03 ± 0.02	$6.89 \pm 0.05*$	$6.97 \pm 0.03*$
PCr: Pi	1.52 ± 0.28	1.39 ± 0.44	1.30 ± 0.29
Hypoventilation			
CBF	27.90 ± 2.80	$189.40 \pm 35.0*$	27.80 ± 2.30
$CMRO_2$	1.02 ± 0.07	$1.49 \pm 0.18*$	1.01 ± 0.16
CMR_{GI}	0.26 ± 0.03	0.24 ± 0.01	0.37 ± 0.07
pH	7.04 ± 0.02	$6.97 \pm 0.02*$	7.02 ± 0.05
PCr: Pi	1.67 ± 0.23	1.30 ± 0.23	1.86 ± 0.45
Trauma + Hypoventilation			
CBF	27.00 ± 1.70	$74.60 \pm 12.9*$	31.00 ± 3.10
$CMRO_2$	1.09 ± 0.13	1.00 ± 0.19	1.03 ± 0.17
CMR_{GI}	0.31 ± 0.03	$1.03 \pm 0.17*$	0.35 ± 0.07
pH	7.06 ± 0.03	$6.64 \pm 0.03*$	$6.95 \pm 0.08*$
PCr: Pi	1.79 ± 0.12	$0.90 \pm 0.23*$	1.81 ± 0.42

[a] CBF = cerebral blood flow (ml/100 g min);
$CMRO_2$ and CMR_{GI} = oxygen and glucose consumption, respectively (µmoles/g min)
PCr: Pi = phosphocreatine: inorganic phosphate ratio.
* Significant difference ($p < 0.01$, or less) when compared with control values

Data taken from [1] and [8].

With *normoventilation after trauma* only tissue-pH was transiently decreased from 7.04 to 6.89 (30 min postinsult). Cerebral blood flow, oxygen- and glucose-consumption, as well as the phosphocreatine/inorganic phosphate-ratio (PCr/Pi) were not significantly altered. At 60 min postinsult tissue-pH had nearly returned to control values.

Hypoventilation without percussion injury revealed a six-fold increase of CBF associated with a moderate rise of oxygen consumption and a slight decrease in tissue-pH. Glucose-consumption and the PCr/Pi-ratio were not affected. After returning to normoventilation all parameters were within normal ranges within 30 min.

On the other hand, in animals with *combined trauma-hypoventilation,* only a moderate rise of CBF was observed during the period of hypoventilation, while tissue glucose-consumption was markedly enhanced and oxygen-consumption slightly decreased indicating that the CBF rise was inadequate to meet tissue demand. This is reflected by a pronounced drop of tissue-pH to 6.64 after trauma during hypoventilation and a significant decrease of the PCr/Pi-ratio. Again, after returning to normoventilation, all parameters showed a nearly complete recovery within 60 min.

The study demonstrates that fluid percussion brain injury produces only moderate metabolic disturbances, if the animals are normally ventilated. This is in conflict with other investigations [4, 9] reporting that fluid percussion injury in rats is accompanied with a significant decrease in phosphocreatine. However, those studies were performed in unventilated rats, and it might be assumed that a respiratory distress following trauma is responsible for the alterations in tissue high energy phosphates.

When mechanical brain injury is followed by hypoventilation, relative cerebral ischemia is produced, and the brain is rendered unable to produce sufficient energy to meet demand. This is a pronounced metabolic derangement and more accurately mimics the metabolic aberrations that may occur in clinical head injury.

Though, there is complete metabolic recovery after returning to normoventilation, the insufficient energy supply and the metabolic disturbances during the acute secondary insult could be of great significance for morbidity and mortality after severe head injury.

Acknowledgements. The technical assistance of Dr. H. Gruemer, Dr. K. Kraft, Nancy Nieling, Kimberly Battista, H. Rittner and Lisa Nugent is highly appreciated.

References

1. Andersen BJ, Unterberg AW, Clarke GD et al. (1988) Effect of posttraumatic hypoventilation on cerebral energy metabolism. J Neurosurg 68:601–607
2. DeSalles AAF, Kontos HA, Becker DP et al. (1986) Prognostic significance of ventricular CSF lactic acidosis in severe head injury. J Neurosurg 65:615–624
3. DeWitt DS, Jenkins LW, Wei EP et al. (1986) Effects of fluid-percussion brain injury on regional cerebral blood flow and pial arteriolar diameter. J Neurosurg 64:787–794
4. Ishige N, Pitts LH, Pogliani L et al. (1987) Effects of hypoxia on traumatic brain injury in rats: Part 2. Changes in high energy phosphate metabolism. Neurosurgery 20:854–858
5. Miller JD, Sweet RC, Narajan R et al. (1978) Early insults to the injured brain. JAMA 240:439–442
6. Petroff OAC, Prichard JW, Behar KL et al. (1985) Cerebral intracellular pH by ^{31}P nuclear magnetic resonance spectroscopy. Neurology 35:781–788
7. Sullivan HG, Martinez J, Becker DP et al. (1976) Fluid-percussion model of mechanical brain injury in the cat. J Neurosurg 45:520–534
8. Unterberg AW, Andersen BJ, Clarek GD et al. (1988) Cerebral energy metabolism following fluid-percussion brain injury in cats. J Neurosurg 68:594–600
9. Vink R, McIntosh TK, Weiner MW et al. (1987) Effects of traumatic brain injury on cerebral high energy phosphates and pH: A ^{31}P MRS study. J Cereb Blood Flow Metab 7:563–571

Effects On Intracranial Pressure In a Clinically Derived Fluid Resuscitation Protocol Following Hemorrhagic Shock with an Accompanying Intracranial Mass

J.M. Whitley, D.S. Prough, D.D. Deal, A.K. Lamb, D.S. DeWitt

Department of Anesthesia, Section on Critical Care, Wake Forest University Medical Center, Winston-Salem, North Carolina (USA)

Introduction

We have previously shown, in a hemorrhagic shock – intracranial mass model, that isotonic crystalloid results in a greater and more rapid increase in ICP immediately following resuscitation than hypertonic crystalloid, colloid or a combination of crystalloid and colloid (Whitley 1988). This rapid increase in ICP may exacerbate the neurological sequelae of the shock episode by decreasing CBF following resuscitation. While the effects of resuscitation on ICP have been extensively studied, they have dealt only with the effects of a single resuscitation fluid bolus, unlike the clinical protocol where systemic hemodynamics are maintained. The present study compared the cerebrovascular effects of resuscitation with isotonic and hypertonic crystalloid, each with and without colloid (10% Pentastarch), while maintaining cardiac output above baseline levels in a hemorrhagic shock – intracranial mass model.

Methods

Twenty-four dogs were anesthetized with thiopental, intubated, and ventilated. Cardiac output (CO) was recorded using a Noninvasive Continuous Cardiac Output Monitor (NCCOM-3). Cerebral blood flow (CBF) was measured using the cerebral venous outflow technique (Rapela and Green 1964). A 18G catheter inserted into the cisterna magna provided continuous intracranial pressure (ICP) monitoring. ICP was increased to 15 mm Hg before shock, by inflation of a subdural balloon overlying the left cortex, and maintained throughout the 30 minute shock period (MAP = 50 mm Hg, CPP = 35 mm Hg). Animals received one of four fluid groups for resuscitation: Group I: isotonic saline (40 ml/kg); Group II hypertonic saline (20 ml/kg, 250 mEq/L Na^+); Group IP: isotonic saline (20 ml/kg) with 10% Pentastarch; Group IIP: hypertonic saline (20 ml/kg) with 10% Pentastarch. Additional fluid was infused as needed to maintain CO at or above baseline. Data were compared at: baseline (BL), elevation of ICP to 15 mm Hg (BI), early (T0) and late shock (T30), following fluid resuscitation (T35), and at 30 minute intervals for two hours.

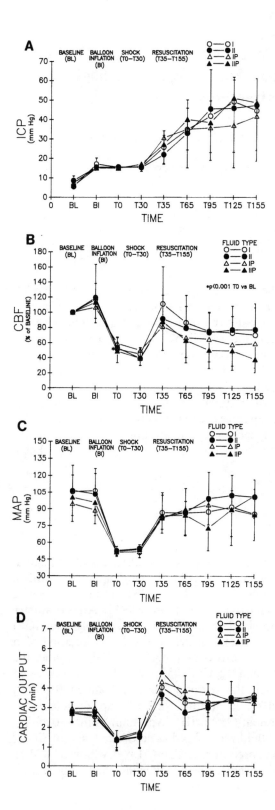

Fig. 1 A–D. Cerebrovascular and systemic hemodynamics following resuscitation from hemorrhagic shock in the presence of a intracranial mass with isotonic (I) and hypertonic (II) crystalloid alone or in combination with 10% Pentastarch (IP, IIP)

Results

Intracranial Pressure

ICP (Fig. 1 A), was increased to 15 mm Hg by balloon inflation (BI) and maintained throughout shock (T0–T30). ICP increased rapidly with the initiation of fluid resuscitation (T35) in all groups. Further increases in ICP occurred as a result of supplemental fluid infusion (T65–T155). No differences between groups were detected.

Cerebral Blood Flow

Induction of hemorrhage resulted in significant reductions in CBF from BL in all groups (Fig. 1 B, $p < 0.001$). Following resuscitation, CBF declined steadily in all groups over time.

Mean Arterial Pressure

During shock (T0–T30), MAP was decreased to 50 mm Hg and maintained for 30 minutes (Fig. 1 C). Following fluid resuscitation, MAP increased and then stabilized for the remainder of the experimental period.

Cardiac Output

CO was maintained following resuscitation by supplemental fluid infusion (Fig. 1 D). Animals resuscitated with crystalloid required a greater fluid volume initiated at an earlier time as compared to animals receiving crystalloid plus colloid.

Discussion

The deleterious effect of increased ICP is its effect on CBF. We have shown that isotonic and hypertonic crystalloid solutions alone or in combination with colloid rapidly increased ICP during the immediate post-resuscitation period. Supplemental fluid infusion, necessary to maintain CO, markedly increased ICP. As a result, CBF declined steadily over time. These results suggest that fluid resuscitation following hemorrhage in the presence of an intracranial mass may exacerbate the neurological sequelae of the shock episode.

References

Rapela C, Green H (1964) Autoregulation of canine cerebral blood flow. Circ Res [Suppl] 15:205–212

Whitley JM, Prough DS, DeWitt DS (1988) Shock plus an intracranial mass in dogs: Cerebrovascular effects of resuscitation fluid choices. Anesth Analg 67:259

Continuous Monitoring of ICP, CPP and BAER

Significance of Concomitant Changes

F. Artru, L, Larrea, Ch. Jourdan, O. Bertrand, J. Pernier, and F. Mauguière

Neurological Hospital, Hospital "Pierre Wertheimer", Lyon Montchat, 69394 Lyon Cedex 03 (France)

Introduction

Continuous monitoring of brainstem evoked auditive responses (BAER) proved to be helpful in evaluating brainstem dysfunction secondary to intracranial hypertension (Garcia-Larrea et al. 1987). The present work focuses on transient changes in BAERs observed during phases of critically elevated ICP or lowered cerebral perfusion pressure (CPP).

Methods

BAERs were sequentially recorded every few minutes by means of a standard evoked potential device controlled in its operations by a microcomputer (Bertrand et al. 1987). Latencies of wave I, III et V were automatically calculated and displayed as trend curves along with curves of ICP and mean arterial blood pressure.

ICP and BAER records were reviewed in 57 patients monitored for periods of 1 to 15 days. The cause of coma was head injury (35 cases), cerebral hemorrhage (20 cases) and cerebral infarction (2 cases). ICP and CPP were considered to reach critical levels when remaining for more than 10 min respectively above and below 40 mm Hg.

A pathological transient change in BAER was constituted of a progressive increase followed by a decrease in the I–V interwave latency over at least five successive BAERs in each phase. Inter-response increment and decrement were to be smaller than 0.2 ms to rule out artefactual changes and a significant correlation between I–V interwave latency and time was also required. Changes in body temperature or anesthetic blood level which could modify BAERs were ruled out.

Results

Influence of Critical ICP/CPP Alterations on BAERs

Critical levels of ICP or CPP were temporary present, at least once, in 22/47 patients. In 11 of them, BAER monitoring shows at that time a transient leng-

		Yes	No	Absent (3) or unreliable (3) BAEPs
Transient modifications of ICP or CPP *	Yes	11	11	4
	No	4	20	1
no ICP monitoring		3	2	1

*ICP > 40 mmHg, CPP < 40 mmHg

** unrelated to hypothermia or drugs

Fig. 1. Tabulation of patients with transient critical alterations of ICP or cerebral perfusion pressure (CPP) and/or transient increase in I–V interpeak latency (IPL) in BAER monitoring

thening of response latencies. In contrast, only 13% of patients whose ICP and CPP remained within the 40 mm Hg threshold had a significant change in BAER. The difference between the two groups was significant ($P < 0.05$).

Prognostic Significance of Transient Changes in BAERs Secondary to ICP/CPP Critical Alterations

Nearly all patients (91%) whose BAERs were transiently modified during phases of critically elevated ICP or lowered CPP ultimately progressed to brain death or persistant vegetative state. This outcome was significantly less frequent (18%) in the patient group with unmodified BAERs ($p < 0.01$).

Discussion

In this series of comatose patients, we demonstrated that continuous monitoring of BAERs over several days is feasible and allows detection of latency changes related to rise in ICP above 40 mm Hg and reduction in CPP below 40 mm Hg. Transient changes in BAERs were considered to reflect phases of brainstem dysfunction only in cases where the influence of non-pathological factors, like hypothermia and increasing lidocaine blood level, has been ruled out (Garcia-Larrea et al. 1988).

Only half critical ICP/CPP episodes induced transient changes in BAERs. It may be assumed that for critical ICP/CPP levels to affect brainstem electrophysiological activity, they must have initiated by transtentorial herniation. Whatever the mechanism, when ICP or CPP critical levels were associated with transient changes in BAERs, prognosis appeared almost desesperate. Conversely, patients who kept stable BAERs had a much better outcome. The question whether early detection of transient changes in BAER latencies could improve the outcome by prompting immediate measures deserves further investigation.

References

Bertrand O, Garcia-Larrea L, Artru F, Mauguière F, Pernier J (1987) Brain stem monitoring. I. Description of a system of sequential BAEP monitoring and feature extraction. Electroencephalogr Clin Neurophysiol 68:433–445

Garcia-Larrea L, Bertrand O, Artru F, Pernier J, Mauguière F (1987) Brain stem monitoring in coma. II: Dynamic interpretation of preterminal BAEP changes observed until brain death in deeply comatose patients. Electroencephalogr Clin Neurophysiol 68:446–457

Garcia-Larrea L, Artru F, Bertrand O, Pernier J, Mauguière F (1988) Transient pharmacological BAEP abolition in coma. Neurology (in press)

The Effect of Posttraumatic Hypoxia on ICP in Rats

N. Ishige, L.H. Pitts, and M.C. Nishimura

Department of Neurological Surgery, University of California, San Francisco, California 94110 (USA)

Hypoxia is almost certainly the most frequent secondary insult in several head-injured patients (Lutz et al. 1982), and its adverse effects on neurological outcome has been confirmed both clinically (Miller 1985) and experimentally (Ishige et al. 1987). We compared changes in intracranial pressure (ICP) after fluid percussion impact injury in rats with and without mild and severe post-traumatic hypoxia. We found that severe hypoxia (PaO_2 of 25 mm Hg for 1 hour) caused a significant increase in ICP up to 36 hours after impact injury and also caused more widespread brain edema compared with either no or mild hypoxia.

Materials and Methods

Sixty-two adult male Sprague-Dawley rats (350–400 gms) were used. ICP was monitored in 30 rats randomly assigned to one of four groups: Group S, sham operated ($n=4$); Group I, fluid percussion impact injury alone ($n=8$); Group IHm, impact injury plus mild hypoxia (PaO_2 of 40 mm Hg for 30 min, $n=8$); and Group IHs, impact injury plus severe hypoxia (PaO_2 of 25 mm Hg for 60 min, $n=10$). The severity and distribution of brain edema was determined using a microgravimetric technique (Marmarou et al. 1982) in an additional 32 rats (8 rats in each group). Under chloral hydrate anesthesia (0.35 mg/kg), IP, an impact injury of 4.9 ± 0.3 atmospheres was applied to the right temporal region of the animal's head through a 4 mm-diameter craniectomy. Hypoxia was given by exposing the spontaneously breathing animal to a low-concentration oxygen gas. Epidural ICP was monitored continuously for 72 hours via a saline-filled polyethylene catheter positioned through left parietal burr holes.

Results

Time courses for changes in ICP are shown in Fig. 1. Group S rats showed minimal fluctuations in ICP throughout the experimental period. In Group I rats, ICP remained between 0 and 4 mm Hg except for the momentary increase after injury.

In Group IHm rats, ICP increased only slightly 12 to 24 hr after injury. Paroxysmal transient increases, which were not seen in Group I, were observed

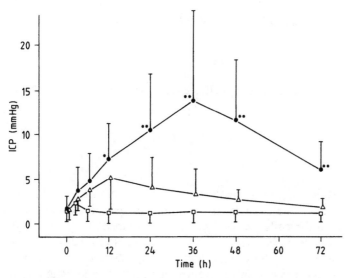

Fig. 1. Time courses of ICP in Group I (*open square*), Group IHm (*open circle*) and Group IHs (*solid circle*). An * indicates the value was significantly higher than Group I ($p<0.01$), and ** that the value was significantly higher than Group I ($p<0.005$)

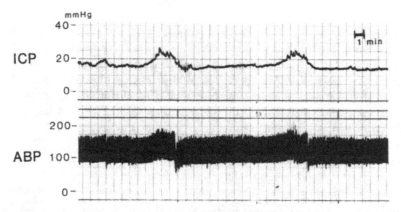

Fig. 2. Lundberg's B-waves associated with changes in arterial blood pressure in Group IHs animals. * $P<0.01$, Group IHs vs. Group I; ** $P<0.005$, Group IHs vs. Group I

in 50% of rats in Group IHm. ICP usually increased by 5–20 mm Hg for 5–25 min, most often 12 to 36 hr after impact.

In Group IHs, a pronounced increase of up to 14 mm Hg in ICP was seen 36 hr after injury, which was significantly greater than that of Group I rats at the same period after injury ($p<0.005$). Moreover, 50% of rats showed additional intermittent small increases in ICP levels above 15 mm Hg between 24 and 48 hr after injury, and increases often were associated with changes in blood pressure

(Fig. 2) and respiration. These findings may correspond to Lundberg's B-waves. Specific gravity of brain tissue, measured 24 hr after injury in another 32 rats, showed that there was more widespread and severe brain edema in rats with impact injury plus severe hypoxia.

Conclusion

The results of the present study show that hypoxic insult increases the incidence of intracranial hypertension after traumatic brain injury. The resulting increased intracranial pressure probably is also due, in part, to brain edema.

References

Ishige N, Pitts LH et al. (1987) The effect of hypoxia on traumatic brain injury in rats: Part 1. Changes in neurological function, electroencephalograms, and histopathology. Neurosurgery 20:848–853

Lutz HA, Becker DP et al. (1982) Monitoring, management and the analysis of outcome. In: Gross RG, Gildenberg PL (eds) Head injury. Basic and clinical aspects. Raven Press, New York, pp 221–228

Marmarou A, Tanaka K et al. (1982) An improved gravimetric measure of cerebral edema. J Neurosurgery 56:246–253

Miller JD (1985) Head injury and brain ischemia. Implication for therapy. Br J Anaesth 57:120–129

Neuro-Intensive Care for Cerebral Herniation in Childhood Meningitis

D.I. Rosenberg[1], J.H. McCrory, M.K. Abhoudon, A.A. Murante, and C.E. Downs

Department of Pediatrics, Division of Pediatric Critical Care Medicine, University Hospital of Jacksonville, Jacksonville, Florida (USA)

[1] Rainbow Babies and Childrens Hospital, Department of Pediatric Pharmacology and Critical Care, 2101 Adelbert Road, Cleveland, Ohio 44106 (USA)

Purpose

To determine the features of cerebral herniation associated with bacterial meningitis in children, including incidence, clinical presentation, relationship to lumbar puncture, CT scan findings, morbidity, mortality and mechanisms of death.

Methods

The population studied consisted of all children between the ages of 6 weeks and 17 years admitted to either University Hospital of Jacksonville or Jacksonville Wolfson's Childrens Hospital during the period 2/1/80 and 10/31/87, with the diagnosis of acute bacterial meningitis. All patients were directly managed by the attendings and fellows of the Pediatric Critical Care Service. The hospital medical charts of those children who suffered cerebral herniation were reviewed retrospectively to obtain the following information: age, sex, clinical presentation, time of lumbar puncture, infectious agent, CT scan results, therapy employed and outcome. Cerebral herniation was defined as: 1) change in pupillary status from equal and reactive to anisocoria, pinpoint, or bilaterally non reactive, and 2) ICP ≥ 20 mm Hg for ≥ 30 minutes with progression to brain death or survival.

Results

A total of 453 cases of bacterial meningitis were identified; 17 of these patients died (3.8%). Of the 17 deaths, 5 resulted from cardiovascular collapse, whereas 12 were from cerebral herniation with elevated ICP. In addition to the 12 who died, 4 children who survived cerebral herniation were identified. (Total number of cases of cerebral herniation 16/453 or 3.5%.) Mean age ($n = 16$) was 42 months (2–168 months), 12 were male and 3 were black. Of those 16 cases complete medical records were available in 15. Nine of whom presented initially with a

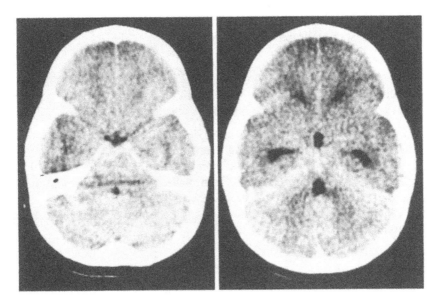

Fig. 1. A 12 month old black female who presented to the Emergency Room after having a seizure. She developed anisocoria 4 hours later and was brain dead upon admission to the Pediatric Intensive Care Unit. Her CT scan demonstrates dilated temporal horns with absent basal cisterns

sudden neurological deterioration [seizures (4) apnea (5),] as opposed to rostro-caudal progression in 6. Five of 15 children had their first pupillary change on presentation to the Emergency Room and the mean time after Emergency Room admission to pupillary change in 10/15 was 6.35 hours (0.3–23). Two of 12 children presented with fixed, dilated pupils (F/D) in the Emergency Room, and the mean time from admission to F/D pupils (brain death) was 11.9 hours (0.3–78) in the remaining 10.

Eight of 14 children for whom information was available had pupillary changes before lumbar puncture (LP). The mean time between LP and pupillary changes in 6/14 was 8.6 hours (2–23 hrs).

CT scans were obtained in 11 children and demonstrated enlarged lateral ventricles with absent basal cisterns in 9 (82%). Fifty children with bacterial meningitis, but without clinical evidence of herniation, also underwent CT scans and 7/50 (14%) had enlarged lateral ventricles, but all had basal cisterns visible (absent cisterns 0/50) (Fig. 1).

Seven patients had dilated, non-reactive pupils and absence of cortical function on admission to the Pediatric Intensive Care Unit. Therapy in the remaining 8 patients who were not brain dead on admission to the Pediatric Intensive Care Unit and for whom information was available consisted of: standard (fluid restriction, head elevation, hyperventilation, mannitol) in 8/8, steroids in 4, and barbiturates (bolus or coma) in 6. ICP monitoring was performed in 8 patients and a ventricular catheter was inserted for decompression in 3 patients; 2 of whom survived. The mortality from cerebral herniation in our series was 75%.

There were 4/16 survivors: 2 are normal, 1 has a resolving cortical blindness and 1 had a spastic quadraparesis with late death.

Conclusion

1. Cerebral herniation from childhood bacterial meningitis presents suddenly in 50% of cases, therefore limiting neuro-intensive care.
2. No relationship between lumbar puncture and herniation was identified.
3. Enlarged lateral ventricles with absent basal cisterns were present in 9/11 cases and appeared predictive of cerebral herniation.
4. A significant male to female ratio was encountered, the cause of which is unknown.

ICP, CSF Outflow Resistance and Brain Edema in Experimental Pneumococcal Meningitis

J. Gyring, E. Gutschik, N. Andersen, and F. Gjerris

Department of General Physiology and Biophysics, The Panum Institute,
University of Copenhagen, DK-Copenhagen 2200 (Denmark)

Introduction

The mortality and morbidity of bacterial meningitis remain high. Clinical observations indicate that increased ICP and brain oedema are the main causes of adverse outcome.

Materials and Methods

Randomly bred albino rabbits (Ssc:CPH) weighing 2.4–3.5 kg with permanent bilateral cerebral ventricular cannulae (Gyring and Brøndsted 1984).

Meningitis was induced by injecting live Streptococcus pneumonia type III into one lateral ventricle followed by flushing with CSF in order to rapidly disperse the bacteriae within the subarachnoid space. The control animals had an infusion of CSF.

We used an innoculum of 1.2×10^8 and 1.2×10^6 colony forming units in order to obtain severe meningitis with a 100% mortality in 30 h and a mild meningitis with a 50% mortality in 48 h in untreated animals.

General procedures and measurement of ICP and CSF outflow resistance (R_{out}) by the constant infusion method were as previously described (Gyring and Brøndsted 1984). ICP and R_{out} was measured at the start of the experiments and 10 and 24 h after induction of meningitis and then at 24 h intervals. In addition ICP was measured at 4, 14 and 18 h. In the control animals ICP and R_{out} was measured at the start, 10, 24 and 96 h.

Brain specific gravity was measured in a linear bromobenzene–kerosene gradient (Marmarou et al. 1978). After sacrifice the brain was removed, wrapped in alufoil and placed on ice in a cooled humidity chamber until it was firm. The brain was then dissected on parafilm on ice and samples weighing 30 to 50 mg were taken sequentially from twelve regions. Animals with severe meningitis were examined at 24 h. In the animals with mild meningitis 11 were examined at 24 h and the remaining animals were sacrificed during the following days.

Intracranial Pressure VII   773
Eds.: J. T. Hoff and A. L. Betz
© Springer-Verlag Berlin Heidelberg 1989

ICP

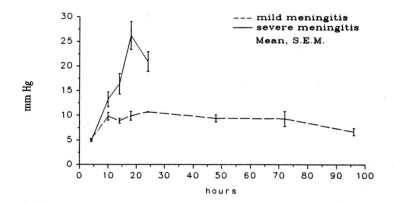

R~out~

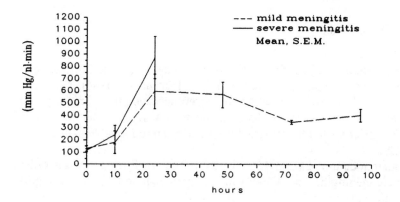

CSF~bacteria~

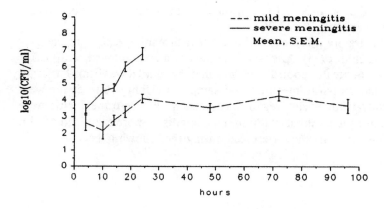

Results

All inoculated animals showed signs of infection and all had bacteriaemia 6 h after the inoculation.

In the nine control animals subjected to repeated measurements the ICP remained stable and the R_{out} was unchanged in seven and showed a temporary increase in two animals. When the specific gravity in these animals with repeated measurements was compared with the nine control animals that had neither ICP nor R_{out} measurements there was no significant difference and the data were pooled.

The results of the ICP measurements and the measurements of R_{out} are shown in the Figure 1. In both infected groups the ICP was stable. We saw A waves in only four animals with severe meningitis, all with baseline ICP above 20 mm Hg and definite B-waves were seen only once in an animal with mild meningitis of 72 h duration.

In nine animals with severe meningitis surviving less than 20 h the peak ICP was 35.4 mm Hg. In seven of these animals it was impossible to measure R_{out} as any infusion even at the lowest rate increased ICP dramatically, worsened ophistotonus and precipitated respiratory ataxia, indicating herniation of the cerebellum at the foramen magnum. In all these animals it was impossible to obtain CSF from the cisterna magna and at autopsy the cerebellar tonsils occluded the cistern. The same picture was also seen in 11 animals with severe meningitis surviving for more than 20 h with ICP in the range of 15 to 45 mm Hg.

In animals with mild meningitis, the ICP reached a peak level within the first 48 h and then decreased during the following days in spite of a significantly increased R_{out}. The measurement of R_{out} was uneventful in all these animals and the cisterna magna was open at autopsy.

In animals monitored until death the ICP remained stable until the appearance of respiratory ataxia at which stage the blood pressure began to fall with a parallel decrease in the ICP.

The specific gravity was significantly decreased in all animals with severe meningitis. In the animals with mild meningitis there was no decrease in specific gravity and there was no difference between animals examined at 24 h and animals examined at 48, 72 and 96 h.

In 18 animals with severe meningitis the pressure in the deep cervical veins was between 2 and 4.5 mm Hg.

Fig. 1. *Upper panel:* The ICP as a function of time after inoculation with Streptococcus pneumonia type III. At ten hours the ICP is significantly elevated but there is no difference between the two groups. At 14, 18 and 24 h the ICP is significantly higher in the severe meningitis group. In the mild meningitis group the ICP does not increase after 10 hours. *Middle panel:* CSF outflow resistance (R_{out}) as a function of time after induction of infection. The R_{out} is significantly increased as early as ten hours after the innoculation but there is no difference between the groups at 10 or 24 hours. *Lower panel:* The concentration of bacteriae (colony forming units/ml) in the CSF as a function of time. After four hours the concentration is significantly higher in the animals with severe meningitis

Discussion

In this experimental meningitis model the ICP increase can be explained partly by the increase in R_{out}, probably due to malfunctioning of the arachnoid villi or occlusion of the subarachnoid space over the hemispheres (Butler et al. 1983). However, very high ICP was seen only in animals with severe meningitis and brain oedema and in these animals the increaed R_{out} could only account for less than 50% of the pressure increase if normal choroidal and extrachoroidal CSF production was assumed. This indicates either an increase in the venous pressure or an increased rate of extrachoroidal CSF formation. As 30 to 50% of the CSF in the rabbit drains into the cervical lymph in the rabbit and the pressure in the cervical veins was normal, we suggest that there could be an increased extrachoroidal CSF formation due to continuous clearance of brain oedema. The highest ICP values were observed in animals in which it was impossible to measure the R_{out} due to herniation at the foramen magnum which was also the cause of death in all animals with severe meningitis monitored through the terminal phase of the disease. In animals without signs of herniation artificially increased ICP up till 50 mm Hg was tolerated without any adverse effects during constant rate CSF infusion. We thus conclude that the main cause of mortality is brain oedema and that the increased ICP is of less importance as long as there is no herniation.

References

Butler AB, Mann JD, Maffeo CJ, Dacey RG, Johnson RN, Bass NH (1983) Mechanism of cerebrospinal fluid absorption in normal and pathologically altered arachnoid villi. In: Wood HJ (ed) Neurobiology of the cerebrospinal fluid, vol 2. Plenum Press, New York, pp 682–695
Gyring JA, Brøndsted HE (1984) Repetitive measurements of intracranial pressure in awake rabbits. Acta Physiol Scand 122:299–305
Marmarou A, Poll W, Shulman K, Bhagavan H (1978) A simple gravimetric technique for measurement of cerebral edema. J Neurosurg 49:530–537

Brain Edema, ICP and CSF Outflow Resistance in Experimental Pneumococcal Meningitis: Effect of Mannitol and Antiinflammatory Drugs

J. Gyring, E. Gutschik, P.S. Sørensen, N. Andersen, and F. Gjerris

Department of General Physiology and Biophysics, The Panum Institute,
University of Copenhagen, DK-Copenhagen 2200 (Denmark)

Introduction

The mortality and morbidity of bacterial meningitis have remained virtually unchanged since the introduction of penicillin 40 years ago.

Materials and Methods

Randomly bred albino rabbits and experimental procedures as described (Gyring et al. 1988).

Meningitis was induced by injecting live Streptococcus pneumonia type III in 300 µl isotonic saline into one lateral ventricle followed by flushing with 500 µl CSF in order to rapidly disperse the bacteriae within the subarachnoid space. The control animals had an infusion of 800 µl CSF. We used two sizes of inocula, $1.2 \times 10^8 \pm 0.1$ (SD) and $1.2 \times 10^6 \pm 0.1$ (SD) colony forming units in order to obtain a severe meningitis with a 100% mortality in 30 h and a mild meningitis with a 50% mortality in 48 h in untreated animals.

Experimental Groups

A: Control animals, rapid infusion of mannitol 1 g/kg; sacrifice after 45 min.
B: Severe meningitis, rapid infusion of mannitol 1 g/kg 24 h after induction of the infection; sacrifice after 45 min.
C: Control animals, no treatment.
D: Mild meningitis, no treatment.
E: Severe meningitis, no treatment.
F: Severe meningitis, penicillin 10 h after induction of infection.
G: Severe meningitis, penicillin plus Indomethacin 12.5 mg/kg and Promethazine 5 mg/kg 10 h after induction of infection.
H: Severe meningitis, penicillin plus dexamethasone 3 mg/kg 10 h after induction of infection.

ICP was measured 10 h after induction of infection in all animals. ICP and outflow resistance were measured at 24 h. The animals were then sacrificed and

BRAIN specific gravity

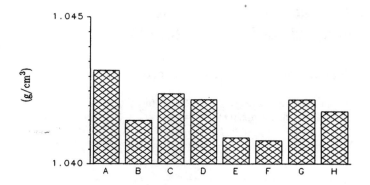

ICP 24 hours

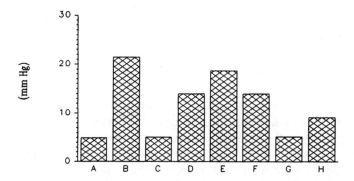

R out

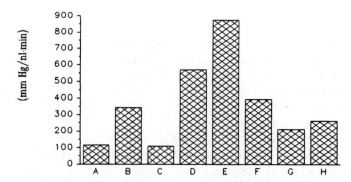

Fig. 1. Brain specific gravity (*upper panel*), ICP (*middle panel*) and CSF outflow resistance (*lower panel*) in experimental groups A to H measured 24 h after induction of infection. For explanation of treatment groups and discussion see text

the brain specific gravity was measured in a linear bromobenzene–kerosene gradient (Marmarou et al. 1978).

Results

The antibiotic treatment sterilised the CSF in all but a few animals. There was no difference in the number of CSF leukocytes in the animals with severe meningitis irrespective of treatment, but the number of leukocytes was significantly lower in the animals with mild meningitis.

The results of the measurements of brain specific gravity, ICP and R_{out} are shown in the Fig. 1. Brain specific gravity was normal in animals with mild meningitis (D) and in animals with severe meningitis treated with penicillin plus indomethacin and promethazine (G). Also in the group G animals the ICP was normal at 24 h in spite of a significantly increased ICP 10 h after the induction of the infection. In the animals treated with penicillin plus dexamethasone (H) the brain specific gravity was slightly but significantly decreased, but it was significantly higher than in group B, E and F animals indicating a beneficial effect which was also seen in the ICP and the R_{out}. The group G animals were all in a good condition at 24 h whereas all the group H animals had signs of severe infection.

In the animals with severe untreated meningitis (E) and animals treated with penicillin only (F) there was a pronounced decrease in specific gravity and in both groups the ICP and R_{out} was significantly increased.

The infused dose of mannitol increased the plasma osmolality to a mean value of 312 mosm/kg and led to a significant increase in the brain specific gravity in both control animals (A) and in infected animals (B). The increase in specific gravity was of the same magnitude in both groups. The relative ICP decrease 30 min after the infusion was not different in the two groups. This indicates that in spite of the leaky blood brain barrier mannitol retains its osmotic dehydrating effect. The R_{out} was also significantly lower in the group B animals when compared to the two untreated groups (D and E). This could be due to either a widening of the subarachnoid space or a direct effect on the arachnoid villi. However the R_{out} was not significantly different from the values in the animals treated with penicillin alone or penicillin plus antiinflammatory drugs.

Discussion

Inhibition of the inflammatory response has a beneficial effect in this experimental meningitis model. Indomethacin or promethazine used alone was not effective (results not reported here) whereas the combination was highly effective, virtually eliminating edema and ICP increase. The combination of a H_1 histamine antagonist with a cyclooxygenase inhibitor should also be more effective than either drug used alone as there is a synergistic effect of histamine/serotonin and prostaglandins in the inflammatory response. That other mediators than the prostaglandins and leukotrienes are active in the inflammatory reaction is also indicated by the less pronounced effect of dexamethasone which blocks the formation of both by inhibiting the phospholipase A_2 through the release of lipocortin.

There was no effect of treatment with antibiotics alone. The infusion of mannitol decreased the ICP and the brain edema significantly. The observation time in these experiments is too short to allow for any conclusion as to whether this effect is lasting or if there is a late rebound in pressure and edema.

References

Gyring JA, Brøndsted HE (1984) Repetitive measurements of intracranial pressure in awake rabbits. Acta Physiol Scand 122:299–305

Gyring J, Gutschik E, Andersen N, Gjerris F (1988) ICP, CSF outflow resistance and brain edema in experimental pneumococcal meningitis. In: Hoff JT (ed) Intracranial pressure VII. Springer, Berlin Heidelberg New York Tokyo

Marmarou A, Poll W, Shulman K, Bhagavan H (1978) A simple gravimetric technique for measurement of cerebral edema. J Neurosurg 49:530–537

Changes of Intracranial Pressure in a Rat Meningitis Model

H.W. Pfister [1], U. Dirnagl [1], R. Haberl [1], F. Anneser [1], U. Ködel [1], P. Mehraein [2], W. Feiden [2], and K.M. Einhäupl [1]

Departments of Neurology [1] and Neuropathology [2], University of Munich, Marchioninistr. 15, D-8000 Munich 70 (FRG)

Introduction

Brain edema formation, raised intracranial pressure (ICP) and alterations of the cerebral blood circulation are thought to be of great importance for the outcome of bacterial meningitis (Dodge and Swartz 1965, Swartz 1984, Igarashi et al. 1984). The purpose of our study was to develop an animal model for the evaluation of secondary brain damage during the course of meningitis. This model should permit continuous monitoring of ICP, brain edema and cerebral blood flow during chemical meningitis with carrageenan (CAR). CAR is reported to induce reproducible and fast acting chemical meningitis in the mouse brain (Gamache et al. 1986).

Methods

Meningitis was induced in 10 Wistar rats by intracisternal injection of 350 µg of CAR. In 10 control animals saline was injected. In a closed cranial preparation the cerebral blood flow, blood volume and blood flow velocity of the brain microcirculation were assessed by Laser-Doppler (LD) spectroscopy (Haberl et al. 1987). Brain edema formation was estimated by electrical impedance measurements (Van der Veen et al. 1973) and brain water content determinations. ICP, systemic arterial pressure, endexpiratory CO_2 and LD parameters were continuously monitored. At baseline and every two hours blood gases and hematocrit were evaluated. The animals were sacrificed 4 hours after CAR-injection. In order to detect meningeal inflammation 5 animals of each group were examined histologically.

Results

In all animals in the CAR group which were examined by light microscopy there was histological evidence of meningitis without signs of brain edema or hydrocephalus. In the CAR group there was a significant increase in ICP from a baseline of 2.6 (± 0.8 SEM) mm Hg to 16.2 (± 3.7) mm Hg at 4 hours after CAR

Intracranial Pressure VII
Eds.: J. T. Hoff and A. L. Betz
© Springer-Verlag Berlin Heidelberg 1989

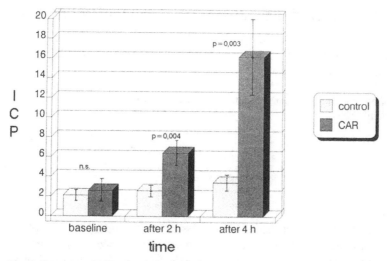

Fig. 1. Increase of ICP after injection of Carrageenan into the Cisterna magna

injection (Fig. 1). Blood flow increased significantly by $82.7 \pm 21.9\%$ in the CAR group, mainly due to an increase in blood velocity, whereas there was only a non-significant tendency for an increase of blood volume ($+10.7 \pm 6.9\%$). Impedance measurements and brain water content determinations did not give evidence of brain edema formation.

Discussion

A new animal model was established for the continuous monitoring of microcirculatory cerebral blood flow, ICP and edema formation during experimental chemical meningitis. The major findings were that ICP and blood flow were significantly increasing following CAR induced meningitis without formation of brain edema or histological evidence of hydrocephalus. The increase in cerebral blood volume was too small to fully account for the ICP elevation. Since no perfusion fixation of the brains was carried out mild acute ventricular dilatation may have been missed in the histological examination. Further studies will use this model to evaluate the role of these factors in the genesis of secondary brain damage in the course of bacterial meningitis as induced by pneumococci.

References

Dodge PR, Swartz MN (1965a) Bacterial meningitis – a review of selected aspects. II. Special neurologic problems, postmeningitic complications and clinicopathologic correlations. N Engl J Med 272:954–960

Dodge PR, Swartz MN (1965 b) Bacterial meningitis – a review of selected aspects. II. Special neurologic problems, postmeningitic complications and clinicopathologic correlations. N Engl J Med 272:1003–1010

Gamache DA, Povlishock JT, Ellis FE (1986) Carrageenan-induced brain inflammation. Characterization of a model. J Neurosurg 65:679–685

Haberl RL, Heizer ML, Ellis EF (1987) Laser-Doppler flowmetry for the evaluation of the brain microcirculation. Circ Res (submitted)

Igarashi M, Gilmartin RC, Gerald B, Wilburn F, Jabbour JT (1984) Cerebral arteritis and bacterial meningitis. Arch Neurol 41:531–535

Swartz MN (1984) Bacterial meningitis: more involved than just the meninges. N Engl J Med 311:912–914

Van der Veen PH, Go KG, Zuiderveen F, Buiter D, van der Meer J (1973) Electrical impedance of cat brain with cold-induced edema. Exp Neurol 40:675–682

Session VI: Free Radicals

Chairmen: A.L. Betz and D.P. Becker

Oxygen Radicals in Experimental Brain Injury
H.A. Kontos

Oxygen Free Radicals in the Genesis of Traumatic Brain Edema
Y. Ikeda, K.L. Brelsford, K. Ikeda, and D.M. Long

Reduction of Intracranial Hypertension with Free Radical Scavengers
R.S. Zimmerman, J.P. Muizelaar, E.P. Wei, and H.A. Kontos

Allopurinol and Dimethylthiourea Limit Infarct Size in Partial Ischemia
R.D. Martz, G. Rayos, G.P. Schielke, and A.L. Betz

The Effect of Superoxide Dismutase on Rabbit Brain Reperfusion Injury
D.P. Christenberry, E. Tasdemiroglu, J.L. Ardell, R. Chronister, P.W. Curreri, and A.E. Taylor

The Role of Catecholamine-Induced Lipid Peroxidation and Histamine
in Ischemic Brain Edema
H. Morooka, H. Sasayama, K. Sakai, S. Namba, and A. Nishimoto

Oxygen Radicals in Experimental Brain Injury

H.A. Kontos

Department of Internal Medicine, Medical College of Virginia. Virginia Commonwealth University, Richmond, Virginia 23 298 (USA)

Introduction

Brain injury remains a serious cause of mortality and morbidity, despite considerable efforts to improve its outcome. In our studies, we have assumed that at least some of its adverse consequences would be potentially reversible with appropriate therapy. We have, therefore, attempted to formulate proper therapies by a systematic approach, which, as an initial step, seeks to identify the mechanisms of the abnormalities in experimental brain injury.

We have used in cats and rats a model of fluid percussion brain injury (Sullivan et al. 1976) which mimics many of the vascular abnormalities seen in human brain injury. Most of the important steps in the mechanisms of the cerebral vascular abnormalities seen in this model are now understood. This paper gives an account of the vascular abnormalities due to experimental fluid percussion brain injury, of their mechanisms, and of their potential significance in human brain injury. We hope that rational approaches to more successful treatment of human brain injury can be based on what we have learned from these animal studies.

Vascular Abnormalities in Fluid Percussion Brain Injury

Experimental fluid percussion brain injury has been best studied in anesthetized and paralyzed cats. This type of injury is associated with increases in arterial blood pressure and in intracranial pressure (Wei et al. 1980). The increase in arterial blood pressure is due to activation of the sympathetic nervous system because of mechanical pressure on the brain stem in the course of fluid percussion brain injury. It subsides within a few minutes. The increase in intracranial pressure in mild to moderate injury is usually transient. In severe injuries where there may be extensive subarachnoid hemorrhage, the increased intracranial pressure persists.

The cerebral vascular abnormalities in fluid percussion brain injury are listed in Table 1. The cerebral arterioles dilate immediately after the occurrence of fluid percussion brain injury (Wei et al. 1980). The degree of dilation is quantitatively related to the severity of injury. With mild injury, the dilation is mild and subsides within a few minutes. With severe injury, sustained dilation occurs which outlasts the duration of the hypertensive episode and may last as long as several hours.

Intracranial Pressure VII
Eds.: J. T. Hoff and A. L. Betz
© Springer-Verlag Berlin Heidelberg 1989

Table 1. Cerebral vascular effects of fluid percussion brain injury

---

Arteriolar dilation
Focal endothelial and vascular smooth muscle lesions
Abnormal vascular reactivity
Absent endothelium-dependent responses
Reduced oxygen consumption of vessel wall
Enhanced platelet agreggability
Hemorrhage
Increased endothelial permeability to macromolecules

Accompanying the arteriolar dilation is abnormal vascular reactivity to both vasodilator and vasoconstrictor responses (Wei et al. 1980). The vasoconstrictor response to arterial hypocapnia is reduced or abolished following experimental brain injury. Autoregulatory vasodilation in response to reductions in arterial blood pressure is reduced after moderate injury and abolished following severe injury. Under these conditions, the vessels behave passively showing a reduction in vessel caliber as the arterial blood pressure is reduced (Wei et al. 1980).

Of particular importance are the abnormalities in response to agents which induce vascular changes via endothelium-dependent mechanisms. It is known that certain agents induce their vascular effects by acting on the endothelium to induce the release of endothelium-derived vasoactive agents which then diffuse to the vascular smooth muscle to induce the appropriate changes in vascular tone and caliber (Furchgott, 1983). The best known such response is the vasodilator response to acetylcholine, which is due to the release of endothelium-derived relaxing factors (EDRFs). In unpublished observations we found that after experimental brain injury, the response to acetylcholine is abolished or converted from vasodilation to vasoconstriction (Fig. 1). The vasoconstrictor response is presumed to be the result of the direct action of acetylcholine on vascular smooth muscle, which becomes unmasked when the dominant endothelium-dependent relaxation is eliminated. Similarly, the response to bradykinin, another agent which dilates cerebral vessels by endothelium-dependent mechanisms, is severely reduced (Fig. 2). Finally, the response to serotonin is converted from the normal vasoconstrictor response to a vasodilator influence (Fig. 2). This may be due to the fact that serotonin releases an endothelium-derived vasoconstrictor factor from the endothelium (EDCF). When this indirect effect is eliminated, the vasodilator effect of serotonin, which presumably represents the direct effect on vascular smooth muscle, is uncovered. The elimination of these endothelium-dependent responses may be due to damage to the endothelium so that it is no longer able to produce vasoactive agents or to destruction of the vasoactive agents after they are released, or to a combination of these mechanisms.

These abnormalities in vessel caliber and vascular reactivity are reflected in changes in cerebral blood flow. Following mild to moderate brain injury, there is initially hyperemia with increases in blood flow and decreases in vascular resistance (DeWitt et al. 1986). Subsequently, blood flow may subside to the resting

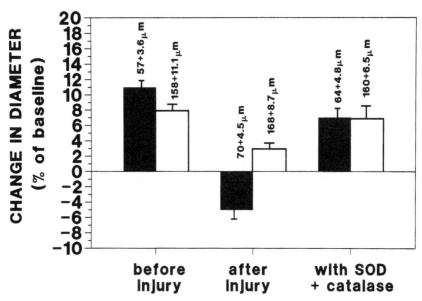

Fig. 1. Effect of topical acetylcholine (10^{-7} M) on small and large cerebral arterioles before injury, 30 min after injury and following the topical application of 60 U/ml of SOD and 40 U/ml of catalase. The values are mean ± standard error. The baseline diameters from which the percentage changes were calculated are given above each bar. Note the elimination or reversal of the normal vasodilator response to acetylcholine after injury and the restoration of the normal response in the presence of SOD and catalase

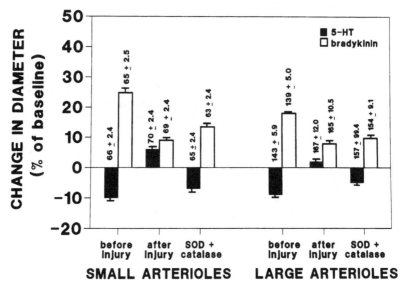

Fig. 2. Changes in vessel caliber induced by topical application of serotonin (5-HT, 10^{-4} M) or bradykinin (5 µg/ml) before injury, 30 min after injury and following the topical application of SOD and catalase in the same doses as in Fig. 1. Note that the normal response to serotonin is vasoconstrictor, that it is converted to vasodilation after injury, and that the normal vasoconstrictor response is restored in the presence of SOD and catalase. The response to bradykinin is significantly reduced after injury and SOD and catalase do not affect it

level. Blood flow increases in response to arterial hypercapnia are reduced following fluid percussion brain injury (Lewelt et al. 1983). Autoregulatory responses are also altered so that the range of effective autoregulation is diminished (Lewelt et al. 1980). In addition, the hyperemic responses to arterial hypoxia are reduced following brain injury (Lewelt et al. 1983).

The cerebral arterioles following brain injury display characteristic lesions when examined by scanning and transmission electron microscopy (Wei et al. 1980). The endothelium shows discrete lesions which appear in two forms, a crater-like lesion and a balloon-like lesion, which projects like a dome into the lumen of the vessel. Their density is approximately $0.5-1.5/100\ \mu m^2$. Examination of a large number of these lesions suggests that they represent the same basic abnormality which begins as a localized destructive lesion of the endothelium, creating a balloon or a bleb-like lesion. When the bleb bursts into the lumen of the vessel, it creates a crater. These lesions are similar to what has been described in cultured hepatocytes in response to oxidant attack on the cells (Orrenius 1988). It is believed that in such cells these lesions are due to oxidation of thiols in the cytoskeleton of the cell which leads to alterations in the actin filaments which then form aggregates and create the blebs.

The dilated vessels following brain injury display biochemical abnormalities. Their oxygen consumption measured in vitro in a microrespirometer is severely reduced, indicative of a severe abnormality in the oxidative machinery of the cell (Wei et al. 1980).

The endothelial injury causes a tendency towards platelet aggregation, although it is by itself usually insufficient to induce overt platelet aggregation (Rosenblum et al. 1987). However, after brain injury, pro-aggregatory stimuli induce platelet aggregation more easily than in control animals (Rosenblum, et al. 1982).

Other abnormalities in endothelial function are reflected in abnormal permeability of the blood-brain barrier to macromolecules (Porlishock et al. 1978). In moderate to severe brain injury, there is extensive extravasation of protein into the vessel wall and into the perivascular compartment. This appears to be due to accelerated transport of the protein via vesicles.

Although lesions of the vascular smooth muscle do occur, they are generally rare and not very severe. They consist of vacuoles or inclusion bodies. Occasionally outright necrosis of the vessel wall may be found (Wei et al. 1980).

Fluid percussion brain injury is associated with a transient abolition of electrical brain activity (Sullivan et al. 1976). The hemispheres do not display any recognizable histological lesions except for the contusion at the site of the attachment of the brain injury device (Wei et al. 1980). The brain stem frequently displays hemorrhage which in severe brain injury may extend into the subarachnoid space (Wei et al. 1980). There is also evidence of axonal disruption in the brain stem (Povlishock et al. 1983).

In anesthetized but not paralyzed rats, fluid percussion injury causes cessation of respiration which may be transient or sustained causing death unless assisted ventilation is provided (Kim et al. unpublished.)

It is unlikely that any one model of experimental brain injury would mimic all the abnormalities seen in human brain injury. This is because human brain injury covers a very wide spectrum of abnormalities which range from direct mechanical disruption of brain tissue to hemorrhage with space occupying lesions and consequent pressure effects on the brain and its blood vessels inducing ischemia, as well as vascular abnormalities which cause edema and abnormal vascular permeability.

Fluid percussion brain injury seen in cats mimics many of the abnormalities of brain injury seen in humans to a sufficiently pronounced degree to render this a suitable model for studying mechanisms of brain injury. For example, this type of experimental brain injury induces alterations in intracranial pressure, vascular caliber, and reactivity similar to those in human disease. The induction of increased intracranial pressure in human brain injury is well known to be due to a major extent to vascular causes. The induction of edema, secondary to abnormalities in blood flow and endothelial permeability, is also a common feature of the disorder in experimental animals and man. Also, in both cat and rat, fluid percussion injury produces signs resembling unconsciousness in humans (Dixon et al. 1987; Hayes et al. 1984). Similar to mild and moderate head injury in humans, fluid percussion produces prolonged vestibular and motor deficits (Binder 1982) as well as memory and attentional deficits (Lyeth et al. 1987), all of which persist after resolution of the disturbed states of consciousness. In addition to these functional and behavioral changes, fluid percussion injury also replicates many of the pathological changes seen in head-injured humans. Importantly, in the cat, mild, moderate and severe fluid percussion injury result in axonal damage (Povlishock et al. 1983; 1986) consistent with that reported in humans (Adams et al. 1987 a; 1987 b; Strich 1961). The damaged axons have been identified in anatomical loci comparable to those described in man. Although there appears to be higher predilection for infratentorial involvement with fluid percussion injury, this most likely reflects differences in brain geometry and alignment rather than differences in pathogenesis. Interestingly, as studies in the cat fluid percussion injury have shown that reactive axonal change requires 12 hours for maximal development; this finding in cat explains why reactive axonal change is not recognized in humans surviving for less than 12 hours after injury (Pilz 1983). In addition to the presence of axonal damage, fluid percussion injury also results in other forms of pathological change similar to that seen in humans. In both rat and cat, fluid percussion causes an increased vulnerability of the CA_1 sector of the hippocampus to secondary insults (Jenkins et al. 1986; in press) and this finding is consistent with comparable observation made in humans (Graham et al. 1988).

Collectively, the above cited findings suggest that fluid percussion injury in both rat and cat provides useful information on many traumatically induced abnormalities recognized in head-injured man. Obviously, fluid percussion cannot replicate every feature of human head injury; yet, when data obtained from fluid percussion studies are placed in the appropriate scientific framework, information relevant to head-injured man can evolve.

Mechanism of Cerebral Vascular Injury in Experimental Fluid Percussion Brain Injury

The important steps in the vascular abnormalities in experimental fluid percussion brain injury are shown in Fig. 3. According to this scheme, the immediate cause of the vascular injury is the generation of oxygen radicals.

We have shown the production of superoxide in the brain of cats as a consequence of fluid percussion brain injury by two techniques. We use the SOD-inhibitable reduction of nitroblue tetrazolium to measure superoxide production (Kontos and Wei 1985). We showed that superoxide is produced both in the immediate post-injury period, and that the generation of this radical continues for at least an hour.

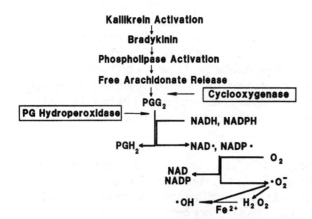

Fig. 3. Suggested mechanism for the vascular effects of fluid percussion brain injury

One of the sites of generation of superoxide was identified by a histochemical technique which is based on the oxidation of manganese by superoxide from the divalent to the trivalent state (Povlishock et al. 1988). The oxidized manganese in turn oxidizes diaminobenzidene which precipitates. The oxidized diaminobenzidine can in turn be identified because it forms an electron dense product when reacted after fixation with osmic acid. Using this technique, we found that superoxide is produced in the wall of cerebral vessels following brain injury. No production of superoxide in the brain parenchyma could be identified by this technique. However, this must be interpreted with caution because the absence of superoxide at this site may be due to incomplete penetration of the reagents.

˙ The mechanism by which superoxide and its products induce tissue injury have been discussed extensively. It appears that superoxide anion itself is not very reactive in aqueous solution (Fridovich 1978). Its preferred reaction under conditions which normally prevail in tissue fluids is the dismutation reaction with itself. The product of this dismutation reaction is hydrogen peroxide. Hydrogen peroxide is not a true radical, but because of its high reactivity and its ability to produce tissue injury is usually considered along with other oxygen radicals. Superoxide and hydrogen peroxide can interact in the presence of catalytic iron or other transition metals, such as copper, via the Haber-Weiss reaction, to produce the highly reactive hydroxyl radical. This radical has a very short half-life

Table 2. Cellular effects of oxygen radicals

1. Lipid peroxidation
2. Increased membrane permeability
3. Inhibition of enzymes
4. DNA damage
5. Release of Ca^{2+} stores
6. Mitochondrial destruction
7. Disruption of cytoskeleton

and a correspondingly short range. It is a very powerful oxidative agent. It is known that cerebrospinal fluid contains enough free iron to support the catalysis of the Haber-Weiss reaction and the production of hydroxyl radical in the presence of superoxide and hydrogen peroxide (Gutteridge et al. 1981; 1982).

Oxygen radicals have a number of cellular effects which are listed in Table 2. One or more of these effects can lead to irreversible tissue injury and death. Most of the emphasis with respect to the destructive effects of oxygen radicals on the central nervous system has centered on the ability of the radicals to induce lipid peroxidation. This effect of the radicals alters the characteristics of cell membranes and leads to abnormal reactivity with sometimes destructive effects.

There is considerable evidence that the generation of superoxide and other oxygen radicals is involved in the pathogenesis of the cerebral vascular abnormalities from experimental brain injury. Pretreatment of the brain with topical agents which scavenge oxygen radicals have a protective effect against the vascular damage induced by fluid percussion brain injury. For example, nitroblue tetrazolium, a dye which reacts with superoxide, superoxide dismutase, an enzyme which converts superoxide anion radical to hydrogen peroxide, mannitol, a scavenger of the hydroxyl radical, or a combination of superoxide dismutase with catalase, an enzyme which eliminates hydrogen peroxide, reduce the sustained dilation seen after brain injury and minimize or eliminate the abnormalities in vascular responsiveness and reduce or eliminate the number of endothelial lesions seen after this type of injury (Wei et al. 1981).

Of great practical significance is the fact that the production of superoxide continues for sometime after the occurrence of brain injury. If one intervenes 30 minutes after injury with topical superoxide dismutase and catalase, then the vasodilation and abnormal reactivity to arterial hypocapnia seen at this time are reversed (Kontos and Wei 1985). Similarly, topical SOD and catalase given 30 minutes after injury restore the normal endothelium-dependent responses to acetylcholine and serotonin (Figs. 1, 2). Clearly then, these abnormalities are in part due to continued production of the radicals and can be reversed after treatment with radical scavengers.

Sources of Oxygen Radicals in Experimental Brain Injury

Superoxide anion radical and other oxygen radicals can be produced from a variety of sources. The most common cellular sources are listed in Table 3.

Table 3. Cellular sources of oxygen radicals

1. Univalent reduction of oxygen in mitochondria
2. Oxidative enzymes (xanthine oxidase)
3. Unsaturated fatty acid oxygenation (cyclooxygenase, lipoxygenase)
4. Hemoglobin, myoglobin
5. Leucocytes

Considerable evidence has accumulated that a major source of superoxide in experimental brain injury is the metabolism of arachidonate and other unsaturated free fatty acids, via PGH synthase. This enzyme is a hemoprotein that has two activities. The cyclooxygenase activity is responsible for the conversion of arachidonate to the endoperoxide PGG_2. The hydroperoxidase activity is responsible for the conversion of PGG_2 to another endoperoxide PGH_2. Purified reconstituted PGH synthase is capable of producing superoxide in vitro under suitable conditions (Kukreja et al. 1986). The production of superoxide by this enzyme is due to its hydroperoxidase activity and requires the presence of suitable reducing cosubstrate such as NADH or NADPH. The mechanism of the production of superoxide under these conditions is similar to what has been described for peroxidases in general (Dunford 1987). It involves the interaction of an unstable intermediate form of the enzyme called compound I with NADH or NADPH. This interaction results in the production of the radical forms of NAD and NADP, which then react by a non-enzymatic means with oxygen to produce superoxide. Thus, it is possible for this enzyme to produce superoxide in one location where it is coupled with the appropriate cosubstrate and not in another where the concentration of these substrates is too low. Agents like arachidonate in high concentration or PGG_2 which can function as substrates of the prostaglandin hydroperoxidase are capable of producing brain vessel injury, similar to what is seen in the course of experimental fluid percussion brain injury (Kontos et al. 1980). In addition, pretreatment with non-steroidal anti-inflammatory agents which inhibit cyclooxygenase and thereby deprive the prostaglandin hydroperoxidase of substrate protect the cerebral vessels from experimental brain injury (Wei et al. 1981).

The production of superoxide by PGH synthase occurs in burst-like fashion with a very fast initial rate which is followed by much less pronounced slower subsequent production (Dunford 1987). In view of this kind of characteristic behavior, the continued production of superoxide from this mechanism would require the sequential activation of accelerated arachidonate metabolism in fresh locations. Alternatively, the initial production of the radical may be due to this mechanism and it may then be sustained by the activation of other mechanisms. The efficiency of production of superoxide from PGH synthase is sufficient to make this a credible mechanism for superoxide production. One mole of superoxide is produced for each 10 moles of arachidonate metabolized under ideal conditions. Soybean lipoxygenase is also capable of producing superoxide in the presence of NADH or NADPH, but the efficiency of production is much lower so that this enzyme is not a credible source of superoxide (Kukreja et al. 1986).

We do not know whether lipoxygenase in mammalian tissue behaves similarly to soybean lipoxygenase.

There is strong evidence that in the course of fluid percussion brain injury there is acceleration of unsaturated fatty acid metabolism via PGH synthase. We know that immediately after brain injury, there is an increase in phospholipase C activity which should release free arachidonate from tissue sources (Wei et al. 1982). In the first few minutes after brain injury, there is an increase in prostaglandin concentration in brain tissue, attesting to the release of arachidonate and the acceleration of arachidonate metabolism via PGH synthase (Ellis et al. 1981).

Less well understood are the initial steps which lead to the activation of phospholipases. It is likely that this step is mediated via the generation of polypeptides such as bradykinin. We found that the topical application of a specific bradykinin antagonist inhibits the vascular reactivity alterations caused by fluid percussion brain injury (Ellis et al. in press). Bradykinin activates phospholipase and thereby accelerates arachidonate metabolism and induces the production of superoxide and other oxygen radicals derived from it (Kontos et al. 1985). Bradykinin as well as arachidonate are capable of reproducing the cerebral vascular abnormalities induced by brain injury (Kontos et al. 1984).

The potential role of other sources of oxygen radicals in fluid percussion injury is virtually unknown. Leucocytes and macrophages are worthy of special consideration, because they accumulate in tissues in response to injury and may be a delayed source of oxygen radicals. Their accumulation in brain in response to injury due to radicals begins 3–4 hours later and peaks at about 24 hours (Kontos et al. 1985).

Hemoglobin produces superoxide by autooxidation (Misra and Fridovich, 1972). It also inhibits endothelium-dependent cerebral arteriolar dilation from acetylcholine (Marshall and Kantos 1986). These effects may be important if there is hemorrhage in the course of brain injury.

Vascular Effects of Oxygen Radicals

Oxygen radicals generated topically on the brain surface by a variety of mechanisms cause vascular abnormalities that are similar to those induced by fluid percussion brain injury (Wei et al. 1985). With a short lasting application, they are capable of causing vasodilation due to vascular smooth muscle relaxation. With prolonged application, there is sustained dilation that outlasts the duration of exposure to the radical generated mechanism. There is abnormal reactivity, elimination of endothelium-dependent responses, depression of arteriolar wall oxygen consumption and increased permeability of the blood-brain barrier to macromolecules (Wei et al. 1986).

It is clear that the generation of exogenous oxygen radicals reproduces well the vascular abnormalities of fluid percussion brain injury. These close similarities support the view that oxygen radicals mediate the vascular consequences of brain injury.

Effects of Therapeutic Interventions Directed Against Oxygen Radicals on Mortality from Experimental Brain Injury

We have tested the effect of therapeutic interventions which interfere with the generation or scavenge oxygen radicals on mortality from experimental fluid percussion brain injury in rats. The results of two such studies are summarized in Table 4 which shows that the initial 1–2 hour mortality following brain injury is markedly reduced by pretreatment by superoxide dismutase or with indomethacin (Kim et al. unpublished; LeVasseur et al. unpublished). These studies suggest strongly that therapeutic interventions that are directed against oxygen radicals may be effective in reducing mortality and morbidity in human brain injury.

In selecting the most appropriate agent for human trials, it must be remembered that in addition to effectiveness and safety, the agent must also be able to reach the site of generation of radicals as rapidly as possible. It is conceivable, in fact likely, that the production of radicals would cease after a period of time following brain injury. If the therapeutic intervention directed against radicals is going to be effective, it must be given during this period of time when there is continued production of radicals, otherwise the tissue injury may have already occurred and therapy may be ineffective.

There is, at present, one human trial designed to attack an oxygen radical mediated mechanism in human brain injury which is at an advanced stage of planning. This is the U.S. Army penetrating wound study in which bovine copper-zinc superoxide dismutase coupled with polyethylene glycol (PEG-SOD) will be used in a randomized trial to treat patients with brain gunshot wounds. This enzyme has been shown to be sufficiently non-toxic so that its administration is considered safe. It is not antigenic. The attachment to polyethylene glycol prolongs its half life, a desirable consequence, and probably allows it to penetrate more easily into cells where it retains its activity. The use of superoxide dismutase is advantageous because it will eliminate superoxide irrespective of its origin. It is possible that in different species the source of superoxide may be different, or

Table 4. Effects of treatments directed at oxygen radicals on short-term mortality in rats from experimental fluid percussion brain injury

A Indomethacin[a]	
Control	50
Indomethacin	8
B SOD[b]	
Control	21
SOD	4

[a] Indomethacin was given 15 min before injury 3 mg/kg. Data are from Kim et al. (unpublished)
[b] SOD was given if 24,000 U/kg 5 min before injury and 96,000 U/kg over the first 60 min following injury. Data are from Levasseur et al. (unpublished). Each group comprised 24 rats. Indomethacin trial is based on 1 hr mortality; SOD trial is based on 2 hr mortality.

that multiple sources may be involved. Hence therapeutic interventions which are effective in one species or a specific source may not be effective under different circumstances where the agent used is acting only via inhibition of the production of oxygen radicals from a specific enzymatic pathway.

Another trial is being planned to test the effect of PEG-SOD in a randomized trial in patients with severe brain injuries at the Medical College of Virginia and the University of Maryland Trauma Center. It is expected that the results of these trials would provide the first test of the significance of the oxygen radical mechanism in the abnormalities seen after human brain injury.

Acknowledgement. Supported by grants NS19316 and NS 12587.

References

Adams J, Graham D, Murray L, Scott G (1982a) Diffuse axonal injury due to nonmissile head injury in humans: an analysis of 45 cases. Ann Neurol 12:557–563

Adams S, Mitchell D, Graham D, Doyle D (1982b) Diffuse damage of immediate impact type: its relationship to 'primary brain-stem damage' in head injury. Brain 100:489–502

Binder LM (1986) Persisting symptoms after mild head injury: A review of the post-concussive syndrome. J Clin Exp Neuropsychol 8(4):323–346

DeWitt DS, Jenkins LW, Wei EP, Lutz H, Becker DP, Kontos HA (1986) Effects of fluid percussion brain injury on regional cerebral blood flow and pial vessel diameter. J Neurosurg 64:787–794

Dixon CE, Lyeth BG, Povlishock JT et al. (1987) A fluid percussion model of experimental brain injury in the rat. J Neurosurg 67:110–119

Dunford HB (1987) Free radicals in iron-containing systems. Free Radical Biology & Medicine 3:405–421

Ellis EF, Wright KF, Wei EP, Kontos HA (1981) Cyclooxygenase products of arachidonic acid metabolism in cat cerebral cortex after experimental concussive brain injury. J Neurosurg 56:695–698

Ellis EF, Holt SA, Wei EP, Kontos HA (1989) Kinins induce abnormal vascular reactivity. Am J Physiol (in press)

Fridovich I (1978) The biology of oxygen radicals. Science 201:875–880

Furchgott RF (1983) Role of endothelium in responses for vascular smooth muscle. Circ Res 53:557–573

Graham DI, Lawrence AE, Adams JH, Doyle D, McLellan D, Gennarelli TA (1988) Pathology of mild head injury. In: Hoff J (ed) Mild head injury, vol 3, Contemporary issues in neurological surgery. Blackwell Scientific Publications, Boston

Gutteridge JMC, Rowley DA, Halliwell B (1981) Superoxide-dependent formation of hydroxyl radicals in the presence of iron salts. Biochem J 199:263–265

Gutteridge JMC, Rowley DA, Halliwell B (1982) Superoxide-dependent formation of hydroxyl radicals and lipid peroxidation in the presence of iron salts. Biochem J 206:605–609

Hayes RL, Pechura CM, Katayama Y et al. (1984) Activation of pontine cholinergic sites implicated in unconsciousness following cerebral concussion in the cat. Science 233:301–303

Jenkins LW, Marmarou A, Lewelt W, Becker DP (1986) Increased vulnerability of the traumatized brain in early ischemia. In: Baethman A, Go KG, Unterberg A (eds) Mechanisms of secondary brain damage. Plenum Press, New York, pp 273–281

Jenkins LW, Moszynski K, Lyeth BG, Lewelt W, DeWitt DS et al. (1989) Increased vulnerability of the mildly traumatized rat brain to cerebral ischemia: The use of controlled second insult as a research tool. Brain Res (in press)

Kim HJ, Levasseur JE, Patterson JL Jr, Madge GE, Povlishock JT, Kontos HA (1989) Reduction in mortality in experimental brain injury by pretreatment with indomethacin. J Neurosurg (submitted)

Kontos HA, Wei EP (1985) Superoxide production in experimental brain injury. J Neurosurg 64:803–807

Kontos HA, Wei EP, Povlishock JT, Dietrich WD, Magiera CJ, Ellis EF (1980) Cerebral arteriolar damage by arachidonic acid and prostaglandin G_2. Science 209:1242–1245

Kontos HA, Wei EP, Jenkins LW, Povlishock JT, Rowe GT, Hess ML (1985) Appearance of superoxide anion radical in cerebral extracellular space during increased prostaglandin synthesis in cats. Circ Res 57:142–151

Kontos HA, Wei EP, Povlishock JT, Christman CW (1984) Oxygen radicals mediated the cerebral arteriolar dilation from arachidonate and bradykinin in cats. Circ Res 55:295–303

Kukreja RC, Kontos HA, Hess ML, Ellis EF (1986) PGH synthase and lipoxygenase generate superoxide in the presence of NADH or NADPH. Circ Res 59:612–619

Levasseur JE, Patterson JL Jr, Kontos HA (1989) Major reduction of mortality in severe experimental brain injury with superoxide dismutase. J Neurosurgery (submitted)

Lewelt W, Jenkins LW, Miller JD (1980) Autoregulation of cerebral blood flow after experimental fluid percussion injury of the brain. J Neurosurg 53:500–511

Lewelt W, Jenkins LW, Wei EP, Lutze H, Becker DP, Kontos HA (1983) Effects of fluid percussion brain injury on regional cerebral blood flow and pial vessel diameter. J Neurosurg 56:332–338

Lyeth BG, Jenkins LW, Hamm RJ et al. (1987) Enduring short-term memory deficits in the absence of hippocampal cell death following moderate head injury in the rat. Soc Neur Abstr 13:1253

Marshall JJ, Kontos HA (1986) Independent mechanisms of blockade of endothelial-dependent and nitroprusside-induced cerebral dilation. FASEB J 2:A1290, 1988

Misra HP, Fridovich I (1972) The generation of superoxide radical during the autooxidation of hemoglobin. J Biol Chem 247:3170–3175

Orrenius S (1988) Mechanisms of oxidant-induced cell damage. J Cell Biochem [Suppl] 12A:34

Pilz P (1983) Axonal injury in head injury. Acta Neurochir (Wien) [Suppl] 32:119–123

Povlishock J (1986) Traumatically induced axonal damage without concomitant change in focally related neuronal somata and dendrites. Acta Neuropathol (Berl) 70:53–59

Povlishock JT, Becker DP, Sullivan HG, Miller JD (1978) Vascular permeability alterations to horseradish peroxidase in experimental brain injury. Brain Res 153:223–239

Povlishock JT, Becker DP, Cheng CLY, Vaughan GW (1983) Axonal change in minor head injury. J Neuropathol Exp Neurol 42:225–242

Povlishock JT, Williams JI, Wei EP, Kontos HA (1988) Histochemical demonstration of superoxide in cerebral vessels. FASEB J 2:A835

Rosenblum WI, Wei EP, Kontos HA (1982) Platelet aggregation in cerebral arterioles after percussive brain trauma. J Texas Heart Inst 9:345–348

Strich S (1961) Shearing of nerve fibers as a cause of brain damage due to head injury. Lancet II:443–448

Sullivan HG, Martinez AJ, Becker DP, Miller JD, Griffith R, Wist AO (1976) Fluid-percussion model of mechanical brain injury in the cat. J Neurosurg 45:520–534

Wei EP, Dietrich WD, Povlishock JT, Navari RM, Kontos HA (1980) Functional, morphologic and metabolic abnormalities of the cerebral microcirculation after concussive brain injury in cats. Circ Res 46:37–47

Wei EP, Kontos HA, Dietrich WD, Povlishock JT, Ellis EF (1981) Inhibition by free radical scavengers and by cyclooxygenase inhibitors of pial arteriolar abnormalities from concussive brain injury in cats. Circ Res 48:95–103

Wei EP, Lamb RG, Kontos HA (1982) Increased phospholipase C activity after experimental brain injury. J Neurosurg 56:695–698

Wei EP, Christman CW, Kontos HA, Povlishock JT (1985) Effects of oxygen radicals on cerebral arterioles. Am J Physiol 248:H157–H162

Wei EP, Ellison MD, Kontos HA, Povlishock JT (1986) O_2 radicals in arachidonate-induced increased blood-brain barrier permeability to proteins. Am J Physiol 251:H693–H699

Oxygen Free Radicals in the Genesis
of Traumatic Brain Edema

Y. Ikeda, K.L. Brelsford, K. Ikeda, and D.M. Long

Department of Neurological Surgery, The Johns Hopkins University, School of Medicine, Baltimore, Maryland 21205 (USA)

Introduction

Oxygen free radicals such as superoxide radical, hydrogen peroxide and hydroxyl radical have been implicated as important deleterious factors in ischemia, trauma and inflammation (Bulkley 1983). Oxygen free radicals may damage endothelial cells disrupting the blood-brain barrier or they may directly injure brain, causing cerebral edema and structural changes in neurons and glia. Therefore, oxygen free radical scavengers can potentially be used to treat brain edema. In this study we investigated the effects of superoxide dismutase (SOD) as a superoxide radical scavenger and dimethylthiourea (DMTU) as a hydroxyl radical scavenger on cold-induced edema.

Materials and Methods

Forty-four cats were anesthetized with ketamine hydrochloride, 25 mg/kg intramuscularly, and anesthesia was maintained with a 0.5 ml bolus of IV thiamylal sodium. Brain edema was produced with a 5 mm diameter, pre-chilled metal probe in a standard fashion. Animals for study at 24 and 48 hours were returned to their cages.

Animals were separated into three groups. 1. Cold-induced edema with sacrifice at 6, 24 and 48 hours. 2. Cold-induced edema with SOD treatment: subgroup-A was pretreated with 10000 U/kg polyethylene glycol (PEG) SOD with sacrifice at 24 and 48 hours; subgroup-B received a bolus injection of free SOD (4 mg/kg) and then 1 mg/kg/min for 20 minutes following the lesion with sacrifice at 6 hours. 3. Cold-induced edema with sacrifice at 6 and 24 hours. This group was pretreated with 500 mg/kg DMTU.

Six cats underwent bilateral craniectomy and double cranial windows were put in place based on the method of Kontos and Wei (1986). Immediately following unilateral cold lesion, nitroblue tetrazolium (NBT) in phosphate-buffered saline (PBS: 2 mg/ml) was applied topically and left in contact with brain surface for 1 hour. Animals were sacrificed by transcardiac perfusion with PBS. Detection of superoxide radicals was based upon reduction of NBT.

Brain water content was measured by the specific gravity (SG) method. Brain samples, approximately 1 mm³, were excised and placed onto a kerosene/

Intracranial Pressure VII   799
Eds.: J. T. Hoff and A. L. Betz
© Springer-Verlag Berlin Heidelberg 1989

monobromobenzene column. The position of brain samples was read 5 minutes after the placement of the sample onto the column. Columns were calibrated with NaCl solutions of known SG.

Results

Cold injured brain showed the deposition of reduced NBT which means that cold injury produced superoxide radicals. Free SOD or PEG-SOD did not reduce the brain's water content of the injured side at 6, 24 and 48 hours following injury (Fig. 1). DMTU reduced the development of brain edema in the adjacent white matter to the lesion at 6 hours, but DMTU did not reduce the brain's water content at 24 hours following injury (Fig. 2).

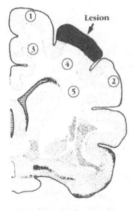

SG Values of 6 Hours Study

Area	SOD Untreated (n=5)	SOD Treated (n=5)
1	1.0466 ± 0.0006	1.0450 ± 0.0026
2	1.0434 ± 0.0026	1.0452 ± 0.0022
3	1.0360 ± 0.0039	1.0354 ± 0.0035
4	1.0344 ± 0.0009	1.0332 ± 0.0013
5	1.0410 ± 0.0027	1.0390 ± 0.0032

SG Values of 24 Hours Study

Area	PEG-SOD Untreated (n=5)	PEG-SOD Treated (n=5)
1	1.0434 ± 0.0027	1.0445 ± 0.0008
2	1.0435 ± 0.0029	1.0434 ± 0.0024
3	1.0340 ± 0.0028	1.0357 ± 0.0045
4	1.0322 ± 0.0012	1.0335 ± 0.0022
5	1.0364 ± 0.0006	1.0374 ± 0.0035

SG Values of 48 Hours Study

Area	PEG-SOD Untreated (n=5)	PEG-SOD Treated (n=5)
1	1.0434 ± 0.0042	1.0429 ± 0.0043
2	1.0448 ± 0.0006	1.0444 ± 0.0016
3	1.0347 ± 0.0031	1.0342 ± 0.0050
4	1.0336 ± 0.0013	1.0317 ± 0.0016
5	1.0370 ± 0.0033	1.0362 ± 0.0036

Values are mean ± SD

Fig. 1. SOD study; Brain sample areas used for specific gravity (SG) measurement and SG values at 6, 24 and 48 hours following cold injury

6 HOURS STUDY

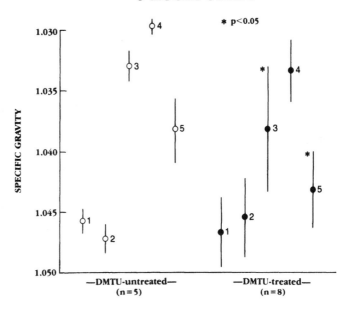

24 HOURS STUDY

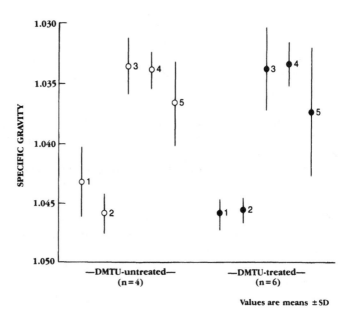

Values are means ± SD

Fig. 2. DMTU study; SG values at 6 and 24 hours following cold injury

Discussion

There is now accumulating evidence that oxygen free radicals play an important role in the pathogenesis of brain edema (Chan et al. 1984; Chan et al. 1987; Kontos and Wei 1986; Long et al. 1972). Such findings suggest that treatment of brain edema with free radical scavengers might have therapeutic significance. This study detected superoxide radicals in the brain following cold-induced injury, but free and PEG-SOD had no beneficial effect on vasogenic brain edema produced by cold-induced injury. Chan et al. (1987) also reported that the intravenous injection of free SOD was not effective. They pointed out several reasons for the failure of free SOD to reduce brain edema. The half-life of free SOD is very short and seems to be unable to cover the prolonged period of development of brain edema. PEG-SOD provides for a prolongation of the half-life of SOD. PEG by itself is a surface active molecule and has been used extensively in molecular biology to promote cell fusion. PEG-SOD consists of free SOD attached to PEG of 5000 daltons. Approximately 36% of PEG-SOD remains in serum after 72 hours and intraperitoneally injected PEG-SOD enters the bloodstream more readily than free SOD. However, PEG-SOD with a prolonged circulation time did not reduce brain edema either. Free SOD with a molecular weight of 31 000 cannot pass through the normal BBB nor penetrate into brain cells. NBT, a polar and water soluble compound, is also unlikely to penetrate into the brain cells.

Kontos and Wei (1986) suggest that superoxide radical is produced by intact cells and escapes into the extracellular space via normal membrane channels. They also emphasized that superoxide radical in the extracellular space is important and necessary for NBT reduction. One can assume that if the Evans blue-albumin complex with a molecular weight of 69 000 could pass the BBB, free SOD with a molecular weight of 31 000 might traverse the BBB and reach the extracellular space, especially in cold injury, and could interact with the postulated superoxide radicals in the extracellular space. Contrary to these expectations, free and PEG-SOD did not reduce brain edema. Oxygen free radicals are produced by both extracellular and intracellular sources: neutrophils, vascular endothelium and mitochondria (Simpson et al. 1987). A major etiology of cell damage is known to be increased intracellular production of oxygen free radicals (Freeman et al. 1983). Chan et al. (1987) showed that free SOD, a negatively charged protein, is almost completely excluded by endothelial cells, but free SOD, when entrapped within liposomes, was taken up by cultured neurons and astrocytes in a time dependent manner. Our data suggest that the lack of intracellular uptake of free or PEG-SOD and the intracellular location of superoxide radicals explain the therapeutic failure. That free and PEG-SOD could not interact with critical intracellular sites of oxygen free radical generation in edema is one possible explanation to be explored. Alternative methods of delivery of free or PEG-SOD into the brain cells must be considered (Chan et al. 1987).

Among oxygen free radicals, the hydroxyl radical is one of the most highly reactive species and is generated from two active oxygen species: superoxide radical and hydrogen peroxide, via the iron-catalyzed Haber-Weiss reaction. Evaluation of role of the hydroxyl radical has been hindered by the fact that there are no oxygen free radical scavenger enzymes and some chemical scavengers available may lack potency or specificity. In this study we used DMTU as a hydroxyl radical scavenger. Bolli et al. (1987) emphasized several favorable effects of DMTU. The effects of DMTU reflect the cytotoxic action of the hydroxyl radical rather than that of superoxide radical or hydrogen peroxide. DMTU is highly permeable and may scavenge oxygen metabolites both intracellularly and extracellularly. DMTU is considerably more effective than other hydroxyl radical scavengers such as mannitol and dimethyl sulfoxide. Pharmacokinetic data demonstrate that DMTU has a relatively long plasma half-life, which seems to be useful in prolonged protection against oxygen free radical-mediated damage. This study showed that DMTU prevented the early development of brain edema in the adjacent white matter to the lesion at 6 hours following the lesion. These findings indicate that oxygen free radicals are generated by the brain following cold injury and the demonstration of these radicals offers an important clue in the genesis of traumatic brain edema.

References

Bolli R, Zhu W-X, Hartley CJ, Michael LH, Repine JB, Hess ML, Kukreja RC, Roberts R (1987) Attenuation of dysfunction in the postischemic stunned myocardium by dimethylthiourea. Circulation 76:458–468

Bulkley GB (1983) The role of oxygen free radicals in human disease processes. Surgery 94:407–411

Chan PH, Schmidler JW, Fishman RA, Longar SM (1984) Brain injury, edema and vascular permeability changes induced by oxygen derived free radicals. Neurology 34:315–320

Chan PH, Longar S, Fishman RA (1987) Protective effects of liposomes entrapped superoxide dismutase on post traumatic brain edema. Ann Neurol 21:540–547

Freeman BA, Young SL, Crapo JD (1983) Liposome mediated augmentation of superoxide dismutase in endothelial cells prevents oxygen injury. J Biol Chem 258:12534–12542

Kontos HA, Wei EP (1986) Superoxide production in experimental brain injury. J Neurosurg 64:803–807

Long DW, Maxwell RE, Choi KS, Cole HO, French LA (1972) Multiple therapeutic approaches in the treatment of brain edema induced by a standard cold lesion. In: Reulen HJ, Schurmann K (eds) Steroids and brain edema. Springer, Berlin Heidelberg New York, pp 87–94

Simpson PJ, Mickelson JK, Lucchesi BR (1987) Free radical scavengers in myocardial ischemia. Fed Proc 46:2413–2421

Reduction of Intracranial Hypertension with Free Radical Scavengers

R.S. Zimmerman[1], J.P. Muizelaar[1], E.P. Wei[2] and H.A. Kontos[2]

[1] Divisions of Neurosurgery and [2] Cardiology, Medical College of Virginia, MCV Station Box 631, Richmond, Virginia 23298 (USA)

Introduction

Intracranial hypertension after severe head injury continues to remain a serious problem affecting morbidity and mortality. Excluding space occupying lesions, the etiology of raised ICP is due to either vascular engorgement (brain swelling) or brain edema. Engorgement occurs when there is a loss of the normal regulation of vascular tone, resulting in cerebrovascular dilatation. Brain edema can occur from increased vascular permeability, producing a vasogenic component of extracellular fluid. Free radical scavengers have demonstrated protective effects against both dilatation and increased permeability of the cerebral vasculature in response to various experimental insults. Based on this evidence, it was postulated that prevention of free radical mediated injury might attenuate the development of intracranial hypertension.

Experiments were performed using a cold lesion model of brain trauma. Previous work has demonstrated that both vasodilatation (Zimmerman et al. 1987) and vasogenic edema (Baethmann 1978, Klatzo 1967) result from this type of injury. A closed cranial window preparation allowed direct observation of the pial microcirculation, and provided a route to administer the free radical scavengers superoxide dismutase (SOD) and catalase.

Methods

Cats were given sodium pentobarbital (30 mg/kg iv) and gallamine triethiodide (5 mg/kg iv) and were placed on a warming blanket at 37° C. Mean arterial blood pressure (MABP), ventricular intracranial pressure (ICP), end-tidal carbon dioxide (ETCO$_2$), and temperature were continuously recorded. Ventilation was controlled using an animal respirator and tracheostomy. Arterial blood gases (ABG) were obtained to assure the presence of physiologic P$_a$O$_2$, P$_a$CO$_2$, and pH.

The animal's head was placed on a stereotactic frame. A left frontal trephination for the cold lesion was made leaving the dura intact. The closed cranial window was situated over the right parietal cortex for visualization of pial vessels and arteriolar diameters were measured with an image-splitting microscope (Levasseur et al. 1975). Thirty minutes before the measurements began, 1 ml of artificial CSF was gently irrigated under the window.

Eds.: J.T. Hoff and A.L. Betz
© Springer-Verlag Berlin Heidelberg 1989

In a control period, normocapnia ($P_aCO_2 = 30$ mm Hg) was maintained and the first set of diameter measurements taken. A 2 minute transdural cold lesion 1 cm^2 in area was then made with a copper rod cooled to $-90\,°C$ with liquid nitrogen. Serial measurements of vessel diameters, MABP, ICP, and P_aCO_2 were taken over the subsequent 3 hours. Animals were sacrificed with an overdose of sodium pentobarbital.

There were 3 groups of animals: (1) control – received no treatment, (2) SOD and catalase – bovine SOD (60 units/ml) and catalase (40 units/ml) (Sigma chemical Co., St. Louis, MO) were added to the artificial CSF instilled under the window, and (3) sham – the rod used to create the lesion was never cooled. The osmolality of both the artificial CSF and the CSF + SOD + catalase solution was 312 mosm/kg.

Statistical Analysis

ANOVA and a Student's t-test were used to analyze differences in vessel diameters and systemic parameters respectively. The chosen alpha level for significance in all tests was $p < 0.05$, and the Bonferonni procedure was used to adjust for multiple comparisons. All values presented refer to a mean ± 1 standard error of the mean.

Results

Heart rate, MABP, and ABG's were equivalent in all groups. Cerebral perfusion pressures (CPP = MABP – ICP) were never less than 80 mm Hg.

No Treatment (13 cats, 105 vessels): At 1 hour ICP had risen significantly from 4.5 to 10.9 mm Hg ($p < 0.05$), and at 3 hours post injury the ICP had a further significant increase to 17.2 mm Hg ($p < 0.05$, Fig. 1). To distinguish the progression of ICP which occurred early vs. late, values of ΔICP were defined as:

Early $\equiv \Delta ICP_{1hr} =$ ICP at 1 hr – ICP pre-injury
Late $\equiv \Delta ICP_{3hr} =$ ICP at 3 hr – ICP pre-injury

The difference between ΔICP_{1hr} and ΔICP_{3hr} (6.4 and 12.7 mm Hg, $p < 0.05$) illustrates that intracranial hypertension late after injury is significantly greater than that which occurs earlier. Significant vasodilatation occurred at 1 hour, with a 13% increase in arteriolar diameter ($p < 0.05$). By three hours, the vessels had recovered from this dilatation, and approximated their baseline diameter (Fig. 2). It appeared that the dilatation in response to injury was brief, in comparison to the changes in ICP, which were persistent and progressive.

SOD/catalase (5 cats, 43 vessels): After 1 hour, ICP had significantly increased from 4.4 to 10.6 mm Hg ($p < 0.05$). 3 hours after injury the ICP was a value not significantly different from that seen at 1 hour (12.6 mm Hg, $p < 0.05$, Fig. 1). In this group, the differences between early and late progression of ICP were

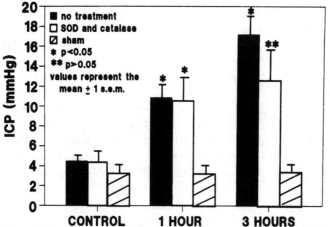

Fig. 1. ICP response post-injury. Values represent the mean ± 1 SEM

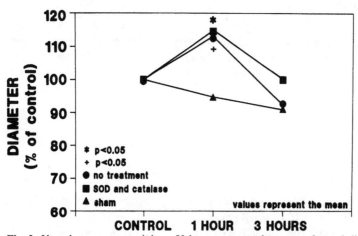

Fig. 2. Vascular response to injury. Values represent the mean of vessel diameters as a percent of control

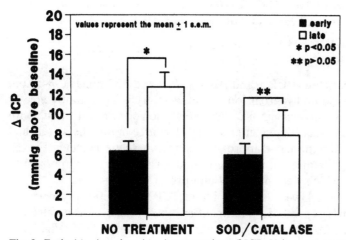

Fig. 3. Early ($\Delta_{1\,hr}$) vs. late ($\Delta_{3\,hr}$) progression of ICP. Values represent the mean ± 1 SEM

not significant, as $\Delta ICP_{1hr} = 6.0$ mm Hg, while $\Delta ICP_{3hr} = 8.0$ mm Hg ($p < 0.05$). Significant vasodilation did occur, with a 15% increase in diameter ($p < 0.05$). Just as in the first group, this dilatation was short-lived, and by three hours after injury, vessel diameters were again at their pre-injury level (Fig. 2).

Comparisons between groups 1 and 2 reveal that there was no differences in the degree of vasodilatation between groups at either 1 or 3 hours (Fig. 2). Figure 3 shows the protection afforded by SOD and catalase late after injury.

SHAM (5 cats, 33 vessels): There was no rise in ICP, and ΔICP_{1hr} and ΔICP_{3hr} were insignificant at 0 and 0.2 mm Hg respectively. No vasodilatation occurred.

Discussion

Elevated intracranial pressure can provide a secondary insult to the traumatized brain. Thus a patient who sustains a primary brain injury will have a poorer prognosis if recovery is marked by significant elevations in ICP (Becker et al. 1977). In a recent study of severe head injury (Marmarou et al. 1987), aggressive measures including mannitol, hyperventilation, CSF drainage, and barbiturates were still unable to control elevations of ICP, and 20% of the population studied died from progressive neurological deterioration.

Current therapies used to reduce elevated ICP address both the intravascular volume and edema components of increased intracranial volume. Hyperventilation, barbiturate coma, and hypothermia are able to reduce ICP by influencing intravascular volume. The former has a direct vasoconstrictor effect via increased pH on the cerebral vasculature, while the latter two reduce the brain's oxygen requirements, causing a reduction in vessel diameter and blood flow when metabolic autoregulation is intact. Mannitol and other osmotic agents are felt to act primarily by reducing the water content of the brain. However, none of the above modalities are prophylactic against the development of intracranial hypertension.

A disruption of the normal cerebrovascular milieu can be seen as a common pathway for the development of intracranial hypertension. In cases where the normal regulation of vascular tone is lost, vasodilatation results. The subsequent lowering of cerebrovascular resistance with an increased cerebral blood flow (CBF) has been regarded by several investigators as hyperemia, and can cause elevated ICP (Langfitt et al. 1966, Miller 1982, Obrist et al. 1984). As well, a breakdown of the blood brain barrier with the resultant "leak" of intravascular fluid and protein into brain tissue occurs after brain injury, and may constitute vasogenic edema (Baethmann 1978, Klatzo 1967). It has been shown that oxygen free radicals can be involved in the genesis of both these events (Chan et al. 1986, Kontos et al. 1984), and are formed after traumatic brain injury (Kontos and Wei 1986). These findings provided the impetus for a trial of free radical scavengers to prevent the development of intracranial hypertension. In the group with no treatment, the amount of ICP elevation which developed after 3 hours (ΔICP_{3hr} was significantly higher than that occurring after 1 (ΔICP_{1hr}). However, when pre-treated with SOD and catalase, there was no significant progression of intracranial hypertension after the first hour.

Gross examination of the brains revealed no mass lesions. Vasodilatation was present as the intracranial pressure began to rise. With an increase in diameter of 13–15%, intracranial blood volume would theoretically increase 30% in the arteriolar bed. Early progression of ICP (ΔICP_{1hr}) is thus due to the increase in intravascular volume plus the effects of early edema formation. However, as the vasodilatation was transient and resolved by three hours, late progression of elevated ICP in this model is likely to be due to the continuing generation of edema. The lack of a significant late progression of ICP in the treated group is, therefore, felt to represent reduction of edema generation caused by free radical damage.

Conclusion

Using the cold lesion model of brain injury, we found a significant transient arteriolar dilatation at 1 hour which resolves by 3 hours. Intracranial pressure was also significantly elevated at 1 hour, but continued to progress throughout 3 hours. It is therefore felt that the early progression in ICP is due to both an increase in intravascular volume and some early edema formation. The late progression of ICP is unaccompanied by vasodilatation, and is thus predominantly due to continued edema generation alone. Pre-treatment with the free radical scavengers SOD and catalase have no protective effect regarding vasodilatation. However, there is a significant reduction in the late progression of ICP when SOD and catalase are administered prior to the injury. It is, therefore, hypothesized that the development and progression of intracranial hypertension in head injured patients may be reduced through the use of agents which scavenge free radicals, most likely by attenuating edema formation.

Acknowledgements. This research has been supported by grants NS-19316, NS-12587, and NS-19364 from the National Institutes of Health.

References

Baethmann A (1978) Pathophysiological and pathochemical aspects of cerebral edema. Neurosurg Rev 1:85–100
Becker DP, Miller JD, Ward JD (1977) The outcome from severe head injury with early diagnosis and intensive management. J Neurosurg 47:491–502
Chan P, Fishman RA, Longar S (1986) Liposome-entrapped superoxide following traumatic brain injury. Soc Neurosci Abst 12:38
Klatzo I (1967) Neuropathological aspects of brain edema. J Neuropathol Exp Neurol 26:1–14
Kontos HA, Wei EP (1986) Superoxide production in experimental brain injury. J Neurosurg 64:803–807
Kontos HA, Wei EP, Povlishock JT, Christman CW (1984) Oxygen radicals mediate the cerebral arteriolar dilation from arachidonate and bradykinin in cats. Circ Res 55:295–303
Langfitt TW, Tannenbaum HM, Kassell NF (1966) The etiology of acute brain swelling. J Neurosurg 24:47–56
Levasseur JE, Wei EP, Raper AJ, Kontos HA, Patterson JL (1975) Detailed description of a cranial window technique for acute and chronic experiments. Stroke 6:308–317

Marmarou A, Maset AL, Ward JD, Choi S, Brooks D, Lutz HA, Moulton RJ, Muizelaar JP, DeSalles A, Young HF (1987) Contribution of CSF and vascular factors to elevation of ICP in severely head-injured patients. J Neurosurg 66:883–890

Miller JD (1982) Disorders of cerebral blood flow and intracranial pressure after head injury. Clin Neurosurg 29:162–173

Obrist WD, Langfitt TW, Jaggi JL, Cruz J, Gennarelli TA (1984) Cerebral blood flow and metabolism in comatose patients with acute head injury: Relationship to intracranial hypertension. J Neurosurg 61:241–253

Zimmerman RS, Muizelaar JP, Wei EP, Kontos HA (1987) Acute cerebral arteriolar responses following cold injury. In: Cervos-Nevarro J, Ferszt R (eds) Stroke and microcirculation. Raven Press, New York, pp 303–309

Allopurinol and Dimethylthiourea Limit Infarct Size in Partial Ischemia

R.D. Martz[1], G. Rayos[1], G.P. Schielke[1], and A.L. Betz[2]

[1] Departments of Surgery, [2] Pediatrics and Neurology, University of Michigan, Ann Arbor, Michigan 48 109-0718 (USA)

Introduction

Toxic oxygen metabolites such as superoxide and hydrogen peroxide are produced as a normal part of cellular metabolism. These compounds, as well as their breakdown products, may act to injury the macromolecular components of the cellular cytoplasm and membrane. Under normal circumstances, adequate intracellular defense mechanisms are present to neutralize these toxic species. However, in settings of tissue ischemia, these buffers may be used up, allowing direct attack of free radicals on cellular constituents. This interaction can result in cell injury and death.

Free radical effects have been well described in organ systems other than the central nervous system. Pretreatment with free radical scavengers prior to ischemic insult has minimized the damage due to ischemia in tissue injury models including kidney (Paller et al. 1984), intestine (Granger et al. 1981) and heart (Jolly et al. 1984). The protective effect is most marked in models of ischemia with reperfusion. Free radical injury in partial ischemia has been less well studied. We will present evidence to suggest a role for free radical mediated injury in central nervous system tissue. Further, our results suggests that free radicals are indeed involved in partial ischemia and that pretreatment with appropriate free radical scavengers can effectively reduce injury in a model of continuous partial ischemia, middle cerebral artery occlusion (MCAO) in the rat.

Methods

Three hundred to 350 gram male Sprague-Dawley rats were treated with dimethylthiourea (DMTU) (750 mg/kg i.p.) one hour prior to occlusion of a 10 mm segment of middle cerebral artery. Fox (1984) has shown that this dose of DMTU results in serum and tissue levels similar to those shown to adequately scavenge the hydroxyl radical in in vitro settings. Control animals received vehicle alone, which in this instance was saline. A second group of animals received allopurinol (100 mg/kg) 48, 24 and one hour prior to MCAO. Allopurinol was delivered intra-gastrically as a suspension in 2% carboxymethylcellulose. Controls received vehicle alone. For each drug, treatment and control groups contained ten animals each.

Intracranial Pressure VII
Eds.: J. T. Hoff and A. L. Betz
© Springer-Verlag Berlin Heidelberg 1989

Twenty-four hours following MCAO, animals were sacrificed by decapitation while under anesthesia with ketamine (30 mg/kg) and xylazine (25 mg/kg). Prior to sacrifice, a femoral artery cannula was inserted for determination of physiological parameters. Treatment and control groups were similar with respect to body temperature, blood pressure, hematocrit, pH and blood gases. After measurement of these parameters, brains were rapidly removed, sectioned and then stained with triphenyltetrazolium chloride (TTC). For sectioning, brains were positioned on a Starrett tissue slicer and 10 consecutive one millimeter sections were taken, beginning approximately 2 mm posterior to the frontal pole. Immediately after sectioning at one millimeter intervals, the slices were removed and placed into phosphate buffered 1% TTC solution. Stained slices were photographed after 45 minutes incubation at room temperature. Volume of infarction was determined by computer assisted planimetry. The area of unstained tissue was compared to total hemisphere area. Since each slice was one millimeter thick, the total infarct volume (mm^3) and hemisphere volume could be calculated by summing the respective area measurements (mm^2) of the ten slices.

Results and Discussion

A variety of free radical generating systems exists (McCord 1985; Demopoulos et al. 1980). Many of these have been shown to contribute to free radical generation in ischemia-reperfusion. The most potent end product of these free radical producing reactions appears to be the hydroxyl radical. It is formed by the combination of superoxide with hydrogen peroxide in a trace metal catalyzed reaction (Halliwell and Gutteridge 1986). Because this species is an end product common to most free radical reactions, we chose DMTU, a scavenger of the hydroxyl radical to test for free radical generation in partial ischemia. Following DMTU pretreatment, the volume of infarcted tissue was reduced by 29%. Data were also compared on a slice by slice basis as shown in Fig. 1. The most significant protection was obtained between five and eight millimeters from the frontal pole. This area is primarily supplied by the middle cerebral artery.

As mentioned above, a number of potential free radical generating systems exist in normal cerebral tissue (Demopoulos et al. 1980). Scavenging of the hydroxyl radical, the end product of these reactions, results in significant tissue salvage in our model. This result implies that free radicals do play a role in situations of continuous partial cerebral ischemia. It has been previously shown that the xanthine oxidase system is important in free radical generation in intestine and heart (Parks et al. 1982; Werns et al. 1986). In situations of ischemia, high energy phosphates are degraded to hypoxanthine and xanthine while xanthine dehydrogenase is converted to xanthine oxidase. When an appropriate amount of oxygen is supplied to the system, superoxide may be produced as a byproduct of the breakdown of hypoxanthine to uric acid (McCord 1985). Xanthine oxidase activity has been shown to be present in normal rat brain. Further, this activity is enriched in the capillary fraction (Betz 1985). Brain capillaries, therefore, contain an enzyme capable of free radical generation. Once produced in the capillary, free radicals could diffuse to injure cerebral tissue directly or cause damage

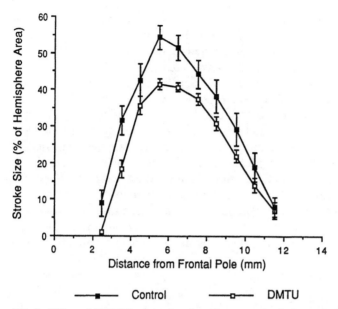

Fig. 1. Effect of DMTU on stroke size. The percent of the cross sectional area of the right hemisphere which did not stain with TTC is shown for each of 10 slices in control or DMTU treated animals. Data are averages of the results from 10 animals in each group and are shown ± standard error

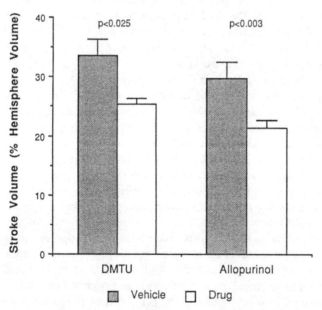

Fig. 2. Effect of DMTU and allopurinol on total stroke volume. The cross sectional area of the hemisphere which did not stain with TTC was determined for each of 10 brain slices one millimeter in thickness. The results were then summed to obtain stroke volume. Data from the 10 vehicle-treated and 10 drug-treated animals in each group were averaged and are shown ± standard error. Statistical significance of differences between control and treated groups were determined with Wilcoxon's rank sum test

indirectly through compromise of capillary function. Because of the previously demonstrated role of xanthine oxidase in ischemia reperfusion injury in other organ systems and its presense in cerebral tissue, we next examined the effect of inhibition of this enzyme on ischemic injury in our model. Protection was similar to that observed for DMTU treated animals. Again, this effect was most prominent in areas of brain supplied by the middle cerebral artery.

As shown in Fig. 2, reduction in infarct size was similar for allopurinol and DMTU treated groups. Stroke volume was reduced approximately 30 percent by both therapies. This finding of similar reduction in stroke volume with a generalized free radical scavenger, dimethylthiourea, and a specific inhibitor of one of the known free radical generating systems implies that, in our model, xanthine oxidase is the primary free radical generating system.

The xanthine oxidase system may not be of equal importance in all species. Studies in rabbit heart, a tissue lacking xanthine oxidase activity, have shown no reduction in infarct size following allopurinol pretreatment. However, in the same system, the generalized scavenger superoxide dismutase reduced infarct size significantly (Downey et al. 1987). Therefore, although the free radical generating system may vary from species to species, the contribution of these toxic compounds to ischemic injury remains significant.

In summary, free radical species appear to be important in injury associated with partial cerebral ischemia. Although several putative free radical generating systems exist, the xanthine oxidase system appears to be of primary importance in the rat model of middle cerebral artery occlusion.

References

Betz AL (1985) Identification of hypoxanthine transport and xanthine oxidase activity in brain capillaries. J Neurochem 44:574–579

Demopoulos HB, Flamm ES, Pietronigro DD, Seligman ML (1980) The free radical pathology and the microcirculation in the major central nervous system disorders. Acta Physiol Scand [Suppl] 492:91–119

Downey JM, Miura T, Eddy LJ, Chambers DE, Mellert T, Hearse DJ, Yellon DM (1987) Xanthine oxidase is not a source of free radicals in the ischemic rabbit heart. J Mol Cell Cardiol 19:1053–1060

Fox RB (1984) Prevention of granulocyte-mediated oxidant lung injury in rats by a hydroxyl radical scavenger, dimethylthiourea. J Clin Invest 74:1456–1464

Granger DN, Rutili G, McCord JM (1981) Superoxide radicals in feline intestinal ischemia. Gastroenterology 81:22–29

Halliwell B, Gutteridge JMC (1986) Oxygen free radicals and iron in relation to biology and medicine: some problems and concepts. Arch Biochem Biophys 246:501–514

Jolly SR, Kane WJ, Bailic MB, Abrams GD, Lucchesi BR (1984) Canine myocardial reperfusion injury: its reduction by the combined administration of superoxide dismutase and catalase. Circ Res 54:277–285

McCord JM (1985) Oxygen-derived free radicals in postischemic tissue injury. N Engl J Med 312:159–163

Paller MS, Hoidal JR, Ferris TF (1984) Oxygen free radicals in ischemic acute renal failure in the rat. J Clin Invest 74:1156–1164

Parks DA, Bulkley GB, Granger DN, Hamilton SR, McCord JM (1982) Ischemic injury in the cat small intestine: role of superoxide radicals. Gastroenterology 82:9–15

Werns SW, Shea MJ, Mitsos SE, Dysko RC, Fantone JC, Schork MA, Abrams GD, Pitt B, Lucchesi BR (1986) Reduction of the size of infarction by allopurinol in the ischemic-reperfused canine heart. Circulation 73:518–524

The Effect of Superoxide Dismutase on Rabbit Brain Reperfusion Injury

D.P. Christenberry, E. Tasdemiroglu, J.L. Ardell, R. Chronister, P.W. Curreri, and A.E. Taylor

Departments of Physiology, General Surgery and Anatomy, University of South Alabama, Mobile, Alabama 36688 (USA)

Damage to the microvasculature after transient ischemia and subsequent reperfusion has been shown in several organ systems (small intestines, heart, skeletal muscle, and liver) to be mediated at least partially through the generation of oxygen-derived free radicals (Granger and Korthuis 1986; Romson et al. 1983; Taylor 1986). Recent data has suggested a similar role for these highly reactive and destructive molecules during states of cerebral hypoperfusion, hypertension or contusion (Cerchiuri et al. 1987; Demopoulos et al. 1980; Kontos et al. 1981; Kontos 1986; Taylor 1986; Wei et al. 1981). Only a limited amount of information, however, is available concerning the vascular injury produced within focal areas of brain rendered ischemic and then subjected to reperfusion. We have developed a rabbit model which measures microvascular damage within the central nervous system by quantitating the amount of albumin-dye complex that crosses the normally occlusive blood-brain barrier (Tasdemiroglu et al. 1988). Using this model, we have begun to study the role of oxygen-derived free radical species in the damage to the brain microvasculature by utilizing the oxyradical scavenging enzyme, superoxide dismutase (SOD).

Materials and Methods

New Zealand white rabbits were anesthetized with 40 mg/kg of ketamine hydrochloride and 25 mg/kg of thorazine given intramuscularly. The animals were then mechanically ventilated on room air via a cervical tracheostomy to maintain arterial blood gases within normal ranges. Intraoperative anesthesia and paralysis were maintained with sodium pentobarbital (20 mg/kg/hr) and pancuronium bromide (0.6 mg/kg/hr) administered intravenously. Cannulas were then placed into the left atrium and into the abdominal aorta for blood pressure monitoring and periodic blood sampling. Cerebral blood flows were calculated by the reference organ technique utilizing a left atrial injection of 15 micron microspheres (Ce 141, Sc 46, Sr 85) during concurrent withdrawal of arterial blood samples from the descending aorta (Granger 1981).

To isolate cerebral vessels for subsequent occlusion, a globe was decompressed and the orbital contents removed unilaterally thereby exposing the optic nerve and its cranial hiatus. The optic hiatus was expanded with a high speed drill to create a retro-orbital defect that exposed the dura mater covering the middle

Eds.: J. T. Hoff and A. L. Betz

cerebral, the (azygous) anterior cerebral and intracranial internal carotid arteries. The dura was incised and reflected and the arachnoid membrane surrounding these vessels was dissected to fully expose them. A control blood flow measurement was then performed by injection of the first radioactive microspheres.

After adequate exposure had been obtained and a control microsphere blood flow determination completed, aneurysm clips were placed on these vessels to occlude them for a period of 60 minutes. A second microsphere injection, and thus blood flow determination, was made 40 minutes into this period to determine cerebral blood flow during the ischemic phase of the experiment. After 50 minutes of ischemia had elapsed (and 10 minutes prior to reperfusion) either copper zinc bovine superoxide dismutase (SOD, 8 mg/kg) or an equal volume of normal saline was infused intravenously. After one hour ischemia, the aneurysm clips were removed and perfusion through these vessels was re-established. Fifteen minutes after clip removal a third and final microsphere injection was performed to determine cerebral blood flow during the reperfusion phase. Twenty minutes after clip removal, Evan's blue dye, in a concentration of 30 mg/kg, was infused intravenously and allowed to circulate for an additional hour. At this concentration, the dye is completely bound to plasma albumin (Rappoport et al. 1972).

Following completion of the 80 minute reperfusion phase, the animals were sacrificed with a bolus of pentobarbital (200 mg/kg) and the kidneys and brain were harvested. After a 48 hr fixation period in sucrose-formalin solution, the brains were frozen and sectioned in a rostral to caudal fashion with alternate 50 and 500 micron sections taken for quantitation of cerebral dye leakage and blood flow, respectively. Renal and cerebral blood flow determinations were made using the reference organ technique, quantitating the levels of gamma radiation in the respective tissues and blood samples (Granger 1981).

The 50 micron sections were mounted and examined under a Lietz microspectrofluorometer. The tissue sections were exposed to light of a wavelength of 530–560 nanometers (nm). This range excites the dye and causes it, in turn, to emit light of a wavelength of 580 nm which is quantitated by the photometer. The amount of light emitted with this wavelength is directly proportional to the amount of dye present in the tissue section. Paired observations were made between occluded and unoccluded hemispheres with results normalized to relative dye leakage (epifluorescence) in the hemisphere with the unoccluded circulation, i.e. [epifluorescence occluded hemisphere/epifluorescence unoccluded hemisphere].

Results

Figures 1 and 2 summarize the induced changes in cerebral blood flow and relative leakage for both the control and SOD treated animals. Arterial blood gases, body temperatures and blood pressures were not different between both experimental groups. In both the control and the SOD treated groups the blood flow during the ischemic period was significantly less within the hemisphere subjected to occlusion relative to the contralateral, non-occluded hemisphere. In

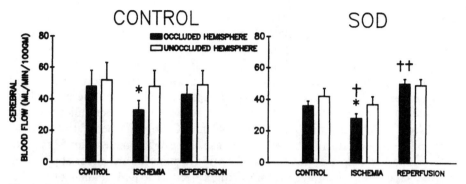

Fig. 1. Cerebral blood flows in the occluded (*filled bars*) and the unoccluded (*open bars*) hemispheres during the control, ischemic and reperfusion periods. *Stars* (*) indicate significant differences ($p < 0.05$) in the flows between occluded hemispheres and unoccluded hemispheres. *Crosses* ($+ = p < 0.1$ and $++ = p < 0.05$) indicate significant differences in the blood flows between control and either ischemic or reperfusion periods within the same hemispheres

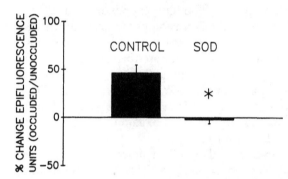

Fig. 2. Comparison of the amount of albumin-dye leakage into the extravascular space as determined by microspectrofluorometric assay. Paired observations were made between the occluded and unoccluded hemispheres with the results normalized to relative dye leakage (epifluorescence) in the hemisphere with the unoccluded arterial inflow. *Star* (*) indicate $p < 0.001$ between control and SOD treated groups

addition to the decrease in blood flow in conjunction with unilateral occlusion, significant changes in regional blood flow were evident upon reperfusion, especially for the SOD group. Note the profound hyperemia in both the occluded and unoccluded hemispheres in the SOD treated animals during the reperfusion period. Such hyperemia was not evident in the control group.

Examination of the brains of the control group with light microscopy revealed the dye to be confined to the intravascular space in the hemispheres not subjected to inflow interruption. This finding was in contrast to the extensive distribution of the albumin-dye complex into the extravascular space within the occluded hemispheres (Fig. 2). Microspectrofluorometric assay for the dye complex confirmed these findings with an increase of approximately 50% in dye extravasation being noted in the occluded, as compared to the unoccluded, hemispheres. In the SOD treated group, however, the dye remained intravascular when examined either macroscopically, with the light microscope, or by microspectrofluorometric techniques.

Conclusions

Transient occlusion of the intracranial internal carotid, middle cerebral and anterior cerebral arteries damages the blood brain barrier. Following 60 minutes of unilateral focal ischemia, the relative transcapillary leakage of the Evan's blue-albumin complex is increased approximately 50%. Administration of the free radical scavenging enzyme superoxide dismutase prevents the increase in cerebral microvascular permeability associated with ischemia/reperfusion injury. SOD also causes an exacerbated hyperemia upon reperfusion.

The brain's microvasculature is damaged by transient ischemia with reperfusion. This damage to the endothelium appears to be mediated to a significant extent through oxygen derived free radicals as reflected by the protective effect afforded by superoxide dismutase.

Acknowledgement. Research supported by the American Heart Association NIH HL-22 549 and GM-08 154.

References

Cerchiuri EL, Hoel TL, Safar P et al. (1987) Protective effects of combined superoxide dismutase and deferoxamine on recovery of cerebral blood flow and function after cardiac arrest in dogs. Stroke 18:869–878

Demopoulos HB, Flamm ES, Pietronigro DD, Seligman ML (1980) The free radical pathology and the microcirculation in the major central nervous system disorders. Acta Physiol Scand 492:91–119

Granger DN (1981) Measurement of blood flow. In: Granger DN, Bulkley GB (eds) Williams and Wilkins, Baltimore

Granger DN, Korthuis RJ (1986) Ischemia-reperfusion injury: Role of oxygen-derived free radicals. In: Taylor AE, Matalon S, Ward PA (eds) Physiology of oxygen radicals. Williams and Wilkins, Baltimore, pp 207–216

Kontos HA (1986) Oxygen radicals in cerebral vascular responses. In: Taylor AE, Matalon S, Ward PA (eds) Physiology of oxygen radicals. Williams and Wilkins, Baltimore, pp 207–216

Kontos HA, Wei EP, Dietrich WD et al. (1981) Mechanism of cerebral arteriolar abnormalities after acute hypertension. Am J Physiol 240:H511–H527

Rappoport SI, Hori M, Klatzo I (1972) Testing a hypothesis for osmotic opening of the blood brain barrier. Am J Physiol 223:323–331

Romson JL, Hook BG, Kunkel SL (1983) Reduction of the extent of ischemic myocardial injury by neutrophil depletion in the dog. Circulation 67:1016–1023

Tasdemiroglu E et al. (1988) Ischemia-reperfusion injury in the rabbit brain. Intracranial pressure and brain injury: The 7th International Symposium

Taylor AE (1986) Physiology of oxygen radicals. In: Taylor AE, Matalon S, Ward PA (eds) Williams and Wilkins, Baltimore

Wei EP, Kontos HA, Dietrich WD et al. (1981) Inhibition by free radical scavengers and cyclooxygenase inhibitors of pial arteriolar abnormalities from concussive brain injury in cats. Circ Res 48:95–103

The Role of Catecholamine-Induced Lipid Peroxidation and Histamine in Ischemic Brain Edema

H. Morooka[1], H. Sasayama[1], K. Sakai[1], S. Namba[1], and A. Nishimoto[2]

Department of Neurological Surgery, [1] Okayama Rosai Hospital, and Okayama University,
[2] Medical School, Okayama 702 (Japan)

Introduction

The purpose of the present study was to investigate the pathogenesis of cerebral microcirculatory disturbances caused by toxic oxygen radicals (O_2^-, $\cdot OH$, H_2O_2) in the dynamics of brain ischemia and subsequent brain edema by simultaneous examination of the role of active oxygen formed in the platelets and the auto-oxidation of catecholamines and the involvement of norepinephrine (NE), acetylcholine (ACh), and histamine in the changes in cerebrovascular permeability.

Materials and Methods

Cerebral ischemia was produced in male Wistar rats by a right intracarotid injection of plastic microspheres (35 μm in diameter) and arachidonic acid (AA, 5 mM, 25 μl). The brain was fixed by freezing with liquid nitrogen before the injection of the microspheres and then 1, 2, 3 and 4 hr after the injection, after which it was subjected to biochemical analysis. Tissue dopamine-β-hydroxylose (DβH) activity was measured by a partial modification of the method of Nagatsu et al. (Morooka 1978). Tissue α-tocopherol, glutathione (GSSG/GSH), malonyl-dialdehyde (MDA), histamine, and ACh concentrations were measured by the method of Abe et al. (1975); Hissin et al. (1975); Ohkawa et al. (1979); Anton et al. (1969); and Asano et al. (1986), respectively. Histochemical demonstration of NE and histamine were by the method of Kimura et al. (1979); and Ehinger et al. (1968), respectively. For the measurement of water content in the brain, the lyophilization method was used.

Rats were divided into three groups. The first was the control group. The second group was treated with 0.2 mg 6-hydroxydopamine (6-OHDA) injected by cisternal puncture 48 hr before the experiment. The third group was treated with bifemelane hydrochloride (Celeport, 25 mg/kg, i.p.) 1 hr before embolization.

Results

The water content of the brain tissue on the embolized side in untreated rats increased gradually after the stroke and 4 h after stroke was $81.5 \pm 1.8\%$, which was significantly higher than that of the controls, $77 \pm 1.0\%$ ($p < 0.05$). DβH activity, NE fluorescence, α-tocopherol concentration, and ACh concentration in

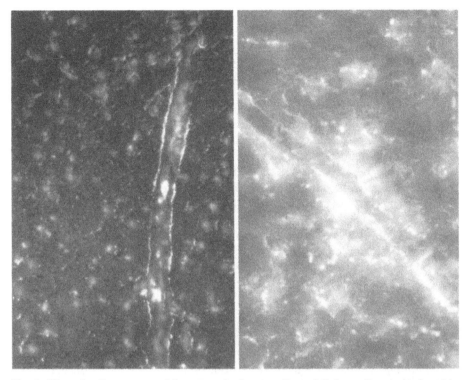

Fig. 1. Histamine fluorescence of the rat cerebral cortex. Control (*left panel*), untreated rat 2 hr after stroke (*right panel*)

the embolized hemisphere decreased immediately after stroke and remained low for the entire 4 hr. MAD concentration and GSSG/GSH in the embolized hemisphere gradually increased up to 2 hr, but had returned to normal by 4 hr after the stroke. Histamine concentration in the embolized hemisphere gradually increased to three times control levels by 4 hr after the stroke. This was associated with increased intensity of histamine fluorescence of the deep penetrating vessels (Fig. 1). Microscopic findings demonstrated marked edema in the untreated rat brain 2 hr after the stroke, while pathological changes in the 6-OHDA-treated rat brain 2 hr after the stroke as well as in the bifemelane hydrochloride-treated rat brain after the stroke were absent or minimal. The increase in MDA level after stroke was attenuated by treatment with bifemelane hydrochloride. The decrease in the ACh level after the stroke as well as that of NE fluorescence, was inhibited by treatment with bifemelane hydrochloride.

Discussion

In our experiment, α-tocopherol and GSH were consumed after ischemia, while MDA in the brain tissue increased for more than 2 hr after ischemia, which suggests that lipid peroxidation by a free radical reaction lasted for more than 2 hr after ischemia, causing membrane damage. TXA_2, ADP, and 5HT are

819

released from platelets by Ca^{2+}-dependent actinomyosin contraction, and platelets aggregate successively in a cascade in cooperation with the active oxygen formed. As a result of an increase in sympathetic activity in the vascular wall, NE and DβH are released from the nerve endings into the blood by exocytosis, and the auto-oxidation of this catecholamine also forms active oxygen (Singal et al. 1983). The oxidation of 6-OHDA is believed to be the basis for its ability to selectively destroy catecholamine nerve terminals. Befemelane hydrochloride has the ability to inhibit the release of NE from the nerve terminals, which may be secondary to the preservation of ACh levels following ischemia (Vanhoutte 1974).

In our experimental model of cerebral infarction caused by platelet aggregation with AA in rats subjected to pretreatment with 6-OHDA or bifemelane hydrochloride, edema in the area of infarction and around the blood vessels were totally absent or slight compared with those in rats with infarction and no treatment.

In addition, it was believed that the formation of histamine was accelerated by free radicals and/or the reduction of sympathetic activity, and increased the macromolecular permeability to the blood-brain barrier (BBB) leading to vasogenic edema.

Summary

Oxidation products of catecholamines may play an important role in microcirculatory damage caused by lipid peroxidation following stroke, and accumulation of histamine in brain tissue may increase the macromolecular permeability of the BBB leading to the vasogenic edema.

References

Abe K, Yukuchi Y, Katui (1975) Quantitative determination of tocopherols by high speed liquid chromatography. J Nutr Sci Vitaminol (Tokyo) 21:183–188

Anton AH, Sayre DF (1969) A modified fluorometric procedure for tissue histamine and its distribution in various animals. J Pharmacol Exp Ther 166:285–292

Asano M, Miyauchi T, Kato T (1986) Determination of acetylcholine and choline in rat brain tissue by liquid chromatography/electrochemistry using an immobilized enzyme post column reactor. J Liq Chromatogr 9:199–215

Ehinger B, Hakanson R, Owmar C (1968) Histochemical demonstration of histamine paraffin sections by fluorescence method. Biochem Pharmacol 17:1997–1998

Hissin P, Hilf R (1979) A fluorometric method for determination of oxidized and reduced glutathione in tissues. Anal Biochem 74:214–226

Kimura H, Nagai T, Iamoto K (1979) A sensitive wet-histo-fluorescence method by glyoxylic acid for central catecholamine terminals. Acta Histochem Cytochem 20th Anniv Meet JSHC Kyoto, p 571

Morooka H (1978) Cerebral arterial spasm I. Adrenergic mechanism in experimental cerebral vasospasm. Acta Med Okayama 32:23–37

Ohkawa H, Ohishi N, Yagi K (1979) Assay for lipid peroxides in animal tissues by tiobarbituric acid reaction. Anal Biochem 95:351–358

Singal PK, Beamish RE, Dhalla NS (1983) Potential oxidative pathways of catecholamines in the formation of lipid peroxides and genesis of heart disease. In: Spitzer JJ (ed) Plenum Publ, New York, pp 391–401

Vanhoutt PM (1974) Inhibition by acetylcholine of adrenergic neuro-transmission in vascular smooth muscle circulation. Circ Res 34:317–326

Session VII: Cerebral Perfusion and Metabolism

Chairmen: M. Rosner and A. Tamura

ICP and PVI with Blood Pressure Alterations and Relation with CBF Autoregulation

J.P. Muizelaar, A. Marmarou, and A. Wachi

Division of Neurosurgery, Medical College of Virginia, Virginia Commonwealth University, Richmond, Virginia 23298-0631 (USA)

Brain compliance is the ability of the cranial contents to accommodate an extra amount of volume (e.g., hematoma, CSF, increased cerebral blood volume, CBV) without much increase in ICP. PVI is a measure of brain compliance and is the calculated volume (in milliliters) required to raise ICP by a factor of 10 (Marmarou et al. 1978). It is thought to be a reflection of the vascular component of the intracranial compartment (Lofgren et al. 1973; Shapiro et al. 1980), also after head injury (Marmarou et al. 1973). Changes in blood pressure or CPP have a major influence upon the intracranial blood vessels, particularly arterioles, the extent and the direction of this influence being in turn dependent on whether autoregulation is (still) operative or not. Thus, several authors, using pento-barbital-anesthetized animals, found that PVI or some other measure of brain compliance did not change with changes in CPP within the range of autoregulation (Avezaath et al. 1980; Leech and Miller 1974; Takagi et al. 1980). Outside the range of autoregulation, brain compliance or PVI became inversely related to changes in CPP in these and other studies (Avezaath et al. 1980; Gray and Rosner 1987; Leech and Miller 1974). However, Gray and Rosner found that within the limits of autoregulation PVI and CPP were related in a linear fashion, with increasing blood pressure being reflected by a rise in PVI (Gray and Rosner 1987). But, this relationship was marked only in cats anesthetized with methohexital and hardly present with pentobarbital anesthesia. They concluded that pentobarbital, because of its own major vasoconstrictory effect, blunted the responses of cerebral blood vessels to changes in CPP and therefore obscured the relationship between PVI and CPP (Gray and Rosner 1987). In the present paper responses of ICP and PVI to changes in blood pressure were investigated in severely head injured patients in whom anesthesia is not necessary at all. Moreover, in some of these patients autoregulation is intact, while in others it is absent (though, for unknown reasons) (Muizelaar et al. 1984).

Materials and Methods

Measurements were performed in comatose patients with severe head injuries ranging in age from 4 to 50 years. All patients were paralyzed with pancuronium bromide and mechanically ventilated, resulting in excellent control of $PaCO_2$. All patients had an intraventricular catheter from which ICP was digitally displayed on a monitor and written on paper tape. PVI was measured by intraventricular injection and withdrawal of 0.5–1.5 ml aliquots of normal slaine, as described before (Marmarou et al. 1987). Each PVI value represents the mean of 3 or 4 measurements. CBF_{15} was measured with a Novo 10-a instrument using i.v. injected $^{133}Xenon$. Autoregulation was tested by i.v. infusion of phenylephrine or trimetaphan camcylate (Arfonad) to raise or decrease MABP by 30%, respectively. We defined autoregulation as being intact if $\%\Delta CPP/\%\Delta CVR \leq 2$, as described before (Muizelaar et al. 1984). During the CBF measurements 2 $AVDO_2$ measurements were performed. $CMRO_2$ was calculated by multiplying CBF and $AVDO_2$ and it serves as a quality control on the CBF measurements, as it is expected that $AVDO_2$ changes in a direction opposite to CBF during a constant $CMRO_2$.

Results

A total of 22 measurements in 20 patients were performed. All the data are shown in Table 1 divided in 2 groups with intact or defective autoregulation and subdivided into tests with blood pressure raised or decreased.

In Table 2 the average changes of MABP, ICP and PVI are represented, again in 2 groups, with intact or defective autoregulation, but now with calculations only as if all the lower blood pressures were baseline and all the higher blood pressures represented the alterations. The changes in ICP in both groups and those in PVI in the group with defective autoregulation were statistically significant (paired Student's t-test). PVI in the group with intact autoregulation remained the same.

Discussion

The present data indicate that within the range of autoregulation of CBF PVI is not dependent on CPP changes. This concurs with findings of most other authors (Avezaat et al. 1980; Leech and Miller 1974; Takagi et al. 1980), but is in contrast to those of Gray and Rosner (1987). In fact, those authors concluded that "with methohexital anesthesia, PVI is almost four times more dependent on CPP changes than with pentobarbital anesthesia. This implies that CPP variation may be even more important in the clinical situation where no anesthesia may be in use." Consequently, the only drug used in our patients was the paralyzing agent pancuronium-bromide (Pavulon®), but this drug is not known to have any influence upon $CMRO_2$. If, indeed, PVI is largely dependent on vascular factors, increased CPP would not be expected to have a large influence on PVI when autoregulation is intact. The higher intraluminal pressure in the larger conductance vessels is probably not transmitted to the brain tissue because of the thick wall of these vessels. In the resistance vessels the intraluminal pressure is higher in the inflow part but unaltered at the outflow portion due to vasoconstriction.

826

Table 1. Data of individual measurements, divided into groups with intact or defective auto-regulation

Patient #	MABP	ICP	PVI	CBF	CMRO$_2$
Autoregulation intact					
142	91–125	21–25	18–25	25–31	1.60–2.00
156	89–106	19–20	21–22	34–36	1.15–1.25
172	98–135	12–15	27–26	39–41	0.98–1.10
175	114–132	36–32	8–6	31–33	0.72–0.95
179	89–105	14–14	17–19	63–64	1.25–1.25
182	100–128	8–6	11–12	35–30	1.01–0.98
192	114–135	12–10	17–17	21–21	–
148*	137–90	26–30	19–17	41–37	1.48–1.38
157*	120–93	21–33	25–16	39–33	0.47–0.32
165*	120–100	19–29	23–31	26–33	0.86–0.94
168*	133–105	6–5	30–30	45–42	1.00–1.00
193*	100–80	16–28	16–19	38–36	1.02–1.27
Autoregulation defective					
134	123–145	8–10	19–10	30–36	2.08–2.05
141	100–130	22–16	9–17	24–31	1.53–2.07
143	105–134	14–20	34–18	39–69	1.35–1.75
151	115–138	23–26	17–9	21–28	0.80–0.80
154	103–131	31–35	22–23	29–41	1.37–1.28
156	84–115	22–30	20–17	34–51	1.35–0.83
168	84–110	6–5	23–19	40–52	1.20–1.20
180	85–120	12–8	21–18	37–50	1.35–1.65
129*	85–70	10–1	10–24	130–50	2.99–2.35
60*	146–116	22–5	30–25	80–65	–

In tests marked with an asterisks, blood pressure was lowered with Arfonad, in all others it was raised with phenylephrine. MABP and ICP in mm Hg, CBF and CMRO$_2$ in ml/100 g/min and PVI in ml

Table 2. Average changes of MABP, ICP and PVI

Autoregulation	MABP	ICP	PVI
Intact	97 ± 10	20.6 ± 10.4	19.3 ± 7.0
$n = 12$	123 ± 13	16.7 ± 7.6	20.0 ± 6.6
		$p < 0.025$	$p < 0.4$
Defective	99 ± 17	14.4 ± 9.7	21.4 ± 6.3
$n = 10$	125 ± 19	18.2 ± 10.1	17.1 ± 6.4
		$p < 0.05$	$p < 0.05$

All data ($\pm$ SD) are those taken at the lower blood pressure, compared to those at other higher blood pressures. Paired Student's t-tests were used

Although this somewhat higher intraluminal pressure might conceivably be transmitted to brain tissue, the vasoconstriction makes the wall thicker, thereby mitigating transmural pressure transfer and compensating for the higher intraluminal pressure. The capillary and venous beds are not affected with either intraluminal pressure changes or diameter (=volume) changes. The whole

827

cascade leads to decreased ICP (decreased volume and unchanged transmural pressure transfer) and unaltered PVI.

The situation is completely different when autoregulation is not intact. Now, the higher pressure in the arterial system is transmitted into the arterioles, capillaries and veins. This leads to increased transmural pressure transfer into the brain parenchyma. This effect may even be magnified by passive dilation of these vessels. This makes their walls thinner, thereby decreasing the barrier to pressure transfer. We speculate that the decrease in PVI is affected mostly by arterial pressure transfer and to a lesser degree by increased venous pressure with its possible effects on CSF outflow resistance. The increase in ICP with higher blood pressure and defective autoregulation is also dependent on the two above mentioned factors plus an increase in CBV because of passive arteriolar and capillary dilation.

References

Avezaat CJJ, van Eijndhoven JMM, Wyper DJ (1980) Effects of hypercapnia and arterial hypotension and hypertension on cerebrospinal fluid pulse pressure and intracranial volume-pressure relationships. J Neurol Neurosurg Psychiatry 43:222–234

Gray WJ, Rosner MJ (1987) Pressure-volume index as a function of cerebral perfusion pressure. Part 1: The effect of cerebral perfusion pressure changes and anesthesia. J Neurosurg 67:369–376

Gray WJ, Rosner MJ (1987) Pressure-volume index as a function of cerebral perfusion pressure. Part 2: The effects of low cerebral perfusion pressure and autoregulation. J Neurosurg 67:377–380

Leech P, Miller JD (1974) Intracranial volume-pressure relationships during experimental brain compression in primates. 2. Effect of induced changes in systemic arterial pressure and cerebral blood flow. J Neurol Neurosurg Psychiatry 37:1099–1104

Lofgren J, von Essen C, Zwetnow NN (1973) The pressure volume curve of the cerebrospinal fluid space in dogs. Acta Neurol Scand 49:557–574

Marmarou A, Shulman K, Rosenda RM (1978) A nonlinear analysis of the cerebrospinal fluid system and intracranial pressure dynamics. J Neurosurg 48:332–344

Marmarou A, Maset AL, Ward JD et al. (1987) Contribution of CSF and vascular factors to elevation of ICP in severely head-injured patients. J Neurosurg 66:883–890

Muizelaar JP, Lutz HA, Becker DP (1984) Effect of mannitol on ICP and CBF and correlation with pressure autoregulation in severely head-injured patients. J Neurosurg 61:700–706

Shapiro K, Marmarou A, Shulman K, (1980) Characterization of clinical CSF dynamics and neural axis compliance using the pressure-volume index: I. The normal pressure-volume index. Ann Neurol 7:508–514

Takagi H, Walstra G, Marmarou A et al. (1980) The effect of blood pressure and $PaCO_2$ upon bulk compliance (PVI). In: Shulman K Marmarou A, Miller JD et al. (eds) Intracranial pressure IV. Springer, Berlin Heidelberg New York, pp 163–166

Cerebral Perfusion Pressure, Autoregulation and the PVI Reflection Point: Pathological ICP

Y. El-Adawy and M.J. Rosner

University of Alabama at Birmingham, Divison of Neurosurgery, University Station, Birmingham, Alabama 35294 (USA)

Introduction

Observations reported by Gray and Rosner (1986, 1987a, 1987b) have demonstrated PVI to be a function of CPP. They used an experimental model in which ICP was normal and the CPP was reduced by gradual SABP decrements using ATP infusion. Cerebral blood flow (CBF) was measured at each CPP decrement which allowed identification of the CPP at which autoregulation was impaired. PVI was found to be a complex function of CPP, varying directly with CPP within the autoregulatory range, and indirectly below the autoregulatory range. The "reflection point" between these two functions was found to correspond with the point at which impairment of autoregulations occurred: about 50 mm Hg.

Because of these observations, we wished to examine similar issues under pathological circumstances. In the presence of high ICP we expected earlier impairment of autoregulation (i.e., at a higher CPP) and in the presence of a mass lesion we expected even earlier impairment of autoregulation (at a still higher CPP) when compared to the "no mass lesion" ICP increase (Lewis and McLaurin 1972; Weinstein and Langfitt 1967; Zierski et al. 1983). Therefore, we expected to find the same qualitative relationship between PVI and CPP in the presence of pathologically high ICP although deviation of the "reflection point" would likely occur at a higher CPP due to earlier impairment of autoregulation.

Methods

Sixteen adult cats, of either sex, weighing 2.5–4.5 kg were used. Group 1 ($n=8$) was the "no brain shift model" and group 2 ($n=8$) was the "brain shift model". Anesthesia was induced in all animals with intravenous methohexital sodium (10 mg/kg). The animals were paralyzed with pancuronium bromide (0.2 mg/kg), intubated endotracheally and ventilated with a 70% nitrous oxide/30% oxygen mixture; surgical anesthesia was obtained with local 2% lidocaine. Details of surgical preparation, placement of arterial and venous catheters, ICP monitoring were the same as previously described (Gray et al. 1986; Gray and Rosner 1987a, 1987b). PaO_2 was kept above 100 mm Hg, $PaCO_2$ at 30–35 mm Hg, hematocrit between 30 and 35% and temperature at 39°C throughout the experiments.

Group 1 (high ICP, no mass group) ICP was increased to 20 mm Hg by continuous cisternal infusion of artificial CSF through a 22 gauge needle. The rate of infusion was approximately 0.06 ml/min and was adjusted to maintain ICP at 20 mm Hg at the start of the experiment. Once the experiment began, the infusion rate remained constant.

In Group 2 (high ICP, mass lesion): an epidural balloon was inserted through a left parietal craniectomy and the hole around the balloon was sealed water tight using acrylic and cyanoacrylic cements. The balloon was inflated slowly (0.06 ml/min) until ICP stabilized at 20 mm Hg. Balloon volume was then held constant.

In both groups, CPP was reduced using a continuous infusion of adenosine triphosphate (ATP) 5 mg/ml in 0.95 NaCl at a rate of 0.2–3.0 mg/min. CPP was allowed to stabilize prior to any PVI measurement.

The pressure volume index (PVI) was calculated from the ICP response to a bolus injection (0.1 ml) of artificial CSF over one second into the lateral ventricle by the equation (Marmarou et al. 1978):

$$PVI = \frac{V}{\log \frac{Pp}{Po}}$$

where V = volume injected (ml)
Pp = peak ICP after injection (mm Hg)
Po = baseline ICP before injection (mm Hg)

In each animal three PVI estimations were made at every CPP after ICP stabilized at the start of the experiment and after CPP stabilization at each decrement level. The mean of three PVI estimations at each specific CPP level was considered the PVI at that CPP in every experiment.

Results

A total of 74 PVI estimations in the first group and 77 in the second group were calculated at different CPP levels from 15 mm Hg to 135 mm Hg. The PVI and corresponding CPP values were analyzed in the two groups using piecewise linear regression analysis. A complex relationship between PVI and CPP was identified. In both groups PVI varied directly with CPP at high CPP's and indirectly at low CPP's. A "reflection point" was identified at a CPP of 64 mm Hg in the cisternal infusion group (no mass lesion group) and 83 mm Hg in the mass lesion group (Fig. 1). At this reflection point the PVI reached its lowest value and the relation of PVI as a function of CPP changed from direct to indirect. The regression equation in the no mass group was:

PVI = 0.73 − 0.008CPP + 0.01 (CPP − 64) x,
where x = 1 if CPP > 62 and x = 0 if CPP < 64
($p < 0.001$)

The regression equation in the mass group was:

PVI = 0.74 − 0.007CPP + 0.01 (CPP − 83) x,
where x = 1, if CPP > 83 and x = 0 if CPP < 83
($p < 0.001$)

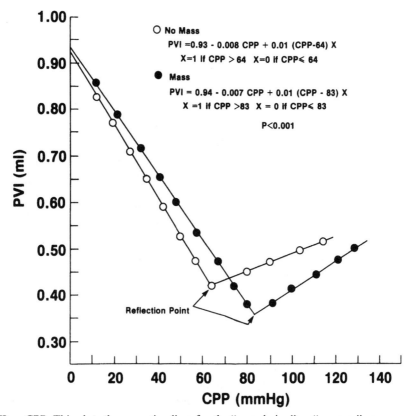

Fig. 1. PVI vs. CPP: This plots the regression lines for the "mass lesion" vs "no mass" groups. The PVI-CPP relation is complex. In normal brain the "reflection point" is at 50 mm Hg. This relationship shifts to the right under pathological circumstances, probably to a degree which is directly proportional to the pathology

Comparison of hematocrit and $PaCO_2$ in the two groups revealed no significant difference (T-Test, $P < 0.05$).

Discussion

In earlier work, we established that, under light anesthesia in healthy brains, there is a direct relationship between PVI and CPP within the autoregulatory range, and an indirect relationship between the same variables below the lower limit of autoregulation (Gray et al. 1986; Gray and Rosner 1987a, 1987b). Using the same methodology our current results were consistent with those previously reported. The same relationship was found between PVI and CPP although the reflection point moved to a higher CPP (64 mm Hg) in the no mass group and higher still (83 mm Hg) in the mass lesion group. This shift of the "reflection point" from 50 mm Hg in healthy brains to 64 mm Hg in the presence of diffuse

ICP increase and to 83 mm Hg in the presence of intracranial mass could be explained by earlier impairment of autoregulation in the latter groups. Impaired autoregulation has been shown to be related to the "reflection point" between the two regression phases (Gray and Rosner 1987b).

Early impairment of CBF autoregulation has been reported to occur in the presence of high ICP and mass lesions (Lewis and McLaurin 1972; Weinstein and Langfitt 1967; Zierski et al. 1983). The absence of significant differences with regard to $PaCO_2$, PaO_2, hematocrit, temperature, and initial ICP suggest these control variables did not account for differences between groups.

From these results we conclude that PVI, as a measure of brain stiffness, if used as a single parameter of impending deterioration is clinically misleading when CPP and autoregulation are not considered. "Improving" PVI values may occur at low CPP's which also does not represent a clinically favorable situation. This error is more likely to occur in the presence of intracranial mass lesions where early impairment of autoregulation (at high CPP) occurs. Our data suggest that PVI will improve as CPP improves and that unusually high values of CPP may be required under pathological circumstances.

Summary

1. PVI remained a function of CPP in the presence of intracranial hypertension.
2. PVI varied with CPP in a manner similar to that in normal brain, with values "improving" as CPP declined or rose above what has been identified as the "reflection point".
3. The reflection point occurred at a higher CPP in mass lesion group when compared to the no mass group; both occurred at higher CPP than in normal brain. This probably represents different autoregulatory characteristics in these groups.

Conclusions

1. CPP and autoregulation must be taken into consideration when interpreting PVI information. "Improving" values may be misleading in the presence of low CPP.
2. If PVI or similar measures of brain stiffness are used to imply clinical improvement or deterioration, the PVI should be varying directly with CPP and multiple measures of PVI at different CPP's should be obtained to define this curve.
3. Artificial elevation of CPP within the autoregulatory range produces a theoretically desirable state characterized by reduced brain "stiffness".
4. Repeated PVI estimations may prove to be useful in estimating the autoregulatory capacity of a given patient.

References

Gray WJ, Rosner MJ (1987a) Pressure-volume index as a function of cerebral perfusion pressure. Part 1: The effects of cerebral perfusion pressure changes and anesthesia. J Neurosurg 67:369–376

Gray WJ, Rosner MJ (1987b) Pressure-volume index as a function of cerebral perfusion pressure. Part 2: The effects of low cerebral perfusion pressure and autoregulation. J Neurosurg 67:377–380

Gray WJ, Rosner MJ, Richmond GH (1986) Pressure-volume index as a function of cerebral perfusion pressure and anesthesia. Neurosurgery 19:152

Lewis HP, McLaurin RL (1972) Regional cerebral blood flow in increased ICP produced by increased cerebrospinal fluid volume, intracranial mass and cerebral edema. In: Brock M, Dietz H (eds) Intracranial pressure: Experimental and Clinical Aspects. Springer, Berlin Heidelberg New York, pp 160–164

Marmarou A, Schulman K, Rosende RM (1978) A non linear analysis of the cerebrospinal fluid system and intracranial pressure dynamics. J Neurosurg 48:332–344

Weinstein JD, Langfitt TW (1967) Responses of cortical vessels to brain compression: Observations through a transparent calvarium. Surg Forum 18:430–432

Zierski J, Kurjay E, Hoffman O, Winkler B (1983) Cerebral blood flow in the brain stem during increased intracranial pressure. In: Ishii S, Negai H, Bralk M (eds) Intracranial pressure V. Springer, Berlin Heidelberg New York Tokyo, pp 452–457

Pressure-volume Index as a Function of Cerebral Perfusion Pressure, Autoregulation and Anesthesia

W.J. Gray and M.J.Rosner

Division of Neurosurgery, MEB 516, University Station, University of Alabama, Birmingham, Alabama 35294 (USA)

Introduction

Using a bolus technique, the pressure-volume index (PVI) of the cranio-spinal axis can be calculated. As the rise in intracranial pressure (ICP) which follows a bolus injection is instantaneous, it is generally accepted that the PVI is mainly a reflection of the response of the intracranial vascular compartment (Avezaat et al. 1980; Shapiro et al. 1980). The vascular compartment itself is influenced by many factors, including the cerebral perfusion pressure (CPP), carbon dioxide tension ($PaCO_2$), blood viscosity and many anesthetic agents. This present study was carried out to test the hypotheses that the PVI will change with changes in CPP and will also be influenced by the type of anesthetic agent employed.

Methods

Eighteen adult cats were used in the study. Anesthesia was induced with methohexital sodium (10 mg/kg) in 12 animals, while pentobarbital (30 mg/kg) was used in the other six. All the animals were paralyzed with pancuronium bromide (0.2 mg/kg) and ventilated with a 70% N_2O/30% O_2 mixture via endotracheal tube. Indwelling polyethylene catheters were placed in the aorta and inferior vena cava under additional local anesthesia for measurement of systemic arterial blood pressure and for administration of drugs.

The animals were then placed in the sphinx position in a stereotactic frame and the ICP measured via a 22 gauge needle placed in each lateral ventricle. In 6 of the methohexital studies, insulated platinum electrodes (platinum 90%/iridium 10%) with a diameter of 0.007 in, and a bare tip of 2 mm were placed in the caudate nucleus and deep frontal white matter bilaterally for cerebral blood flow (CBF) study. The temperature, O_2, pH and hematocrit were maintained constant within the normal range. Ventilation was adjusted to keep the CO_2 constant at 30 mm Hg.

The CPP was either raised using a norepinephrine infusion (3–15 µg/min) or lowered by an infusion of adenosine triphosphate (ATP) (0.2–2 mg/min). The PVI was calculated by injecting a bolus of 0.1 ml of 0.9% saline into one lateral ventricle and recording the ICP baseline and rise from the contralateral ventricle. The PVI was estimated at baseline CPP levels in all animals, and then CPP was either raised or lowered by increments of 20 mm Hg and the PVI estimated at each new steady state. In the 6 pentobarbital animals, CPP was increased in 3 and decreased in three. In the methohexital animals, CPP was increased in 3 and decreased in nine. In 6 of these 9, CBF was estimated using the hydrogen clearance method and calculated from the equation: CBF (ml/100 gm/min) = $69.3/T_{1/2}$ where $T_{1/2}$ = the time in minutes for the electrode current to fall to half of its original value.

Results

1. Non CBF Measurement Series

A total of 222 PVI measurements were made in animals in which CBF was not measured, 102 in the methohexital group, and 120 in the pentobarbital group. When the variables in each group were examined, it was found that the difference in $PaCO_2$ levels was less than 1 mm Hg, there was no difference in the baseline ICP levels before bolus injection, and the hematocrit did not vary by more than $\pm 3\%$ in all animals.

In both the pentobarbital and methohexital groups, the PVI varied with changes in CPP. In the pentobarbital group, 2 of the animals showed a slight decrease in PVI as CPP was increased, one animal showed a slight increase in PVI as CPP increased, and in the other 3 animals there was no change in PVI with changes in CPP. As a total group there was a slight overall increase in PVI with increasing CPP. (PVIml = 0.37 ± 0.0005 CPPmm Hg, $p < 0.05$). The scatter of results is shown in Fig. 1 a.

In contrast, in the methohexital group, each of the 6 animals showed an increase in PVI with increasing CPP. When taken as a group, this relationship (PVIml = 0.14 ± 0.0019 CPPmm Hg, $p < 0.001$) was much more positive than in the pentobarbital group. The scatter of results is shown in Fig. 1 b.

2. CBF Measurement Group

In these 6 animals, in which CPP was reduced from the normal level to well below the lower limit of autoregulation, a total of 76 PVI estimations were made. When CBF changed by less than 15% of baseline level with falling CPP, the PVI was considered to fall within the autoregulatory range. There were 41 such measurements. When CBF fell by more than 15% of baseline value with further falls in CPP, the PVI was considered to lie below the autoregulatory range. There were 35 PVI estimations in this category.

Within the autoregulatory range, CBF fell slightly as CPP decreased (CBF = 31 ml/100 gm/min ± 0.079 CPPmm Hg). In this range the PVI decreased with decreasing CPP in a similar way to the previous methohexital group (PVIml = 0.24 ± 0.0013 CPPmm Hg, $p < 0.001$) (Fig. 2a). Below the autoregulatory range, the CBF fell quickly with further reductions in CPP (CBF =

Pentobarbital

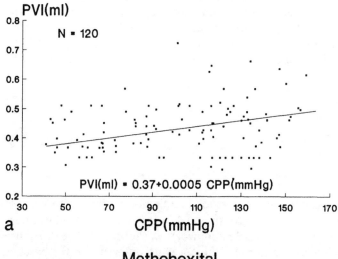

PVI(ml)

N = 120

PVI(ml) = 0.37+0.0005 CPP(mmHg)

CPP(mmHg)

a

Methohexital

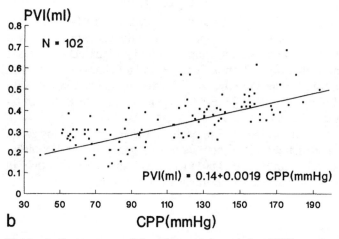

PVI(ml)

N = 102

PVI(ml) = 0.14+0.0019 CPP(mmHg)

CPP(mmHg)

b

Fig. 1a, b. Scattergrams of the pressure-volume index (*PVI*), results as a function of cerebral perfusion pressure (*CPP*). **a** Results obtained in the pentobarbital group are shown. Note the large scatter of results and the small positive slope. The results in the methohexital group (no cerebral blood flow measurement) are shown in **b**. Note the more positive slope and smaller scatter

7 ml/100 gm/min ±0.53 CPPmm Hg). In this range of CPP there was an opposite relationship between PVI and CPP, with the PVI increasing with decreasing CPP (Fig. 2b). There was no difference between the resting ICP level, $PaCO_2$ or hematocrit within or below the autoregulatory range.

Autoregulatory Range

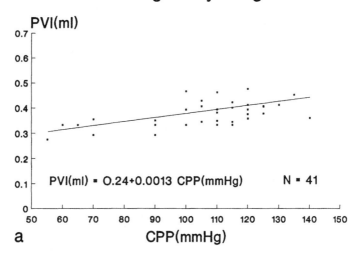

PVI(ml) = 0.24+0.0013 CPP(mmHg)   N = 41

a

Below Autoregulatory Range

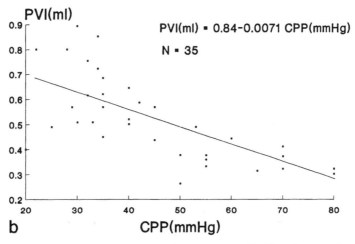

PVI(ml) = 0.84-0.0071 CPP(mmHg)

N = 35

b

Fig. 2 a, b. This shows the effect of reducing cerebral perfusion pressure (*CPP*). **a** (Autoregulatory range), while cerebral blood flow (CBF) remains relatively constant, a similar relationship between PVI and CPP is demonstrated as was seen in *1 b*. When the CPP is reduced below the lower limit of autoregulation, **b** the opposite relationship was found with PVI increasing with further reduction in CPP. Note the marked negative slope in this range

Discussion

Previous studies have suggested that brain 'stiffness' is not influenced by changes in CPP when autoregulation is intact, but will change with CPP beyond the limits of autoregulation (Leech and Miller 1974; Lofgren et al. 1973). However, most previous studies have been carried out under deep barbiturate anesthesia. Our results establish that under deep barbiturate anesthesia. Our results establish that under deep barbiturate anesthesia (pentobarbital) there is a slight, but significant, change in PVI with changing CPP in the range 50–160 mm Hg. We suggest that with this type of anesthesia, the cerebral vascular resistance (CVR) is held at a relatively constant and increased level. Reduction in CPP will have little effect on CVR, with little resultant change in the vascular intracranial compartment, and this is expressed as a relatively constant PVI response.

Under light anesthesia (methohexital) a different response is seen. The CVR is not held constant, but is able to change with changes in CPP throughout the autoregulatory range. As CPP falls, the vessels progressively dilate, and the cerebral blood volume increases. This is expressed by a PVI which decreases as CPP decreases. This relationship has previously been suggested in the canine model under methohexital anesthesia (Schettini and Walsh 1983).

In the animals in which CBF was measured, there was a change in this direct relationship between PVI and CPP when the CPP was reduced below the lower limit of autoregulation. At these levels of CPP, the PVI increased with further reductions in CPP. At the lower limit of autoregulation the vessels have dilated maximally and the cerebral blood volume is at its maximum. This is the point of the lowest PVI measurement. As CPP is reduced even further, blood volume will start to decrease and the PVI will start to increase. If we extrapolate the PVI/CPP relationship below the autoregulatory range to a CPP of zero, we have a calculated PVI of 0.84 ml. This is close to the PVI which we recorded in 2 dead animals (0.93 ml, 0.68 ml).

These results indicate that PVI is a complex function of CPP in the normal cranio-spinal axis. Interpretation of PVI values without due account of the CPP may, in many instances, be impossible. As the relationship between PVI and CPP in the normal animals is different within and below the autoregulatory range, it may be even more complex in injury models where autoregulation is impaired. It is also clear that PVI measurement made under deep anesthesia will be much different from the PVI measured under light anesthesia.

References

Avezaat CJJ, Van Eijndhoven JHM, Wyper DJ (1980) Effects of hypercapnia and arterial hypotension and hypertension on cerebrospinal fluid pulse pressure and intracranial volume-pressure relationships. J Neurol Neurosurg Psychiatry 43:222–234

Leech P, Miller JD (1974) Intracranial volume-pressure relationships during experimental brain compression in primates. 2. Effect of induced changes in systemic arterial pressure and cerebral blood flow. J Neurol Neurosurg Psychiatry 37:1099–1104

Lofgren J, Von Essen C, Zwetnow NN (1973) The pressure-volume curve of the cerebrospinal fluid space in dogs. Acta Neurol Scand 49:557–574

Schettini A, Walsh EK (1983) Brain elastance parameters and cerebral hemodynamics in hemorrhagic hypotension. In: Ishii S, Nagai H, Brock M (eds) Intracranial pressure V. Springer, Berlin Heidelberg New York, pp 282–285

Shapiro K, Marmarou A, Shulman K (1980) Characterisation of clinical CSF dynamics and neural axis compliance using the pressure-volume index: 1. The normal pressure-volume index. Ann Neurol 7:508–514

A Cerebral Perfusion Pressure Greater than 80 mm Hg is More Beneficial

C.P. McGraw

University of Louisville, School of Medicine, Louisville, Kentucky 40292 (USA)

Introduction

The issue of determining the most beneficial CPP was a topic of considerable discussion during the last ICP meeting. From that discussion, it was apparent that the data gathered over the last 9 years at the University of Louisville Trauma Center could best answer that question.

Methods

We graphed Glasgow Outcome Scale (GOS) versus Cerebral Perfusion Pressure (CPP) and observed that 80 mm Hg is a critical point at which mortality and morbidity changed grossly. We then compared whether a CPP of 60–80 and 81–101 mm Hg is most beneficial to patients with respect to four parameters: mortality and three different indications of morbidity. The frequency of Glasgow Coma Scale (GCS) (n=104) deteriorations or improvements in patients with a GCS of 5 or 6, Glasgow Outcome Scale (GOS) (n=180), and the neurophysiolo-

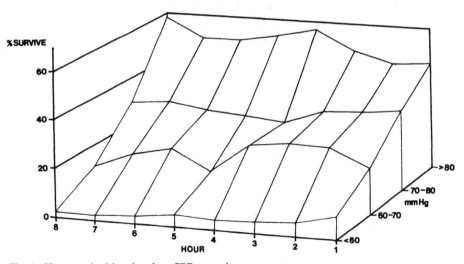

Fig. 1. How survival is related to CPP over time

Intracranial Pressure VII
Eds.: J.T. Hoff and A.L. Betz
© Springer-Verlag Berlin Heidelberg 1989

gical outcome ($n = 30$) 1 year or more post-injury. In each instance, the observation was made and then tested on a totally separate group of patients for validity. The decrease in GCS deteriorations and increase in improvements when the CPP was maintained above 80 mm Hg during the first 48 hr of monitoring was first observed on 88 patients and verified on another 16. The decrease in mortalities and increase in good outcomes (GOS = 4 or 5) when the CPP was kept above 80 mm Hg during the first 48 hr of monitoring was first observed in 136 patients and verified in another 44. The association between neurophysiological outcome 1 year or more post-injury and CPP during the first 48 hr of monitoring was first observed in 17 patients and verification was attempted in another 13.

The monitored data of 221 closed head injuries was then analyzed by comparing follow-up information with a designated level of CPP such as 60, 70 and 80 mm Hg. For example, the first time the CPP was below 60 mm Hg for 6 consecutive hr could be examined with respect to outcome. This data was then used to construct graphs of how depressed CPP overtime was associated with outcome. These same data were used in discriminant analysis in determining at what depressed CPP for how long, death or poor outcome could be predicted accurately (100% sensitivity). That was to discriminate from such data the patients who would die without any false calls.

Results

With mortality, GOS, and GCS deteriorations we observed a semi-linear relationship with a predominant step at 80 mm Hg CPP. With each of these parameters of outcome, there was a natural break observed in the data at a CPP of 80 mm Hg. This consistent correlation between whether a patient previously had a CPP above or below 80 mm Hg and a significant change in the incidence of mortality and morbidity in three separate studies was examined. The outcomes were observed to be more favorable when the CPP was kept above 80 mm Hg. Thus, we observed with a CPP kept above 80 mm Hg a decrease in the percent mortality ($p < 0.01$), an increase in the percent good outcomes (GOS = 4 of 5) ($p < 0.02$) and a decrease in the number of GCS deteriorations ($p < 0.02$). This association was real and repeatedly present. The positive increase in Wechsler memory scores ($p < 0.02$) did not hold true in the second group of patients or in a combination of the groups.

This 80 mm Hg point was a specific point at which mortality or good outcome significantly ($p < 0.001$) increased as determined by Fisher exact analysis. This point was statistically significant ($p < 0.02$) for the 44 additional patients tested for reliability who were not used in the initial observation. Thus, the percent mortality increased when the CPP was below 80 mm Hg, and the percent of good outcome increased when the CPP was above 80 mm Hg (Table 1).

A time relationship was not observed with CPP unless the categories of 60–70 mm Hg CPP were compared to the 80–90 mm Hg CPP. With increased time, these categories had opposite effects on the percentage of survivals. While the 70–80 mm Hg category remained unchanged with increasing time up to 8 hr.

Table 1. Critical cerebral perfusion pressure (by Fisher-Exact-Test)

Critical point	Outcome	Group I p	Group II p value
ACPP < 80 mm Hg	Mortality	< 0.0001	< 0.0074
ACPP > 80 mm Hg	Good outcome	< 0.0001	> 0.0142

That is to say that when the CPP averaged below 70 mm Hg, there was a decrease in survivals and good outcomes the longer the CPP was allowed to remain in that range. An apparent drop was noted when the CPP remained in the 60–70 mm Hg range for more than 5 hr. When the CPP averaged above 80 mm Hg, there was an increase in survivals and good outcomes proportionate to the length of time the CPP was allowed to remain within that range.

When the CPP remained below 60 mm Hg for 6 hr, death could be predicted with the highest accuracy (a 100% sensitivity and 37% specificity by discriminant analysis). Therefore, once the CPP was, on the average, below 60 mm Hg for more than 5 hr, there would be no predicted patient deaths, by discriminant analysis, who had subsequently survived. It was also observed that 36% of these patients had a drop in GCS within 24 hr after the beginning of a CPP depression that lasted more than 5 hr, and this drop in GCS occurred 6.5 ± 5.2 hr after the first hr of the 5 hr depression in CPP.

Discussion

There is an effect of CPP independent of neurological status. Even though in some patients, it may not be possible to maintain a CPP above 80 mm Hg, the remaining patients should have their CPP maintained above 80 mm Hg with diligence; thus, mortality and morbidity can be kept to a minimum. Apparently, patients can withstand acute drops in CPP to much lower levels; however, a sustained drop of 6 hr is less tolerable. This information supplies us with an idea of the time window faced in working with getting CPP above 80 mm Hg and maintaining the CPP above that point. The critical time is 5 hr or under for depressions in CPP below 60 mm Hg. Otherwise, these pressure variations for their associated time periods produce a significant secondary injury that is distinguishable in discriminant analysis predictions of either survival or good outcomes. Also these abnormal pressure variations for their associated time periods are associated with drops in the GCS.

Vasodilatory Cascade:
ICP Response to CPP Level and Reduction Rate

Y. El-Adawy and M.J. Rosner

University of Alabama at Birmingham, Division of Neurosurgery, University Station, Birmingham, Alabama 35294 (USA)

Introduction

Previous work has suggested that CSF pressure waves are in large part the result of an unstable blood pressure acting upon a more or less intact autoregulating cerebral vascular bed in the face of pathologically increased ICP and/or increased brain stiffness. The "vasodilatory cascade" model for CSF pressure wave generation was subsequently developed. This model suggests decrements in CPP will stimulate vasodilatation which will tend to increase cerebral blood volume (CBV). The increase will increase ICP which will further reduce CPP. Unless there is a response in the systemic arterial blood pressure (SABP) side of the CPP equation, the cycle will continue leading to more vasodilatation, increased CBV and a further increase in ICP which will further reduce CPP until vasodilatation is maximal. We have undertaken a series of experiments to further validate this ICP wave model.

Hypotheses

1. An indirect relationship will exist between SABP and ICP when CPP is high (above the lower limit of autoregulation).
2. A direct relationship will exist between SABP and ICP when CPP is low (at or below the lower limit of autoregulation).

Methods

Mongrel cats, 2.5–4.5 kg of either sex were used. Anesthesia was induced by IV methohexital (10 mg/gm IV), and after endotracheal intubation the cats were placed on $N_2O:O_2$: 70:30. Pancuronium bromide 0.1 mg–0.2 mg/kg IV was used to obtain muscle relaxation for adequate respiratory and $ET\text{-}CO_2$ control. Lidocaine (2%) was used locally for surgical placement of femoral arterial and venous catheters as well as all other surgical preparation. Cats were placed on Harvard respirators with $V_t =$ to 15 cc/kg. Continuous records of SABP and CVP via strain gauge transducers were displayed on a Gould 2800 S polygraph. Tem-

Eds.: J. T. Hoff and A. L. Betz

perature was continously monitored via a rectal probe and controlled via Yellow Springs temperature controller and radiant heating lamp. ET-CO_2 was continuously monitored and displayed on the polygraph. ICP was monitored by a 22 gauge intraventricular needle placed stereotaxically. The animals were held in a DKI stereotaxic headholder with all pressures referenced to the level of the ear bars. Arterial blood gases and hematocrit were monitored frequently. ET-CO_2 was maintained constant at 4.5–5.0%, FiO_2 was approximately 0.30 and PaO_2's were maintained above 100 mm Hg. Hematocrit was maintained constant by withdrawal of red cells or infusion of packed RBC's. pH was maintained at 7.35–7.40 by sodium bicarbonate infusion. Intracranial pressure was elevated by means of a 22 gauge cisternal needle and infusion of mock CSF. This typically required an 0.06 ml/min infusion rate. As ICP reached 20 mm Hg this infusion rate was then held constant for the remainder of the experiment. SABP/CPP was reduced in decrements using an intravenous infusion of a fresh solution of adenosine triphosphate (ATP) 5 mg/cc in NaCl 0.9%.

Summary of Results

When CPP was within the range where pressure autoregulation can act, and ICP was pathologically high, variation in SABP resulted in *active* ICP waves. These were characterized by:

a) indirect variation of ICP with SABP
b) some degree (5–30 sec ±) of latency between the SABP change before the ICP responded
c) large changes in CPP

When CPP was outside the range where pressure autoregulation was intact, variation in SABP yielded *passive* ICP waves, characterized by:

a) direct variation of ICP with SABP
b) zero latency between SABP change and ICP response
c) little to no change in CPP

Rapid changes in CPP which crossed the lower limit of autoregulation led to the generation of complex intracranial pressure wave phenomena which had both active and passive characteristics.

These results were consistent with predictions made from the vasodilatory cascade model or the interaction of relatively intact autoregulation interacting with increased intracranial pressure and an unstable systemic arterial blood pressure.

Conclusions

1. These findings were consistent with the "vasodilatory cascade" model of intracranial pressure wave generation as well as the reciprocal "vasoconstriction cascade" model.

2. Manipulation of this cascade is useful in:

a) control of intracranial pressure
b) maintenance of cerebral perfusion pressure
c) prevention of intracranial pressure waves
d) identification of "optimal" SABP-CPP levels for a given patient/clinical situation.

Experimental Study of the Correlation Between Evoked Potentials (SEP and AEP) and the Perfusion Pressure

T. Yokoyama, K. Uemura, H. Ryu, K. Sugiyama, T. Miyamoto, S. Nishizawa, and I. Shimoyama

Department of Neurosurgery, Hamamatsu University School of Medicine, 3600 Handa-Cho, Hamamatsu 431-31 (Japan)

Inflating a balloon in the supratentorial epidural space (Nagao et al. 1979; Tsutsui et al. 1986) and infusing solutions (Foltz et al. 1987) into the lateral ventricle have been used to study increased intracranial pressure (ICP) experimentally. However, the balloon technique is not biological because the inflated balloon itself could damage the underlying cerebral cortex. We developed a new technique for production of increased ICP to overcome this problem.

Somatosensory evoked potentials (SEP) and auditory evoked potentials (AEP) were recorded serially to determine correlations with the cerebral perfusion pressure (PP) (Sohmer et al. 1983; Sohmer et al. 1984).

Method

Six adult cats weighing 3–4 kg were anesthetized with intraperitoneal sodium pentobarbital (40 mg/kg). The femoral artery was cannulated for continuous arterial pressure monitoring. The cat was mounted on a stereotactic frame. A 16 gauge catheter was inserted into the epidural space and mineral oil was infused at a rate of 3 ml/hr by infusion pump (Atom, Type 201). The pressure transducer (Gaeltec) was placed in the contralateral epidural space and ICP was monitered continuously.

The median nerve was stimulated with 0.1 msec duration. 4 Hz, 0.6–1.0 mA pulses for SEP and ears were stimulated bilaterally with 0.1 msec duration; 10 Hz, 90 dB clicks through hollow ear bars for AEP. Each response was summated 500 times and analyzed for up to 20 msec after the stimulation (Nihonkohden, Neuropack 4). SEP and AEP were recorded every 5 minutes throughout the experiment. After completion of the experiment the animal was prepared for histological study.

Results

The cerebral hemisphere on the infused side showed a concave shape and histological examination revealed edema with microhemorrhages.

Intracranial Pressure VII   845
Eds.: J. T. Hoff and A. L. Betz
© Springer-Verlag Berlin Heidelberg 1989

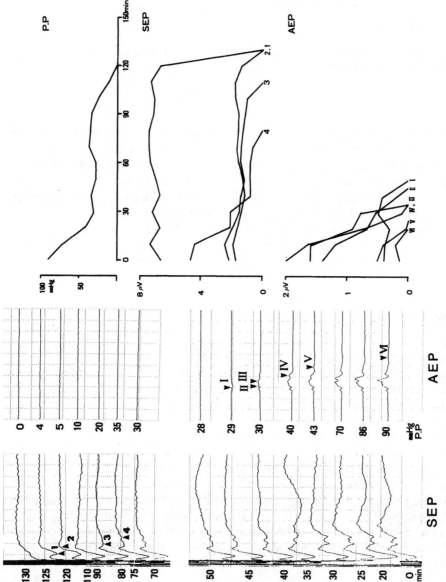

Fig. 1. This figure shows serial SEP, AEP recordings, the PP and amplitudes of the respective components of the SEP and AEP in type I

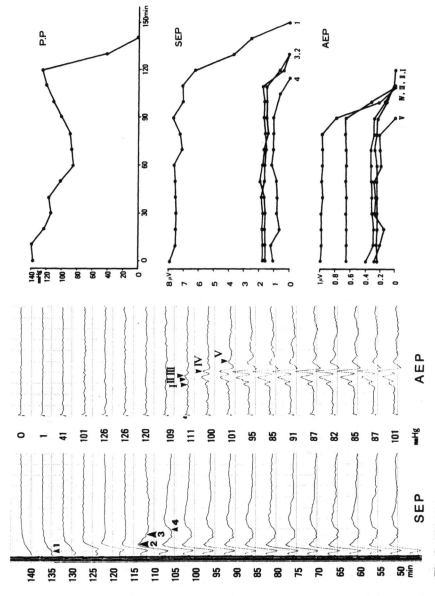

Fig. 2. This figure shows serial SEP, AEP recordings, the PP and amplitudes of the respective component of the SEP and AEP in type II

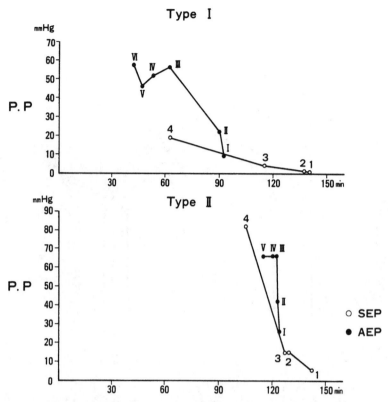

Fig. 3. This figure shows the relationships between the PP and the time when each wave of the SEP and AEP disappeared

Wave 1 to 4 and wave I to VI were identified according to latencies for components of the SEP and AEP, respectively.

The cats were classified into two groups according to ICP and the PP patterns. In type I, ICP increased gradually and the PP rapidly fell to 40 mm Hg and remained below this level (Fig. 1). In type II, ICP never exceeded 90 mm Hg and the PP remained above 40 mm Hg up to the final stage (Fig. 2).

Compared to the SEP, susceptibility of the AEP in type I and that in type II was quite different. In type I the components of the SEP and AEP disappeared successively from the late component. The components of the AEP disappeared earlier than those of the SEP. Wave 1 to 3 of the SEP disappeared in the late stage when the PP reached around 10 mm Hg which was far below the range of auto-regulation of cerebral blood flow (Fig. 3). However, in type II all components of the SEP and AEP were kept intact until the late stage when the PP began to decrease rapidly. The waves of both evoked potentials disappeared quickly from the late component. Wave I of the AEP and wave 1 to 3 of the SEP disappeared when the PP fell below 30 mm Hg (Fig. 3).

Summary

The present study revealed that:
1. The epidural infusion method was adequate to study the effects of increased intracranial pressure on the central nervous system.
2. In type I, the AEP was more susceptible to increased ICP than the SEP.
3. In type II, components of the AEP and SEP disappeared simultaneously.
4. Disappearance of wave 1 to 3 of the SEP indicated complete loss of autoregulation of cerebral blood flow.

References

Foltz EL, Blanks JP, McPherson DL (1987) Hydrocephalus: Increased intracranial pressure and brain stem auditory evoked responses in the hydrocephalic rabbit. Neurosurg 20:211–218

Nagao S, Roccaforte P, Moody RA (1979) Acute intracranial hypertension and auditory brain-stem responses. Part 2: The effects of brain-stem movement on the auditory brain-stem responses due to transtentorial herniation. J Neurosurg 51:846–851

Sohmer H, Gafni M, Goitein K, Fainmesser P (1983) Auditory nerve-brain stem evoked potentials in cats during manipulation of the cerebral perfusion pressure. Electroencephalogr Clin Neurophysiol 55:198–202

Sohmer H, Gafni M, Havatselet G (1984) Persistence of auditory nerve response and absence of brain-stem response in severe cerebral ischemia. Electroencephalogr Clin Neurophysiol 58:65–72

Tsutsui T, Nitta M, Ladds A, Symon L (1986) Effects of an expanding supratentorial mass on the auditory brain-stem responses in baboons. Acta Neurochir (Wien) 79:132–138

Correct Measurement of Cerebral Perfusion Pressure (CPP)

D. Woischneck, M.R. Gaab, E. Rickels, H.E. Heissler, and A. Trost

Medizinische Hochschule Hannover, Neurosurgical Department, Konstanty Gutschow Str. 8, D-3000 Hannover 61 (FRG)

Introduction

For the monitoring of patients with intracranial mass lesions, the measurement of intracranial pressure (ICP) is an essential parameter. Therapy of brain swelling, indication for CT or even neurosurgical operations are often based on the use of the ICP. In addition, using arterial pressure (AP), the cerebral perfusion pressure (CPP) can be calculated ($CPP = AP - ICP$). CPP is important in considering extracranial factors, such as changes in blood volume or arterial pressure, resulting in secondary brain swelling and ischemia. In contrast to ICP-monitoring, where hydrostatic level is easily standardized to the foramen of Monro, there exist various methods of measuring AP. It is usually not registered at the level of skull base, but in peripheral arteries with structural and functional differences (Gauer 1965). Previous investigations on CPP used varying mathematical methods for calculation of the mean arterial pressure, and the optimal grade of head elevation in intracranial hypertension is still under discussion.

Patients and Methods

The study group included 13 patients with ages from 18 to 66 years (mean: 45) with a spontaneous or traumatic intracranial hemorrhage (Glasgow Coma Scale 4–9). In each patient, we registered epidural ICP (Gaeltec minitransducer, referenced to the foramen of Monro) and AP in a peripheral artery (A. radialis, A. dorsalis pedis, A. femoralis). In addition, all patients underwent catheterization of A. temporalis superficialis (in 6 cases, the catheter position at the level of the jaw angle was proved by x-ray). In 5 cases, where out of diagnostic reasons angiography was performed, we could measure AP in the A. carotis interna for comparison. In the horizontal position ("O"), the arterial transducers were positioned at heart level. During head elevation (in 30° increments), the transducers were, at each position, referenced either to the heart or to the skull base in distinct periods of measurement. AP and ICP curves were continuously registered by monitor and video printer. Calculations of mean AP was done arithmetically according to van Eijndhoven and Avezaat (1983).

Results

The ICP up to head elevation of 30° in all patients fell 24.24% (mean) compared to the horizontal position (Fig. 1). Further elevation resulted in inconsistent changes: From 30° to 60° and from 60° to 90° respectively, the ICP in 6 cases increased, in 7 cases it decreased. Statistically, head elevation up to 90 resulted in a fall of ICP in 19.70% (relative to the 0° position), but a constant was only reached up to 30°.

The mean arterial pressure (MAP) in the internal carotid artery showed a difference to the MAP in A. temporalis superficialis from 0.28 to 6.25 mm Hg. This shows that the arterial pressure in the superficial temporal artery is practically identical to the AP at skull base. The comparison between MAP in A. temporalis superficialis and MAP in peripheral arteries revealed marked differences: We found MAP in the periphery to be, on average, 12% higher than in A. temporalis when the transducers of both had been placed at heart level. This cannot be explained by simple hydrostatic differences. Then the temporal artery transducer was at the level of the skull base, the difference to the MAP in the periphery increased further (due to the addition of the hydrostatic error). The difference now was registered between 25% (30°) and 103% (90° of head elevation).

When calculating cerebral perfusion pressure, we found three different curves (Fig. 2): 1. By using the AP measured in A. radialis (dors. pedis, femoralis), CPP increased up to 30° of head elevation and again, between 60° and 90° (transducers

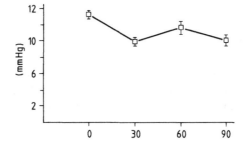

Fig. 1. ICP and Head Elevation. In all cases a fall of ICP up to 30°. Further elevation results in inconsistent changes (due to rotation of the head and compression of jugular veins)

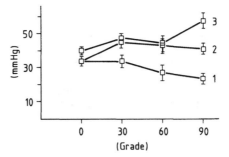

Fig. 2. CPP and Head Elevation. Real pressure at skull base is calculated by using AP in A. temporalis superficialis (referenced to the head)

at heart level). 2. By using AP in A. temporalis superficialis, the curve up to 60 degrees was parallel to the first one, but CPP was averaged 16% lower (transducers still referenced to heart level). 3. Analyzing CPP calculated by AP in A. temporalis superficialis and referenced to the skull base, we found it nearly constant between the horizontal position and 30°, but a marked decrease up to 60° (20% of 30° value) was noticed.

Discussion

The finding of a decrease in ICP by head elevations up to 30° corresponds to other investigations (Rosner and Coley 1986). For the first time, however, it is shown that AP measurement in A. temporalis superficialis is a practical method for calculating the real CPP at the level of skull base. Previous authors (Rosner and Coley 1986) were able to show that, in contrast to older concepts, CPP declines by head elevation when AP registration is referenced to the skull. But by using arteries of different anatomy and function far away from the head, their results could not be correlated to the real pressure in the carotid circulation. We were able to show identical results at our point of measurement (A. temporalis and A. carotis interna). Another critical point is the use of different mathematical models for gaining MAP. A first comparison of our arithmetical results to planimetric methods revealed a deviation of 30% for A. radialis and, far better, of 15% for A. temporalis superficialis. This deviation seems to be constant with head elevation.

Conclusion

1. Measurement of AP in A. temporalis superficialis (referenced to the head), is a practical method for determining the real CPP at the skull base.
2. The optimal grade of head elevation is up to 30°.
3. Up to 30° of head elevation, ICP consistently decreased, while CPP remains unchanged. Further elevation leads to a decrease of CPP.

References

Gauer OH (1965) Postural changes in the circulation. In: Handbuch der Physiologie, vol. 3. Baltimore, pp 2409–2439
Rosner J, Coley IB (1986) Cerebral perfusion pressure, intracranial pressure and head elevation. J Neurosurg 65:636–641
Van Eijndhoven JHM, Avezaat JJ (1983) Cerebrospinal fluid pulse pressure as parameter of intracranial elastence. In: Wood JH (ed) Neurobiology of cerebrospinal fluid, vol 2. Plenum, pp 643–660

Critical Thresholds of Rebound of ICP
After Cerebral Compression

K.E. Jakobsson[1], J. Löfgren[1], and N.N. Zwetnow[2]

[1] Department of Neurosurgery, Gothenburg University, Sahlgrenska Hospital, S-41345 Göteborg (Sweden), [2] The Division of Experimental Neurosurgery, The National Hospital, Rikshospitalet, Oslo (Norway)

Introduction

Deflation of an epidural balloon after a period of brain compression is sometimes followed by a rapid and sustained rise in ICP and brain swelling (Clubb et al. 1980; Ishii 1966; Langfitt et al. 1965). The characteristics and nature of this rebound phenomenon, which has obvious clinical correlations, remain yet to be clarified. A main feature is the inconsistency of the response, occurring in some cases and not in others under apparently similar conditions. We have continued previously reported studies (Jakobsson et al. 1986) to define the critical mechanical conditions under which the rebound response is generated, including measurements of regional CBF.

Methods

Seventy-five mongrel dogs, anesthetized with pentobarbital sodium (30 mg/kg supplemented as needed), were intubated, paralyzed and artificially ventilated with room air. The right brachial artery and both femoral arteries were cannulated with polyethylene catheters used for blood gas sampling and measurement of systemic arterial and venous pressures. In some of the animals a catheter was advanced into the left ventricle for injection of radioactive microspheres. The EEG was recorded by means of biparietal electrodes. Fluid pressures were recorded in the lateral ventricle and cisterna magna.

ICP was raised either by inflation of a rubber balloon inserted into the epidural space through a burrhole in the left temporo-parietal region or by infusion of artificial CSF at body temperature into the cisterna magna from a pressure reservoir. The increase in ICP was maintained for periods of 5, 15, 30, 45 and 60 min. After discontinuation of the period of compression the course of ICP was followed for 2–3 h.

Regional CBF was measured in a group of dogs (n = 8) during the period of increased ICP by the radioactive microsphere technique using 15 μm diameter microspheres.

Intracranial Pressure VII
Eds.: J.T. Hoff and A.L. Betz
© Springer-Verlag Berlin Heidelberg 1989

Results

The course of ICP after decompression falls into either of two groups. In one group a rebound occurred within 10–20 min to values of 30–96 mm Hg. In the other group ICP remained below 20 mm Hg. Intermediate behaviour was rarely observed.

Multiple linear regression analysis revealed that duration and degree of compression, the latter expressed as mean perfusion pressure (MPP), were critical factors determining the occurrence of rebound of ICP. The curve in Fig. 1 based on 50 balloon compression experiments describes the relationship between MPP, duration of compression and the rebound response. The values of the asymptotes of the pressure-time curve may be regarded as thresholds for the occurrence of a rebound. Thus, there is a minimum duration of about 5 min in order to produce a rebound and a critical MPP of about 50 mm Hg. Within these narrow limits, the pressure-time threshold function is described by the curve.

Among 21 dogs subjected to hydrostatic compression, only one showed a rebound of ICP and in this case the MPP had been below 10 mm Hg for one hour. In the others MPP was 20.0 ± 10.8 mm Hg, which is actually lower than in the balloon compression experiments, where MPP was 38.0 ± 18.3 mm Hg. The amplitude of the rebound response was correlated to the duration of the preceeding period of compression ($r = 0.62$; $p < 0.001$).

The hemodynamic correlations to the ICP rebound were studied by measuring changes in regional CBF induced by the compression (Fig. 2). Balloon compression with a supra- and infratentorial MPP of 32 ± 5 mm Hg and 55 ± 9 mm Hg respectively, resulted in significant flow reductions within the supratentorial compartment. An extremely low flow was seen adjacent to the balloon. With absolute flow values in the temporal cortex and white matter of 6.4 ± 3.4 and 1.1 ± 0.9 ml/100 g/min respectively. Hydrostatic compression (MPP

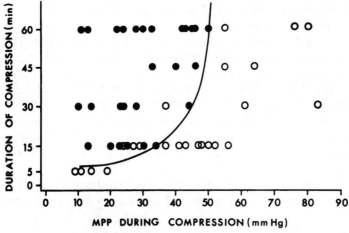

Fig. 1. Plot of duration of balloon compression against mean supratentorial perfusion pressure during compression. *Dots* denote rebound of ICP, *open circles* absence of rebound response

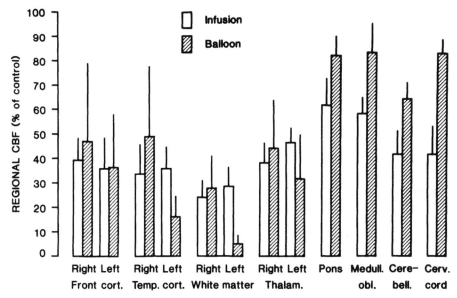

Fig. 2. Changes in regional CBF expressed in percent of control

22 ± 6 mm Hg) on the other hand resulted in a uniform flow reduction within both the supra- and infratentorial compartments to approximately 45% of control.

The hemodynamic changes were further defined by calculation of cerebrovascular resistance. Hydrostatically raised ICP was associated with a generalized vasodilatation. Balloon compression produced more complex effects on the vascular bed. Obviously the vasodilatory effect was counteracted by a direct and distributed compression of the vascular bed by the balloon, resulting in a marked increase in the flow resistance ipsilateral to the balloon and to a lesser degree on the contralateral side.

Discussion

A preliminary study (Jakobsson et al. 1986) showed that a severe reduction in the perfusion pressure was necessary to produce a rebound in the present sense and that the frequency with which the response occurred was proportional to the duration of the compression. These findings have been amplified and can now be explained by a refined concept of a sensitive dependence of the rebound response on a narrow compression-time threshold.

Apparently a rebound of ICP takes place when two critical conditions are fulfilled. The compression has to produce an ICP high enough to result in a perfusion pressure below about 50 mm Hg. This is not a sufficient condition, however, which was our earlier contention. The compression has to be maintained for a period of time which is a function of the perfusion pressure in accordance with the discriminant function showed in Fig. 1. A minimum duration of compression can be defined of about 5 min to elicit a rebound response, i.e. with zero perfusion pressure. A perfusion pressure of about 50 mm Hg represents a state of compression which may go on, in theory, for an infinite period of time without resulting in a rebound of ICP on release.

When a rebound of ICP occurs, CBF has characteristically been reduced during the period of compression to values below established thresholds for infarction (Symon 1985) in extensive regions of the brain within the supratentorial compartment, especially ipsilateral to the balloon. Thus, it is probable that the marked rise in ICP and brain swelling which may develop after a period of compression are due to the mass effect of wide spread barrier damage and cerebral infarction. A vasodilatation and an increase in CBF and cerebral blood volume may contribute but can not explain adequately the rebound effect as it develops only in exceptional cases after hydrostatic compression in spite of hemodynamic changes of similar magnitude.

The explanation of this absence of a rebound in hydrostatic compression is that the CBF is reduced to considerably and critically lower values in balloon compression experiments in spite of actually somewhat higher perfusion pressures. This is evidently due to differences in the flow resistance, which is much higher in balloon compression because of a direct effect of vascular compression and distortion. This effect overrides the vasodilatation which is otherwise the response to an increase in ICP.

There is consequently no evidence that rebound of ICP develops on the basis of neurogenic mechanisms. The apparently arbitrary and unpredictible appearance of a rebound after decompression in both clinical cases and experimental animals, which may suggest a neural effect, can be interpreted as related to the exquisite sensitivity to the initial conditions which is a characteristic of the rebound response.

The rebound of ICP is another example of threshold phenomena in intracranial pathophysiological processes which are ultimately related to the existence of ischemic flow thresholds for various metabolic and functional effects (Symon 1985; Kuroiwa et al. 1982). The fact that the detrimental effects of a mass lesion in some respects is not proportional in a simple linear fashion to the time or degree of compression, but distinctly dependent on critical thresholds have certainly important clinical implications, e.g. in understanding the effects of therapeutic measures.

Conclusions

1. Rebound of ICP after a period of brain compression is a strict threshold phenomenon sensitively dependent on the degree and duration of compression.
2. Brain compression by a mass lesion results in a restriction of cerebral blood flow due to the combined effect of an elevation of ICP and a direct compressional effect on the vascular bed causing a rise in cerebrovascular resistance.
3. In the final analysis rebound of ICP is related to a reduction in CBF during the period of compression below the ischemic flow threshold for cerebral infarction.

856

Acknowledgements. This work was supported by grants from: Radman och fru Ernst Collianders Stiftelse; The Göteborg Medical Society; Anders Jahres Foundation for the Advancement of Medical Science; Norwegian Society for Fighting Cancer; Norwegian Association against Cancer; The Medical Faculty, University of Oslo; Norwegian Research Council for Science and the Humanities.

References

Clubb RJ, Maxwell RE, Chou SN (1980) Experimental brain injury in the dog. J Neurosurg 52:189–196

Ishii S (1966) Brain swelling: studies of structural, physiologic and biochemical alterations. In: Caveness WF, Walker AE (eds) Head injury. Conference Proceedings Philadelphia: J.B. Lippincott, pp 276–299

Jakobsson KE, Löfgren J, Zwetnow NN (1986) Determinants of intracranial pressure rebound after brain compression. In: Miller JD, Teasdale GM, Rowan JO, Galbraith SL, Mendelow AD (eds) Intracranial pressure VI. Springer, Berlin Heidelberg New York Tokyo, pp 161–165

Kuroiwa T, Ting P, Suzuki R, Fenton I, Klatzo I (1982) The relationship of the blood-brain barrier (BBB) opening to the thresholds of regional blood flow (rCBF) in cerebral ischaemia. J Neuropathol Exp Neurol 41:352–359

Langfitt TW, Weinstein JD, Kassell NF (1965) Cerebral vasomotor paralysis produced by intracranial hypertension. Neurology 15:622–641

Symon L (1985) Flow thresholds in brain ischemia and the effect of drugs. Br J Anaesth 57:34–43

Critical Thresholds of ICP and Cerebral Perfusion Pressure (CPP) for Cerebral Blood Flow and Brain Functions – Noninvasive Study

M. Shigemori, T. Moriyama, H. Nakashima, T. Tokutomi, N. Nishio, K. Harada, and S. Kuramoto

Department of Neurosurgery, Kurume University School of Medicine, 67 Asahi-machi, Kurume City, Fukuoka 830 (Japan)

Introduction

Neuronal damage in intracranial hypertension is closely related to brain ischemia, and therefore, the critical thresholds of ICP and CPP (cerebral perfusion pressure) for cerebral circulatory disturbance and brain dysfunction have important clinical significance. To ascertain these thresholds, extra- and intracranial hemodynamic phenomena and brain function were studied noninvasively in intracranial hypertension.

Clinical Materials and Methods

We studied 50 patients with severe head injury (GCS scores of 8 or lower) in which extradural ICP was monitored using ICT/b catheter tip transducer (Gaeltec) and systemic arterial pressure was also recorded simultaneously in order to calculate CPP. The mean age of the patients was 46 years. For the evaluation of cerebral circulation, blood flow velocities in the middle cerebral artery (MCAFV) and in the common carotid artery (CBFV) as well as the pressure pulse wave of the common carotid artery (CA-PW) were recorded under endotidal CO_2 monitoring by use of transcranial Doppler ultrasonography (TC2-64, EME) (Aaslid et al. 1982), ultrasonic Doppler flowmeter (QFM, Nihonkhoden) and pulse wave transducer (TF-601, Nihonkhoden), respectively. The means of MCAFV and CBFV were calculated by averaging over 5 trials. The mid-diastolic flow velocity (Md) in CBFV and the elasticity index (EI) of CA-PW were also calculated.

Brain function was evaluated with multimodality evoked potentials (MEPs) consisting of auditory evoked brainstem response (ABR), cortical somatosensory evoked potential (SEP), and visual evoked potential (VEP) recorded by Neuropack (MEP-3200, Nihonkhoden). The responses of the patients were classified into 4 grades (Shigemori et al. 1987).

Eds.: J. T. Hoff and A. L. Betz

Results

The mean MCAFV remained within the normal range (67 ± 13 cm/s, n: 25) until ICP reached 30 mm Hg. When ICP increased to 31–40 mm Hg, the mean velocity decreased to 57.3 ± 26.0 cm/s which was significantly lower than the normal level (n: 57, $P < 0.05$). When ICP increased to 41–60 mm Hg, it was 47.9 ± 21.0 (n: 38, $P < 0.01$). The further increase of ICP induced a rapid fall of the mean velocity

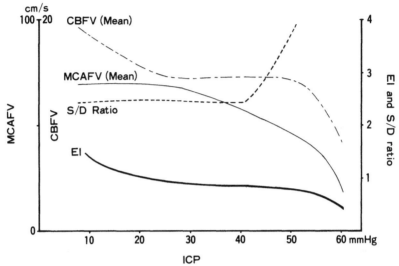

Fig. 1. The changes in mean MCAFV, CBFV, and EI of CA-PW in intracranial hypertension in 50 patients with severe head injury. S/D ratio indicates the ratio of the amplitudes of systolic and diastolic flow velocity in MCAFV

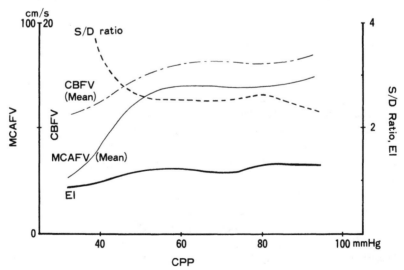

Fig. 2. The changes in mean MCAFV, CBFV, S/D ratio, and EI when CPP decreased due to ICP elevation

859

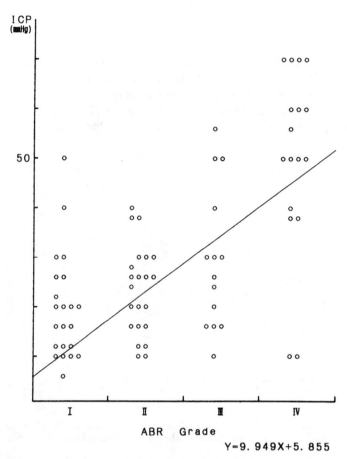

Fig. 3. The relationship between ICP level and ABR grade in patients with severe head injury (*n*: 75)

with disappearance of diastolic flow velocity. When CPP decreased to less than 41 mm Hg, the mean MCAFV decreased to 42.1 ± 24 cm/s (*n*: 55, $P < 0.01$). When ICP increased to 21–40 mm Hg, the mean CBFV and Md decreased to 12.82 and 9.54 cm/s (*n*: 52, $P < 0.01$) which was significantly lower than the normal level (19.48 ± 3.52 and 15.98 ± 2.01 cm/s (*n*: 44) (Shigemori et al. 1986). When CPP decreased to less than 51 mm Hg, they were 12.37 and 8.21 cm/s (*n*: 52, $P < 0.01$), respectively. EI of CA-PW was also decreased to less than 1.0 as ICP increased to 21 mm Hg or higher and as CPP decreased to 51 mm Hg or lower (Fig. 1, 2).

The frequency and degree of abnormalities on MEPs were also proportional to the rise of ICP and the reduction of CPP. ABR, SEP, and VEP showed normal or mildly abnormal grades in more than 62.7% of the recording when ICP was less than 30 mm Hg (*n*: 51). In contrast, when ICP increased to higher than 31 mm Hg, MEPs were classified as moderately or severely abnormal (*n*: 24) in more than 76% of the recordings (Figs. 3–5).

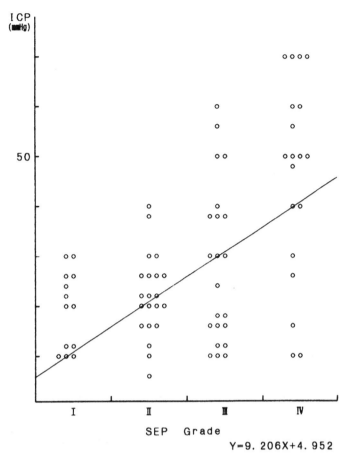

Fig. 4. The relationship between ICP level and SEP grade in patients with severe head injury
(*n*: 75)

Discussion

Transcranial doppler ultrasonography has now been widely used in the detection of intracranial hemodynamic phenomena (Aaslid et al. 1982). The principles of CBFV measurement and its clinical values have also been well documented (Shigemori et al. 1986). MEPs consisting of several sensory evoked potentials can provide a useful index of the global brain function (Shigemori et al. 1987). In the present study, the critical thresholds of ICP and CPP which induce severe brain ischemia and brain dysfunction were studied by using these techniques in patients with severe head injury.

It was found that the mean MCAFV as well as CBFV exhibited the flow patterns which changed monotonously depending on the changes of ICP and CPP. The extra- and intracranial blood flow velocities were decreased when ICP increased to 20–30 mm Hg and when CPP decreased to 40–50 mm Hg. The wave

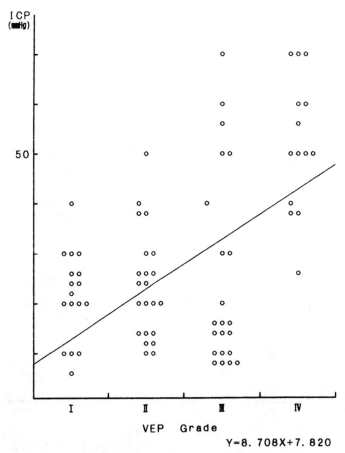

Fig. 5. The relationship between ICP level and VEP grade in patients with severe head injury (*n*: 75)

V of ABR has been thought to be generated by neural activity in the auditory pathways in the midbrain, and it is suppressed by transtentorial herniation (Shigemori et al. 1987). The alterations of SEP and VEP have been reported to be caused not only by primary injury of the pathways but also by the secondary effect of raised ICP or brain ischemia (Sutton et al. 1986, York et al. 1981). In our study, the high incidence of severe abnormalities of MEPs in intracranial hypertension over 30 mm Hg of ICP indicate the secondary effects of the raised ICP on the upper brainstem and global brain ischemia.

Noninvasive study by use of Doppler ultrasonography and MEPs can provide valuable information on critical intracranial hemodynamic phenomena and brain dysfunction in patients of severe head injury with raised ICP.

References

Aaslid R, Markwalder TM, Nornes H (1982) Noninvasive transcranial Doppler ultrasound recording of flow velocity in basal cerebral arteries. J Neurosurg 57:769–774

Shigemori M, Tokutomi T, Kawaba T, Nakashima H, Kuramoto S (1986) Analysis of epidural pressure pulse wave (EDP-PW) and common carotid blood velocity (CBFV) in acute intracranial hypertension. Neurol Res 8:105–108

Shigemori M, Yuge T, Kawasaki K, Tokutomi T, Kawaba T, Nakashima H, Watanabe M, Kuramoto S (1987) Evaluation of brain dysfunction in hypertensive putaminal hemorrhage with multimodality evoked potentials. Stroke 18:72–76

Sutton LN, Cho BK, Jaggi J, Joseph PM, Bruce DA (1986) Effects of hydrocephalus and increased intracranial pressure on auditory and somatosensory evoked responses. Neurosurgery 18:756–761

York DH, Pulliam MW, Rosenfeld JG, Watts C (1981) Relationship between visual evoked potentials and intracranial pressure. J Neurosurg 55:909–916

Flow Threshold in Increased Intracranial Pressure

J. Izumi, S. Toya, T. Kawase, S. Okui, and Y. Iizaka

Department of Neurosurgery, Keio University Hospital, 35 Shinanomachi, Shinjuku-ku, Tokyo 160 (Japan)

During increased intracranial pressure (ICP), decreased cerebral perfusion pressure (CPP) causes reduction of cerebral blood flow (CBF). In experimental cerebral ischemia, the flow threshold level to maintain brain function and the time threshold for duration of ischemia to recover brain function have been reported previously (Bell et al. 1985; Branston et al. 1974; Jones et al. 1981; Lesnick et al. 1984; Yamagata et al. 1982). The purpose of the present study was to clarify whether those thresholds exist during increased ICP, as seen in experimental cerebral ischemia.

Materials and Methods

Thirty adult cats were anesthetized with ketamine hydrochloride and paralyzed with pancuronium bromide. Arterial PCO_2 was maintained at between 35 and 45 mm Hg. Epidural pressure (EDP) was measured with a Gaeltec pressure transducer placed on the left occipital region (contralateral side to the balloon). Cortical local cerebral blood flow (ICBF) was measured by the hydrogen clearance technique. Needle type electrodes were inserted into the cortex of the ectosylvian gyrus of each hemisphere through small burr holes. Increased ICP was produced by an epidural balloon placed on the right occipital region. The balloon was inflated at a rate of 0.033 ml/min using an auto injector. Changes in SAP, EDP, CPP, SEP and ICBF were continuously monitored.

In 21 animals, the inflation of the balloon was discontinued when the SEP was flattened, and the EDP was kept at that level. The balloon was deflated 0–40 min after the flattening of the SEP. The duration of the maintained critical CBF level was defined as compression time in the present study. Those parameters were monitored until 120 min after the deflation of balloon.

Results

The control value of ICBF in the left hemisphere was 46.1 ± 8.8 ml/100 g/min and that of the right hemisphere was 44.8 ± 10.7 ml/100 g/min (mean $\pm$ SD, $n = 30$).

Following inflation of the balloon, EDP increased and CPP decreased gradually. ICBF began to decrease in the early stage without a significant change in

Eds.: J. T. Hoff and A. L. Betz
© Springer-Verlag Berlin Heidelberg 1989

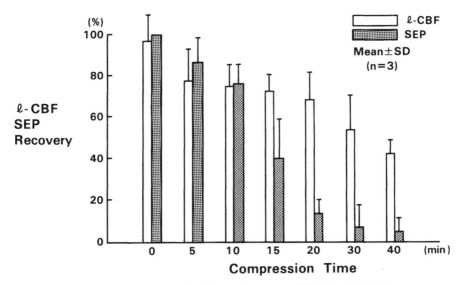

Fig. 1. Relationship between compression time and recovery of ICBF and SEP. The percentage of control value for ICBF and amplitude of the SEP on the side contralateral to the balloon at 120 min after the deflation of balloon are shown. The compression time is the duration of maintained critical CBF level between the abolishment of SEP and deflation of the balloon

SEP. Then the amplitude of the SEP abruptly began to decrease (attenuation of SEP). Local CBF continued to decrease and SEP became flattened (abolishment of SEP).

At the attenuation of SEP, EDP was 61.7 ± 5.3 mm Hg, CPP was 72.1 ± 5.8 mm Hg, ICBF in the left hemisphere was 29.2 ± 6.5 ml ($62.0 \pm 7.3\%$ of control), and ICBF in the right hemisphere was 27.6 ± 10.2 ml/100 g/min ($60.2 \pm 10.3\%$ of control). At the abolishment of the SEP, EDP was 83.5 ± 9.7 mm Hg, CPP was 49.0 ± 5.6 mm Hg, ICBF in the left hemisphere was 19.6 ± 3.9 ml/100 g/min ($44.2 \pm 7.0\%$ of control) and ICBF in the right hemisphere was 19.4 ± 4.3 ml/100 g/min ($43.1 \pm 7.3\%$ of control).

After deflation of the balloon, some animals showed transient hyperemia. Local CBF reduced thereafter to value lower than the control value and continued at that level for up to 120 min. Recovery of the SEP on the balloon side was usually unfavorable and is not discussed here. Recovery in the amplitude of the SEP and ICBF of the contralateral side 120 min after deflation of the balloon are shown in Fig. 1. Recovery of SEP was favorable when deflation was carried out within 10 min and unfavorable when deflation was carried out after more than 20 min. SEP showed moderate recovery in animals with compression time of 15 min. The local CBF subsequently decreased when the compression time was longer. In animals with compression time of 15 and 20 min, a discrepancy was seen between recovery of ICBF and SEP.

Discussion

The flow threshold of cortical ICBF in the present study was 19.6 ± 3.6 ml/ 100 g/min in the left hemisphere and 19.4 ± 4.3 ml/100 g/min in the right hemisphere. The critical CBF level reported in experimental ischemia is 10–20 ml/ 100 g/min (Branston et al. 1974; Jones et al. 1981; Yamagata et al. 1982) or 40–45% of the control CBF (Bell et al. 1985; Lesnick et al. 1984). The time threshold for recovery of neural function indicated by the SEP was 15 min in the present study. A time threshold of 15–20 min has been reported with increased ICP by infusion into the cisterna magna (Kramer,ä et al. 1967), and in ischemia (Miller et al. 1970; Yamagata et al. 1982). In animals with 15–20 min of compression time, recovery of the SEP was unfavorable despite a relatively favorable recovery of the ICBF. This result suggests that ischemic damage during compression itself inhibits recovery of the SEP.

References

Bell BA, Symon L, Branston NM (1985) CBF and time thresholds for the formation of ischemic cerebral edema, and effect of reperfusion in baboons. J Neurosurg 62:31–41

Branston NM, Symon L, Crockard HA, Pasztor E (1974) Relationship between the cortical evoked potential and local cortical blood flow following acute middle cerebral artery occlusion in the baboon. Exp Neurol 45:195–208

Jones TH, Morawetz RB, Crowell RM, Marcoux FW, FitzGibbon SJ et al. (1981) Thresholds of focal ischemia in awake monkeys. J Neurosurg 54:773–782

Kramer W, Tuyman JA (1967) Acute intracranial hypertension – An experimental investigation. Brain Res 6:686–705

Lesnick JE, Michele JJ, Simeone FA et al. (1984) Alteration of somatosensory evoked potentials in response to global ischemia. J Neurosurg 60:490–494

Miller JR, Myers RE (1970) Neurological effects of systemic circulatory arrests in the monkey. Neurology 20:715–734

Yamagata S, Carter LP, Erspamer R (1982) Cortical ischemia: Effect upon direct response. Stroke 13:680–686

Influences of Intracranial Pressure on Regional Cerebral Blood Flow

T. Kojima, K. Iwata, H. Yuasa, and T. Sugiyama

Department of Neurological Surgery, Aichi Medical University, Aichi-ken 480-11 (Japan)

Cerebral function during acutely increased ICP as well as during the recovery period were evaluated using visual evoked potential (VEP) and regional blood flow (rCBF) monitoring.

Methods

Forty adult cats, weighing 2.5 to 3.5 kg were used. They were anesthetized with intramuscular ketamine chloride (5–10 mg/kg) and tracheostomized. The femoral artery and vein were cannulated with polyethylene tubing for arterial blood pressure monitoring and maintaining of general anesthesia with pancuronium bromide. Experimental animals were placed on an artificial respirator. ICP was monitored in two ways: 1) supratentorial pressure through a sealed parietal burr hole and 2) infratentorial pressure through a catheter in the cisterna magna via polyethylene tubing from a lumbar laminectomy. ICP was experimentally increased by infusion of artificial cerebrospinal fluid through the second polyethylene tubing (1.0 mm) introduced through the lumbar laminectomy. The lumbar dural sac was ligated as previously described with the 2 tubes in place to prevent the leakage of CSF and to maintain the desired ICP level for study.

Visual evoked potentials were recorded at two places, one from the visual cortex and another from the lateral geniculate body. Concentric electrodes of 0.8 mm diameter were inserted according to Snider's stereotaxic atlas. The reference electrode was placed at the ear. Stimulation of the visual pathway by xenon flash was given by Nihonkodenvisual stimulation system. The intensity of flash stimulation was 2 Hz in frequency. Evoked electrical activities were recorded from cortical and depth electrodes, amplified, and filtered through a bandpass of 30 Hz to infinity. These potentials were averaged by computer. rCBF was monitored from the visual cortex by the heat clearance method and blood flow to the lateral geniculate body was obtained using a stereotactically, introduced needle electrode and the hydrogen clearance method.

Results

1) In our study, the control value of rCBF at the visual cortex and lateral geniculate body were measured 56.1 ± 14.6 ml/100 g brain/min and 48.1 ± 7.44 ml/100 g

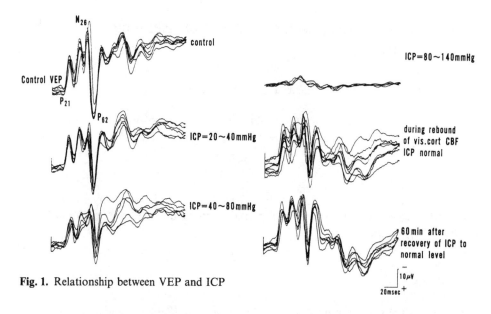

Fig. 1. Relationship between VEP and ICP

brain/min respectively. 2) Wave components of the potential evoked by flash stimulation can be summarized at the visual cortex, latency of P wave 21.0 ± 1.93 msec, N 26.4 ± 2.81, P 61.5 ± 6.67 and N 80.3 ± 7.89 in sequence. At the lateral geniculate body, the evoked potential was seen as a positive single wave at 26.4 ± 2.34 msec. 3) When ICP was experimentally increased diffusely by infusion of artificial CSF and then when cerebral perfusion pressure remained between 40 and 60 mm Hg, VEP and rCBF of both cortex and lateral geniculate body did not show a significant change in our study. When CPP was reduced less than 20 mm Hg, VEP became flat, while the electroretinogram retained its electrical activity. At this time rCBF of the visual cortex measured 16.7 ± 3.59 ml/100 g brain/min and we believe this is the critical pressure and critical rCBF for the cerebral cortex. It is interesting to note that the rCBF of the lateral geniculate body remains 24.6 ± 3.13 ml/100 g brain/min in this situation. 4) When ICP was reduced from the severe increase, there is a group in which the VEP reappeared after severely increased ICP of 15 min duration. In these instances, reductions of rCBF in the lateral geniculate body and the visual cortex were 50% and 70% respectively, and the rCBF showed increases following release of ICP elevation 20% and 80% respectively. When the disappearance of VEP lasted for an average of 25 min and the reduction in rCBF to the lateral geniculate body was reduced about 70%, no more recovery was found in neural activity. 5) As Figure 1 shows, the critical ICP to abolish VEP activity to the cortex appeared to be 80 mm Hg in this study. 6) We investigated the recovery of the VEP after release of the ICP elevation and found recovery began in the N_{26} component of the VEP which had been considered to be derived from the lateral geniculate body while the P_{62} component, which we assume comes from the cortex, showed poor recovery (Table 1).

Table 1. Average VEP wave latencies and standard deviations under different experimental conditions ($n = 17$)

VEP wave latencies	Visual cortex			LBG
	P_{21}	N_{26}	P_{62}	P
Control	21.0 ± 1.93	26.4 ± 2.81	61.5 ± 6.67	26.4 ± 2.34
15 min	24.5 ± 4.49	32.8 ± 7.99	67.2 ± 8.80	33.4 ± 7.21
	4[a]	9[a]	10[a]	9[a]
60 min	25.4 ± 3.98	35.1 ± 7.04	68.1 ± 8.03	33.5 ± 7.86
	1[a]	3[a]	4[a]	2[a]

VEP wave latencies which was recorded 15 min or 60 min after ICP was returned to control level. During increased ICP, VEP waves kept almost flat.

[a] represents animal number which did not show recovery of VEP, these VEP wave flat even after recovery of ICP.

Discussion and Conclusion

In a previous communication, we reported changes of ABR in diffusely and acutely increased ICP experiment (Iwata et al. 1986). We found that the auditory brain stem response showed a high tolerance to a decrease in CPP. In this study, we focused on the VEP – visual path way system – to investigate the brain stem activity above the cerebellar tentorium. We found 20 mm Hg of CPP was the critical level to abolish the VEP. If CPP was kept above 60 mm Hg (or above 40 mm Hg in some animals), the VEP showed no change. When CPP was reduced to the 20 mm Hg level and the VEP became flat, the rCBF to the lateral geniculate body was reduced by about 50% while rCBF to the visual cortex showed a 70% reduction. When the ICP was reduced to a normal level after acute elevation, the VEP returned as long as the duration of the ICP elevation was limited to 15 min. When the ICP was elevated high enough to abolish the VEP for more than 25 min, the blood pressure began to fall and CPP became zero or negative and then the VEP would no longer return. In the latter situation, no possibility of cerebral recovery could be expected. Our data provides a critical value for an acute rise of ICP in relation to upper brain stem function and its recovery.

References

Greenberg RP, Stablein DM (1981) Noninvasive localization of brain-stem lesions in the cat with multimodality evoked potentials. J Neurosurg 54:740–750

Iwata K, Yamazaki A, Yuasa H (1986) Auditory brain stem evoked response in increased intracranial pressure produced by infusion method in cats. Intracranial Pressure 6:351–354

Kuschinsky W, Wahl M (1978) Local chemical and neurogenic regulation of cerebral vascular resistance. Physiol Rev 58:656–689

Sutton LN, Byung-KYZ Cho (1986) Effect of hydrocephalus and increased intracranial pressure on auditory and somatosensory evoked responses. Neurosurgery 756–761

Circulatory Disturbances of Cerebral Blood Vessels During Increased Intracranial Pressure

J. Izumi, S. Toya, T. Kawase, S. Okui, and Y. Iizaka

Department of Neurosurgery, Keio University Hospital, Shinjuku-ku, Tokyo 160 (Japan)

Introduction

Under increased intracranial pressure (ICP), decreased cerebral perfusion pressure (CPP) causes a reduction in cerebral blood flow (CBF). In a previous study of increased ICP (supratentorial balloon inflation) by the authors (Izumi et al. 1986), decreased local CBF to the cerebral cortex was recorded. However, the three-dimensional development of disturbances of the cerebral circulation, especially in the brain stem could not be determined. Therefore, in the present study we used perfusion of a carbon black solution during increased ICP by supratentorial balloon inflation.

Methods

Nine adult cats were used under ketamine anesthesia. Epidural pressure (EDP), somatosensory evoked potential (SEP), and cortical local cerebral blood flow (ICBF) using the hydrogen clearance technique were monitored in the left hemisphere. A right occipital epidural balloon was inflated at a rate of 0.033 ml/min. The details of the method are described in another paper.

A bolus of 40 ml of carbon black solution was injected into a femoral artery catheter during the increased ICP. The carbon was perfused at the time of SEP abolishment (4 animals), at the stage when ICBF was further decreased (4 animals) and when ICBF could not be measured (1 animal). Animals were sacrificed and brains were removed and fixed in 10% formalin solution. The brain was cut with a midline sagittal section and two coronal sections at the level of the chiasma and the superior colliculus. The distribution of the defect in carbon perfusion was observed macroscopically.

Results

In animals with carbon perfusion at the time of SEP abolishment, the low perfused area was localized to the ipsilateral cerebral hemisphere and brain stem. Blood flow was still preserved in the contralateral hemisphere and also in the

Intracranial Pressure VII
Eds.: J. T. Hoff and A. L. Betz

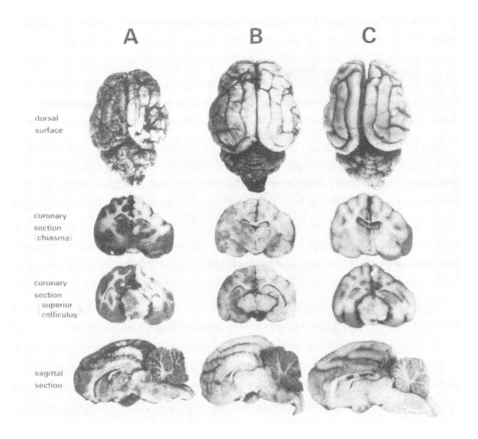

Fig. 1 A–C. Perfusion of carbon black during increased ICP. Carbon black was perfused at three different stages: at the time of SEP abolishment (**A**), at the stage when compression of brain was advanced and ICBF was further decreased (**B**), and when ICBF could not be measured (**C**)

brain stem. In animals with carbon perfusion at the stage when ICBF was further decreased, the low perfused area extended into the contralateral side and the upper pons, but not the lower pons and the cerebellum. In animals with carbon perfusion at the stage when ICBF could not be measured, the hemisphere, the midbrain, the upper pons and even the lower pons were not perfused. These observations are shown in Fig. 1.

Discussion

In the present study, carbon perfusion showed that ischemia began around the balloon and spread to the upper brain stem and finally to the lower brain stem. In a dye injection study, Weinstein et al. (1968) reported that vascular compression and ischemia spread in an essentially circumferential manner from the subdural supratentorial balloon. Eventually almost the entire brain became ischemic and only the cerebellum was spared. Hekmatpanah (1970) reported similar results.

In a CBF study, Zierski et al. (1983) observed a marked drop of CBF in most of the regions at the beginning of balloon inflation. In the lower brain stem, the reduction in CBF was smaller and less rapid than in other regions. Nagao et al. (1984) reported that concomitant with supratentorial balloon expansion, the local CBF in the thalamus started to decrease first, then in the inferior colliculus, and finally in the medulla oblongata.

The results of the present study and these reports suggest that in increased ICP by supratentorial balloon expansion, ischemia begins around the balloon side and progresses to the upper brain stem, and finally to the lower brain stem. Thus, in this model of increased ICP, dysfunction of the brain stem may not precede reduced excitability of the supratentorial cerebrum in abolishment of SEP.

Carbon perfusion in the contralateral hemisphere was still preserved at a time when the SEP was abolished. Increased ICP that caused the defect in carbon perfusion was a much more severe insult than the threshold for abolishment of SEP, but at this stage, a blood flow disturbance could be shown in postmortem examination after carbon black perfusion. Although brain stem function was not examined in the present study, decreased CBF of the supratentorial compartment of the cerebrum may play a primary role in abolishment of the SEP.

References

Hekmatpanah J (1970) Cerebral circulation and perfusion in experimental increased intracranial pressure. J Neurosurg 32:21–29

Izumi J, Kawase T, Okui S, Iizaka Y, Toya S (1986) Relationship between cerebral blood flow and somatosensory evoked potential in increased intracranial pressure in cats. In: Miller JD, Teasdale GM et al. (eds) Intracranial pressure VI. Springer, Berlin Heidelberg New York Tokyo, pp 369–372

Nagao S, Sunami N, Tsutsui T, Honma Y, Momma F, Nishiura T, Nishimoto A (1984) Acute intracranial hypertension and brain-stem blood flow. An experimental study. J Neurosurg 60:566–571

Weinstein JD, Langfitt TW, Bruno L, Zaren HA, Jackson JLF (1968) Experimental study of patterns of brain distortion and ischemia produced by an intracranial mass. J Neurosurg 28:513–521

Zierski J, Kurzaj E, Hoffmann O, Winkler B (1983) Cerebral blood flow in the brain stem during increased ICP. In: Ishii S, Nagai H, Brock M (eds) Intracranial pressure V. Springer, Berlin Heidelberg New York, pp 452–457

Two Dimensional Analysis of Microcirculation, Vascular Permeability, Energy Metabolism, Ion Exchanges in the Intracranial Hypertension

S. Kimura, N. Hayashi, and T. Tsubokawa

Department of Neurosurgery, Nihon University, Itoboshi 173, Tokyo (Japan)

Introduction

In this paper, changes in dendrite and cell soma specific high molecular protein: MAP2 (microtubule associated protein 2) (Matus et al. 1981) following cerebral compression are presented. In addition, the effect of changes in vascular permeability, energy metabolism, ion metabolism and microcirculation on changes in MAP2 were also studied.

Method

Experiments were performed on 45 Sprague Dawley rats weighing 250–350 gm. The animals were anesthetized with nembutal (18 mg/kg). Intracranial hypertension was produced by epidural compression with 3, 5 and 7 mm lengths of 3 mm diameter dual-hole silastic tube. After 24, 48 and 72 hr, intracranial pressure was measured. At the end of the experiment, changes in energy metabolism (ATP, NADH), vascular permeability (Na-fluorescein), tissue potassium and microcirculation (using 1 μ and 7 μ diameter fluoresbright microspheres, single dye passage method) were studied simultaneously. Alterations in neuronal function were evaluated with MAP2 (using immunohistochemical technique).

Results and Discussion

Three different levels of intracranial hypertension (20–30, 30–45, 50–60 mm Hg) were produced by epidural compression with silastic tubes.

(A) Pathological Changes. 1. 20–30 mm Hg intracranial hypertension: Metabolic changes, such as loss of ATP, increased vascular permeability, low tissue potassium and disturbances of the microcirculation were localized just under the compressed brain tissue. These metabolic changes gradually recovered by 72 hr. 2. 30–45 mm Hg intracranial hypertension: Increased vascular permeability and aerobic metabolic changes such as increased NADH and microcirculatory disturbances, were observed more severely and deeper than with 20–30 mm Hg

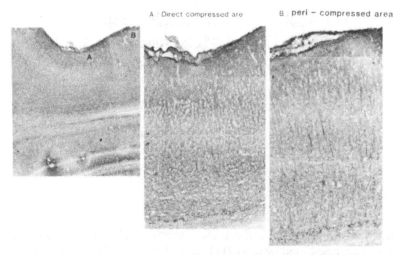

A : Direct compressed are   B : peri − compressed area

Fig. 1. Alterations of dendrite specific high molecular protein (MAP2) at 48 hr following epidural compression (ICP: 20−30 mm Hg)

ICP. 3. 50−60 mm Hg intracranial hypertension: Loss of ATP and tissue potassium extended to deep brain tissue and medial basal ganglia, correlating with microcirculatory changes. However, increased vascular permeability was limited to the cortex under the compression site.

(B) Changes in MAP2 in the Neuron: The changes in MAP2 were studied during the most severe stage 48 hr after cerebral compression. In the range of 20−30 mm Hg intracranial hypertension, changes of MAP2 were localized just under the compressed brain tissue. The staining of MAP2 disappeared most prominately in layers 1 and 2 of the cortex. In cortical layers 3 to 6, mild heterogeneous changes were observed. However, large cells connected to dendritic MAP2 were maintained. This result shows that dendrite dysfunction occurs even with reversible metabolic changes (Fig. 1). In the 30−45 mm Hg range of intracranial hypertension, absence of staining for MAP2 extended to the deeper layer 6, correlating well with changes in tissue potassium. In the 50−60 mm Hg intracranial hypertension, severe loss of MAP2 was observed in all layers of the compressed cortex and extended beyond directly compressed areas. In this stage, loss of MAP2 was observed in the contralateral cortex in layer 3.

Previous studies about the role of cerebral MAP2 documented dendrite sprouting (Bernhart and Matus 1982) and longterm cAMP-mediated effects on the electrical activity of neurons (Furmanski 1971). Furthermore, a critical ICP of 40 mm Hg resulted in changes of MAP2 in the dendrite (Hayashi et al. 1988). From these results, high sensitivity of dendrite MAP2 in the cerebral compression area was documented.

Conclusion

Specific patterns of neuronal dendrite dysfunction following cerebral compression were elucidated through changes in energy metabolism, vascular permeability, microcirculation and tissue potassium.

References

Bernhart R, Matus A (1982) Initial phase of dendrite growth; evidence for the involvement of high molecular weight microtubule associated protein (HMWP) before the appearance of tubulin. J Cell Biol 92:589–593

Furmanski P (1971) Expression of differentiated functions in mouse neuroblastoma mediated by dibutyl-cyclic adenosine monophosphate. Nature 233:413–415

Hayashi N, Tsubokawa T et al. (1988) Changes of CSF migration, energy metabolism and high molecular protein of the neuron in the hydrostatic intracranial hypertension (in press, in this book)

Matus A, Bernhart R et al. (1981) HMWP proteins are preferentially associated with dendritic microtubules in brain. Proc Natl Acad Sci USA 78:3010–3014

Intracranial Pressure (ICP) Correlation with Cytochrome a, a₃ and Hemoglobin Redox State Measured by Noninvasive Near Infrared Spectrophotometry

M. Dujovny, C. Wasserman, A. Martinez-Coll, J.I. Ausman, A. Perlin, M. Stewart, and G. Lewis

Henry Ford Neurosurgical Institute, 2799 W. Grand Blvd., Detroit, Michigan 48202 (USA)

Introduction

Change in cytochrome a, a_3 and hemoglobin redox state were assessed using nearinfrared (NIR) spectrophotometry in an animal model during normal and increased intracranial pressure.

Material and Method

Twenty mongrel dogs, weighing 15–25/kg were anesthetized with pentobarbital sodium (25 mg/kg) I.V. A femoral artery and vein were cannulated to allow injection of drugs, monitoring of arterial pressure and withdrawal of arterial blood for pO_2, pCO_2, and pH determination. The animals were intubated and then connected to a Harvard ventilator. The dog's heads were mounted in a stereotactic holder and a midline incision was made through the scalp to allow the reflection of the extracranial muscle to expose the skull. A microprocessor driven ICP fiberoptic monitor was implanted in the right frontal lobe. A noninvasive fiber optic probe was placed over the left parietal region in order to transluminate the brain through the skull with light in the NIR range (500–1300 nm), (Somanetics, Troy, MI.). Computerized calculation of photon absorption at well defined wavelengths for cytochrome a, a_3 (600 nm) and Hb (780 nm) was studied (Kariman and Burkhart 1985). ICP was increased by total global ischemia or by extradural balloon inflation during short and long periods of time.

Results

Increased intracranial pressure was accomplished with significant reduction in oxidation of both systems. The correlation coefficient between I.C.P. and oxidation was significant. Also observed was a very early response to a decrease of the cytochrome a, a_3 redox state measured before the acute change in intracranial pressure.

Eds.: J.T. Hoff and A.L. Betz
© Springer-Verlag Berlin Heidelberg 1989

Discussion

Near infrared optical spectroscopy is used to measure intracranial oxygen delivery and cellular metabolism in vivo (Jobsis and Vander 1985). The technique immediately reveals changes in concentration of Hb and HbO_2, and the redox state of the enzyme cytochrome a,a_3. The latter is a direct measure of aerobic cellular metabolism; 90% of aerobic electron/oxygen transfer occurs through this enzyme, and a decrease in the oxidized concentration indicates a decrease in the level of aerobic metabolism.

The principle of optical spectroscopy is that molecules absorb light energy by varying amounts, depending upon the wavelength. Many substances have unique, characteristic patterns of absorption across the light spectrum. Concentration of such substances can be measured by metering the light attenuation at several wavelengths and isolating the effects of the target substance. Animal tissue is relatively transparent to NIR light in the wavelength range of 600 nm to 1100 nm, with which Hb, HbO_2, and cytochrome a, a_3 have useful spectral characteristics of absorption (Keizer 1985). NIR optical spectroscopy calculates parameters from directly measured variables, it is temperature independent over a wide range, and is independent of intensity of the light source. Although, the information obtained by NIR monitoring is mainly qualitative, the possibility of a non-invasive brain monitor of metabolic change closely related with ICP variation, is valuable. The redox energy state and oxygen transport monitoring could be of significant value in neuroscience. The early detection of changes on Hb, or HbO_2 and cytochrome aa_3 provides a better understanding of the early change that occurs during increased intracranial pressure. Further development on computer science, light source, fiber optics, and light absorption may provide a better technique to evaluate cerebral metabolism in a simple and non invasive way.

References

Jobsis FF, Vander V (1985) Non-invasive, near infrared monitoring of cellular oxygen sufficiency in vivo. Adv Exp Med Biol 191:833–841

Kariman K, Burkart DS (1985) Non-invasive in vivo spectrophotometric monitoring of brain cytochrome a, a_3 revisited. Brain Res 360:203–231

Keizer HH (1985) The near infrared (NIR) absorption bank of cytochrome aa3 in purified enzyme, isolated mitochondria, and the intact brain in situ. Adv Exp Med Biol 191:823–832

Cerebral Hemodynamics in Benign Intracranial Hypertension Studied with PET

L. Junck

Department of Neurology, University of Michigan, Ann Arbor, Michigan 48109 (USA)

The pathogenesis of benign intracranial hypertension (BIH) remains poorly understood. Many investigators suspect the disorder to be caused by obstruction of CSF outflow at the arachnoid villi (Johnston 1973), but this same mechanism is also suspected to cause an entirely different syndrome, normal pressure hydrocephalus. In 1985, I proposed that BIH might be caused be weakness in the walls of the dural venous sinuses, resulting in compression of the venous sinuses, partial venous outflow obstruction, and elevated ICP (Junck 1986).

In order to gain insight into the pathogenesis of BIH, we measured CBV and CBF in three women with BIH at both high pressure (before lumbar puncture) and at low pressure (immediately after lumbar puncture).

Methods

The subjects of this study were three obese women, aged 32 to 48, who presented with headaches. All had papilledema, and one had optic atrophy and visual field deficits, but neurological examinations were otherwise normal. All had normal X-ray computed tomography and magnetic resonance scans. All had sustained pressure elevation at multiple lumbar punctures.

Each patient underwent scans of cerebral blood volume (CBV) and cerebral blood flow (CBF) before and after pressure reduction by lumbar puncture. Either two or three sets of CBV scans at different brain levels and a single set of CBF scans were performed. Lumbar puncture was then performed and approximately 20 ml CSF were removed to reduce to 40–75 mm CSF. The entire set of scans was then repeated over approximately the next hour.

PET scans were performed using a PCT 4600A tomograph, which has a resolution of $1.1 \times 1.1 \times 0.9$ cm and scans five planes simultaneously. Cerebral blood volume (CBV) was determined from 5-min scans starting 1 min after inhalation of approximately 30 mCi $[^{15}O]CO$. Cerebral blood flow (CBF) was determined by the weighted integral approach (Alpert et al. 1984) from a 6-min dynamic series of scans after injection of approximately 25 mCi $[^{15}O]H_2O$.

Table 1. CBV and CBF results in BIH patients

Variable measured	High ICP	Low ICP	High ICP / Low ICP
CBV (ml hg^{-1})			
Whole brain	3.87±0.55	3.49±0.14	1.11±0.12
Sup. sag. sinus	- - - - - -	- - - - - -	0.98±0.08
Straight sinus	- - - - - -	- - - - - -	1.04±0.03
Transverse sinus	- - - - - -	- - - - - -	0.94±0.20
Sigmoid sinus	- - - - - -	- - - - - -	1.03±0.23
CBV (ml hg^{-1} min^{-1})			
Whole brain	44±8	49±6	1.11±0.09

Results and Discussion

Pressure at lumbar puncture in the 3 patients was 240, 520, and 275 mm CSF.

CBV in cerebral parenchyma (avoiding major veins and venous sinuses) aver-aged 3.87±0.53 ml hg^{-1} at high ICP and 3.49±0.14 ml hg^{-1} at low ICP (differ-ence not significant). This result suggests that intravascular pressure is increased in parallel with CSF pressure in BIH, because decreased CBV would have been expected at high ICP if intravascular pressure were normal. Increased intravascu-lar pressure would be expected with partial collapse of the dural venous sinuses. It could also occur when CSF outflow resistance is increased if the terminal veins collapse by a Starling resistor mechanism (Shapiro 1977). In either case, the 11% increase in CBV at high ICP could be due to relative vasodilatation in compen-sation for the decreased cerebral perfusion pressure. This finding argues against CSF outflow obstruction as the cause of BIH in the absence of increased resis-tance at some point in the venous system.

CBV in dural venous sinuses was unchanged between the high ICP and low ICP measurements. This finding is consistent with collapse of the dural venous sinuses, if the site of collapse is at the jugular foramen. It is also consistent with obstruction of CSF outflow as the primary cause of BIH.

CBF was 10% lower at high ICP (44±8 ml hg^1 min^{-1}) than at low ICP (49±6 ml hg^1 min^{-1}). While this trend is not significant, it could possibly indi-cate a slight impairment of CBF due to the low cerebral perfusion pressure at high ICP.

Conclusions

1. In BIH, we found CBV in the cerebral parenchyma to be unchanged or slightly increased at high ICP compared to low ICP. This result suggests that intra-vascular pressure is increased in BIH, and that resistance to blood flow must be increased at some point in the venous system.

2. CBV in the dural venous sinuses was unchanged at high ICP compared to low ICP. This result suggests that collapse of the dural venous sinuses, if present, is likely to occur at the jugular foramen.
3. CBF was unchanged or slightly reduced at high ICP compared to low ICP. This result suggests that CBF is little affected by the high ICP, but could be slightly reduced as a result of reduced cerebral perfusion pressure.

Acknowledgment. This work was supported by NIH grants # NS 15655 and 5 KO7 NS00908.

References

Alpert NM, Eriksson L, Chang JY, Bergstrom M, Litton JE, Correia JA, Bohm C, Ackerman RH, Taveras JM (1984) Strategy for the measurement of regional cerebral blood flow using short lived tracers and positron emission tomography. J Cereb Blood Flow Metab 4:28–34
Johnston I (1973) Reduced C.S.F. absorption syndrome. Reappraisal of benign intracranial hypertension and related conditions. Lancet II:418–420
Junck L (1986) Benign intracranial hypertension and normal pressure hydrocephalus: Theoretical conditions. In: Miller JD, Teasdale GM, Rowan JO, Galbraith SL, Mendelow AD (eds) Intracranial pressure VI. Springer, Berlin Heidelberg New York Tokyo, pp 447–450
Shapiro A (1977) Steady flow in collapsible tubes. J Biomech Eng 99:126–147

CBF-Studies in Patients with NPH: The Frontal Flow Pattern

J. Meixensberger, A. Brawanski, and W. Ullrich

Department of Neurosurgery, University of Würzburg, Josef-Schneider-Str. 11, 8700 Würzburg (FRG)

Introduction

Since the description of the NPH by Hakim and Adams (1965), many CBF-studies and ICP-measurements have been performed in order to evaluate the possible benefit of a shunt-operation to these patients (Mamo et al. 1987). However, the results are equivocal. Therefore, we studied the mean CBF as well as the frontal flows in patients with suspected NPH in order to find additional criteria which could help to predict the success of a shunt operation.

Patients and Methods

We studied 31 patients with suspected NPH (18 male and 13 female) with a mean age of 50.5 (21 to 86) years. As a control group, we used CBF-data of 11 normal subjects (8 male and 3 female) with a mean age of 42.8 (33 to 50) years. We performed a detailed clinical examination of each patient and noted symptoms such as vertigo, headaches, and neurological deficits according to the classical triad of NPH. All patients had a CT-scan from which we calculated the Evans-ratio (Gyldensted 1977) as a measure of ventricular dilatation. All patients had a continuous epidural ICP recording for a mean time of 48 hr. We determined the mean ICP and duration of nightly B-waves. After lumbar bolus- and infusion tests we calculated the pressure volume index and the outflow resistance according to the Marmarou model (Marmarou 1978). Based on the ICP-data, we formed two groups; one with normal and one with abnormal ICP-data. Both groups were subdivided again into groups with and without neurological deficits. The cerebral blood flow studies were performed with the noninvasive two-dimensional CBF method by the inhalation of Xenon 133 using a helmet of 32 detectors. We calculated the F1 (%ml/100 g/min) according to the two-compartment model by Obrist (Obrist 1975). The mean hemispheric flow and the mean frontal flow pattern (Geraud 1987) was calculated.

Results

Comparing the hemispheric mean flow of the two main groups to normal flow values, a significant decrease was observed for both groups. However, we could

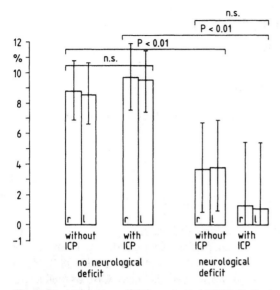

Fig. 1. Frontal pattern (%) is suspected NPH. Patients are grouped according to clinical and ICP-data. Differences were analyzed for statistical significance by unpaired t-test; *ns* = not significant

not see any significant absolute and interhemispheric flow difference within the groups. Evaluating the patients without neurological deficits irrespectively of their ICP data, we found no significant difference to the control CBF. Looking at the patients with neurological deficits in the same subdivision, we found a significant flow decrease in comparison to the control group. Furthermore, the patients with additional pathological ICP data had the lowest CBF levels. Studying the frontal pattern, we found no loss of hyperfrontality in the group without neurological deficits independent of the ICP-recordings. However, neurological symptoms caused a significant loss of hyperfrontality (Fig. 1).

Conclusion

Our data indicate that neurological deficits are the leading parameter for a flow decrease in NPH patients. The ICP level seems only to be of partial influence. Similarly, a loss of hyperfrontality is not primarily dependent on pathological ICP values in NPH. Thus, CBF-studies are a helpful tool in the evaluation of hydrocephalic patients. However, this technique is not a primary indicator for shunting.

References

Geraud G, Arne-Bes MC, Güell A, Bes A (1987) Reversibility of hemodynamic hypofrontality in schizophrenia. J Cereb Blood Flow Metab 7:9–12

Gyldensted C (1977) Measurement of the normal ventricular system and hemispheric sulci of 100 adults with computed tomography. Neuroradiology 14:183–192

Hakim S, Adams RD (1965) The special clinical problem of symptomatic hydrocephalus with normal cerebrospinal fluid pressure. Observation on cerebrospinal fluid hydrodynamics. J Neurol Sci 2:307–327

Mamo HL, Meric PC, Ponsin JC, Rey AC, Luft AG, Seylauz JA (1987) Cerebral blood flow in normal pressure hydrocephalus. Stroke 18:1074–1080

Marmarou A, Shulman K, Rosende RM (1978) A nonlinear analysis of the cerebrospinal fluid system and intracranial pressure dynamics. Neurosurgery 48:332–344

Obrist WD, Thomson HK, Wang HS (1975) Regional cerebral blood flow estimated by 133 Xenon inhalation. Stroke 6:245–256

Perioperative Intracranial Hypertension in Patients with Supratentorial Tumors: Role of CBF Changes vs Importance of Mass Effect

N. Shah, G. DiResta, E. Arbit, C. Long, W. Marx, and R. Bedford

Departments of Anesthesiology, Medical Physics and Neurological Surgery, Memorial Sloan-Kettering Cancer Center, and Cornell University Medical College, New York, NY 10021 (USA)

Introduction

Intracranial hypertension is a well-recognized complication in the perioperative management of patients with malignant supratentorial brain tumors of every cell-type, and this always is a serious concern with regard to optimal anesthetic care (Bedford et al. 1982). The compromised intracranial compliance caused by these tumors could be based on at least two possible mechanisms. One possibility is that the tumor causes an expanding mass lesion that gradually exhausts the pressure-volume reserves of the cranial compartment such that a relatively small increase in cerebral blood volume within normal brain can produce a large increase in ICP. An alternative possibility is that impaired cerebrovascular reactivity in the tumor mass might result in large increases in cerebral blood flow and consequent intracranial hypertension whenever arterial blood pressure or CO_2 tension increases. To our knowledge the relative role of these two possible mechanisms for intracranial hypertension have not been studied in a systematic fashion, although both are often invoked whenever ICP problems are discussed in managing malignant supratentorial tumors.

Recently, the availability of Laser-Doppler Flowmetry (LDF) has facilitated the measurement of regional cerebral blood flow in a variety of pathological states. LDF is an optical method that derives local blood flow from the mean Doppler shift imparted to laser light as erythrocytes move through a capillary network. Its output is a "flow index" that reflects the mean frequency of the Doppler-shifted light and is linearly related to tissue blood flow.

We have applied this technology to correlate changes in blood flow in brain tumors with normal brain blood flow during general anesthesia for craniotomy and tumor excision.

Methods

Six patients with malignant supratentorial tumors (4 gliomas, 2 metastatic lesions) were the subjects of this investigation. The protocol was approved by the local Institutional Review Board and informed consent for the study was given by the patient or their nearest relative. General anesthesia was induced with a thiopental-nitrous oxide-vecuronium sequence supplemented with either fentanyl, 3–8 µg/kg, or isoflurane, 0.4% end-tidal concentration. Controlled venti-

Table 1

Blood pressure (mm Hg)	PaCO$_2$ (mm Hg)	Normal cortex	Tumor
88 ± 5	39 ± 1	100%	16 ± 7%
83 ± 4	27 ± 1	78 ± 34%	25 ± 16%
136 ± 2	39 ± 1	100 ± 8%	16 ± 10%

All values: Mean ± S.E.; * $P < 0.05$.

lation was instituted to maintain P$_{ET}$CO$_2$ at approximately 25 mm Hg. After a wide craniotomy flap had been turned and the brain cortex had been exposed, a laser-spectroscopy flow probe was alternately placed over normal brain and over the brain tumor.

Blood flow determinations were made during the following sequence of perturbations: 1) During hypocarbia with blood pressure normal; 2) During normocarbia with blood pressure normal; 3) During normocarbia with blood pressure elevated by infusion of 0.1% phenylephrine solution. Statistical comparisons between normal brain and tumor blood flow were performed using Student's t-test for paired data. $P < .05$ was regarded as significant.

Results

Our results are summarized in Table 1. Since the numerical factor for converting LDF output to cerebral blood flow has not yet been determined for human brain, all data for tumor blood flow are tabulated as a percentage of the flow determined in the same patient's normal cortex during normotension and normocarbia.

Discussion/Conclusions

These observations indicate that blood flow through malignant supratentorial brain tumors is often only a small fraction of normal cortical cerebral blood flow. Furthermore, in the tumors examined thus far, blood flow does not change markedly with increases in arterial pressure above normal values, nor does it change with reduction of arterial CO$_2$ tension. In contrast, cerebral cortex in the vicinity of malignant brain tumors appears to retain both autoregulatory capacity and CO$_2$ responsiveness. These data support the thesis that intracranial hypertension occurring before and during operations for malignant supratentorial tumor resection results from compromised intracranial compliance due to the mass effect of the tumor, and not because of impaired vascular reactivity to CO$_2$ or arterial pressure within the tumor itself.

Reference

Bedford R, Morris J, Jane JA (1982) Intracranial hypertension during surgery for supratentorial tumors: Correlation with preoperative computed tomography scans. Anesth Analg 61:430–433

Local Brain Pressure, Microcirculation and pH During Neurosurgical Operations

M.R. Gaab, K. Ehrhardt, and H.E. Heissler

Neurosurgical Department, Hanover Medical School, Konstanty-Gutschow-Str. 8, D-3000 Hannover 61 (FRG)

Introduction

Already our daily neurosurgical experience demonstrates the adverse effects of locally increased brain pressure. If forced spatula retraction severely disturbs the microcirculation in the underlying brain tissue, a focal brain edema will rapidly follow, often associated with subarachnoid hemorrhage. The tissue damaged by the spatula pressure will undergo necrosis and large cystic defects are often the deplorable result of a careless neurosurgical technique with comfortable spatula retraction. High local brain pressures caused by spatula retraction have already been reported at the first international ICP symposium (Rivano et al. 1972) and special spatulas with automatic recording of retraction force have been designed by Albin and Bunegin (Codman Surgical Products Catalog 1985). Avoiding excessive spatula pressures is one of the main goals of microneurosurgery (Yasargil 1984) and various devices for self-retaining retractors have been developed in order to minimize the retraction force (Greenberg, "LEYLA", Yasargil 1977). However, little is known about the quantitative effects of spatula pressures on local tissue blood flow and metabolism and exact thresholds of tissue tolerance have not been established.

We therefore investigated the effects of spatula pressure on local cortical microcirculation (parameter: laser doppler) and on local tissue pH during neurosurgical operations.

Patients and Methods

The effects of spatula pressure were investigated in 9 patients during microsurgical operations. Diagnoses were glioma (4 pts.), meningiomas (2 pts.), aneurysm (1 pt.), and frontobasal trauma (2 pts.) operated by parasagittal (Rosenblum et al. 1987), transcallosal (Codman Surgical Products Catalog 1985), pterional (Rosenblum et al. 1987), and frontolateral approach (Rivano et al. 1972). According to the CT scan, the tissue edema in the area of the operative retractor position was graded.

A special spatula was designed with integrated pressure sensor, pH electrode and laser doppler probe. The stainless steel spatula is 12 mm in width, it contains a special flat pressure transducer (manufactured by GAELTEC Ltd., Scotland)

Intracranial Pressure VII
Eds.: J. T. Hoff and A. L. Betz

coplanarly mounted in the round tip. This transducer (strain gauge) with a membrane diameter of 10 mm gives a perfect frequency resolution up to 20 Hz. Next to the transducer a laser doppler head (3 mm diam.) is mounted connected with a PERIFLUX II control unit. Although the local tissue flow measured by laser doppler can by calculated in absolute values (Rivano et al. 1972), we use arbitrary units (%) for our investigation. The cortical pH is measured with a macro-pH electrode (Beetrode® manufactured by WPI) next to the pressure probe. With a length of 2 mm and a diameter of only 100 μ this micro-pH sensor measures the cortical pH directly below the tip of the spatula.

For evaluating the pressure distribution during tissue retraction, a miniature pressure sensor (GAELTEC ICT/b) was inserted subdurally below the bony margin of the trephination. It was positioned in the direction of the pressure exerted by the retractor in order to measure the "counterpressure".

All data were written on a paper recorder and evaluated by computer (HP VECTRA). As the spatula pressure decreases slowly after retraction ("pressure relaxation"), the data platted by the computer (Fig. 1) represent the average 1-s-values during 30 s (one point = 30 sec).

For comparison with the operative situation, the retractor effects were classified by the operating surgeon (M.R.G.) into "sufficient for microsurgery", "optimal for microsurgery" and "sufficient for macrosurgery" (Table 1), without knowledge of the actual spatula pressures which were noted by the engineer (K.E.).

Results

In all patients, the cortical laser-doppler-flow rapidly decreases with spatula pressures exceeding 15 mm Hg. With spatula pressures of 35–40 mm Hg, the cortical microcirculation usually collapses completely. With relaxing the retractor, the microcirculation does not recover again at spatula pressures of ≦15 mm Hg; the normalization of the microcirculation requires a complete release of the spatula ("hysteresis") (Fig. 1). Then an overproportional increase

Table 1. Retraction force and surgical requirements: Low spatula pressure without risk of structural brain damage only with careful microsurgery (n = 7)

Approach	Mean spatula pressures
Microsurgical approach – sufficient	10 ± 3 mm Hg
Microsurgical approach – "comfortable"	15 ± 4 mm Hg
Macrosurgical approach (headlight)	22 ± 7 mm Hg

Fig. 1 a–f. Retraction pressure, microcirculation, pH and counterpressure in a patient with (e–f) and without (a–c) brain edema: Decrease in cortical ICBF at ≧10–15 mm Hg, earlier with edema (a/d); simultaneous drop in pH. "Hysteresis" in ICBF with release of retraction, post-retraction hyperemia only without edema, with pH remaining low. "Counterpressure" (c/f) only slightly elevated. *pH scale:* Add +7./+6. resp. ▶

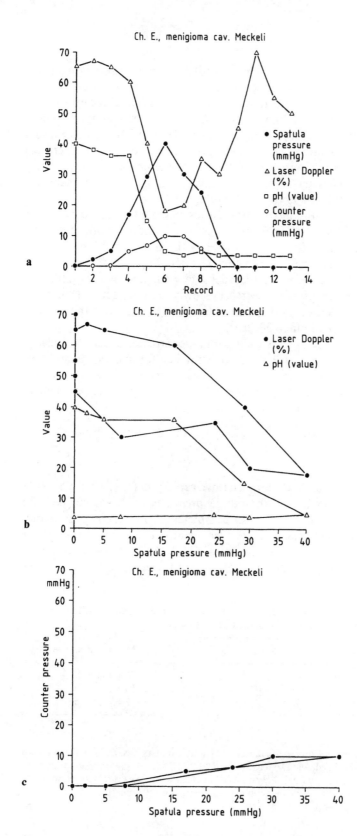

888

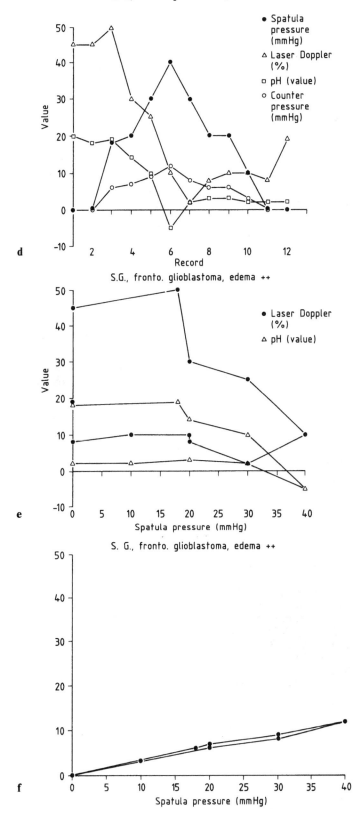

S. G., fronto. glioblastoma, edema ++

- Spatula pressure (mmHg)
△ Laser Doppler (%)
□ pH (value)
○ Counter pressure (mmHg)

d

S.G., fronto. glioblastoma, edema ++

- Laser Doppler (%)
△ pH (value)

e

S. G., fronto. glioblastoma, edema ++

f

in the laser doppler signal (= postischemic hyperemia) is often seen (Fig. 1). The pH immediately falls with decreasing cortical microflow, it may even decrease below pH 7.0 with retractor pressures of ≥ 40 mm Hg. In contrast to microflow, the pH does usually not normalize within the observation period of 10 min after release of the spatula. This low pH may explain the "relaxation hyperemia" (acidotic vasodilatation).

The "counterpressure" measured below the opposite skull margin increases only slightly with forced retraction (linear regression). This demonstrates the existence of considerable pressure differences ("gradients") within the brain during spatula retraction, a further factor for tissue damage (Fig. 1 c−f).

In edematous brain tissue, some differences were noted: The microcirculation and the pH already decrease at lower retraction pressures, the pH being lower from the beginning (Fig. 1 d−f). A postrelaxation hyperemia is usually missing.

Conclusions

Retraction pressures which will damage the local cortical blood flow and the cortical metabolism (shown by the drop in pH) may easily be exceeded during neurosurgical operations. An uncritical use of spatula retraction will then result in considerable tissue necrosis. Edematous brain tissue is even more sensitive to any retraction force.

The use of spatula retraction should therefore be avoided whenever possible (positioning, microsurgery!).

Careful microsurgical approaches require less retraction. If required, spatulas should be used with the lowest pressure which is sufficient for preparation, and the retraction would completely be released as soon as possible in short intervals.

The perioperative use of CSF drainage and/or osmotherapy may be useful in preventing excessive retraction forces.

References

Codman surgical products catalog (1985) Codman and Shurtleff Inc., pp 213
Rivano C, Rossi GF, Zattoni J (1972) Variations of intraventricular and local brain pressures during neurosurgical procedures. In: Dietz H, Brock M (eds) Intracranial pressure. Springer, Berlin Heidelberg New York, pp 343−347
Rosenblum BR, Bonner RF, Oldfield EH (1987) Intraoperative measurement of cortical blood flow adjacent to cerebral AVM using laser Doppler velocimetry. J Neurosurg 66:396−399
Yasargil MG (1977) Technical adjuncts neurosurgery. Surg Neurol 8:331−336
Yasargil MG (1984) Microneurosurgery, vol 1. Thieme/Stratton, Stuttgart New York, pp 211

Effects of Barbiturate Anesthesia and Hyperventilation on CBF in Patients with Brain Tumors

L. Junck [1], A.S.L. Van Der Spek [2], M.S. Aldrich [1], S.S. Gebarski [2], and H.S. Greenberg

Departments of [1] Neurology, [2] Anesthesiology, and [3] Radiology,, University of Michigan, Ann Arbor, Michigan 48109 (USA)

Barbiturate anesthesia and hyperventilation are both used for treatment of increased ICP. Their effectiveness for increased ICP may be related to their vascular effects, including reduction of cerebral blood volume (CBV) which directly removes volume from the head, and reduction of cerebral blood flow (CBF) which makes the Starling forces more favorable for fluid removal from the brain.

We are utilizing barbiturate anesthesia and hyperventilation to decrease CBF and increase tumor drug exposure during intra-arterial bischloroethylnitrosourea (BCNU) chemotherapy for gliomas. Drug infusion is followed by a brief period of hypercarbia to expedite drug washout from brain. It can be shown that treatment with this approach has the potential to increase tumor drug exposure nearly two-fold, while drug exposure elsewhere in the distribution of the infused artery is less affected, compared to intraarterial treatment without barbiturate anesthesia or CO_2 changes (Eckman et al. 1974).

Prior to treatment, CBF is measured in each patient using positron emission tomography (PET) in the awake resting state, during voluntary hyperventilation, and during methohexital anesthesia with normocarbia, hypocarbia, and hypercarbia.

Methods

Five patients aged 32–48 were studied. All had pathologically confirmed gliomas of grade III (2 patients), IV (2 patients), or indeterminate grade (1 patient). All had failed external beam radiotherapy. Three had tumors confined to the distribution of one carotid artery, and two had tumors confined to the distribution of the vertebrobasilar system. All patients had minimal or no mass effect from their tumor and were good candidates for anesthesia.

Positron emission tomography was performed with a PCT 4600A tomograph, which has a resolution of $1.1 \times 1.1 \times 0.95$ cm and scans 5 planes simultaneously. Cerebral blood flow (CBF) was measured by dynamic scanning for 6 min after intravenous injection of 25–30 mCi $[^{15}O]H_2O$. Parameter estimation was performed by the weighted integral lookup table approach (Alpert 1984).

Patients underwent CBF scans in 5 states: (1) awake and resting; (2) voluntary hyperventilation (P_aCO_2 ~20 mmHg); (3) barbiturate anesthesia (P_aCO_2 ~40 mmHg); (4) barbiturate anesthesia with hypocarbia (P_aCO_2 ~20 mmHg);

and (5) barbiturate anesthesia with supplemental CO_2 (P_aCO_2 ~60 mm Hg). Anesthesia was induced and maintained with methohexital. Vecuronium was used for muscle relaxation, and respirations were controlled. The depth of anesthesia was gauged by electroencephalography (EEG), and the methohexital infusion was regulated to achieve a burst-suppression pattern with interburst intervals averaging 10–15 s.

Results and Discussion

Our results indicate that CBF is markedly affected by barbiturate anesthesia and by changes in P_aCO_2, even in patients with gliomas involving the brain who have previously undergone radiation therapy (Table 1). The relative effect of barbiturate anesthesia on tumor blood flow was significantly reduced compared to the effect on remote brain (Table 2). In contrast, the CO_2 responsiveness of tumor was equal to that of brain.

Table 1. Blood flow results

	$PaCO_2$ mm Hg	Blood flow in remote brain ml hg^{-1} min^{-1}	Blood flow in tumor ml hg^{-1} min^{-1}
Awake, resting	40 ± 6	34 ± 8	25 ± 8
Awake, hyperventilation (% of awake)	22 ± 5	22 ± 2 ($64\pm14\%$)	15 ± 9 ($63\pm23\%$)
Barbiturate, normocarbic (% of awake)	42 ± 5	18 ± 3 ($54\pm5\%$)	19 ± 8 ($76\pm13\%$)
Barbiturate, hypocarbic (% of awake)	20 ± 2	12 ± 2 ($37\pm6\%$)	13 ± 7 ($50\pm14\%$)
Barbiturate, hypercarbic (% of awake)	68 ± 15	50 ± 14 ($170\pm67\%$)	40 ± 20 ($140\pm39\%$)

All values are expressed as mean ± SD.
Values in parentheses represent the percentage of the awake, resting values.

Table 2. Barbiturate and CO_2 effects on blood flow are additive

Region	Barbiturate effect (Blood flow barbiturate/awake)		CO_2 effect (%/mm Hg)	
	Normocarbia ($PaCO_2$ ~40)	Hypocarbia ($PaCO_2$ ~20)	Awake	Barbiturate
Remote brain	0.52 ± 0.05**	0.59 ± 0.05*	2.4 ± 0.6	1.8 ± 0.4
Tumor	0.74 ± 0.13**	0.78 ± 0.12*	2.5 ± 1.5	2.0 ± 1.0

All values are expressed as mean ± SD.
CO_2 effect was calculated over the normocarbic-hypocarbic range.
  * $P=0.10$, tumor vs. remote brain.
** $P<0.05$, tumor vs. remote brain.

Our results indicate that the effects of barbiturate anesthesia and CO_2 changes on blood flow are nearly additive. The relative effect of barbiturate anesthesia on blood flow in brain and tumor was only slightly less at hypocarbia than at normocarbia (Table 2). The CO_2 responsiveness under barbiturate anesthesia was 75% and 78% of that in the awake state in brain and tumor, respectively. These differences were not significant.

We were able to reduce blood flow to profoundly low levels of $10-15$ ml hg^{-1} min^{-1} without sequelae during barbiturate anesthesia with hypocarbia. Barbiturate anesthesia is known to reduce cerebral metabolism approximately in proportion to the reduction in blood flow, and as a result the brain does not suffer ischemic consequences.

Both barbiturate anesthesia and hypocarbia are used in the treatment of increased ICP. If decreases in CBF underlie the effectiveness of hypocarbia and barbiturate anesthesia on ICP, then our results suggest that both modalities should be effective for ICP reduction in patients with focal brain lesions, and their effects on ICP should be approximately additive.

Conclusions

1. In brain tumors, blood flow responses to barbiturate anesthesia are attenuated compared to remote brain, but responses to changes in P_aCO_2 are intact.
2. Brief reduction of CBF to profoundly low levels can be performed safely with barbiturate anesthesia and hypocarbia.
3. Effects of barbiturate anesthesia and hypocarbia on CBF are additive.
4. If changes in CBF underlie changes in ICP, then hypocarbia and barbiturate anesthesia should have additive effects on ICP.

Acknowledgements. This work was supported by Grants # NS 15655, 5 K07 NS00908, and 5 M01 RR00042 from the National Institutes of Health.

References

Alpert NM, Eriksson L, Chang JY, Bergstrom M, Litton JE, Correia JA, Bohm C, Ackerman RH, Taveras JM: Strategy for the measurement of regional cerebral blood flow using short-lived tracers and emission tomography. J Cereb Blood Flow Metab 4:28–34
Eckman WW, Patlak CS, Fenstermacher JD (1974) A critical evaluation of the principles governing the advantages of intraarterial infusions. J Pharmacokinet Biopharm 2:257–285

Barbiturates, Cerebral Blood Flow and Intracranial Hypertension

Z.L. Gokaslan, C.S. Robertson, R.K. Narayan, and C.F. Contant

Department of Neurosurgery, Baylor College of Medicine, Houston, Texas 77030 (USA)

Introduction

Although their efficacy in improving outcome from severe head injury is difficult to prove (Ward et al. 1985; Schwartz et al. 1984; Miller 1979), it has conclusively shown that in certain patients barbiturates can reduce intracranial hypertension (ICH) refractory to conventional measures (Marshall et al. 1979; Rockoff et al. 1979; Rea and Rockswold 1983; Eisenberg et al. 1988). The mechanism of this effect remains unclear. It has been demonstrated that under normal physiological conditions, barbiturates in anesthetic doses, decrease cerebral blood flow (CBF) (Michenfelder and Milde 1975) and cerebral metabolic rate of oxygen ($CMRO_2$) (Michenfelder and Milde 1975) and lactate (CMRL) (Carlsson et al. 1975). This prospective study was undertaken to ascertain the effects of barbiturates on these parameters in patients with ICH with the aim of deriving mechanistic insights and possibly identifying features that would characterize patients responsive to barbiturates (responders).

Clinical Materials and Methods

Ten patients with closed head injury who had developed intracranial hypertension (ICH) refractory to conventional measures, and eventually required barbiturate coma (BC) for control of intracranial pressure (ICP), were studied prospectively.

The demographic characteristics, admission Glasgow Coma Scores (GCS) and outcome scores of these patients are illustrated in Table 1. Ages ranged between 20 and 49, and there was a male predominance. Six out of 10 patients had intracranial mass lesions such as epidural hematoma (EDH) and subdural hematoma (SDH), 3 patients had diffuse brain injury (DBI), and one demonstrated only intraventricular hemorrhage (IVH). Only one patient had a GCS of 11 on admission, the rest ranged from 3 to 7.

Conventional measures for ICP control included proper positioning of the neck, sedation, ventricular drainage, hyperventilation and mannitol administration. In those who did not respond to these measures, BC was instituted for ICP control. Serial barbiturate levels were obtained to assure satisfactory blood concentrations (3–4%). Mean arterial pressure (MAP), cerebral blood flow (CBF), cerebral metabolic rate for lactate (CMRL) and for oxygen ($CMRO_2$) were

Table 1. Demographic characteristics of the patients

Case #	Age	Sex	Injury[b]	GCS[c]	Outcome[d]
1	41	F	ICH	6	D
2	20	M	EDH	4	D
3	35	F	ICH	6	D
4	21	M	DBI	6	D
5	22	F	ICH	6	MD[a]
6	24	M	SDH	6	V[a]
7	(unknown)	M	DBI	3	V
8	41	M	IVH	4	V
9	(unknown)	M	DBI	11	D
10	49	F	SDH	7	D

[a] Responders (ICP elevation controlled with barbiturate coma);
[b] Injury types; EDH: Epidural hematoma; SDH: Subdural hematoma; ICH: intracerebral hematoma. DBI: Diffuse brain injury; IVH: Intraventricular hemorrhage;
[c] GCS: Glasgow Coma Score on admission;
[d] GOS: Glasgow Outcome Scale (*GR*–Good recovery; *MD*–Moderate disability; *SD*–severe disability; *V*–vegetative; *D*–dead) at 3 months and/or discharge.

measured before and after the institution of BC. CBF was measured by the Kety-Schmidt technique using nitrous oxide as the indicator. Simultaneously with measurement of CBF, arterial and jugular venous blood samples were obtained for determination of blood gases, oxygen saturation, hemoglobin and lactate concentrations. $CMRO_2$ and CMRL were calculated by multiplying the CBF by the arterial-jugular venous difference of oxygen content and lactate, respectively.

Results

Only 2 out of 10 patients responded to BC with a satisfactory control of ICH. ICP control was defined as being able to keep the mean ICP below or equal to 20 mm Hg. Although the groups were small, no clear differences were noted between the responders and non-responders in terms of age, initial GCS, type of injury, and MAP. All of the patients required vasopressors to correct barbiturate-induced hypotension. Eventual outcome was poor in the non-responders (vegetative – 2; dead – 6) and not much better in the responders (moderately disabled – 1; vegetative – 1).

All patients, regardless of ICP response, showed a decrease in $CMRO_2$ after the administration of barbiturates (responders 1.22 to 0.72; non-responders 0.86 to 0.57 µmol/g/min) except for those with very low initial $CMRO_2$ values (<0.60) (Fig. 1). Similarly, most of the patients showed a decrease in CMRL with treatment (−0.044 to −0.036 µmol/g/min) independent of ICP response (Fig. 2). Both responders had higher CBF values than non-responders before barbiturate administration, and only responders demonstrated significant decrease in CBF following BC (responders 60.2 to 34.4; non-responders 36.7 to 34.7 ml/100/g/min) (Fig. 3).

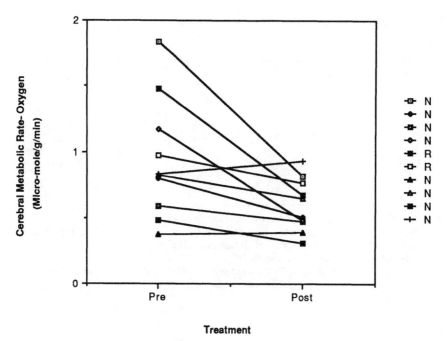

Fig. 1. Pre and post treatment values for $CMRO_2$

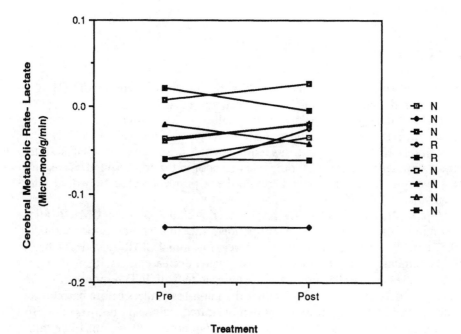

Fig. 2. Pre and post treatment values for CMRL

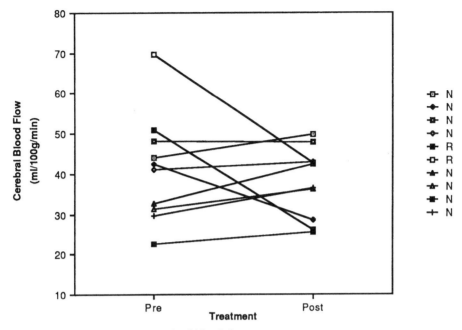

Fig. 3. Pre and post treatment cerebral blood flow

Conclusions

Based on our findings the following conclusions can be made:

1. Barbiturates reduce both aerobic and anaerobic metabolism regardless of their effect on ICP.
2. Patients with high CBF values are more likely to respond to barbiturates than those with low values.
3. CBF measurements can be used to select out a subset of patients with ICH who are more likely to benefit from barbiturates.

References

Carlsson C, Harp JR, Siesjö BK (1975) Metabolic changes in the cerebral cortex of the rat induced by intravenous pentothalsodium. Acta Anaesthesiol Scand [Suppl] 57:7–17

Eisenberg HM, Frankowski R, Contant CF (1988) CNS Trauma Centers: High dose barbiturates control ICP in patients with severe head injury. J Neurosurg (in press)

Marshall LF, Smith RW, Shapiro HM (1979) The outcome with aggressive treatment in severe head injuries: Acute and chronic barbiturate administration in the management of head injury. J Neurosurg 50:26–30

Michenfelder JD, Milde JH (1975) Influence of anesthetics on metabolic, functional and pathological responses to regional cerebral ischemia. Stroke 6:405–410

Miller JD (1979) Barbiturates and raised intracranial pressure. Ann Neurol 6:189–193

Rea GL, Rockswold GL (1983) Barbiturate therapy in uncontrolled intracranial hypertension. Neurosurgery 12:401–404

Rockoff MA, Marshall LF, Shapiro HV (1979) High-dose barbiturate therapy in humans: A clinical review of 60 patients. Ann Neurol 6:194–199

Schwartz ML, Tabor CH, Towed DW et al. (1984) The University of Toronto head injury treatment study: A prospective randomized comparison of pentobarbital and mannitol. Can J Neurol Sci 11:434–440

Ward JD, Becker DP, Miller JD et al. (1985) Failure of prophylactic barbiturate coma in the treatment of severe head injury. J Neurosurg 65:383–388

Cerebral Vasoconstriction is Not Maintained with Prolonged Hyperventilation

J.P. Muizelaar and H.G. van der Poel

Division of Neurosurgery, Medical College of Virginia, Virginia Commonwealth University, Richmond, Virginia (USA)

It is generally accepted that hyperventilation reduces ICP by reducing cerebral blood volume (CBV) through constriction of the pial and cerebral arterioles. As CO_2 readily crosses the blood-brain barrier, a decreased $PaCO_2$ is immediately reflected in a reduced PCO_2 in interstitial brain fluid. This, in turn, leads to a reduction in H^+ concentration in the vicinity of the cerebral blood vessels. Because the H^+ ion is one of the most potent relaxants of smooth muscles of cerebral arterioles, a reduction in its concentration will lead to rapid vasoconstriction. Thus, vasoconstriction is not dependent on low CO_2 and can be maintained only if the increased perivascular pH can be maintained (Kontos et al. 1977; Wahl et al. 1970). It has been shown, however, that pH in blood and cerebrospinal fluid (CSF) returns to normal during prolonged hyperventilation, despite sustained hypocapnia (Christensen 1974; Levasseur et al. 1979; McDowall and Harper 1968). The purpose of the present investigation was to examine whether the return to normal pH during prolonged hyperventilation would be accompanied by vaso-relaxation.

Materials and Methods

New Zealand white rabbits of either sex, weighing between 2 and 4 kg, were used in this study. A cranial window was installed three weeks prior to the actual experiment. Pial arteriolar diameters on the parietal surface of the brain was measured with a Vickers image-splitting device connected to a Leitz microscope (Levasseur et al. 1975). On the day of the experiment, anesthesia was induced by injection of 25 mg/kg pentobarbital. Next, the animal was intubated and lines were introduced into the femoral artery and vein. A 20-gauge i.v. needle was stuck into the cisterna magna for withdrawing of the CSF samples. For the duration of the experiment, the animals were infused with an i.v. solution of 5% dextrose in half normal saline, 3 ml/kg/hr, containing pentobarbital sodium for a dose of 1 mg/kg/hr and gallamine triethiodide 2 mg/kg/hr. The animals were semi-covered with a heating pad and their rectal temperature was maintained at 38°C.

The animals were ventilated with a respirator in which a small amount of oxygen was bled to obtain an inspiratory pO_2 of 25–30%. End-expiratory CO_2 was measured constantly. The rate and volume of the respirator were adjusted to give an end-expiratory PCO_2 equal to 38 mm Hg (corresponding to 38 mm Hg in the blood gases measurements) during baseline measurements and of 25 during hyperventilation. pH, HCO_3^- and PCO_2 were measured in blood and CSF every four hours in a microblood gas analyzer.

To obtain stable baseline readings, 4 hr were allowed to elapse from the beginning of anesthesia. The vessel diameters at this point, taken at a $PaCO_2$ of 38 mm Hg were considered 100%, all subsequent diameters of each individual vessel were calculated as a percentage of its own baseline value. In the control group of 3 rabbits, $PaCO_2$ was maintained at 38 mm Hg for 52 hr. Every 4 hr vessel diameters and blood and CSF gases and pH were measured; then, CO_2 reactivity was assessed by hyperventilation to a $PaCO_2$ of 25 mm Hg for 10 min and measuring vessel diameters again. Next, $PaCO_2$ was allowed to return to baseline for another 4 hr. The experimental group consisted of 7 rabbits. After baseline measurements, the animals were hyperventilated to a $PaCO_2$ of 25 mm Hg. Every 4 hr vessel diameters and blood and CSF gases and pH were measured; then, CO_2 reactivity was assessed by allowing $PaCO_2$ to return to 38 mm Hg for 10 min and measuring vessel diameters again. Next, the animals were hyperventilated again for another 4 hr, for a total duration of hyperventilation of 52 hr.

Results

In the three rabbits in the control group, baseline pH in blood and CSF were 7.42 ± 0.02 and 7.36 ± 0.01, respectively. This remained constant and at the end of the experiment values of 7.40 ± 0.06 and 7.35 ± 0.02 were found. Baseline values of HCO_3^- were 24.9 ± 3.7 mmol/l and 26.0 ± 1.0 mmol/l, respectively, and also did not change significantly, being 22.0 ± 2.8 mmol/l and 25.3 ± 2.9 mmol/l at the end of the experiment. Of course, $PaCO_2$ remained at 38 mm Hg. PCO_2 in CSF was 46.3 ± 2.5 mm Hg at the beginning and 45.8 ± 7.6 mm Hg at the end of the experiment. Diameter of 16 vessels (average diameter 70.9 ± 16.5 μm, range 49–97 μm) was measured. Diameter at $PaCO_2$ of 38 mm Hg did not change during the experiment, while constriction with temporary hyperventilation to $PaCO_2$ of 25 mm Hg remained constantly around 9% of the baseline diameter.

The experimental group consisted of 7 rabbits. Mean arterial blood pressure remained virtually unchanged throughout the experiment. $PaCO_2$, pH and HCO_3^- in arterial blood are shown in Fig. 1. Baseline pH was 7.47 ± 0.05, going up to a maximum of 7.57 ± 0.06 at 30 min after the start of hyperventilation, and then precipitously falling again, with return to baseline at 20 hr. From then on some nonsignificant variation in pH occurred, but at the end of the experiment pH was exactly the same as in the beginning: i.e., 7.47 ± 0.09. In contrast, arterial HCO_3^- remained decreased throughout the experiment. Figure 1 also shows PCO_2, pH and HCO_3^- in CSF. For PCO_2 and pH the trends are similar as they are in blood, albeit somewhat slower: maximum pH and lowest CO_2 in CSF are reached at 8 hrs, but at 30 min there is already a significant change of both values. The reason for these slower changes is probably that we mesured pH and PCO_2 in CSF from the cisterna magna where it takes some time for the extracellular

900

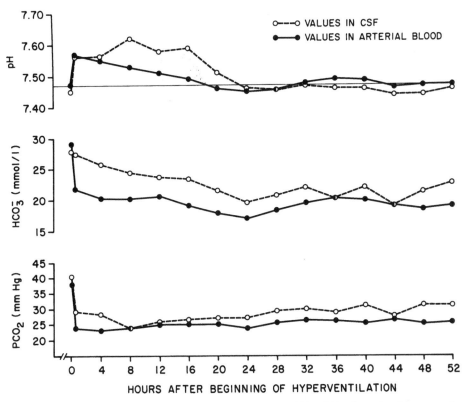

Fig. 1. pH, bicarbonate and PCO_2 values in CSF and arterial blood 30 min and at 4-hr intervals after beginning of hyperventilation in experimental group. Only means are given, *SEM's* were too small to be drawn

fluid to "sink in." In CSF, HCO_3^- did not decrease quickly, and minimum concentration was reached only at 24 hr.

Vessel diameter in the experimental group is shown in Fig. 2. Within 30 min, hyperventilation constricted the vessels by almost 14%. However, from that time on vessel diameter at $PaCO_2$ of 25 mm Hg slowly increased, crossing baseline at 20 hr, concomitant with the return of pH of arterial blood to baseline. From 24 hr on vessels were larger than at baseline, but this was not statistically significant at all 4 hr intervals; however, in cases where diameter was not statistically significantly larger than baseline, p-values were around 0.07 (paired T-test), so that we consider the diameter increase to be real. The vessel relaxation with the temporary return of $PaCO_2$ to 38 mm Hg ranged from 9–13% the first 20 hr and from 12–18% after 24 hr (p<0.01, Student's *T*-test).

Discussion

This paper shows that in the rabbit, pial arteriolar vasoconstriction is not maintained with prolonged hyperventilation. This is due to the return to normal of

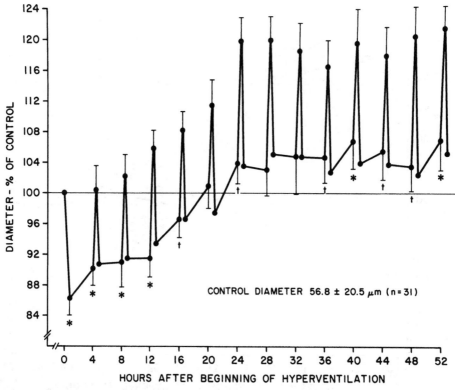

Fig. 2. Diameter of pial arterioles in experimental group, 30 min and at 4-hr intervals after beginning of hyperventilation. The percentages of control values are shown (mean ± *SEM*). Lower values taken at $PaCO_2$ of 25 mm Hg, peak values taken during brief normoventilation to $PaCO_2$ of 38 mm Hg. Values marked with an *asterisk* are significantly different from control ($p < 0.05$), values marked with a *cross* have $p < 0.1$

CSF pH. Moreover, the responses to similar changes in $PaCO_2$ tended to increase in time during prolonged hyperventilation. This is due to the decrease in bicarbonate ion concentration in CSF, so that changes in CO_2 are buffered less adequately, resulting in larger changes in pH with equal CO_2 changes.

Several authors have shown that pH of blood and CSF returns to normal during prolonged hyperventilation (Christensen 1974; Levasseur et al. 1979; McDowall and Harper 1968). In blood this is effected mainly through renal adjustment, in the CSF probably through diminished secretion of bicarbonate by the choroid plexus (Siesjö 1977). It has been shown that with prolonged hyperventilation changes in brain pH in response to CO_2 changes are larger than those to equal CO_2 changes during normal ventilation, and this was found to be accompanied by increased CO_2 reactivity of pial arterioles (Levasseur et al. 1979). These findings were ascribed to diminished buffer capacity as a consequence of decreased bicarbonate concentration. Conversely, in rabbits breathing air rich in CO_2 during 6 days, an increasing concentration of bicarbonate in CSF was found, accompanied by diminishing CO_2 reactivity of pial arterioles (Levasseur et al.

1979). The gradual increase in relative CO_2 reactivity in the present paper can also be ascribed to this increased magnitude of extracellular pH changes with similar CO_2 changes. It is true that the increase in CO_2 reactivity is small: from 12% at 4 hr to 16% at 52 hr, but this corresponds to an increase in volume in these vessels of 25% and 35% respectively. In fact, at the end of the experiment vessel diameter at $PaCO_2$ of 38 mm Hg was 122% of baseline, an increase in blood volume in those vessels of 49%.

The implications of this study are two-fold. First, the results support the hypothesis that (extracellular) pH is more important in so-called CO_2 reactivity than CO_2 itself. Second, and more important, these findings indicate that hyperventilation is effective in reducing cerebral blood volume for less than 24 hours and that it should be used only during actual ICP elevations. If used preventively, as is sometimes advocated (Bruce et al. 1981), its effect may have worn off by the time ICP starts to rise for other reasons and further decreases in $PaCO_2$ are difficult to obtain. Moreover, the reduction in buffer capacity with lower bicarbonate concentration renders the vessels more sensitive to changes in $PaCO_2$. This could lead to more pronounced and dangerous ICP elevations during transient rises in $PaCO_2$, such as during endotracheal suctioning of severely head injured patients.

References

Bruce DA, Alavi A, Bilaniuk L et al. (1981) Diffuse cerebral swelling following head injury in children: The syndrome of "malignant brain edema." J Neurosurg 54:170–178

Christensen MS (1974) Acid-base changes in cerebrospinal fluid and blood, and blood volume changes following prolonged hyperventilation in man. Br J Anaesth 46:348

Kontos HA, Raper AJ, Patterson JL Jr (1977) Analysis of vasoactivity of local pH, PCO_2 and bicarbonate on pial vessels. Stroke 8:358–360

Kontos HA, Wei EP, Raper AJ et al. (1977) Local mechanism of CO_2 action on cat pial arterioles. Stroke 8:226–229

Levasseur JE, Wei EP, Raper AJ et al. (1975) Detailed description of a cranial window technique for acute and chronic experiments. Stroke 6:308–317

Levasseur JE, Wei EP, Kontos HA et al. (1979) Responses of pial arterioles after prolonged hypercapnia and hypoxia in the awake rabbit. J Appl Physiol 46:89–95

McDowall DG, Harper AM (1968) CBF and CSF pH in the monkey during prolonged hyperventilation. J Lab Clin Invest [Suppl] 102

Siesjö BK (1972) The regulation of cerebrospinal fluid pH. Kidney Int 1:360–374

Wahl M, Deetjen P, Thuran K et al. (1970) Micropuncture evaluation of the importance of perivascular pH for the arteriolar diameter on the brain surface. Pflugers Arch 316:152–163

The Effect of High Frequency Ventilation on Cerebral Blood Flow and Cerebrovascular Autoregulation in Rabbits

B. Bissonnette[1], E.A. Hagen[2], C.A. Richardson[2], G.A. Gregory[2]

[1] Department of Anesthesia and the Research Institute, The Hospital for Sick Children, Toronto, Ontario (Canada) [2] Department of Anesthesia and Cardiovascular Research Institute, University of California, San Francisco (USA)

Introduction

The hemodynamic effects of conventional mechanical ventilation are well known. Investigation of high frequency jet ventilation has revealed unique cardiovascular effects (baroreflex, brain surface vessel movement). Although several studies have examined cerebral blood flow and intracranial pressure during high frequency jet ventilation, none have made these measurements across a wide range of blood pressures to determine if high frequency jet ventilation alters cerebrovascular autoregulation and none have controlled for changes in intrathoracic volume that may occur when changing from conventional mechanical ventilation to high frequency jet ventilation. We hypothesized that under the same blood pressure and intrathoracic volume, cerebrovascular autregulation and, therefore, cerebral blood flow were different during high frequency jet ventilation when compared with conventional mechanical ventilation.

Methods and Materials

With the approval of the Committee on Animal Research, we studied 5 New Zealand White Rabbits (2.5–3.5 kg) and continuously measured systemic arterial pressure, intracranial pressure, central venous pressure, and regional cerebral blood flow. Regional cerebral blood flow was measured by the H_2 clearance technique (Aukland et al. 1964). Electrodes were cut from 25 µm diameter teflon coated platinum (Pt) iridium (Ir) wire. One end was briefly held over an alcohol lamp to remove the teflon and allow connection to the preamplifiers. After polarizing the platinum electrodes as anodes ($+0.3$ V) and waiting 20 min for stabilization, H_2 (10%) was delivered for two to five breaths. A nonlinear regression routine estimated the parameters of an exponential function by the least squares method. Measurments were made during conventional mechanical ventilation and compared to measurements during high frequency jet ventilation. The comparisons were made over a wide range of blood pressures (40–175 mm Hg) so that pressure dependent changes in flow (which would indicate changes in cerebrovascular autoregulation) could be determined. To achieve the different blood pressure levels, an intravenous infusion of either trimethaphan or epinephrine was used. Both of these vasoactive drugs do not cross the blood-brain barrier and,

Eds.: J.T. Hoff and A.L. Betz
© Springer-Verlag Berlin Heidelberg 1989

therefore, do not have any direct cerebrovascular effect. A jacket plethysmograph (Cartwright et al. 1983) was used to measure intrathoracic volume so that by adjusting ventilator pressure, the intrathoracic lung volume could be kept constant to avoid changes in venous return and central venous pressure which could effect intracranial pressure and/or cerebral blood flow. The animals were anesthetized with urethane and paralyzed with metocurine. Baseline measurements at normal blood pressure were obtained during conventional mechanical ventilation (rate 35 breaths per minute) and then repeated during high frequency jet ventilation (rate 600 breaths per minute). High frequency jet ventilator pressure was adjusted to maintain the mean lung volume equal to that during conventional mechanical ventilation by using the plethysmograph volume as a guide. After measurements during high frequency jet ventilation the animal was returned to conventional mechanical ventilation and the measurements were repeated. The type of ventilation to start the experiment and to determine the sequence was initially determined in a random manner to avoid any biases. This sequence was repeated across the range of blood pressures for each animal. Finally, at the end of the experiment, two measurements were done outside the range of autoregulation, one hypercarbic (CO_2 equal to 100 ± 5.6 mm Hg) and one hypotensive (mean arterial pressure equal to 30 ± 4.0 mm Hg) as reference. Analysis of cerebral blood flow data for all animals at all blood pressures were analysed by the Wilcoxon Sign test. Differences were considered statistically significant when $p < 0.05$.

Results

In 2 of the 5 animals, regional cerebral blood flow was always greater during high frequency jet ventilation than during conventional mechanical ventilation at the same blood pressures and intrathoracic volume (Fig. 1). In 2 of the remaining 3 animals, regional blood flow during high frequency jet ventilation was not always greater, but in all animals the intracranial pressure during high frequency jet ventilation was always greater than during conventional mechanical ventilation

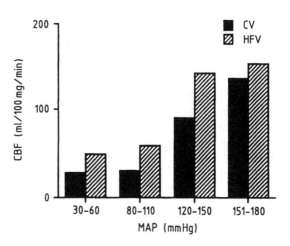

Fig. 1. For rabbit #1 the regional cerebral blood flow during high frequency jet ventilation is greater than conventional ventilation at the same blood pressures and intrathoracic volumes

905

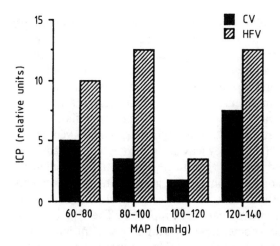

Fig. 2. In all animals the intracranial pressure during high frequency jet ventilation is greater than during conventional mechanical ventilation at the same blood pressures and intrathoracic volumes

(Fig. 2). This result suggests that the total cerebral blood flow may have been greater during high frequency jet ventilation, although the measurement of local blood flow in this instance did not reflect the global blood flow changes. In the one remaining animal, regional blood flow during high frequency jet ventilation was similar to conventional mechanical ventilation and intracranial pressure did not suggest a consistent change in total cerebral blood flow. Analysis of cerebral blood flow data for all animals at all blood pressures shows a statistically significant increase in cerebral blood flow during high frequency jet ventilation compared to cerebral blood flow during conventional ventilation ($p < 0.002$).

Discussion

These results indicate that high frequency jet ventilation can increase total, as well as local, cerebral blood flow when compared to conventional mechanical ventilation at the same blood pressure and intrathoracic volume. This increase in flow can be reflected in an increase in intracranial pressure. The increased flow may be the result of dilation of the cerebral vessels rather than a change in cerebrovascular autoregulation since flow during high frequency jet ventilation was higher at all blood pressures, even during hypotension. Increased cerebral blood flow would be particularly dangerous in individuals with diminished autoregulation (e.g. during hypercarbia), head-injured patients or in neonates whose autoregulation is absent and who have fragile cerebral vessels placing them at risk for spontaneous intracranial hemorrhage.

References

Aukland K, Fowler BF, Berliner RW (1964) Measurement of local blood flow with hydrogen gas. Circ Res 14:164–187
Cartwright DW, Gregory GA, Willis MM (1983) A respiratory function jacket for measuring tidal volume and changes in FRC. J Appl Physiol 55:263–266

Effects of Glycerol on Cerebral Blood Flow and Oxygen Metabolism

M. Ishikawa[2], H. Kikuchi[2], S. Nishizawa[1], Y. Yonekura[1], A. Kobayashi[2], and W. Taki[2]

Department of Neurosurgery and Nuclear Medicine[1], Faculty of Medicine, Kyoto University and Department of Neurosurgery, National Cardiovascular Center[2], Kyoto 606 (Japan)

Introduction

Glycerol, as well as mannitol, reduces intracranial pressure and increases cerebral blood flow. However, the effects of glycerol on regional cerebral oxygen metabolism and its correlation with cerebral blood flow have not been thoroughly investigated. In the present study, using positron emission tomography (PET), regional changes in cerebral blood flow (CBF), cerebral blood volume (CBV), cerebral oxygen consumption ($CMRO_2$) and cerebral oxygen extraction (OEF) after administration of glycerol to normal volunteers and patients with meningioma were studied. A portion of this study had been reported elsewhere (Kobayashi et al. 1985).

Methods

Regional CBF and cerebral oxygen metabolism were studied by continuous inhalation of ^{15}O-labeled O_2 and CO_2 gases with a PET scanner. The unextracted intravascular activity was corrected by separately measuring cerebral blood volume (CBV) after ^{15}O-labeled CO gas inhalation. After the control study with inhalation of CO, O_2 and CO_2 gases in that order, 0.4 g/kg of 10% glycerol was given intravenously for 20 min. The postinfusion study was then started 5 min later and proceeded for about 40 min.

Five normal volunteers and 6 patients with meningiomas with perifocal edema on CT were studied. In the meningioma patients, a single section at the level of perifocal edema was selected and the 4 regions-of-interest were placed on the peritumoral cortex and white matter, and corresponding contralateral cortex and white matter. Values for each parameter were obtained in the 4 regions-of-interest.

Results

Blood gases and mean blood pressure were within normal levels and there were no differences between the control and the postinfusion studies. Modest, but statistically significant decreases in hematocrit and hemoglobin were noted.

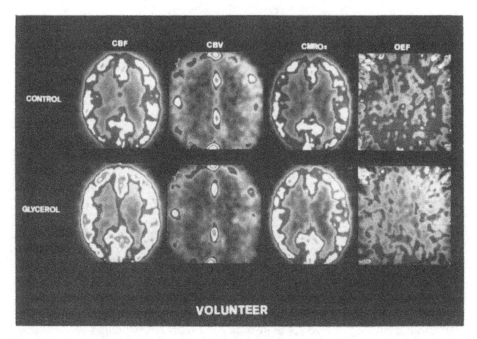

Fig. 1. Cerebral blood flow and oxygen metabolism after glycerol administration in a normal volunteer. Abbreviations: CBF, cerebral blood flow; CMRO$_2$, cerebral metabolic rate for oxygen; OEF, oxygen extraction fraction; CBV, cerebral blood volume

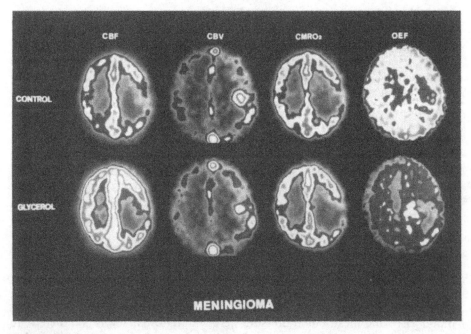

Fig. 2. Cerebral blood flow and oxygen metabolism after glycerol administration in a patient with meningioma. See abbreviation in Fig. 1

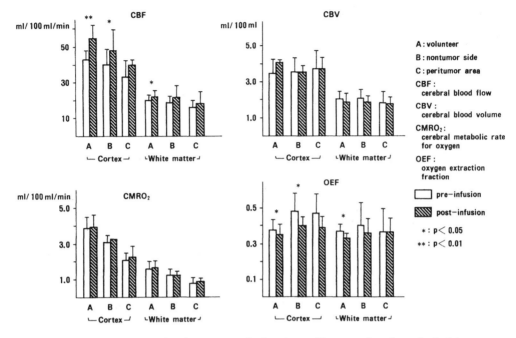

Fig. 3. Regional changes of each parameter in 4 regions-of-interest after glycerol administration. See abbreviation in Fig. 1

Table 1. Physiological parameters before and after glycerol infusion

	Volunteer ($n = 5$)		Meningioma ($n = 6$)	
	Pre	Post	Pre	Post
Ht (%)	41.6 ± 3.1	$39.7 \pm 2.6^*$	39.5 ± 2.6	$37.8 \pm 1.9^*$
Hb (g/dl)	13.3 ± 0.9	$13.5 \pm 1.0^*$	13.3 ± 0.7	$13.2 \pm 0.7^*$
$PaCO_2$ (mm Hg)	37.3 ± 1.3	36.9 ± 1.8	39.0 ± 0.8	38.9 ± 1.6
PaO_2 (mm Hg)	92.3 ± 3.3	96.2 ± 11.2	97.8 ± 9.0	97.3 ± 6.0
O_2 CT (%)	19.3 ± 1.5	19.3 ± 1.4	18.3 ± 0.9	18.3 ± 1.1
BP mean (mm Hg)	92.0 ± 11.9	95.6 ± 13.9	95.7 ± 10.4	99.9 ± 8.1

* $p < 0.05$.

After administration of glycerol, the regional CBF increased in all 5 normal volunteers (Fig. 1) and in 5 of the six with meningioma (Fig. 2). About a 20% increase in CBF was noted throughout an extensive area including the peritumoral area. Quantiatively (Fig. 3), significant increases were noted in the cortex and white matter of normal volunteers, and in the cortex contralateral to the tumor in the meningioma patients. The trend toward CBF increase was also noted in the peritumoral cortex and white matter. In contrast, regional CBV did not change after glycerol administration in either the cortex or white matter in the normal volunteers or the meningioma patients. Regional $CMRO_2$ increased to a modest degree. It was less than the increase in CBF and no statistical differences were noted in all areas examined. This resulted in significant decreases in OEF in the cortex and white matter of the normal volunteers and the cortex contralateral to the meningioma.

Discussion

The present study has revealed that glycerol increases CBF extensively, even in peritumoral edema areas and the overlying cortex. It does increase CBF in the cortex and white matter of normal volunteers. In contrast, however, CBV did not change. $CMRO_2$ was extensively increased to a modest degree and this resulted in a diffuse decrease in OEF. The significant increase in CBF corresponded well with that by mannitol, also a hyperosmolar agent. Mannitol increases perfusion pressure and decreases blood viscosity (Muizellar et al. 1983). These changes favor the increase in CBF. The decrease in the hematocrit, which is closely related to the blood viscosity, was noted after glycerol infusion. Although it decreased by about 2% systemically, the hematocrit in the brain may be reduced by much more. Meyer et al. (1975) reported a decrease in hemispheric oxygen consumption in the infarcted hemisphere. The present study revealed that cerebral oxygen consumption did not decrease, but rather increased slightly in patients with meningioma. This excluded the possible mechanism of an increase in CBF coupled with an increase in oxygen metabolism. Whatever the mechanism of CBF increase, the decrease in OEF indicates that glycerol improves the functional reserve for oxygen metabolism in the brain.

References

Kobayashi A, Hajime H et al. (1985) Changes in local cerebral blood flow and oxygen metabolism with glycerol infusion in various pathologic states: In: Inaba Y, Klatzo I, Spatz M (eds) Brain edema. Springer, Berlin Heidelberg New York Tokyo, pp 272–276
Meyer JS, Ito Y et al. (1975) Circulatory and metabolic effects of glycerol infusion in patients with recent cerebral infarction. Circulation 51:701–712
Muizellar JP, Weil EP et al. (1985) Mannitol causes compensatory cerebral vasoconstriction and vasodilation to blood viscosity changes. J Neurosurg 59:822–828

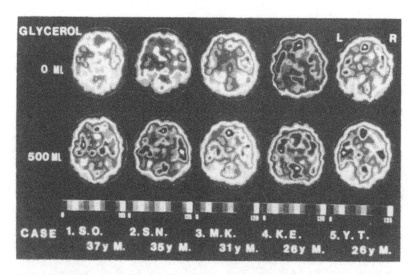

Fig. 1. Change in regional cerebral blood flow before and after glycerol infusion. *Upper:* Before glycerol infusion. Lower: After glycerol infusion. Regional cerebral blood flow (*rCBF*) measured by SPECT increases in every case after 500 ml of glycerol infusion.

Table 1. Change in cerebral blood flow after glycerol infusion. The hemispheric mean cerebral blood flow is almost equal in every case. The hemispheric mean cerebral blood flow increases significantly by 18.0% after 500 ml of glycerol infusion. (Paired *t*-test, $P < 0.04$)

| Case | Hemispheric mean CBF (ml/100 g/min) | | | |
| | Before glycerol | | After glycerol | |
	Left	Right	Left	Right
1	64	66	82	86
2	59	59	77	79
3	55	53	62	61
4	71	69	72	71
5	64	63	73	70
Mean	63	62	73	73

graphic EEGs of the control group did not show distinct changes, those of the drug infusion group showed increases in alpha 1 in the entire area of the brain after 250 ml of glycerol infusion, and decreases in alpha 2 in the occipital region. All the frequency bands decreased after 500 ml of glycerol infusion. As for SPMs, in the control group, delta and theta decreased significantly in the frontal region in comparing SPMs before saline infusion with those after 250 ml infusion. Delta and theta increased significantly in comparing SPMs after 250 ml of saline infusion with those after 500 ml infusion. No significant change was observed between SPMs before saline infusion and after 500 ml infusion. Alpha and beta frequency bands did not change significantly. In the drug infusion group, theta decreased significantly in the frontal region and beta 1 increased significantly in

912

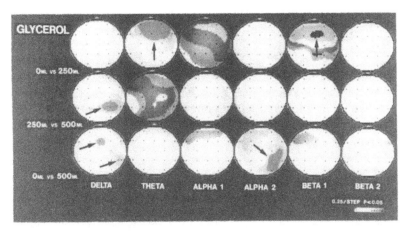

Fig. 2. Change in t-statistic significance probability mapping in the drug infusion group. *Upper:* SPMs comparing the topographic EEGs before glycerol infusion with those after 250 ml infusion. *Middle:* SPMs comparing the topographic EEGs after 250 ml of glycerol infusion with those after 500 ml infusion. *Lower:* SPMs comparing the topographic EEGs before glycerol infusion with those after 500 ml infusion. Theta decreases significantly (*arrow*) and beta 1 increases significantly (*crossed arrow*) in the upper SPMs. The middle SPMs show a significant decrease in delta (*arrow*) and the lower SPMs show significant decreases in delta and alpha 2 (*arrows*). (Paired t-test, $P < 0.05$)

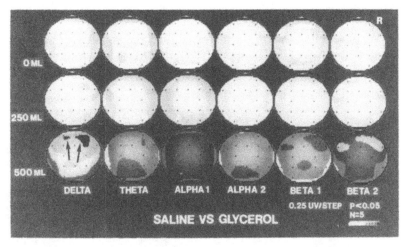

Fig. 3. Change in t-statistic significance probability mapping between the control group and the drug infusion group. *Upper:* SPMs comparing the topographic EEGs before saline infusion with those before glycerol infusion. *Middle:* SPMs comparing the topographic EEGs after 250 ml of saline infusion with those after 250 ml of glycerol infusion. *Lower:* SPMs comparing the topographic EEGs after 500 ml of saline infusion with those after 500 ml of glycerol infusion. The upper and the middle SPMs show no significant differences between both groups. The lower SPMs indicate a significant difference of delta (*arrows*). Delta is higher in the control group than in the drug infusion group, which suggests that 500 ml of glycerol infusion suppresses the appearance of delta wave. (Non-paired t-test, $P < 0.05$)

the frontal region in comparing SPMs before glycerol infusion with those after 250 ml infusion. Delta decreased significantly in the parieto-occipital region in comparing SPMs after 250 ml of glycerol infusion with those after 500 ml infusion. Delta decreased significantly in the frontal region and alpha 2 in the right temporo-parieto-occipital region when SPMs before glycerol infusion were compared with those after 500 ml infusion (Fig. 2). In comparing SPMs of the drug infusion group with those of the control group, delta was significantly suppressed in the drug infusion group when 500 ml of glycerol was infused (Fig. 3).

Discussion

There are some reports of increased cerebral blood flow following glycerol infusion. Glycerol, one of the hyperosmolar agents, is assumed to deprive perivascular glial cells of water and draw it into the vascular lumen, resulting in enlargement of the perivascular space and improvement of microcirculation by lowering hematocrit and viscosity of blood in the capillaries. In positron emission CT (PET) study, the rCBF and cerebral metabolic rate for oxygen ($CMRO_2$) increased (Kobayashi et al. 1985). Glycerol has been reported to pass the blood-brain barrier (BBB) and to be metabolized in the brain to some degree. Therefore, cerebral metabolism has been suspected to be influenced by glycerol infusion. There are a few reports concerning the EEG after glycerol administration showing that the EEG improved both experimentally and clinically. No report, however, could be found about the effects of glycerol on normal brain observed by topographic EEGs.

We have found that rCBF increased, that the amplitude of the EEG became lower, that waves of EEG became faster and that delta waves were suppressed by glycerol infusion.

References

Duffy FH, Bartels PH, Burchiel JL (1981) Significance probability mapping: an aid in the topographic analysis of brain electrical activity. Electroencephalogr Clin Neurophisiol 51:455–462
Kobayashi A, Handa H, Ishikawa M et al. (1985) Changes in local cerebral blood flow and oxygen metabolism with glycerol infusion in various pathologic states. In: Inaba Y, Klatzo I, Spatz M (eds) Brain edema. Springer Berlin Heidelberg New York Tokyo, pp 273–276

Intracranial Pressures in Conscious Sheep During 72 Hours of Hypoxia

D.C. Curran-Everett and J.A. Krasney

Department of Physiology, SUNY-Buffalo, Buffalo, New York 14214 (USA)

Introduction

High altitude cerebral edema (HACE) may occur within several days after a rapid ascent to altitude; it is believed to contribute to the neurological manifestations of acute mountain sickness such as headache, vomiting, and ataxia (Hamilton et al. 1986). Despite centuries of symptoms and studies, the actual mechanisms that produce high altitude cerebral edema are unclear although hypoxia, not hypobaria, appears to be the precipitating factor.

The sheep has been used to study cardiopulmonary responses to hypoxia (e.g., Krasney et al. 1984). In this experiment, we directly measured superior sagittal sinus and lateral ventricular pressures in conscious sheep before, and for 72 hours of, normobaric hypoxia to evaluate the sheep as a model for the study of high altitude cerebral edema.

Methods

Animals and Surgery

Twenty-two ewes, 9–12 months old and weighing 30–35 kg, were used. Catheters were implanted in each sheep under halothane anesthesia. Three days prior to data collection, a Tygon catheter (0.16 cm ID, 0.32 OD) was advanced into the descending aorta to the level of the renal arteries (to measure arterial pressure and withdraw blood samples). The distal tip of a Swan-Ganz thermodilution catheter (# 7-Fr) was positioned in the inferior vena cava (to measure blood temperature). Each catheter was routed subcutaneously, exteriorized, and protected within the pocket of a jacket worn by the sheep (Byron Medical Jackets, Buffalo, NY).

One day before data collection, the superior sagittal sinus was exposed through a burr hole in the skull; a PVC catheter (0.9 cm ID, 0.14 OD; Martech Medical Products, Inc.) was introduced into the sinus so that its tip was roughly 1 cm rostral to the confluence of the sinus. A lateral ventricular catheter (Cordis Corp.) was inserted, through a second burr hole, into the left lateral ventricle; this catheter was attached to a length of Tygon microbore tubing. These catheters were also routed and exteriorized.

Intracranial Pressure VII
Eds.: J. T. Hoff and A. L. Betz
© Springer-Verlag Berlin Heidelberg 1989

Experimental Protocol

The sheep was moved into a lucite environmental chamber when it had regained consciousness after the second surgery. This chamber has been described previously in detail (Krasney et al. 1984). The salient characteristics of the chamber are: 1) F_{ICO_2} was maintained below 0.005 (Beckman Medical Gas Analyzer LB-2), 2) temperature within the box was thermoneutral for the sheep, and 3) the sheep had *ad libitum* access to water and a commercial grain mixture (Early Market Lamb Pellets, Agway, Inc.).

Arterial, superior sagittal sinus, and lateral ventricular pressures were recorded on a Grass Instruments polygraph; all Statham pressure transducers were referred to the level of the right atrium of the standing sheep (6–10 cm dorsal to the sternum). Arterial blood gas values (ABL II, Radiometer) were corrected to the sheep's blood temperature.

After 24 hr of normoxia, the sheep was made hypoxic, over 30–60 min, by nitrogen dilution ($Pa_{O_2} = 40$ mm Hg, $Sa_{O_2} = 50\%$). For 72 hours, chamber F_{IO_2} was adjusted (Beckman Oxygen Analyzer OM-11) to maintain Pa_{O_2} at 40 mm Hg.

Arterial, superior sagittal sinus, and lateral ventricular pressures were measured and arterial blood samples were taken after 20 hr of normoxia and at 24 hr intervals of hypoxia. At each time period, intracranial capillary hydrostatic pressure ($P_{cap\ calc}$) was calculated from arterial (P_a) and sagittal sinus (P_{sag}) pressures using arterial to sagittal sinus resistance ratios (R_a/R_{sag}) ranging from 1 to 20 $[P_{cap\ calc} = (P_a + (P_{sag}*R_a/R_{sag})) / (1+R_a/R_{sag})]$. The data were analyzed by repeated measures analysis of variance (SAS Institute, Inc., 1985).

Results

Pa_{O_2} decreased from 103.8 mm Hg during normoxia to daily means of 43.7–44.6 mm Hg over the 72 hr of hypoxia; Pa_{O_2} decreased from 37.8 mm Hg during normoxia to means of 28.2–29.6 mm Hg. Arterial pressure (P_a) did not change during the first 48 hr of hypoxia (normoxic $P_a = 91.8$ mm Hg); however, at 72 hr of hypoxia, P_a had increased (97.6 mm Hg, $p < 0.001$).

Sagittal sinus, lateral ventricular, and intracranial capillary hydrostatic pressures are shown in the accompanying figure. These pressures increased during hypoxia, attaining zeniths at 48 hr of hypoxia. The increases, however, were not statistically greater than their respective normoxic pressures ($p > 0.10$). Assuming that R_a/R_{sag} did not change between normoxia and hypoxia, $P_{cap\ calc}$ increased by 1–3 mm Hg during hypoxia. This increase in $P_{cap\ calc}$ probably underestimates the "true" increase in $P_{cap\ calc}$ as R_a/R_{sag} decreases during hypoxia. Our estimate of the theoretical increase in $P_{cap\ calc}$ (Fig. 1) assumes that R_{sag} and resting brain oxygen consumption remained constant between normoxia and hypoxia.

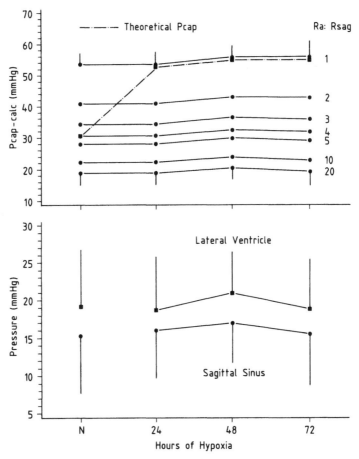

Fig. 1. Superior sagittal sinus, lateral ventricular, and calculated intracranial hydrostatic ($P_{cap\ calc}$) pressures during normoxia (*N*) and hypoxia. The values represent means $\pm$ S.E. The *dashed line* represents the increase in P_{cap} if R_a/R_{sag} declines during hypoxia

Discussion

The increases in sagittal sinus und lateral ventricular pressures that occurred in these sheep over 72 hr of hypoxia coincide with peak cerebral blood flow during 72 hr of hypoxia (Krasney et al. 1984); they are also consistent with the increases in cerebrospinal fluid pressure that occur during HACE (Hamilton et al. 1986). The small increases in sagittal sinus and lateral ventricular pressure are physiologically important as they contribute to a substantial rise in intracranial capillary hydrostatic pressure during hypoxia. The rise in intracranial capillary hydrostatic pressure may contribute to, or result from, the increases in sagittal sinus and lateral ventricular pressures in conscious sheep during hypoxia. We conclude that the sheep is an appropriate model for the further study of high altitude cerebral edema. (This work was supported by HL-36126.)

References

Hamilton AJ, Cymmerman A, Black PM (1986) High altitude cerebral edema. Neurosurgery 19:841–849

Krasney JA, McDonald BW, Matalon S (1984) Regional circulatory responses to 96 hours of hypoxia in conscious sheep. Respir Physiol 57:73–88

SAS Institute Inc (1985) SAS User's Guide: Statistics, Version 5 Edition. SAS Institute Inc., Cary, NC

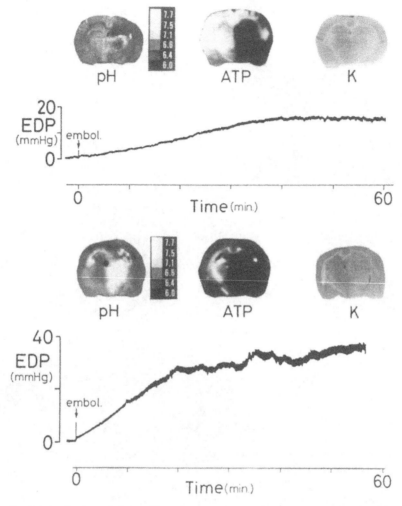

Fig. 1. Distribution of tissue pH, ATP, potassium and recording of EDP. *Upper:* A case with mildly elevated EDP. *Lower:* A case with highly elevated EDP. Note the alkalotic area in the highly elevated case is more extensive than that in the mildly elevated case

lation of the percentage of alkalotic area in the occluded hemisphere at 4 coronal sections (about 160 μm intervals) demonstrated that alkalotic area in the severely elevated group was more extensive than that in the other groups (Fig. 1). Luminescence of ATP and staining for potassium seriously decreased in the highly elevated group. Exudation of trypan blue was frequently detected in the same area of alkalosis.

Discussion

From this study, brain swelling in the embolized rat appeared to be closely related to the alkalotic change in the deep cerebrum. Acidosis due to accumulation of lactic acid is generally accepted in the ischemia, on the other hand, alkalosis in ischemic models has been reported in only a few papers. Kogure et al. (1980) reported alkalosis in the rat following embolization with microspheres 30 min after injection. We also observed alkalosis 30 min after embolization. The mechanism of alkalosis has not been clarified so far. The embolization model was reported to produce severe ischemic damage compared to the trapping model (Okada et al. 1983), therefore, alkalosis may be related to the severe ischemic damage.

Coincidence of alkalosis and trypan blue exudation in the same area implies that alkalotic changes may be induced by the plasma exudation through the cerebral vessels. Normal brain tissue pH has been reported to be about 7.1 and plasma pH is about 7.4. Therefore, tissue pH in the area with plasma exudation may be elevated nearly to the plasma pH which exhibits alkalosis by the bioluminescence method.

References

Csiba L, Paschen W, Hossmann K-A (1983) A topographic quantiative method for measuring brain tissue pH under physiological and pathophysiological conditions. Brain Res 289:334–337

Kogure K, Alonso OF (1978) A pictorial representation of endogenous brain ATP by a bioluminescent method. Brain Res 154:273–284

Kogure K, Busto R, Schwarzman BSciRJ, Scheinberg P (1980) The dissociation of cerebral blood flow, metabolism, and function in the early stages of developing cerebral infarction. Ann Neurol 8:278–290

Mies G, Kloiber O, Drewes LR, Hossmann K-A (1984) Cerebral blood flow and regional potassium distribution during focal ischemia of gerbil brain. Ann Neurol 16:232–237

Okada Y, Shima T, Yokoyama N, Uozumi T (1983) Comparison of middle cerebral artery trunk occlusion by silicone cylinder embolization and by trapping. J Neurosurg 58:492–499

Ischemia-Reperfusion Injury in the Rabbit Brain

E. Tasdemiroglu, D.P. Christenberry, J.L. Ardell, R. Chronister, P.W. Curreri, and A.E. Taylor

Departments of Physiology, General Surgery and Anatomy, University of South Alabama, Mobile, Alabama 36688 (USA)

In response to transient cerebral ischemia there is an increase in microvascular permeability and a corresponding loss of parenchymal function. The increase in vascular permeability can result in vasogenic cerebral edema and subsequent prolonged hypoperfusion of affected CNS regions thereby exacerbating regional cerebral damage (Chan et al. 1984). The mechanisms resulting in the endothelial damage are not well defined. Therefore, to characterize the specific changes in the cerebral circulation during focal ischemia/reperfusion we have developed a model in the rabbit to simultaneously evaluate regional CNS blood flow and microvascular integrity.

Materials and Methods

New Zealand white rabbits, weighing from 2.5 to 3 kg were premedicated with 25 mg/kg chlorpromazine and 30 mg/kg ketamine, i.m. Animals were anesthetized with pentobarbital (Na, 25 mg/kg), paralyzed with pancuronium bromide (0.2 mg/kg) and ventilated mechanically with room air. A femoral artery was cannulated for blood pressure measurements and for blood sampling. The left atrium was cannulated via a left thoracotomy for radioactive microsphere injections. Animals then underwent unilateral eye enucleation. The globe was decompressed (O'Brien and Waltz 1973), small bilateral incisions of the lateral ends of the palpebral fissure were made, the eyelids retracted, and the orbital contents dissected subperiosteally and removed at the apex of the intraorbital muscular cone and the optic nerve. The orbital insertion of the temporalis muscle was dissected, coagulated, and removed. A bone flap (1×1 cm) of the sphenoid bone and lesser sphenoid wing was removed rostrally and superomedially of the optic foramen. The dura mater was then opened and the arachnoid membrane dissected anteriorly and medially exposing the middle cerebral, the (azygous) anterior cerebral, and intracranial internal carotid arteries. Focal CNS ischemia/reperfusion was produced by a 60 min occlusion of the three isolated cerebral vessels using microaneurysm clips (Yamamoto et al. 1958). Microspheres were injected 10 min prior to occlusion, at 40 min of occlusion, and 15 min following removal of the aneurysm clips. Evan's blue dye (30 mg/kg) was then injected i.v. and allowed to circulate for an additional hour. At this concentration, Evan's blue is completely bound to albumin. Animals were then sacrificed and the brain fixed in formaldehyde-sucrose for 48 hr. The brains were frozen and sectioned in a rostral to caudal fashion with alternate 50 and 500 micron sections taken for quantifying regional cerebral dye leakage and blood flows, respectively. Blood flow determinations were made using the reference organ technique. Microvascular integrity was quantified using microspectrofluorometry (excitation wavelength of 530–560 nanometers, emission of 580 nanometer light quantified). Using this method the amount of albumin-Evan's blue dye extravasation was measured.

Results

Table 1 summarizes the simultaneous changes in regional CNS blood flow and relative dye leakage in response to 60 min of unilateral focal ischemia/reperfusion. Note the significant reduction in regional cerebral blood flow in the

Table 1

	Blood flow (ml/min/100)						Protein
	Occluded (O)			Unoccluded (UO)			Leakage
	Cont	Occl	Reper	Cont	Occl	Reper	(O/UO)
Rostral	51 ± 10	$32 \pm 4*$	$41 \pm 5*$	57 ± 13	56 ± 13	55 ± 11	46% *
Middle	53 ± 10	37 ± 7	50 ± 7	52 ± 10	47 ± 8	49 ± 9	48% *
Caudal	$41 \pm 9^+$	$31 \pm 6^+$	41 ± 6	47 ± 11	41 ± 9	43 ± 9	45% *

Stars (*) indicate significant differences ($p < 0.05$) between occluded and unoccluded hemispheres. Crosses (+) indicate differences with $p < 0.1$.

occluded versus the unoccluded hemispheres. All CNS regions demonstrated reperfusion following release of the occlusion. Microvascular integrity, following reperfusion, was assessed by measuring the relative leakage of Evan's blue-albumin complex into the extravascular space. In the unclipped hemisphere the albumin-dye complex was restricted to the CNS capillaries. Within the hemisphere subjected to 60 min of occlusion, dye leakage across the damaged endothelium was evident on microscopic examination and dye fluorescence was increased by approximately 50% within these same regions.

Conclusions

Transient occlusion of the internal carotid, middle cerebral and (azygous) anterior cerebral arteries produces a rapid and reproducible cerebral ischemia that is restricted to the affected hemisphere. Following clip removal, regional CNS blood flows return to preocclusion levels. One hour of focal ischemia is associated with a significant increase in microvascular damage as assessed by regional leakage of the albumin-dye complex.

Acknowledgement. Research supported by the American Heart Association NIH HL 22549 and GM 08154.

References

Chan PH, Schmidley JW, Fishman RA, Jongar SM (1984) Brain injury, edema, and vascular permeability changes induced by oxygen-derived free radicals. Neurology 34:315–320
O'Brien M, Waltz AG (1973) Transorbital approach for occluding the MCA without craniectomy. Stroke 4:210–216
Yamamoto K, Yoshimimo T, Yanagihara T (1985) Cerebral ischemia in rabbit: A new experimental model with immunohistochemical investigation. J Cereb Blood Flow Metabol 5:529–536

Changes in Vascular Permeability
to FITC-Dextran Following Temporary Occlusion
of Middle Cerebral Artery in CAT

H. Ishiguri and H. Kuchiwaki

Department of Neurosurgery, Komaki City Hospital and Nagoya University School of Medicine (Japan)

Introduction

Reperfusion after severe cerebral ischemia usually produces disruption of the blood-brain barrier (BBB) and causes marked brain edema. However, the mechanism responsible for the increase in vascular permeability is not well understood.

The present study was undertaken to examine whether various-sized macromolecules extravasate at the same time, or whether smaller macromolecules extravasate more readily than larger ones, during recirculation after temporary cerebral ischemia.

Materials and Methods

Fourteen adult cats, weighing between 1.9 and 4.1 kg, were anesthetized with ketamine and mechanically ventilated. The right middle cerebral artery (MCA) and internal carotid artery were transorbitally occluded with aneurysm clips for three hours, followed by a two-hour reperfusion period. Local cerebral blood flow (LCBF) was measured hourly by the hydrogen clearance method at the cortex of the bilateral ectosylvian gyrus. For a morphological study, 100 mg/kg fluorescein thiocarbamoyl dextran (FITC-dextran) with a mol. wt. of 20,000 (size 6.4 nm, $n=5$), 70,000 (size 11.6 nm, $n=5$) or 150,000 (size 17.4 nm, $n=4$) was given intravenously and allowed to circulate for thirty minutes prior to sacrifice of the animals. At the same time, Evans blue (60 mg/kg) was injected into all animals as an albumin (mol. wt. 70,000, size 8 nm) tracer.

The brains were fixed in neutral formalin in 70% alcohol for 5 to 7 days and embedded in paraffin wax, and the sections were viewed by fluorescence microscopy (Tripathi and Tripathi 1977).

Moreover, arterial blood pressure, pH, $PaCO_2$ and PaO_2 were maintained within the physiological range.

Results

1. Correlation Between Ischemia and Leakage of Evans Blue

The animals were divided into two groups according to the presence or absence of Evans blue extravasation. In the former group ($n=8$), LCBF (pre-ischemic value: 57.4 ± 7.7 ml/100 g/min) decreased to below 10 ml/100 g/min just after occlusion, and did not improve before reperfusion. Evans blue leaked out into the cortex and/or basal ganglia in the MCA region of the right ischemic hemisphere. The LCBF of the contralateral hemisphere did not change significantly throughout the experiment. In the latter group ($n=6$), however, LCBF was maintained at a value of between 15 and 35 ml/100 g/min during ischemia, and Evans blue did not extravasate after reperfusion.

2. Extravasation of Evans Blue and FITC-Dextrans

Leakage of any size of FITC-dextran closely corresponded with that of Evans blue: in three of five animals (mol. wt. 20,000), two of five (mol. wt. 70,000), and three of four (mol. wt. 150,000), FITC-dextrans and Evans blue extravasated together. However, no graded increase in vascular permeability according to the different sizes of dextrans was demonstrated. In contrast, in the other six animals, neither of the tracers leaked out of the vessels.

3. Histological Findings of Extravasated Dextrans

The dextran leaked out of the vessels and was diffusely taken up into the cytoplasm of neuronal and glial cells in the same lesions into which Evans blue had extravasated (Fig. 1). Moreover, in some animals granular fluorescent materials accumulated in the perikaryon of cells located around the ischemic lesions.

Discussion

It has been reported that recanalization occurs in more than 50% of stroke patients at an early stage of the clinical course, generally within 4 days after the insult. Moreover, even if the obstructed main trunk of the artery does not reopen, collateral pathways may develop and restore the blood flow to the ischemic lesions. If the duration and degree of ischemia is excessively long and severe, prominent brain edema develops after the return of circulation. Many experimental studies have reported increased vascular permeability to various tracers of different sizes, but few studies have examined the correlation between vascular permeability and the size of extravasating macromolecules.

FITC-dextrans are suitable tracers for investigating this correlation, since several tracers of different sizes between 6.4 nm and 17.4 nm are available. In the

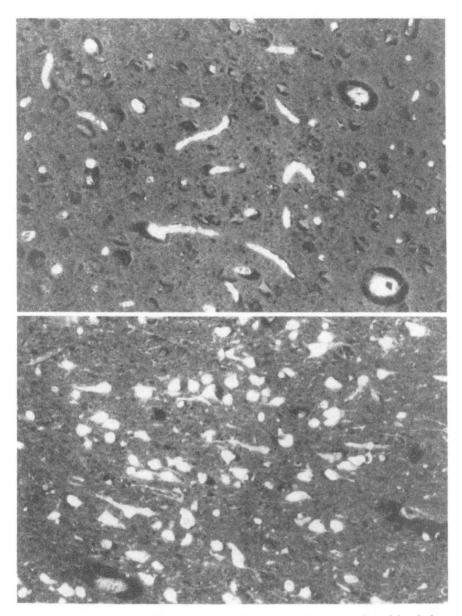

Fig. 1. Fluorescence micrographs. *Upper panel:* The cortex of the contralateral hemisphere. FITC-dextran is located only in the lumen of the vessels. *Lower panel:* The cortex with the extravasation of the tracer. The dextran is diffusely taken up in glial and neuronal cells

927

present experiment, three different-sized dextrans each extravasated together with Evans blue during reperfusion after temporary severe ischemia (LCBF < 10 ml/100 g/min for three hours). However, no differences in extravasation of these tracers were observed in any of the animals. These findings suggest that the plasma, containing various macromolecules, leaks out of the vessels in bulk after the return of circulation to the lesions where the BBB has already been disrupted by severe ischemic injury.

Finally, with regard to histological findings of FITC-dextrans, Hultstrom et al. (1984) have reported two types of tracer accumulation, diffuse and granular labelling, in brain edema produced by a focal cryogenic injury. In the present study, two such types of FITC-dextran uptake were also observed. We consider that diffuse labelling is due to direct uptake of the tracers through the disrupted cell membrane, while granular accumulated fluorescent materials may be distributed from the central lesions as a result of retrograde axonal transport (Tengvar and Olsson 1987).

References

Hultström DC, Tengvar C et al. (1984) Distribution of exudated FITC-dextrans in experimental vasogenic brainedema produced by a focal criogenic injury. Acta Neuropathol (Berl) 63:13−17

Tengvar Ch, Olsson Y (1982) Uptake of macromolecules into neurons from focal vasogenic cerebral edema and subsequent axonal spread to other brain regions. Acta Neuropathol (Berl) 57:233−235

Tripathi RC, Tripathi BJ (1977) A new method for light and electron microscopic localization of fluorescein-labelled dextran in ocular tissue using epoxy-resin embedding. Exp Eye Res 25:259−264

Oxidative Metabolism of 6-(^{14}C)-Glucose During Normoxia, Hypoxia, and Recovery

J.H. Fitzpatrick and J.K. Carmi

Department of Anesthesiology, University of Wisconsin Medical School, University Hospitals and Clinics, B6/387 CSC, Madison, Wisconsin 53796 (USA)

Brain glucose metabolism is altered from its normal pathways during hypoxia and normoxic recovery. In studies of moderate hypoxia (PaO$_2$ 30 or 40 torr) and reoxygenation in the isolated dog brain, up to 40% of the glucose entering the brain is metabolized by pathways that remain to be identified (Kintner 1983). In a previous series of experiments utilizing U-(^{14}C)-glucose as an infusion during normoxia, PaO$_2$ 30 torr hypoxia for 30 min, and normoxic recovery following hypoxia, it was found that during normoxia, about 35% of the labeled glucose was metabolized to ^{14}CO$_2$ during a 30 min infusion. During hypoxia there was a rise to 21% of the label being metabolized to ^{14}CO$_2$ over 30 min, while during normoxic recovery following 30 min of hypoxia there was a slow gradual rise during the 30 min period of recovery to 32%. During early recovery, the amount of labeled glucose metabolized to ^{14}CO$_2$ was considerably less than during normoxia or hypoxia (Fitzpatrick 1987). It is concluded that a significant portion of glucose entering the brain during hypoxia and early recovery is utilized in metabolic processes other than energy production, and that a significant amount of CO$_2$ produced during this period comes from sources other than exogenous glucose, probably lactate produced during hypoxia. We have followed these experiments with a study of the oxidative metabolism of 6-(^{14}C)-glucose under similar conditions.

Materials and Methods

Brains were isolated from 14 dogs anesthetized with halothane and nitrous oxide in oxygen. Perfusion was accomplished via the internal carotid arteries and the anastomotic branch of the internal maxillary arteries by a membrane oxygenator-roller pump system. Venous return was accomplished via a threaded connector placed into the confluence of sinuses. Two separate pump-oxygenator systems were used and were connected by a rotary valve which permits switching between systems without loss of flow or pressure. One system was maintained at normal pH, PO$_2$, PCO$_2$, glucose and T, while the other was similar except for a PO$_2$ of 30 torr. Brains were continuously labeled with 10 μCi of 6-(^{14}C)-glucose infused directly into the arterial perfusion line without venous recirculation. Paired arterial and venous samples were taken every 3 minutes and analyzed for blood gases, glucose, oxygen content and hematocrit. Samples were analyzed for

6-(^{14}C)-glucose specific activity on a Beckman liquid scintillation counter. $^{14}CO_2$ content was analyzed by injecting 1 ml portions through a gas tight rubber cap unto an Erlenmeyer flask containing 0.5 ml ethanolamine:methoxyethanol (1:3 v:v). The samples were acidified, incubated overnight at 37 deg C and counted in the scintillation counter. Four experiments were performed during 30 min of normoxia, 3 during 60 min of normoxia, 3 during 30 min of hypoxia, and 3 during 30 min of normoxic recovery following hypoxia.

Result

Percent of 6-(^{14}C)-glucose metabolized to $^{14}CO_2$

Time (min)	Normoxia (N)	Hypoxia (N)	Recovery (N)
15	3.0±0.6 (7)	0.2±0.1 (3)	0.4±0.3 (3)
30	13.1±2.2 (7)	2.4±0.8 (3)	0.8±0.8 (3)
48	23.1±1.1 (3)		
60	36.3±2.1 (3)		

Discussion

Experiments in cerebral metabolism in intact animals utilizing isotopic tracers are complicated by metabolism in non cerebral tissues, anesthetic effects, indirect measurement of blood flow, and recirculation of tracer and its metabolites. Isolated organ systems avoid these problems as well as permit precise control of experimental conditions and perfusate parameters. These studies confirm that little exogenous glucose is metabolized to CO_2 via the tricarboxylic acid cycle during moderate hypoxia and early recovery. Indeed, less $^{14}CO_2$ is produced from the 6 position during recovery than hypoxia itself. It thus appears that major energy substrates utilized during recovery are already present in the brain following the hypoxic insult. Hawkins et al. (1985) have previously shown that loss of $^{14}CO_2$ during ^{14}C-glucose labeling experiments under normoxic conditions was lowest in the 6-position, followed by the 1-, 2-, and U-labeled analogs. We have demonstrated that there is even less loss of label during hypoxia and recovery. This may give an advantage to the use of 6-(^{14}C)-glucose during studies under non-steady state conditions, which would avoid the long equilibrium process required with 2-deoxyglucose analogs and with little correction being necessary for the loss of $^{14}CO_2$.

References

Fitzpatrick J et al. (1987) Brain U-(^{14}C)-glucose metabolism during moderate hypoxia and recovery. J CBF Metab 7:486
Hawkins RA et al. (1985) Cerebral glucose use measured with (^{14}C) glucose labeled in the 1, 2, or 6 position. Am J Physiol 248:C170–C176
Kintner D et al. (1983) Cerebral glucose metabolism during 30 minutes of moderate hypoxia and reoxygenation. Am J Physiol 245:E365–E372

The Effect of Cerebral Edema on Reperfusion Blood Flow Deficit in Ischemic Animals

D. Cowen, D.J. Combs, and J.R. Dempsey

Division of Neurosurgery, University of Kentucky, College of Medicine, Lexington, Kentucky 40502 (USA)

Transient cerebral ischemia has been shown to result in a series of interrelated pathologic changes in brain physiology with the resumption of blood flow. After a significant period of ischemia, the brain shows ischemic cerebral edema, increased intracranial pressure, and reperfusion decreases in regional cerebral blood flow. Deficits in neuroelectrical functioning and the abnormal generation of metabolic by-products have also been noted. The exact relationship of these processes with one another is not completely understood. The specific effect of the generation of regional cerebral edema on cerebral blood flow is not known. Edema may cause constriction of arteriolar diameter resulting in decreased blood flow, or the two processes may be related only in that both are caused by some other effect of the initial ischemic insult.

The objective of this study was to determine the effect of cerebral edema on reperfusion cerebral blood flow (CBF) in gerbils subjected to bilateral carotid artery occlusion (BCO) with reperfusion. Groups were followed with and without reduction in the postischemic edema and observed for alterations in the reperfusion blood flow deficit.

Methods

Twenty-five adult Mongolian gerbils (Tumblebrook Farms) were divided into four groups. Half received 40 minutes of bilateral carotid artery occlusion and half received sham surgery. Half of the animals received I.V. Mannitol infusion 0.8 gm/kg/hr and half received an equivalent volume normal saline. All animals were monitored for body temperature, blood pressure, arterial blood gases, hydrogen clearance, regional cerebral blood flow, somatosensory evoked potentials and specific gravity regional cerebral edema measurements.

Surgical Preparation

Animals were anesthetized with ketamine 120 mg/kg and maintained with constant infusion of ketamine 60 mg/kg/hr. Twenty-five um platinum/iridium cerebral blood flow electrodes were placed in the cortical surface using a stereotactic micro-manipulator and secured in place with rubber-based impression material. Tracheostomy and carotid artery isolation were done through a mid-line incision. The femoral artery and vein were cannulated for intravenous access and arterial monitoring and a Ag/AgCl subcutaneous reference electrode and a rectal temperature probe were also placed.

Somatosensory evoked potential was monitored using Grass E2 platinum/ iridium needle electrodes placed subcutaneously in the submandibular fossa and abdominal wall. A head screw electrode was used for the active lead. Stimulating electrodes were placed over the left median nerve. Signals were amplified using a Grass 7P511 EEG Amplifier and averaged using a Nicolet 12/70 Signal Analyzer System. Resulting wave forms were displayed and recorded in a plot of voltage vs time.

Cerebral Blood Flow

Hydrogen clearance technique was used using platinum/iridium cerebral blood flow electrodes polarized to $+200$ mV. Hydrogen (approximately 8%) was administrated through the endotracheal tube for a period of 5 min. Once hydrogen administration ceased, the resulting exponential curve expressing decline in local hydrogen as a function of time allowed cerebral blood flow calculation.

Cerebral ischemia was produced for 40 min by occlusion of both carotid arteries using microcerebral aneurysm clips followed by 4 hrs of reperfusion prior to sacrifice. Cerebral edema was determined by specific gravity using a kerosene/ bromobenzene gradient column. Cortical tissue samples from both hemispheres were taken, allowed to equilibrate for one minute at which time readings were taken.

Animals received saline infusion (0.004 cc/gm) or 20% Mannitol, (0.004 cc/gm) intravenously at the time of occlusion, 10 min, 1, 2, and 3 hrs after release of occlusion.

Specific gravity, blood pressure, blood gases, hematocrit at 4 hrs and regional cerebral blood flow were analyzed by 1-way analysis of variance (ANOVA). Fisher PLSD post-hoc testing was employed to determine significant differences between specific groups where ANOVA was significant. All values were expressed as group means $\pm$ standard error of the mean.

Results

Ischemia significantly decreased specific gravity from 1.0479 ± 0.0006 to 1.0448 ± 0.0005 among saline treated gerbils ($P \leq 0.05$). Mannitol treatment eliminated edema formation in ischemic animals without significantly changing the specific gravity of control animals. Bilateral carotid artery occlusion significantly decreased cerebral blood flow in both ischemic groups to less than 2 cc/100 gm/min ($P \leq 0.05$). Postischemic cerebral blood flow was characterized

932

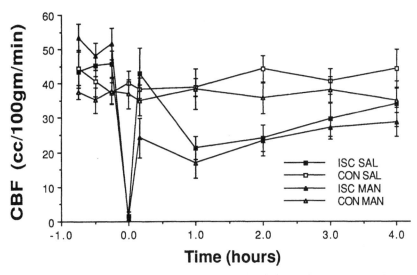

Fig. 1. Plot of cerebral blood flow (*CBF*) vs. time. CBF during ischemia is plotted at 0.0 hours. Ischemia significantly decreased CBF ($P \leq 0.05$). There was no significant difference between group means at 10 min, 3 hrs. or 4 hrs. postischemia. At 1 hour postischemia, ischemic groups were significantly lower than control groups ($P \leq 0.05$). At 2 hours postischemia, ischemic saline and ischemic mannitol gerbils were significantly lower than control saline animals ($P \leq 0.05$). At no time was a significant difference between ischemic saline and ischemic mannitol gerbils detected. *ISC* = ischemia, *CON* = nonischemic, *SAL* = saline infusion, *MAN* = mannitol infusion

by an early hypoperfusion deficit between ischemic and non-ischemic animals. At 1 hr postischemia, CBF in both ischemic groups was 21.2 ± 3.4 in saline and 16.9 ± 4.3 in mannitol. While saline control CBF was 38.8 ± 2.7 and mannitol control CBF was 38.3 ± 5.9 cc/100 gm/min ($P \leq 0.05$). By 4 hr reperfusion, no significant difference in cerebral blood flow was detected between any of the groups (*See* Fig. 1). No clinically significant differences in arterial blood pressure and gases existed between groups.

Discussion

These data demonstrate that 40 min of bilateral artery occlusion in the Mongolian gerbil results in the generation of cerebral edema and a reperfusion deficit in cerebral blood flow. Intravenous mannitol infusion during the ischemic and reperfusion periods results in significant reduction of ischemic edema. However, eleimination of the edema following bilateral carotid artery occlusion, does not improve post-ischemic cerebral blood flow significantly. We conclude that the presence of ischemic edema is not obligatory for the development of a reperfusion deficit in cerebral blood flow after transient ischemia. This implies that other factors such as local metabolic products may play a significant role in post-ischemic cerebral vascular pathophysiology.

Critical Time After Reversible Brain Ischemia for Pentobarbital Administration in the Gerbil

B.B. Mršulja, B.J. Mršulja, B.M. Djuričič, W.D. Lust[1], and M. Spatz[2]

Section on Pathological Neurochemistry and Neuropharmacology, Institute of Biochemistry, School of Medicine, Belgrade (Yugoslavia), [1] Laboratory of Experimental Neurosurgery, CWR University, Cleveland (USA), and [2] LNNS, NINDS, National Institutes of Health, Bethesda, Maryland (USA)

Recently, we found that pentobarbital (PENTO) delayed but did not prevent depletion of energy metabolites and accumulation of lactate in the ischemic brain (Mršulja et al. 1984). However, barbiturates have been reported to possess a protective effect against some pathological sequelae which arise following an ischemic/anoxic episode; nevertheless, the specific mechanism for the protective effect of barbiturates against brain ischemia remains unclear (Shapiro 1985). Barbiturates are the drugs of choice for the inhibition of synaptic transmission (Astrup 1982). Also, it has been shown that barbiturates decrease the excitability of the brain by intensifying the GABAergic system (Richter and Holtman 1982) and by affecting calcium homeostasis (Heyer and MacDonald 1982). Since PENTO given before or immediately after 5 min of ischemia prevents or amelio- rates destruction of hippocampal CA1 sector neurons in the gerbils at 4 days of recirculation after 5 min bilateral carotid occlusion, which was not seen when the drug was administrated 2 hr after ischemia (Mršulja et al. 1987), we were interest- ed in the possible biochemical background of this phenomenon.

In this report we confirm our previous findings that PENTO given before or immediately after transient ischemia indeed ameliorates the loss of neurons in the CA1 sector of hippocampus induced by 5 min of bilateral ischemia in gerbils. In addition, PENTO reverses the reduction of cyclic GMP induced by ischemia which might be the clue for the beneficial influence of PENTO.

Experimental

All experiments were conducted on Mongolian gerbils. PENTO (40 mg/kg, i.p.) was administrated (1) 40 min before ischemia, (2) at the end of 5 min of ischemia, and (3) 2 hr after the ischemia was terminated. Animals were exposed to different periods of ischemia (from 2 sec to 5 min) and varying periods of recirculation. Ischemia was produced by bilateral carotid occlusion and for biochemical investi- gations gerbils were sacrificed by microwave irradiation and tissue analyses per- formed as described previously (Mršulja et al. 1986). Utilization rate of immedi- ate energy reserves (URIER) was estimated (Mršulja et al. 1985).

Separate groups of animals were prepared for the morphologic observation of CA1 sector of the hippocampus after 5 min of ischemia according to the method of Kirino (1982).

Statistical analysis (ANOVA) and Bonferronni's technique were performed and a *p* value less than 0.05 was considered significantly different from the control.

Results

Energy Metabolites and Glycogen

There is no difference between the levels of ATP, P-creatine and glycogen at the end of 5 min of ischemia between PENTO-ischemic and only ischemic group of gerbils; however, already 1 min after reflow was established in PENTO group, ATP and P-creatine are significantly ($p < 0.01$) enhanced in comparison to non-PENTO group (data not shown).

Glycogen accumulates at 6 hr after 5 min of ischemia but not when PENTO is administrated before or at the end of ischemia; this effect of PENTO is lacking when the drug is given 2 hr after ischemia (data not shown).

Utilization Rate of Immediate Energy Reserves

URIER (t/2) at 6 hr after 5 min of ischemia is doubled in comparison to control; t/2 values are 23.0 sec and 49.3 sec in control and ischemic gerbils, respectively.

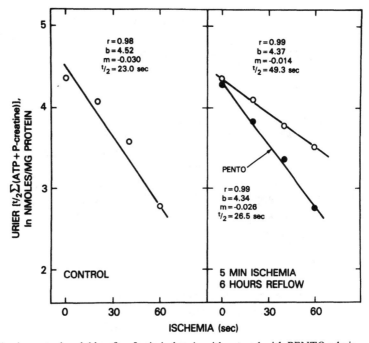

Fig. 1. URIER index in control and 6 hr after 5 min ischemia without and with PENTO administered at the end of the ischemia

935

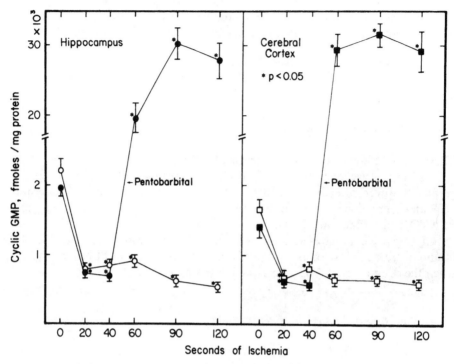

Fig. 2. Changes in cyclic GMP levels during first 2 min of ischemia

In PENTO pretreated and PENTO post-treated groups t/2 values are 24.1 sec and 26.5 sec, respectively (Fig 1); nevertheless, if PENTO is administrated 2 hr after 5 min of ischemia the t/2 value is again 51.6 sec.

Cyclic GMP

Concentrations of cyclic GMP are significantly depressed by 20 sec of ischemia. Since the steady-state levels of cyclic GMP are higher in the hippocampus than in the cortex, the relative decrease is greater in this structure. During 40 sec of ischemia there is no difference between ischemic not treated and PENTO-ischemic animals; however, thereafter sudden and highly significant enhancement of cyclic GMP appears (Fig 2). PENTO was without influence on cyclic GMP levels when administrated 2 hr after 5 min of ischemia.

Comments

The predictable loss of CA1 neurons of the hippocampus has proved to be the model for biochemical investigations of the events that lead up to cell death induced by ischemia. Interest in the pathometabolism of selected neuronal vulner-ability to ischemia has grown with the demonstration of this phenomenon in the gerbil (Kirino 1982). The restoration of energy metabolism has been, for a long

936

time, thought to be a prerequest of the recovery of brain function following ischemia. However, the restoration of high-energy phosphates following ischemia seems not to be an indicator of functional restoration; at a time of normal level of energy sources (ATP and P-creatine), cells of not only CA1 sector, but of the whole hippocampal region are not capable to utilize energy sources at a normal rate (Mršulja et al. 1985). Thus, just the measurement of the levels of metabolites seems not to be as adequate for the judgement of the functional state of the cell, as is the measurement of URIER. Hence, URIER is an index to express tissue ability to utilize available energy reserves and is particularly valid in pathologic conditions. It is obvious that delayed PENTO administration fails to improve URIER index; the same lack of PENTO effect is evident on glycogen accumulation in advanced periods following reversible (from the CBF standpoint) ischemia. Thus, the mechanism(s) leading to the selective destruction of the hippocampus after brief ischemia is operative during the early postischemic period.

It is increasingly apparent that excitatory amino acids play a role in the delayed loss of hippocampal CA1 neurons, probably as a result of lesion in the GABAergic interneurons; it is likely that barbiturates express a protective effect by the mechanism(s) involving a greater expression of the GABAergic system (Richter and Holtman 1982). This is supported by the increase in cyclic GMP levels during ischemia in gerbils protected by PENTO which is contrary to the phenomenon known during ischemia (Mršulja et al. 1986). Previously, we have found an increase of cyclic GMP in young (3 weeks old) gerbils whose hippocampus is also resistant to 5 min of ischemia (Mršulja et al. 1985b).

References

Astrup J (1982) Energy-requiring cell function in the ischemic brain. J Neurosurg 56:482–497

Heyer EJ, MacDonald RI (1982) Barbiturate reduction of calcium-dependent action potentials: correlation with anesthetic action. Brain Res 236:151–171

Kirino T (1982) Delayed neuronal death in the gerbil hippocampus following ischemia. Brain Res 239:57–69

Mršulja BB, Ueki Y, Wheaton A, Passonneau JV, Lust WD (1984) Release of pentobarbital-induced depression on metabolic rate during bilateral ischemia in the gerbil brain. Brain Res 309:152–155

Mršulja BB, Djuričič BM, Ueki Y, Cahn R, Cvejić V, Martinez H, Mićić DV, Stojanović T, Spatz M (1985a) Cerebral blood flow, energy utilization, serotonin metabolism, (Na, K)ATPase activity and postischemic brain swelling. In: Inaba Y, Klatzo I, Spatz M (eds) Brain edema. Springer, Berlin Heidelberg New York Tokyo, pp 170–177

Mršulja BB, Martinez H, Cahn R, Ueki Y, Lust WD, Klatzo I (1985b) Ischemic brain damage. I. Metabolic rate and cyclic nucleotides in young and adult gerbils during ischemia. In: Meyer JS, Lechner H, Reivich M, Ott EO (eds) Cerebral vascular disease 5. Excerpta medica, Amsterdam New York Oxford, pp 241–247

Mršulja BB, Ueki Y, Lust WD (1986) Regional metabolite profile in early stage of global ischemia in the gerbil. Metab Brain Dis 1:205–220

Mršulja BB, Mršulja BJ, Lust WD (1987) Delayed pentobarbital administration fails to protect ischemic damage in gerbils and the critical time after transient ischemia. In: Meyer JS, Lechner H, Reivich M, Ott EO (eds) Cerebral vascular disease 6. Excerpta Medica, Amsterdam New York Oxford, pp 303–308

Richter AJ, Holtman JR (1982) Barbiturates: their in vivo effects and potential biochemical mechanism. Prog Neurobiol 18:275–319

Shapiro HM (1985) Barbiturates in brain ischemia. Br J Anaesth 57:82–87

Recovery Rates of Evoked Potentials, Intracellular pH and Bicarbonate Ion After ICP-Induced Ischemia

M.K. Nishijima, R.C. Koehler, S.M. Eleff, P.D. Hurn, S. Norris, W.E. Jacobus, and R.J. Traystman

Department of Anesthesiology/Critical Care Medicine, The Johns Hopkins Medical Institutions, Baltimore, Maryland 21205 (USA)

Intracellular acidosis is thought to be one of the major factors that contribute to cerebral injury during ischemia. Upon reperfusion, intracellular pH (pHi) eventually recovers, but normalization is not immediate (Smith et al. 1986). The speed of recovery of pHi is probably slower than the speed at which pHi drops during the onset of ischemia because regeneration of intracellular buffers requires a finite time. We postulated that the rate of recovery of pHi may be a marker of cerebral injury because it may reflect the brain's ability to restore ionic gradients necessary for conductive function. In addition, persistent acidosis during reperfusion may further augment injury.

To characterize how the rate of recovery of pHi varies with different degrees of injury, we varied the duration of ischemia as a means to titrate the dose of injury. Complete global cerebral ischemia was produced by intracranial hypertension. Recovery of somatosensory evoked potentials (SEP) was used as an on-line indicator of the degree of injury, while pHi was measured by ^{31}P NMR spectroscopy. Cerebral venous PCO_2 was measured to differentiate components of pHi recovery due to CO_2 washout and to bicarbonate regeneration.

Methods

Dogs weighing $7-10$ kg were anesthetized with intravenous fentanyl (50 µg/kg) and low dose pentobarbital (6 mg/kg plus 3 mg/kg/hr). Arterial blood gases were maintained at normal levels throughout the study by mechanical ventilation. A sagittal sinus catheter was placed through a burr hole to obtain cerebral venous samples for blood gas analysis. A silastic ventricular drain catheter was inserted into the lateral ventricle to infuse artificial cerebrospinal fluid during ischemia and to measure intracranial pressure (ICP) during recovery. SEP were generated with foreleg stimulation and were recorded with electrodes placed in small burr holes in the skull near the somatosensory cortex.

The animal was placed in a 1.9 Tesla magnet with a 25 cm bore. Rectal temperature was maintained with a warm water-perfused blanket under the animal. With scalp and temporalis muscle retracted, and inductively-coupled, two-turn surface coil (3.5 cm diameter) was placed on the skull to obtain ^{31}P NMR spectra. The pulse interval was 4 seconds. Spectra were analyzed from 4 minute collection periods during transient changes and from 16 minute periods

Eds.: J.T. Hoff and A.L. Betz
© Springer-Verlag Berlin Heidelberg 1989

during steady state recovery. The chemical shift in inorganic phosphate was used to measure pHi. Sagittal sinus PCO_2 was assumed to be within a few mm Hg of intracellular PCO_2 during reperfusion. Intracellular bicarbonate was estimated from pHi and sagittal sinus PCO_2 by the Henderson-Hasselbalch equation.

In three groups of eight dogs, complete ischemia was produced for either 3, 12 or 30 minutes by elevating ICP above systolic arterial pressure and by using controlled hemorrhage to prevent increases in arterial pressure. To start reperfusion, ventricular fluid infusion was stopped. Cerebral perfusion pressure recovered to baseline levels within a few minutes. Animals were studied for 4 hours of reperfusion. Steady state recovery was calculated as the average of values obtained between 2 and 4 hours of reperfusion. Values are presented as mean $\pm$ SE.

Results

Baseline pHi was 7.05 ± 0.04 and it decreased to 6.37 ± 0.15, 5.96 ± 0.08 and 6.05 ± 0.08 at the end of 3, 12 and 30 minutes of ischemia, respectively. The values in the 12 and 30 minute groups were not different. Steady state recovery values were similar in all three groups, i.e. 7.00 ± 0.03, 6.99 ± 0.03 and 6.91 ± 0.04 in the 3, 12 and 30 minute groups, respectively. However, the speed of recovery differed.

All groups showed a rapid component of pHi recovery equivalent to about 0.4 pH units during the first 10 minutes of reperfusion. This rapid component was related to CO_2 washout. At 10 minutes of reperfusion, sagittal sinus PCO_2 was below baseline values due to hyperemia, and as hyperemia subsided, venous PCO_2 recovered to baseline values. The time for pHi to recover to within 90% of steady state values was less in the 3 minute ischemic group (15 ± 4 minutes) than in the 12 minute group (36 ± 9 minutes) and 30 minute group (33 ± 6 minutes).

The prolonged recovery of pHi in the latter groups was related to prolonged recovery of intracellular bicarbonate. Baseline bicarbonate was 14 mM. At 10 minutes of reperfusion, bicarbonate was 9.3 ± 1.6, 4.0 ± 0.8 and 2.7 ± 0.7 mM in the 3, 12 and 30 minutes ischemic groups, respectively. At 30 minutes of reperfusion, the corresponding values were 12.2 ± 0.9, 7.6 ± 0.9 and 5.0 ± 1.2 mM. Thus, bicarbonate regeneration required considerable time and depended on ischemic duration.

The primary cortical wave of SEP rapidly became flat during ischemia in all groups. Steady state recovery of SEP amplitude during reperfusion was 70 ± 5, 41 ± 4 and $12 \pm 5\%$ of baseline in the 3, 12 and 30 minute groups, respectively. Steady state SEP recovery amplitude correlated with the time required for pHi to recover 90% ($r = 0.60$) and with the time required for intracellular bicarbonate to return above an arbitrary value of 8 mM ($r = 0.71$).

Discussion

Extending the duration of ischemia augments brain damage. Our data show that prolonging the duration of complete ischemia produced by elevated ICP results in graded reductions in the recovery of SEP amplitude associated with prolonged recovery rates of pHi and intracellular bicarbonate. In pooling data from the three groups of ischemic durations, there was an overall correlation between SEP recovery and the rate of pHi or bicarbonate recovery. Much of the strength of these correlations derived from extending the ischemic duration from 3 to 12 minutes, which lowered the pHi attained at the end of the ischemic period and doubled the recovery time. However, when ischemic duration is extended to 30 minutes, there was no further reduction in pHi at the end of ischemia and no further increase in its recovery speed. Thus other factors may contribute to the further decrement of SEP recovery after 30 minutes of complete ischemia. On the other hand, the speed of pHi recovery appears to provide a physiological marker of functional recovery when ischemic duration is between 3 and 12 minutes.

Delayed recovery of pHi was related to delayed recovery of intracellular bicarbonate rather than tissue PCO_2. Bicarbonate remained below half of the baseline value at 30 minutes of reperfusion following 12 and 30 minutes of ischemia despite maintenance of arterial pH above 7.3. Whether this delayed recovery of intracellular bicarbonate is due to abnormal transport mechanisms or is limited by bicarbonate regenerated through carbonic anhydrase catalyzation is uncertain. It is also possible that enhanced lactic acid production persists for a considerable time into the reperfusion period. Whatever the mechanism, persistent acidosis over the first half hour of reperfusion is likely to impede functional recovery and may contribute to the injury.

These baseline studies demonstrate the power of phosphorus NMR spectroscopy in characterizing the dynamic recovery of physiological processes after cerebral ischemia. This experimental approach will allow one to investigate a variety of interventions on recovery dynamics and gain insight into the mechanisms of cerebral ischemic injury.

Acknowledgement. Supported by grants from the National Institutes of Health (NS-24394 and NS-20020).

Reference

Smith M-L, von Hanwehr R, Siesjö BK (1986) Changes in extra- and intracellular pH in the brain during and following ischemia in hyperglycemic and in moderately hypoglycemic rats. J Cereb Blood Flow Metab 6:574–583

An Experimental Model of "Brain Tamponade".
Preliminary Observations on ICP Dynamics, Carotid Blood Flow Velocitometry and EEG Activity

C. Anile, A. Rinaldi, R. Roselli, M. Visocchi, A. Ferraresi, M. Sericchio, A. Dal Lago, S. Bradariolo, R. Calimici, F. Della Corte, and G. Maira

Institute of Neurosurgery, Institute of Physiology, Department of Internal Medicine, Institute of Anaesthesiology and Resuscitation, I-00168 Roma (Italy)

Introduction

Brain tamponade (BT) represents a condition of cerebral blood flow (CBF) arrest due to a progressive or often sudden increase in intracranial pressure (ICP) up to values close to the corresponding systemic arterial pressure values. This situation, peculiar to an anatomical configuration characterized by the presence of an incompressible organ within a rigid envelope, as the brain substance within the skull, can induce as its final step a diffuse or compartmental brain ischemia. Considering the scarce metabolic autonomy of the CNS, this could produce irreversible damages. Implicated in this process are the direct relationships between cerebral blood volume changes and vascular impedances. To investigate the hemodynamic mechanisms underlying BT we have carried out an experimental study in the rabbit because its cerebral blood supply is analogous to the human (Meyer et al. 1986).

Experimental Protocol

During the experiments, performed on 23 animals using general anaesthesia and assisted ventilation, we recorded the following parameters: 1) the diastolic and pulsatile ICP values, through a 18G needle inserted by sterotactic parameters into the ventricular space; 2) the internal carotid blood pressure (ICBP), at the level of the common carotid artery, previous bilateral external carotid exclusion and one side insertion of a known caliber bypass; 3) the internal blood flow velocity (ICBFV) by means of a continuous wave 8 MHz Doppler probe secured at the common carotid artery or at the bypass wall for CBF calculations; 4) the EEG, through screw electrodes applied on the cranial vault. The protocol of each trial has been schematically subdivided in 7 consecutive phases (I to VII), according to the modifications observed on the Doppler recording. The ICP increment was induced by intraventricular infusion of mock CSF at a constant speed until BT and maintained for varying periods of time (few sec to 60 min).

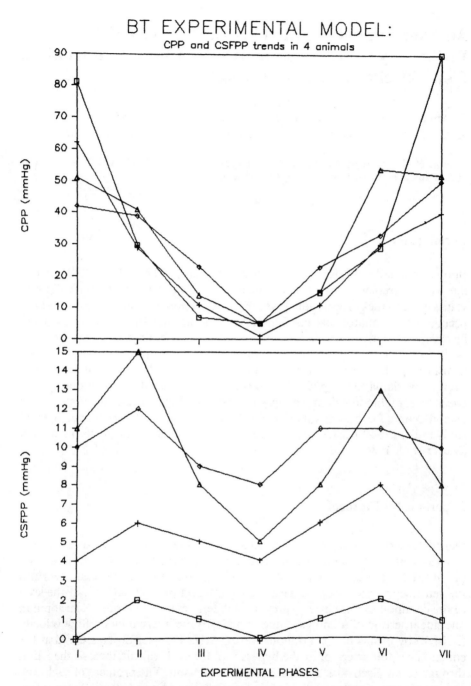

Fig. 1. Simultaneous trends of cerebrospinal fluid pulse pressure (CSFPP) and cerebral perfusion pressure (CPP), during the consecutive phases of a complete trial in 4 of the 23 animals

Results

During each experiment the Doppler recording showed an almost constant trend, characterized by a first phase of relatively stable values (I) until the cerebral perfusion pressure (CPP) remained within the autoregulatory range; below that point (II) the diastolic flow velocity progressively reduced, to disappear at CPP = 5–15 mm Hg (III) a simultaneous decrease of EEG amplitude was observed during the same period. In the following phase a "reverberating wave" (RW) appeared reaching its complete configuration within a few cardiac cycles (IV); 10 to 20 sec after that point the EEG became flat. This state occurred when diastolic ICP was maintained close to ICBP values. Stopping the intraventricular infusion, the last phases (V–VI–VII) showed an inverse symmetric trend to the former. The CSF pulsatile pressure (CSFPP), with respect to CPP modifications, reached its highest value at the limit of the autoregulatory range (II), after which it decreased in most of the cases in phase III, demonstrating then an inverse trend at reversal (Fig. 1). The EEG tracing restored, at hemodynamic stabilization, at a rate and time proportional to the BT period, in all but 3 out of the 4 animals, in which after 60 min BT persisted.

Conclusions

In evaluating CSFPP as a brain elasticity index, our results seem not to confirm what was previously stated in a recent article (Van Eijndhoven and Avezaat 1986): namely, a rapid increase of CSFPP accompanied the first ICP rise within the autoregulatory limits, whereas it showed a progressive decrease in parallel with the configuration of the RW on the Doppler tracing. The CSFPP behavior could be explained by the corresponding Doppler change itself, demonstrating the passage from a volume compliant vascular system (phases I–II) to a stiff one (phases III–IV), as characterized by the RW (Lindegaard et al. 1980). In this context, as further confirmed by obtaining the same results after several trials in one animal, cerebral vasoregulation could be considered as being firstly conditioned by mechanical factors such as blood volume compensation and venous outflow impedance (Portnoy et al. 1983).

References

Lindegaard KF, Grip A, Nornes H (1980) Precerebral haemodynamics in brain tamponade. Part 2: experimental studies. Neurochirurgia (Stuttg) 23:187–196
Meyer FB, Anderson RE, Sundt TM, Yaksh TL (1986) Intracellular brain pH, indicator tissue perfusion, EEG and histology in severe and moderate focal cortical ischemia in the rabbit. J Cereb Blood Flow Metab 6:71–78
Portnoy HD, Chopp M, Branch C (1983) Hydraulic model of myogenic autoregulation and the cerebrovascular bed: the effects of altering systemic arterial pressure. Neurosurgery 13:482–498
Van Eijndhoven JHM, Avezaat CJJ (1986) Cerebrospinal fluid pulse pressure and the pulsatile variation in cerebral blood volume: an experimental study in dogs. Neurosurgery 19:507–522

Cerebral Microvascular Flow Measured by Laser Doppler

A.I.R. Maas and D.A. de Jong

Department of Neurosurgery, Academic Hospital Rotterdam, NL-3015 GD Rotterdam
(The Netherlands)

Raised ICP is often caused by changes in cerebral blood flow. Continuous monitoring of cerebral blood flow (CBF) is not possible with conventional methods, such as Xenon CBF determinations. Moreover it may be doubted whether general or even regional CBF measurements accurately reflect flow disturbances at the microvascular level. We decided to evaluate the applicability of Laser Doppler flow measurements as a method for continuous monitoring of brain microvascular flow. It was hoped to gain more insight in the contribution of microvascular flow disturbances to ICP changes, and in the relation between large vessel flow and microvascular flow.

Material and Methods

The studies were performed in 10 dogs and 6 cats, all anesthetized and artificially ventilated. In the dogs, interest was focussed on the technique of measuring MVBF, the relation of flow to ICP, the correlation between microvascular flow and vertebral artery flow, and on changes in microvascular flow during hypoxic episodes.

In the cats, interest was focussed on changes in microvascular flow induced by variations in arterial pCO_2 (hypocapnia, hypercapnia and hypercarbic normoxic ventilation).

Vertebral artery flow was measured during the experiments with an electromagnetic flow sensor placed on the left vertebral artery. For measurements of the microvascular blood flow, a Laser Doppler device was applied on the parietal dura. The device responds to movements of cells, passing the laser bundle and displays arbitrary units scaled in percentages. For "calibration" only the sensitivity of the optoelectric circuit can be adjusted.

Results

Technique of Laser Doppler Flow Measurements

The signal obtained from the Laser Doppler device showed variations simular to those of ICP-tracings: cardiac and respiratory pulsations are present. In some cases waves, similar to B-waves were noted; these however were not accompanied by B-waves on the ICP recording. Frequently, during the experiments, problems were encountered due to instability of the recorded signal. This was caused mainly by small blood accumulations between the sensor and the dura, despite all attempts to prevent this. Furthermore, the signal appeared to change due to slight pressure variations of the sensor on the dura. The method therefore did not provide absolutely stable recordings, but for the observation of the trend towards short acting flow variations, the method seems to be useful.

Increased ICP and Microvascular Flow

Forty seven volume pressure tests were performed in the 10 dogs. To our surprise the MVBF, increased in 9 instances, decreased in 23 and remained unchanged during 15 tests. This variable response was not only noted between different animals, but even within one animal, undergoing various tests. No relation existed between the direction of MVBF change and the degree of intracranial pressure rise. Despite evident changes in the MVBF, vertebral artery flow remained unchanged but for two cases.

Hypoxia and Microvascular Flow

Twenty-three episodes of hypoxia of varying severity (art. pO_2 17–63 mm Hg) were induced in the 10 dogs. In 9 instances MVBF increased, in 13 MVBF decreased and in 1 instance it remained unchanged. A compensatory increase of MVBF after restitution of normoxic conditions (overshoot) was seen in 7 instances. Despite changes in microvascular flow, vertebral artery flow only twice showed a small increase. The ventricular fluid pressure was increased in 18 cases, also when MVBF decreased.

Table 1. Microvascular blood flow and arterial pCO_2

	Mean PaO_2 mm Hg $\pm SD$	Mean $PaCO_2$ mm Hg $\pm SD$	Mean ICP mm Hg $\pm SD$	Mean MVBF % $\pm SD$
Reference conditions	124.7 8.0	37.8 3.1	9.2 3.6	43.8 13.5
Hyperventilation	137.5 17.0	21.3 1.3	6.5 1.5	41.0 12.1
Hypoventilation	91.4 9.1	53.4 3.0	18.5 9.6	60.4 14.9
Hypercarbic normoxic ventilation	121.7 6.3	63.1 5.4	17.3 7.6	71.4 19.0

The results of the 6 cat-experiments studying this aspect are summarized in Table 1.

Discussion

The Laser Doppler signal does not provide an absolute, but rather a relative value. The tissue volume from which the signal reading is obtained cannot be described exactly due to the inhomogeneity of subdural structures concerning light scattering, reflection and absorption. The width of the subarachnoid space varies with the pressure of the probe and therefore the laser Doppler signal can be influenced by changes of the width of the subarachnoid space during the experimental procedures. This may be one of the possible explanations for the variable changes in microvascular blood flow observed during increased intracranial pressure. It remains a point of debate whether the pulsatile character of the Laser Doppler signal is caused by pulsatile microvascular flow, or by pulsatile movements of the entire brain.

We were surprised to note that microvascular blood flow did not always increase during hypoxia. We would have expected vasodilatation and increased microvascular blood flow during all instances of hypoxia. Apart from the technical limitations of the device used, sludging of the blood flow due to deformation of the erythrocytes during hypoxia could be the explanation for decreased blood flow sometimes occurring during hypoxia.

The fact that a compensatory increase of microvascular blood flow after ending hypoxia was not noted in all cases may be due to nonlinearity of the Laser Doppler flow signal at higher flow levels.

One of the major points obtained from the experiments is that microvascular flow may change very significantly, while the vertebral artery flow remains constant. This finding strengthens our hypothesis that microvascular flow changes may not be reflected by changes in large vessel flow.

The results of the studies reported perhaps raise more questions than they have answered, but certainly stimulate us in our search for more basic understanding of the relation between microvascular cerebral blood flow and ICP levels.

Vasomotor Response and Blood-Brain Barrier Function of Rat Brain Studied in a Closed Cranial Window Preparation

L. Schürer, S. Kawamura [1], B. Schmucker, A. Goetz, and A. Baethmann

Institute for Surgical Research, Ludwig-Maximillians-University of Munich,
Klinikum Großhadern, D-8000 München 70 (FRG) and [1] Department of Surgical Neurology,
Research Institute for Brain and Blood Vessels Akita, Akita 010 (Japan)

Introduction

Many studies on vasomotor control of brain surface vessels using a closed cranial window preparation have been conducted in large animals. The use of small animals, such as rats is technically demanding. Maintenance of normal blood-brain barrier function seems to be particularly difficult after opening of the skull and the dura mater (Oleson 1987). However, an intact blood-brain barrier under controlled conditions is indispensable to study a given pathophysiological condition.

We developed an improved closed cranial window technique in rats which allows for the simultaneous assessment of barrier function and vasomotor control of pial vessels at normal or deliberately changed intracranial pressure.

Methods

Male Sprague-Dawley rats were anesthetized with alpha-chloralose, tracheotomized and artifically ventilated under blood gas control. A tail artery and vein as well as a femoral artery and a jugular vein were cannulated for blood pressure recording, blood sampling and infusion of drugs and of the fluorescence dye Na^+ fluorescein. The animals were then fixed in a stereotactic frame, the skull was exposed, and a rectangular window was made over the left parietal cortex leaving a thin bone layer.

Catheters for superfusion and for measurement of intracranial pressure were embedded in a circular wall of acrylic cement surrounding the window. A funnel (10 cm high) was then placed over the exposed skull of the rat and filled with paraffin oil. Final opening of the skull, incision and reflection of the dura mater as well as sealing of the preparation with a cover glass was made under oil. The funnel was removed after closure of the window, and the preparation was superfused with artificial cerebrospinal fluid (CSF). The CSF outflow catheter was adjusted to obtain an intracranial pressure of 5 mm Hg.

Changes of pial vessel diameters and blood-brain barrier permeability were studied after i.v. injection of Na^+-fluorescein using a modified Leitz-Orthoplan fluorescence-microscope, xenon illumination, a low-light TV camera and video recorder.

Intracranial Pressure VII
Eds.: J. T. Hoff and A. L. Betz
© Springer-Verlag Berlin Heidelberg 1989

Results

Blood-Brain Barrier Function

Blood-brain barrier function was investigated in 16 rats for up to 6.5 hrs. The barrier indicator Na^+-fluorescein (MW 376) was strictly confined to the intra-vascular space during the control phase, indicative of an intact BBB. Superfusion of pial vessels with 2000 mOsmol l^{-1} D-)-mannitol dissolved in CSF resulted in diffuse, gross opening of the barrier to i.v. Na^+-fluorescein 5 min after the start of superfusion. Barrier leakage was stage III according to the classification of Wahl et al. (1985).

Vascular Reactivity

In four rats, the effect on brain surface vessels of continuous superfusion for 180 min was studied using buffered artificial cerebrospinal fluid. As seen in Table 1 continuous superfusion of rat pial arterioles and venules did not affect their diameters. Arterioles displayed slight dilatations and the venules had a tendency to reduce diameters temporarily. The BBB was not opened for Na^+-fluorescein and the intracranial pressure was not increased above 5 mm Hg during the entire observation period.

Table 1. Effect of continuous CSF superfusion on rat pial vessel diameter

Time (min)	Arterioles change of vessel diameter (%)±SEM	Venules change of vessel diameter (%)±SEM
0	100.0±0 (n=50)	100.0±0 (n=46)
30	97.5±1.3 (n=50)	96.8±1.5 (n=46)
60	102.5±1.5 (n=41)	98.0±1.6 (n=46)
90	102.7±1.4 (n=40)	95.9±1.7 (n=46)
120	102.4±1.4 (n=50)	95.9±1.7 (n=46)
150	100.8±1.4 (n=50)	96.9±1.9 (n=46)
180	102.7±1.5 (n=50)	101.0±1.6 (n=46)

Discussion and Conclusion

An improved closed cranial window preparation was established in rats. Continu-ous superfusion of pial vessels with buffered CSF did not lead to significant changes of the vessel diameters and the blood-brain barrier did not open for Na^+-fluorescein used as a vessel marker. Superfusion of the preparation with a hyperosmolar solution according to Rapaport et al. (1972) led to gross opening of the blood-brain barrier immediately. Barrier disruption became visible only five min after the start of superfusion. This is in agreement with findings of Wahl et al. (1985). Opening of the barrier commenced about 1 min later than in similar studies in cats (Wahl et al. 1985), which may indicate a somewhat more resistant blood-brain barrier in rats.

Contrary to earlier experimental techniques (Auer 1987 in press); Haberl et al. 1987; Morii et al. 1986), the present model allows simultaneous investigations of brain surface microhemodynamics and blood-brain barrier function under controlled conditions and during deliberate changes of the intracranial pressure for the first time. The model appears suitable to study pertinent aspects of the cerebral microcirculation and blood-brain-barrier function under various physiological and pathophysiological conditions, providing promising experimental perspectives for a variety of pertinent clinical problems.

Acknowledgement. The competent technical assistance of U. Goerke and H. Fuderer is gratefully acknowledged.

References

Auer LM (1987 in press) Measurement of pial vessel hemodynamics. In: Boulton AA, Baker GB, Boisvert DPJ (eds) Physico-chemical techniques. Neuromethods, vol I. Clifton, NJ, Humana Press

Habert RL, Heizer ML, Elis EF (1987) Effects of the thromboxane A_2 mimetic U46619 on pial arterioles of rabbits and rats. Stroke 18:796–800

Morii S, Ngai AC, Winn HR (1986) Reactivity of rat pial arterioles and venules to adenosine and carbon dioxide: With detailed description of the closed cranial window technique in rats. J Cereb Blood Flow Metab 6:34–41

Olesen S-P (1987) Leakiness of rat brain microvessels to fluorescent probes following craniotomy. Acta Physiol Scand 130:63–68

Rapoport SI, Hori M, Klatzo I (1972) Testing of a hypothesis for osmotic opening of the blood-brain-barrier. Am J Physiol 223:323–331

Wahl M, Unterberg A, Baethmann A (1985) Intravital fluorescence microscopy for the study of blood-brain barrier function. Int J Microcirc Clin Exp 4:3–18

Session VIII: Edema

Chairmen: A. Baethmann and H. Nagai

Effect of the Pressure Gradient on Hydrostatic Brain Edema
H. Umezawa, K. Shima, H. Chigasaki, and S. Ishii

Preservation of Tissue Samples for Measurement of Cerebral Edema
A.M. Kaufmann, E.R. Cardoso, and E. Bruni

A CT Study on Formation, Propagation and Resolution of Brain Edema Fluid
in Human Peritumoral Edema
U. Ito, H. Tomita, H.-J. Reulen, T. Maehara, Y. Kohmo, and Y. Ito

Statistical Analysis of Changes in Topographic EEG on Brain Tumor Cases
with Peritumoral Edema
Y. Katoh, S. Oki, K. Kurisu, A. Nakahara, and T. Uozumi

The Blood: Brain Osmotic Gradient in Ischemic Brain Injury
S. Hatashita, J.T. Hoff, and S.M. Salamat

Brain Biomechanics and Focal Ischemic Injury
S. Hatashita and J.T. Hoff

The Role of Oxidative Reactions in Decompression Ischemic Edema
A. Schettini, B.W. Gibbs, and E.K. Walsh

Fatal Brain Edema After Total Cerebral Ischemia in Man
H. Nihei, A. Tamura, and K. Sano

Effect of Mannitol on Ischemic Brain Edema
A. Tamura, T. Kamiura, H. Kanemitsu, H. Nihei, N. Tomukai, and K. Sano

Colloid Volume Expansion and Brain Edema
B. Tranmer, R. Iacobacci, and G. Kindt

The Effect of IV Fluids on Cerebral Edema After Experimental
Blunt Head Trauma
Y. Shapira, M. Muggia-Sullam, H.R. Freund, and S. Cotev

The Effects of Nonsteroid Anti-Inflammatory Agent BW755C on Traumatic
and Peritumoral Brain Edema
Y. Ikeda, K.L. Brelsford, and D.M. Long

Effect of the Pressure Gradient on Hydrostatic Brain Edema

H. Umezawa, K. Shima, H. Chigasaki, and S. Ishii

Department of Neurosurgery, National Defense Medical College, Department of Neurosurgery, Juntendo University, Saitama 359 (Japan)

Introduction

Recent study has revealed that many factors contribute to the pathogenesis of brain edema, especially hydrostatic pressure gradient produced by the change in intracranial pressure and intracranial arterial pressure (Kogure et al. 1981; Hatashita et al. 1987). This study is designed to identify the effect of the pressure gradient on hydrostatic brain edema. For this purpose, two hydrostatic factors, hypertensive insult and decompressive craniectomy, were chosen and assessed for the development of hydrostatic brain edema.

Materials and Method

Adult Sprague-Dawley rats weighing 300–400 g were anesthetized with thiopental. After transoral intubation, animals were immobilized with pancuronium bromide and ventilated with a respirator. Under aseptic technique, the left common carotid and external carotid arteries, femoral artery and vein were cannulated with a polyethylene tube (PE-50). Animals were divided into two groups, one with craniectomy (Group A) and the other without craniectomy (Group B). In Group A, the area of craniectomy was confined to the coronal suture anteriorly, the rhomboid suture posteriorly. The medial and lateral borders were the sagittal suture and superior temporal line, respectively. Hypertensive insult was added via the left common carotid artery with a bolus injection of heparinized blood (2 ml). Infusion pressure was recorded via the left external carotid artery. ICP was monitored during each experiment using a catheter inserted into the cisterna magna. Physiological parameters such as blood gas pH, paO_2 and $paCO_2$ were controlled within normal range. For the tracer of BBB, 2% EB (2 ml/kg) was injected intravenously as follows: Group 1, prior to the hypertensive insult: Group 2, 24 hours after the hypertensive insult. Rats of Group 1 were sacrificed immediately, 24 and 48 hours after the insult and those of Group 2 were sacrificed 48 hours later. Brains were removed and cut in serial coronal setions about 1 mm thickness. The extent of EB extravasation was examined. A small piece of tissue (1 mm^3) was taken for the measurement of water content from frontal cortex, caudate nucleus and thalamus for gray matter and internal capsule for white matter, pons and medulla oblongata. Water content of the tissue samples was determined with the gravimetric method. Rats with the left common carotid arteries ligated were used for sham controls.

Results

The infusion pressure of both Groups A and B was 395.4 ± 12.30 mm Hg (mean $\pm$ SEM) and 408.2 ± 10.05 mm Hg (mean $\pm$ SEM), respectively. Statistically, there was no significant difference. In Group 1, the extravasation of EB was recognized in nearly all animals of both Groups A and B as patchy spots over the frontoparietal cortex, predominantly at the watershed areas of the anterior and middle cerebral arteries, and thalamus, caudate-putamen complex and the hippocampus. Twenty-four and 48 hours after the insult, the extravasation of EB was more diffusely and uniformly distributed. This effect was more pronounced with the passage of time. The extravasated EB spots were more dense and widely distributed in Group A as compared with Group B. In Group 1, there was no EB extravasation in Group B. However, in Group A, EB spots were faintly recognized in the parietal cortex, confined to the area behind the craniectomized portion.

In a resting state, the ICP in Group A was significantly lower than that in Group B ($p < 0.005$). During the hypertensive insult, the ICP value of Group A was 9.0 ± 1.65 mm Hg, whereas that of Group B reached 22.1 ± 5.38 mm Hg ($p < 0.025$) (Table 1). After the hypertensive insult, the same tendency was recognized ($p < 0.05$).

Specific gravities of Group B were not significantly different from those of sham controls in all portions examined. On the other hand, the values for frontal cortex and thalamus in Group A were significantly lower at 48 hours after the insult (frontal cortex: $p < 0.005$ vs sham control and $p < 0.025$ vs Group B, thalamus: $p < 0.05$ vs sham control and Group B). In the caudate nucleus the increment in water content was noted immediately after the insult and prolonged up to 48 hours later (Fig. 1).

Table 1. Result of ICP measurement in case of unilateral hypertensive insult

	SBP (mm Hg)			ICP (mm Hg)		
	Resting value	During maneuver	After maneuver	Resting value	During maneuver	After maneuver
Cr (−) group (n=5)	127.4 ± 2.98	145.8 ± 6.24	133.8 ± 4.44	6.4 ± 0.83	22.1 ± 5.38	7.6 ± 0.97
Cr (+) group (n=5)	126.8 ± 6.03	130.4 ± 6.37	129.0 ± 4.28	$2.6 \pm 0.68*$	$9.0 \pm 1.65**$	$3.0 \pm 0.54*$

* $P < 0.005$ VS Cr (−) group.
** $P < 0.025$ VS Cr (−) group.

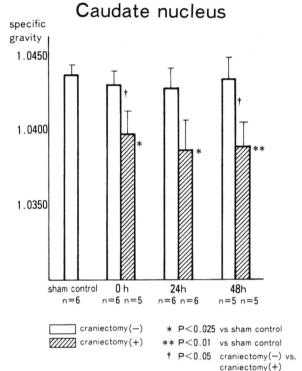

Caudate nucleus

specific
gravity

1.0450

1.0400

1.0350

sham control 0 h 24h 48h
n=6 n=6 n=5 n=6 n=6 n=5 n=5

☐ craniectomy (−)
▧ craniectomy (+)

* P<0.025 vs sham control
** P<0.01 vs sham control
† P<0.05 craniectomy(−) vs, craniectomy(+)

Fig. 1. The change of specific gravity after hypertensive insult. Water content of both group A (*craniectomy +*) and group B (*craniectomy −*) immediately, 24 and 48 hours after hypertensive insult

Discussion

Arterial hypertension is commonly used as a method for reversible opening of BBB. The mechanism of EB extravasation is thought to be caused by the opening of tight junctions due to forced dilatation of the vessels (Johansson and Linder 1978) or increase of pinocytic vesicle formation (Hansson and Johansson 1980). Extravasated plasma-like fluid seems to propagate through extracellular space possibly with bulk flow (Reulen et al. 1977). In our cases, extravasated EB patchy spots tended to be uniformly distributed and extended to the surrounding tissue with the passage of time. The main mechanism of this phenomenon is thought to be bulk flow, but the reopening of the BBB, recognized in Group A between 24 and 48 hours after the hypertensive insult, may to some extent contribute to the peripheral extension of the edema. Many have said that BBB opening is brief and transitional, occurring only during hypertension, or that the BBB is closed within 30 min after the insult (Johansson and Linder 1978). However, Kuroiwa et al. (1985), reported that a biphasic opening of BBB is recognized in the case of temporary middle cerebral artery occlusion, and a second barrier opening occurs as extravasated protein aggravates preexisting cytotoxic edema or a substance released from damaged tissue causes further brain edema as it alters permeability of blood vessels.

In our cases, extravasation of plasma-like fluid was induced in essentially normal brain. There was no significant change of water content in Group B despite EB extravasation. This finding coincides with Kogure's (1981) theory that the extravasation of a macromolecule in itself does not cause brain edema so long as cerebral metabolism remains normal. In our Group A, EB extravasation was not only more dense, but the increment in water content occurred progressively and lasted for 48 hours after insult. After craniectomy, the pressure-volume index is said to increase (Hatashita and Hoff 1987). In Group A, the rise of ICP during the hypertensive insult was significantly lower and there was no difference in infusion pressure so that the hydrostatic pressure gradient between blood vessels and brain tissue was amplified during the insult. Under these conditions EB extravasation might occur more extensively. Blood vessels are thought to be compressed by the extravasated fluid and cerebral blood flow is decreased. As a result, cerebral metabolism might be impaired secondarily so that the preexisting edema is aggravated (Koike 1983). Also, a reopening of the BBB might result from metabolic damage of blood vessels.

References

Hansson H, Johansson B (1980) Induction of pinocytosis in cerebral vessels by acute hypertension and by hyperosmolar solutions. J Neurosci Res 5:183–190

Hatashita S, Hoff JT (1987) The effect of craniectomy on the biomechanics of normal brain. J Neurosurg 67:573–578

Hatashita S, Koike J, Ishii S (1987) Effect of surgery on brain edema associated with intracerebral hematoma and arterial hypertension. Neurol Med Chir (Tokyo) 27:11–17

Johansson B, Linder L (1978) Reversibility of the blood-brain barrier dysfunction induced by acute hypertension. Acta Neurol Scand 57:345–348

Kogure K, Busto R, Scheinberg P (1981) The role of hydrostatic pressure in ischemic brain edema. Ann Neurol 9:273–282

Koike J (1983) Permeability change of cerebral vessels in acute hypertension and external decompression. Neurol Med Chir (Tokyo) 23:325–335

Kuroiwa T, Ting P, Klatzo I (1985) The biphasic opening of the blood-brain barrier to proteins following temporary middle cerebral artery occlusion. Acta Neuropathol (Berl) 678:122–129

Reulen HJ, Graham R, Spatz M, Klatzo I (1977) Role of pressure gradients and bulk flow in dynamics of vasogenic brain edema. J Neurosurg 46:24–35

Preservation of Tissue Samples for Measurement of Cerebral Edema

A.M. Kaufmann, E.R. Cardoso, and E. Bruni

Cerebral Hydrodynamics Laboratory, Departments of Surgery and Anatomy, University of Manitoba (Canada)

The gravimetric technique is a means to determine the specific gravity (SG) and water content (WC) of small cerebral samples. It has been widely used to study alterations of human cerebral edema related to neoplasms, trauma, and mannitol infusion. Measurements of tissue SG have also been correlated with CT and NMR image estimations of human brain edema.

Cerebral samples may be obtained at neurosurgical procedures. The samples must then be immersed in a gravimetric column within 30 sec in order to avoid significant loss of water content by evaporation (Nelson et al. 1978). However, immediate measurement is impractical, as it is difficult to manufacture and employ a gravimetric column in an operating room. Therefore, various means of transporting cerebral samples to a laboratory have been proposed. These include cool humidified chambers, wrapping in plastic, and immersion in lipid or formalin solutions. The efficacy and reliability of these methods have not been formally verified.

The purpose of the present study was to devise a method of sample preservation which prevents alteration of cerebral water content. The effects of formaldehyde fixation and deep-freezing upon SG measurements of cerebral samples were investigated. We described a technique of preserving cerebral tissue which may facilitate delayed SG and WC determinations of human cerebral samples.

Methods and Results

Cerebral tissue was removed from healthy and water intoxicated anesthetized adult mice. Samples were immersed in a gravimetric column to determine SG (Marmarou et al. 1978). Other cerebral samples from the same animals were preserved by either formaldehyde fixation or freezing. The SG was measured after 1 hr to 90 days and compared to corresponding fresh samples.

Formaldehyde Fixation. Non-edematous cerebral samples were stored in 2.5 to 40% formaldehyde solutions for 7 days. Preservation in 2.5 to 10% concentrations caused a decrease in tissue SG, compared to fresh controls. Higher fixative concentrations had the opposite effect. Furthermore, a linear correlation existed between SG and fixative concentration ($r = 0.997$). This suggests that the SG of samples was directly altered and dependent on the formaldehyde concentration.

Intracranial Pressure VII
Eds.: J. T. Hoff and A. L. Betz
© Springer-Verlag Berlin Heidelberg 1989

Osmotic exchange likely occurred between the cerebral samples and the fixative solution. Therefore, formaldehyde fixation is not a suitable technique for preservation of tissue for delayed SG measurements.

Rapid Freezing Technique. Samples were sealed within 0.5 ml microcentrifuge tubes and immersed in liquid nitrogen for 1 to 4 hr. Some samples were then stored at $-80°C$ for up to 90 days. Frozen samples were removed from the microcentrifuge tubes and immediately immersed in a gravimetric column.

The SG of fresh samples and those frozen up to 7 days did not significantly differ ($p < 0.05$). The mean SG of fresh non-edematous samples was 1.0483 ± 0.0001 ($n = 65$), and after freezing for 1 to 4 hr and 2 to 7 days was 1.0486 ± 0.001 ($n = 52$) and 1.0480 ± 0.0002 ($n = 57$), respectively. However, the SG after 90 days of freezing was 1.0475 ± 0.0002 ($n = 12$), which differed significantly from fresh samples ($p = 0.016$). This may reflect water condensation on cerebral tissue during the prolonged storage at $-80°C$.

The mean SG of fresh edematous cerebral samples obtained from 18 water intoxicated mice was 1.0433 ± 0.0005. Edematous samples obtained from the same animal and frozen for 1 or 7 days had mean SG values of 1.0439 ± 0.0004 ($n = 18$) and 1.0430 ± 0.0004 ($n = 9$), respectively. There was no significant difference among these values.

Rapid freezing of cerebral specimens probably prevents alterations of tissue water content by freezing brain solids and water before evaporation occurs. The low storage temperature, small volume of the sealed containers, and immediate immersion of frozen samples into a gravimetric column minimize alterations of tissue water content.

Conclusions

Our results indicate that the SG of formaldehyde fixed tissue reflects the storage solution concentration, rather than the actual tissue SG. Therefore, formaldehyde fixation is not a useful method to preserve tissue for subsequent WC determination. Our proposed method of rapid freezing, followed or not by deep-freeze storage, does not alter SG measurements for up to 7 days. This will allow delayed SG measurements of human cerebral samples obtained in the operating room, and thereby may facilitate clinical brain edema research.

Acknowledgements: We wish to thank Dr. Marc Del Bigio for his contribution, and the St. Boniface Hospital Research Foundation for funding of this project.

References

Marmarou A, Poll W, Shulman K, Bhagavan M (1978) A simple gravimetric technique for measurement of cerebral edema. J Neurosurg 49:530–537
Nelson SR, Mantz ML, Maxwell JA (1971) Use of specific gravity in measurement of cerebral edema. J Appl Physiol 30:268–271

A CT Study on Formation, Propagation and Resolution of Brain Edema Fluid in Human Peritumoral Edema

U. Ito[1], H. Tomita[1], H.-J. Reulen[2], T. Maehara[1], Y. Kohmo[1], and Y. Ito[1]

[1] Department of Neurosurgery, Musasino Red-Cross Hospital 1-26-1, Kyonon-Cho, Musasinocity, Tokyo 180
[2] Department of Neurosurgery, University of Bern, Bern (Switzerland)

Introduction

In the previous studies (Ito et al. 1988), CT was used to examine the time course of the propagation of extravasated contrast medium from small brain metastases into the peritumoral edematous white matter, following infusion of 200 ml of meglumine amidtrizoate for 3 hours. A contrast-enhanced area was observed surrounding clearly delineated tumors, expanding gradually in a circulation fashion into the peritumoral white matter edema.

The area of expanding circular enhancement was measured planimetrically. From these values the increase in volume per hour was calculated assuming a spherical geometry. These data enabled us to determine the formation rate of edema fluid from the tumor, the speed of edema fluid propagation and the resolution rate of edema fluid during tissue passage.

In the present study, increasing volume of peritumoral enhancement was calculated by integrating the volume enhanced areas, planimetrically measured on each CT slice, multiplied by the slice thickness (0.5 cm). This enabled us to estimate peritumoral expansion of contrast medium around non-spherical brain tumors such as meningiomas.

Materials and Methods

Six patients with various kinds of brain tumor were investigated (Patient 1; parietal convexity meningioma, Patient 2; recurrent malignant meningioma, Patient 3; sphenoid ridge meningioma, Patient 4; glioblastoma, Patient 5; malignant lymphoma, Patient 6; metastatic tumor). Except for Patient 3, all patients showed white matter edema of Grade II or III by Lanksh (1982) around the brain tumor. No peritumoral white matter edema was found in Patient 3. Renal and liver functions were normal in all 6 patients from whom informed consent for examinations were obtained. GE 9000 was used for the CT scan. Axial slices of 0.5 cm in thickness were scanned, including whole tumor mass and expanding peritumoral contrast-enhancement. The initial scan was taken at the end of a one-hour continuous i.v. infusion of 200 ml Iopamidol (300 mgI/ml). Second and third scans were obtained 3–6 hr and 6–11 hr after the start of contrast infusion, respectively. The area of contrast enhancement (including tumor) was measured planimetrically in each scan, using a digital planimeter KP-90 (UCHIDA, Tokyo). All measurements were adjusted to the scale in each CT picture.

The volume of contrast-enhancement was calculated by integrating the measured volumes of contrast-enhanced area in each scan (V_1, V_2, V_3) on contiguous slices with 0.5 cm in thickness. The increasing volume from 1st to 2nd (ΔV_1) and 2nd to 3rd (ΔV_2) scan was calculated, respectively. To calculate the formation and resolution rate of edema fluid, the following assumptions were made: a) the concentration of Iopamidol in the extravasated edema fluid was similar to that in the plasma, b) Iopamidol distributes only in the extracellular space, and c) the extracellular space in the peritumoral edematous tissue is about 30% (Fenske et al. 1973).

The value of newly formed edema fluid from the tumor tissue is a summation of values of edema fluid which propagates into the peritumoral region (ΔV_1) during the interval between the first and second scan (t_1), and the volume of edema fluid reabsorbed within ΔV_1 ($=\Delta V_1 - \Delta V_2$) multiplied by the extracellular space (30%). The tumor volume is approximated to the measured volume of enhancement in the 1st scan (V_1). The formation rate (ΔV_F) of edema fluid from one cm^3 of tumor per hour can be calculated as follows:

$$\Delta V_F = \frac{2\,\Delta V_1 - \Delta V_2}{V_1 \cdot t_1} \times 0.3 \text{ ml/hr/cm}^3 \text{ tumor}$$

ΔV_2 was smaller than ΔV_1 in each patient. This decline of ΔV could be explained by reabsorption of edema fluid during its passage through white matter. Otherwise, the increasing rate of volume in adjacent scan interval (ΔV_1 and ΔV_2) per hour should remain constant. Thus, the resolution rate of the ΔV_R per hour during passage in 1 cm^3 of white matter between contiguous time intervals were calculated in each patient, according to the following formula:

$$\Delta V_R = \frac{\Delta V_1 - \Delta V_2}{\Delta V_1 \cdot t_1} \times 0.3 \text{ ml/hr/cm}^3 \text{ white matter}$$

Following this study, all 6 patients received dexamethasone (8–12 mg/day, i.v.) for 4–7 days. The same study was then repeated.

Results

A well defined contrast enhancement of the tumor, with a clear delineation of its border, was observed in all 6 patients after 1 hour of contrast infusion (Fig. 1). At the second scan, 3 to 6 hours after the start of contrast infusion, a halo of peritumoral contrast enhancement expanded gradually around the tumors, except for the meningioma in Patient 3 which did not show peritumoral white matter low density (Fig. 1). The contrast density in the tumor decreased at the 3rd scan, but the circular border of contrast enhancement could still be nicely delineated within the area of white matter low density (Fig. 1). The expanding grade

960

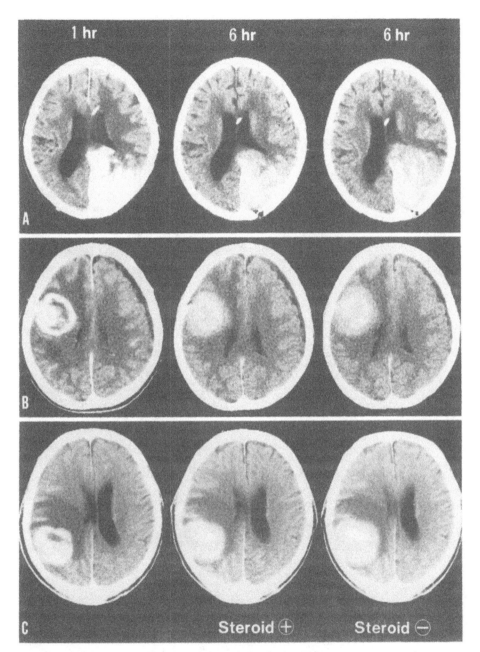

Fig. 1 A–C. Comparison of peritumoral contrast enhancement before and after treatment with dexamethasone, 6 hours following start of contrast infusion. Approximate tumor size represented at 1 hour. **A** malignant meningioma (Patient 2). **B** glioblastoma (Patient 4). **C** Malignant lymphoma (Patient 5)

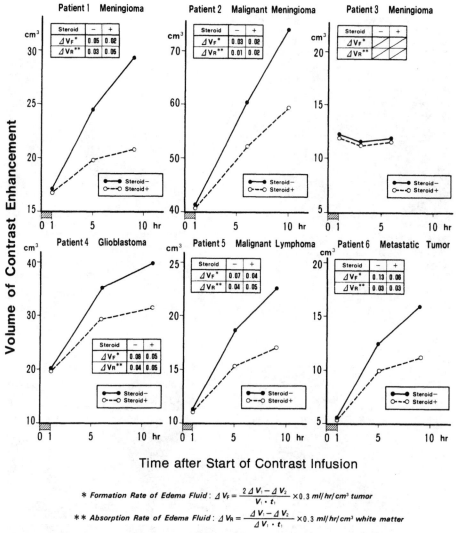

Fig. 2. Increasing volume of the contrast enhancement. Calculated formation rate (ΔV_F) and resolution rate (ΔV_R) of edema fluid

of peritumoral contrast enhancement was obviously reduced in size after dexamethasone treatment (Fig. 1).

The measured volume of expanding peritumoral enhancement at 1st, 2nd and 3rd scan is presented in Fig. 2. All tumors, except for Patient 3, showed a curved increase of volume, of which increasing grade was remarkably reduced by steroid treatment. In each tumor, the formation rate of edema fluid was calculated to 0.03–0.13 ml/hr/cm³ tumor before, and 0.20–0.06 after steroid treatment. The formation rate was obviously reduced by dexamethasone treatment in all tumors except for the meningioma in Patient 3 (Fig. 2).

The absorption rate of edema fluid during passage of 1 cm^3 of white matter per hour ranged between 0.01 to 0.04 before, and 0.02 to 0.05 after steroid treatment. The absorption rate was slighlty increased by dexamethasone treatment in meningiomas (Patient 1 and 2), glioblastoma (Patient 4) and malignant lymphoma (Patient 5, Fig. 2).

Discussion

In experimental brain tumor models, spreading edema fluid which extravasates from leaky vessels within the tumor into the extracellular space of the surrounding white matter, was investigated by labelling the edema fluid with Evans blue or with radioactive marker (Ausman et al. 1977; Blasberg et al. 1979; Hossmann et al. 1980; Yamada et al. 1984; Yen et al. 1985). In this CT study of different kinds of human tumor, lopamidol, a contrast medium (Mol. weight 777,09) was used to label the newly formed edema fluid in the brain tumor. The assumption was made that this substance moves with a similar speed to other solutes with the edema fluid movement (Reulen et al. 1977).

It is generally accepted from experimental studies that, in brain tumors, edema fluid, including serum proteins and macromolecules, extravasates from leaky vessels within the tumor into the extracellular space of the surrounding white matter (Ausman et al. 1977; Blasberg et al. 1979; Long 1970; Yamada et al. 1984), with transcapillary hydrostatic pressure as the driving force (Reulen et al. 1977). In the present study, the formation rate of edema fluid from tumor was similar in different tumors, which showed peritumoral white matter edema of Lanksch (1982), Grade II to III. These values were decreased to 40 to 60% by dexamethasone treatment.

Various mechanisms of edema production has been reported for brain edema surrounding meningiomas including compression of surrounding tissue by tumor, venous congestion by sinovenous occlusion, biological differences depending on histopathology, edema inducing factors, etc. (Stevens 1983). In the present study, the meningiomas of Patient 1 and 2 showed prominent peritumoral white matter edema on CT. Direct contact of tumor to the peritumoral white matter tissue was confirmed by operative microscopy. While the sphenoid ridge meningioma of Patient 3 showed no peritumoral white matter edema on CT, a thin subarachnoid CSF space was confirmed around the tumor which had grown into the proxymal portion of the Sylvian fissure. Therefore, transmission of edema fluid into the extracellular space of the contacted white matter could induce peritumoral white matter edema (Bradac 1986; Stevens 1983).

There have been controversies on the effect of steroids on peritumoral edema associated with meningioma (Hatam et al. 1983). In the present study of a limited number of patients, meningothelial meningioma (Patient 1) and malignant meningioma (Patient 2, recurrence) showed marked reduction of the formation rate and increase of the resolution rate of edema fluid by dexamethasone treatment.

Foncin et al. (1978) reported electron microscopic evidence that edema fluid originates from malignant glioma tissue and propagates into the extracellular space of the surrounding white matter. Dexamethasone was also effective to reduce formation rate and increase absorption rate, both in glioblastoma and malignant lymphoma (Hatam et al. 1983).

In metastatic brain tumor from breast cancer the formation rate of edema fluid was remarkably reduced by dexamethasone; however, steroids did not increase the absorption rate of edema fluid. This observation coincides with data from our previous paper (Ito et al. 1988).

Following treatment of patients with dexamethasone, the rate of expansion of the contrast medium was reduced in all 5 patients who showed peritumoral white matter edema. The main cause of the reduction is supposed to be a reduced formation rate of edema fluid, thus reduced permeability of the tumor vessels. This is consistent with findings of decreased contrast enhancement, and decreased radioactive uptake of the tumor following steroid treatment (Crocker et al. 1976; Fletcher et al. 1975; Hatam et al. 1983). Yamada et al. (1984) found a significant reduction of capillary permeability in an experimental brain tumor following steroid treatment, using ^{14}C-alpha-aminobutylic acid as a tracer. There remains the possibility that dexamethasone alters the structure and compliance of the extracellular space in the white matter around the tumor and thereby increases the resistance of the extracellular space to propagating edema (Ito et al. 1986; Yen et al. 1985).

No adverse effects were noted in any of our patients to whom 200 ml of Iopamidol was infused during one hour (Ito et al. 1986; Ito et al. 1988).

Summary

Propagation of contrast medium which extravasated from different kinds of brain tumor (meningioma, malignant meningioma, glioblastoma, malignant lymphoma, metastatic brain tumor) was imaged via CT, following continuous infusion of 200 ml of Iopamidol for 1 hour. Changing volume of expanding peritumoral contrast enhancement was measured by integrating the volumes of planimetrically measured CT slices of 0.5 cm in thickness. Behavior of the expanding peritumoral contrast enhancement was similar among all tumors which showed peritumoral white matter edema of Grade II to III. The main cause of the steroid effect on peritumoral edema was reduction in the formation rate of edema fluid from each tumor. The above data are compatible with our previously reported results obtained from spherical geometry in small round metastatic tumors (Ito et al. 1988). However, further quantitative data are required to specify behaviors of the peritumoral edema in different kinds of tumor.

References

Ausman JI, Levin VA, Brown WE, Rall DP, Fenstermacher JD (1977) Brain tumor chemotherapy. Pharmacological principles derived from a monkey brain-tumor model. J Neurosurg 46:155–164

964

Blasberg R, Patlak C, Shapiro W, Fenstermacher J (1979) Metastatic brain tumors: local blood flow and capillary permeability. Neurology (Minneap) 29:547

Bradac GB, Ferszt R, Bender A, Schörner W (1986) Peritumoral edema in meningiomas. A radiological and histological study. Neuroradiol 28:304–312

Crocker EF, Zimmerman RA, Phelps ME, Kuhl DE (1976) The effect of steroids on the extravascular distribution of radiographic contrast materials and Technetium pertechnetate in brain tumors as determined by computed tomography. Radiology 119:471–474

Fenske A, Samii M, Reulen H-J et al. (1973) Extracellular space and electrolyte distribution in cortex and white matter of dog brain in cold induced edema. Acta Neurochir (Wien) 28:81–94

Foncin JE, Beau JLe (1978) The brain surrounding malignant gliomas: An ultrastructural study. Acta Neurochir (Wien) 42:33–43

Fletcher JW, George EA, Henry RE, Donati RM (1975) Brain scans, dexamethasone therapy and brain tumors. JAMA 232:1261–1263

Hatam A, Bergström M, Yu ZY, Granholm L (1983) Effect of dexamethasone treatment on volume and contrast enhancement of intracranial neoplasms. J Comput Assist Tomogr 7:295–300

Hirano A, Matsui T (1975) Vascular structure in brain tumors. Hum Pathol 6:611–621

Hossmann KA, Blanik M, Wilmes F, Wechsler W (1980) Experimental peritumoral edema of the cat brain. In: Cervos-Navarro J, Ferszt R (eds) Brain edema. Advances in neurology, vol 28. Raven Press, New York, pp 323–340

Ito U, Reulen H-J, Huber P (1986) Spatial and quantitative distribution of human peritumoral brain edema in computerized tomography. Acta Neurochir (Wien) 81:53–60

Ito U, Tomita H, Kito K, Ueki Y, Inaba Y (1986) CT enhancement after prolonged highdose contrast infusion in the early stage of cerebral infarction. Stroke 17:424–430

Ito U, Reulen H-J, Tomita H, Ikeda J, Saito J, Maehara T (1988) Formation and propagation of brain oedema fluid around human brain metastases. A CT study. Acta Neurochir (Wien) 90:35–41

Lanksch WR (1982) The diagnosis of brain edema by computed tomography. In: Hartmann A, Brock M (eds) Treatment of cerebral edema. Springer, Berlin Heidelberg New York, pp 43–80

Long DM (1970) Capillary ultrastructure and the blood-brain barrier in human malignant brain tumors. J Neurosurg 32:127–151

Reulen H-J, Graham R, Spatz M, Klatzo I (1977) Role of pressure gradients and bulk flow in dynamics of vasogenic brain edema. J Neurosurg 46:24–35

Stevens JM, Ruiz JS, Kendall BE (1983) Observations on peritumoural oedema in meningioma. Part II; Mechanisms of oedema production. Neuroradiology 25:125–131

Yamada K, Hayakawa T, Ushio Y, Kato A, Yamada N, Mogami H (1984) Peritumoral brain edema: Effects of methyl-prednisolone on local cerebral blood flow, glucose utilisation and capillary permeability. In: Go KG, Baethman A (eds) Plenum Press, New York London, pp 345–354

Yen MH, Wright D, Nakagawa N, Blasberg R, Patlak C, Fenstermacher J (1985) Effects of dexamethasone on the blood-brain distribution of [125]J-albumine and ^{14}C-alphaamino-isobutyric acid in vasogenic cerebral edema. In: Inaba Y, Klatzo I, Spatz M (eds) Brain edema. Springer, Berlin Heidelberg New York, pp 638–645

Statistical Analysis of Changes in Topographic EEG on Brain Tumor Cases with Peritumoral Edema

Y. Katoh, S. Oki, K. Kurisu, A. Nakahara, and T. Uozumi

Department of Neurosurgery, Hiroshima University School of Medicine, 1-2-3, Kasumi, Minami-ku, Hiroshima 734 (Japan)

Introduction

EEG is one of the best methods for estimating brain function. Topographic EEG is made by analyzing the power spectrum of EEG as equivalent potential (EP). In this study, the changes in topographic EEG after glycerol administration were observed by statistic calculation of EP in brain tumor patients.

Materials and Methods

A total of 30 cases with supra-tentorial tumors were examined. These 30 cases were divided into three groups: 10 primary malignant brain tumor cases, 10 primary benign brain tumor cases, and 10 metastatic brain tumor cases. All the cases were diagnosed histologically by surgery. 10% glycerol solution was administered intravenously. Topographic EEGs were obtained three times, i.e. before glycerol administration, after administration of 250 ml of glycerol, and after administration of 500 ml of glycerol. Monopolar EEG was recorded from 12 electrodes placed over the scalp according to the 10–20 international system. Topographic EEG was obtained by analyzing the EEG with the Signal Processor (NEC San-ei Instruments, Ltd., Japan) according to Ueno-Matsuoka's method (Ueno et al. 1976). Paired t-test of the affected hemisphere between the topographic EEGs obtained before and after administration of glycerol was conducted on each case. The EPs of seven points of the affected hemisphere were calculated and the change in topographic EEG on each frequency band were estimated statistically ($p < 0.05$).

Results

1. Total Cases. When 250 ml of glycerol was administered, the percentage of the number of increased EP cases was high in beta 1 and beta 2. When 500 ml of glycerol was administered, the percentage of the number of increased EP cases was high in beta 2 and the percentage of the number of decreased EP cases was high in delta, theta and alpha 1 (Table 1).

Table 1. Change in topographic EEG after glycerol administration (brain tumor cases, affected hemisphere), $n = 30$

Tumor	Glycerol (ml)	δ	θ	α_1	α_2	β_1	β_2
Primary malignant tumor	250						
	500		↓				
Benign brain tumor	250				↓		▲
	500	↓	↓	↓			▲
Metastatic brain tumor	250	↓				▲	▲
	500	▼	↓	▼	↓		
Total	250					↑	▲
	500	↓	↓	↓			↑

↑↓   Increase of decrease in EP from 30 to 50%
▲▼ Increase or decrease in EP over 50%

2. Histological Classification and Topographic EEG. In primary malignant brain tumor cases, the changes in topographic EEG were indefinite, but by administration of 500 ml of glycerol, the percentage of the number of decreased EP cases was high in theta. In benign brain tumor cases, by administration of 250 ml of glycerol, the percentage of the number of decreased EP cases in alpha 2 was high and the percentage of the number of increased EP cases in beta 2 was markedly high By administration of 500 ml of glycerol, the percentage of the number of decreased EP cases in delta, theta and alpha 1 was high. In metastatic brain tumor cases, by administration of 250 ml of glycerol, the percentage of the number of increased EP cases in beta 1 and beta 2 was markedly high. By administration of 500 ml of glycerol, the percentage of the number of decreased EP cases in delta, theta, alpha 1 and alpha 2 was high (Table 1).

3. Brain Edema and Topographic EEG. Brain edema was divided into two groups by size. In the small edema group, the size of the edema was smaller than that of the tumor (18 cases). In the large edema group, the size of the edema was larger than that of the tumor (12 cases). By administration of 250 ml of glycerol, the increase in EP of beta 2 was greater in the large edema group than in the other. By administration 500 ml of glycerol, the decrease in EP of delta and alpha 1 was greater in the large edema group than in the other (Fig. 1).

Discussion

Focal slow wave is one of the characteristic findings of EEG in brain tumor patients. In the topographic EEG, increased EPs of slow wave bands are frequently observed at the same site over the brain tumor especially when the tumor exists cortically or subcortically (Matsuoka et al. 1978). In this study, a small amount of glycerol administration (250 ml) increased EP in the fast wave bands,

967

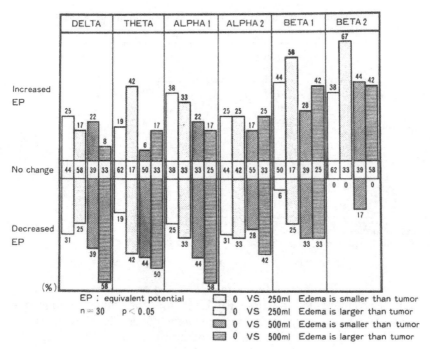

Fig. 1. Brain edema and topographic EEG after glycerol administration

and a large amount of glycerol administration (500 ml) decreased EP in the slow wave bands. These results suggest that glycerol activates brain function in brain tumor patients. These effects of glycerol are more obvious in the large edema group than in the small edema group, and appear to differ according to the kind of brain tumor. In metastatic brain tumor cases, these effects are most apparent, but in primary malignant brain tumor cases, the effects are poorly defined.

Conclusions

It is suggested that the severity of brain edema and the developmental pattern of brain tumor determine whether brain function will be reversible or irreversible in brain tumor patients.

References

Matsuoka S, Arakaki Y, Numaguchi K, Ueno S (1978) The effects of dexamethasone on electroencephalograms in patients with brain tumors. With specific reference to topographic computer display of delta activity. J Neurosurg 48:601–608

Ueno S, Matsuoka S (1976) Topographic computer display of abnormal EEG activities in patients with brain lesions. In: Digest of the 11th international conference on medical and biological engineering, Ottawa, pp 218–219

The Blood: Brain Osmotic Gradient in Ischemic Brain Injury

S. Hatashita[1], J.T. Hoff[2], and S.M. Salamat[2]

[1] Neurosurgery, Tokyo Metropolitan Hiroo Hospital 2-34-10 Ebis, Shibuya-ku, Tokyo 150 (Japan)
[2] Department of Neurosurgery, University of Michigan, Ann Arbor, Michigan (USA)

Introduction

The pathophysiology of ischemic brain edema depends primarily on the duration and severity of ischemia. Cerebrovascular permeability as well as hydraulic conductivity of capillaries, hydrostatic and osmotic pressure gradients, and tissue compliance and resistance are also associated with the ischemic edema process.

Earlier, we demonstrated that a hydrostatic pressure gradient across the capillary develops soon after the ischemic onset and is the driving force for early accumulation of edema fluid (Hatashita and Hoff 1986a, b). Our study of biomechanics has also shown that, as ischemic injury progresses, edema fluid accumulates in highly compliant brain parenchyma, then migrates through highly conductive tissue into the CSF spaces, driven by the hydrostatic pressure gradient between the edematous tissue and the CSF (Hatashita and Hoff 1988a).

The present experiment was designed to study whether BBB permeability and an osmotic gradient across the capillary are associated with the development of ischemic brain edema. We sought to clarify the relationship between brain osmolality, brain water content, tissue sodium and potassium, and the integrity of BBB in focal cerebral ischemia.

Materials and Methods

Adult male Sprague-Dawley rats (300–400 g), were anesthetized by an intramuscular injection of ketamine hydrochloride (40 mg/kg) and xylazine (10 mg/kg). The middle cerebral artery (MCA) was occluded by the transretro-orbital approach, without damage to the zygomatic bone. Sham operation was performed in the same way except for the occlusion. After surgery, the animals were returned to their cages and permitted free access to food and water. Then, the animals were reanesthetized and sacrificed by decapitation at 1 h, 3 h, 6 h, 12 h, 24 h, 48 h and 72 h after MCA occlusion.

Brain tissue osmolality was measured by a vapor pressure osmometer (M 5100C, Wescor, Inc.) (Tornheim 1980). The head was frozen in situ with liquid nitrogen and stored in dry-ice at −70° C. Two slices of cortex supplied by the MCA were dissected from both frozen hemispheres. The slice on dry-ice was transferred immediately to the osmometer and osmolality was measured. Water content of adjacent brain tissue was measured by the wet and dry weight method. Then the concentrations of sodium and potassium ions in the same samples were determined by flame photometry with lithium as an internal standard, and expressed as mEq/kg dry weight.

The permeability of the blood brain barrier (BBB) was evaluated by intravenous injection of either 2% Evans blue (2.5 cc/kg) or Na-Fluorescein (2.5 cc/kg) dye 30 min before sacrifice. The degree of extravasation of dye tracers was evaluated grossly. The incidence of BBB damage was calculated as a percentage of the number of animals sacrificed at each time interval.

Quantitative evaluation of BBB permeability was also done by the brain tissue uptake of radioactive tracers. ^{125}I-bovine serum albumin (15 µci) or ^{14}C-sucrose (15 µci) was given intravenously 30 min before sacrifice. Tissue samples were taken from the cortex supplied by the MCA in both hemispheres. Radioactivity in arterial blood and brain samples was determined with a gamma scintillation counter or beta-scintillation spectrometer. The passage of these tracers from the blood into brain was calculated by dividing the radioactivity of brain tissue by the blood, expressed as a percentage of the contralateral side. The water content of adjacent brain tissue was also measured by the specific gravity method.

Statistical significance of results was determined by Student's t test. All values were expressed as mean ± SEM.

Results

Brain Tissue Osmolality

Brain tissue osmolality in control animals was 311.3 ± 2.2 mOsm/kg ($n=6$). After MCA occlusion the osmolality in ischemic brain tissue increased progressively and reached a maximum of 329.6 ± 1.9 mOsm/kg ($n=7$, $P<0.01$) at three hours, then plateaued for the next three hours. Osmolality returned to control values 12 hours after occlusion and was maintained at about the same level thereafter (Fig. 1). Plasma osmolality was 303.3 ± 1.0 mOsm/l ($n=6$) in control animals and did not change in animals with MCA occlusion.

A significant increase in the osmotic gradient between ischemic brain tissue and blood was found only at three and six hours after MCA occlusion. The gradient values at three and six hours were 25.4 ± 2.6 and 26.1 ± 2.9 mOsm/kg ($n=7$, $P<0.01$), respectively.

Brain Water, Sodium and Potassium Contents

Water content increased significantly as early as one hour after occlusion ($80.28 \pm 0.28\%$, $n=7$, $P<0.05$). The increase in water content progressed and reached $86.39 \pm 0.47\%$ ($n=7$, $P<0.01$) at its maximum 24 hours of occlusion. Then the increase in water content remained at about the same level within 72 hours.

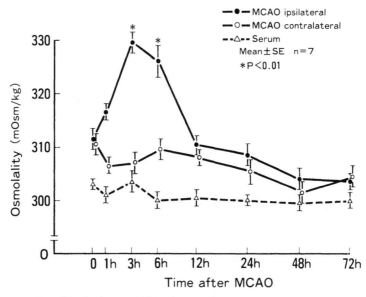

Fig. 1. Changes in osmolality of brain tissue and blood serum from 1 to 72 hours after middle cerebral artery occlusion (*MCAO*). Brain osmolality increases significantly at three and six hours after MCAO

After MCA occlusion reciprocal changes in brain tissue sodium and potassium contents occurred concomitantly. The sodium content in ischemic brain tissue increased progressively until 2 days of occlusion while potassium content decreased. There was no increase in sodium plus potassium content of brain tissue within 6 hours of occlusion.

Brain Osmolality and Water Content

After the ischemic insult the osmolality of brain tissue increased significantly until the increase in water content reached about 20 mg/g brain. When water content increased above about 40 mg/g brain, the increase in osmolality no longer correlated with that of water content (Fig. 2).

BBB Permeability to Evans Blue and Na-Fluorescein

There was no extravasation of Evans blue within six hours of MCA occlusion. Extravasation of Evans blue was observed in only one of 11 animals killed 12 hours of occlusion and in 10 of 81 animals within 72 hours. EB extravasation was mostly faint staining, and located only in the proximal portion of the core of the MCA territory.

In contrast, extravasation of Na-Fluorescein was first found in one of 10 animals killed six hours of occlusion. The staining was seen in 10 of 70 animals within 72 hours. The extent and location of NaFl extravasation into ischemic brain tissue was more extensive than Evans blue.

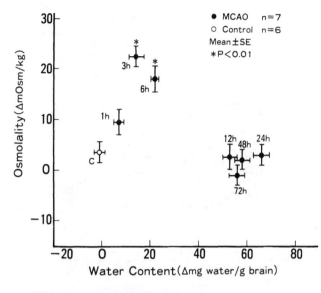

Fig. 2. Relationship between changes in brain osmolality and water content within 72 hours of middle cerebral artery occlusion (*MCAO*). Brain osmolality increases significantly until the increase in water content reaches about 20 mg/g brain

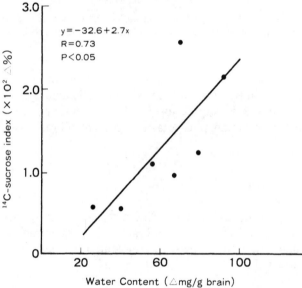

$$y = -32.6 + 2.7x$$
$$R = 0.73$$
$$P < 0.05$$

Fig. 3. Relationship between changes in ^{14}C-sucrose index and water content within 72 hours of middle cerebral artery occlusion (*MCAO*). There is a significant correlation between increases in ^{14}C-sucrose and water content

BBB Permeability to ^{125}I-BSA and ^{14}C-Sucrose

Brain uptake of ^{125}I-BSA and ^{14}C-sucrose tracers did not increase significantly within six hours of MCA occlusion. A significant increase in these tracers was first found at 12 hours after occlusion. The index in ^{14}C-sucrose increased from $1.09 \times 10^2 \pm 0.06$ to $2.20 \times 10^2 \pm 0.21\%$, whereas ^{125}I-BSA from $1.15 \times 10^2 \pm 0.12$ to $1.95 \times 10^2 \pm 0.38\%$ ($n = 8$, $P < 0.05$). Then, the uptake of ^{14}C-sucrose increased gradually up to 72 hours after MCA occlusion and reached $3.66 \times 10^2 \pm 0.34$ ($n = 10$, $P < 0.05$). In contrast, the increase in ^{125}I-BSA index was maintained about the same level up to 72 hours after occlusion.

When changes in mean values of the ^{125}I-BSA or ^{14}C-sucrose index was correlated with water content, there was a significant correlation between increases in water content and ^{14}C-sucrose within 72 hours of occlusion (Fig. 3). The increase in the ^{125}I-BSA index did not correlate with water content.

Discussion

We have demonstrated that a significant increase in osmolality of ischemic brain tissue is found three and six hours after MCA occlusion. The osmotic gradient between ischemic brain tissue and blood is about 26 mOsm/kg. The increment in brain osmolality correlated with that of water content until water content increased to about 20 mg/g brain. These findings indicate that the osmotic pressure gradient which develops between ischemic brain and blood is a fundamental factor in the early accumulation of edema fluid after ischemic injury.

A significant increase in tissue osmolality was not found 1 hour after MCA occlusion despite an increase in water content. We have recently demonstrated that, in ischemic tissue, water passage is related to a hydrostatic pressure gradient between arterial blood and brain (Hatashita and Hoff 1986 a, b). However, this hydrostatic pressure gradient dissipates as tissue pressure in the ischemic cortex rises with time. Our findings suggest that ischemic brain edema is associated with a hydrostatic pressure gradient between blood and brain soon after the onset of ischemia and is later followed by the development of an osmotic pressure gradient as the ischemic injury progresses.

This study has also shown that the radioactive indicators, ^{125}I-BSA and ^{14}C-sucrose, are not significantly detected in ischemic brain within 6 hours of MCA occlusion. The extravasation of Evans blue or Na-Fluorescein did not extend diffusely into ischemic brain tissue. This confirms previous work which showed that BBB injury is not found during the acute stage of cerebral ischemia (Klatzo 1980). Our findings also indicate that BBB permeability to serum protein or small molecules remains nearly intact during the early stage of cerebral ischemia.

We have further shown that a breakdown of BBB to small and large molecules is found in the ischemic tissue 12 hours after MCA occlusion. The increase in BBB permeability to ^{14}C-sucrose correlates with the rise of water content within 72 hours of MCA occlusion, whereas ^{125}I-BSA does not. This implies that accumulation of edema fluid is associated with BBB disruption to small molecules during the late stages of ischemic brain edema formation.

Conclusion

We conclude that the accumulation of edema fluid is related to a hydrostatic pressure gradient which develops soon after the onset of ischemia. Then, an osmotic pressure gradient develops as the ischemic injury progresses. Further accumulation of edema fluid is associated with BBB disruption to small molecules at the later stages of ischemic edema formation.

References

Hatashita S, Hoff JT (1986a) Cortical tissue pressure gradients in early ischemic brain edema. J Cereb Blood Flow Metab 6:1–7

Hatashita S, Hoff JT (1986b) Role of a hydrostatic pressure gradient in formation of early ischemic brain edema. J Cereb Blood Flow Metab 6:546–552

Hatashita S, Hoff JT (1988a) Biomechanics of brain edema in acute cerebral ischemia. Stroke 19:91–97

Hatashita S, Hoff JT, Salamat SM (1988b) Ischemic brain edema and the osmotic gradient between blood and brain. J Cereb Blood Flow Metab (in press)

Klatzo I (1983) Disturbance of blood-brain barrier in cerebrovascular disorders. Acta Neuropathol [Suppl] (Berl) 8:81–88

Tornheim AP (1980) Use of a vapor pressure osmometer to measure brain osmolality. J Neuroscience Methods 3:21–35

Brain Biomechanics and Focal Ischemic Injury

S. Hatashita[1] and J.T. Hoff[2]

[1] Neurosurgery, Tokyo Metropolitan Hiroo Hospital, 2-34-10 Ebis, Shibuya-ku, Tokyo 150 (Japan)
[2] Department of Neurosurgery, University of Michigan, Ann Arbor, Michigan (USA)

Introduction

Many factors modify the edema process, including cerebrovascular permeability, capillary hydraulic conductivity, hydrostatic and osmotic pressure gradients, and tissue compliance and conductivity.

We have recently demonstrated that a hydrostatic pressure gradient across the capillary develops within minutes after the onset of ischemia and is the driving force of early accumulation of edema fluid (Hatashita and Hoff 1986a, b). As the ischemic injury progresses, an osmotic pressure gradient develops which contributes to the formation of ischemic edema (Hatashita et al. 1988).

We have recently reported a difference between biomechanical properties of normal cortical gray and white matter (Hatashita, Hoff 1987). However, the biomechanics of ischemic brain tissue, particularly tissue elastic compliance and hydraulic resistance, remain poorly understood.

The present experiment was designed to clarify the relationship between brain tissue pressure, tissue compliance, tissue resistance, ischemic edema and blood flow in adjacent cortical gray matter made variably ischemic.

Material and Methods

Focal cerebral ischemia was produced for six hours by left middle cerebral artery (MCA) occlusion in 22 anesthetized cats. Tissue pressure (TP) was measured by our modified needle system, regional cerebral blood flow (rCBF) by hydrogen clearance and water content by specific gravity. Tissue compliance (TC) and tissue resistance (TR) were measured by a bolus injection of saline (0.63 – 0.73 µl/min) into brain tissue, using the same TP needles (Marmarou et al. 1976).

Tissue compliance is defined as the volume increase per change in pressure and was calculated by dividing the change in infusion volume by the observed increase in pressure (ml/mm Hg). Tissue resistance is defined as change in pressure per change in flow and was calculated by the increase in pressure by the change in infusion rate (mm Hg/ml/min).

TC and TR were measured from the same regional cortex in the central core "the sylvian gyrus" and peripheral margin "the anterior lateral gyrus" of the MCA territory. Intracranial pressure was continously recorded as ventricular

Intracranial Pressure VII
Eds.: J.T. Hoff and A.L. Betz
© Springer-Verlag Berlin Heidelberg 1989

fluid pressure (VFP) from the right lateral ventricle. Five additional cats served as sham-operated controls.

All values were expressed as mean ± SEM. Statistical significance of results was determined by Student's t test.

Results

One hour after occlusion, rCBF fell from 44.15 ± 1.05 to 6.27 ± 0.32 ml/ 100 mg/min in the core and 17.65 ± 0.73 ml/100 mg/min in the periphery. The reduction of rCBF in the core was greater than that in the periphery. The flow in both areas did not fall further over the next five hours.

Water content increased significantly in the core one hour after occlusion. The increase of water content progressed at three and six hours after occlusion, reaching $82.83 \pm 0.18\%$ ($n=7$, $P<0.01$) at its maximum. In contrast, there was a significant increase in water content six hours after occlusion in the periphery, but not before.

TP in the core increased progressively after two hours of occlusion and then the rate of rise slowed. The value of TP was 14.3 ± 0.4 mm Hg ($n=7$, $P<0.01$) six hours after occlusion. In contrast, TP in the periphery rose from 6.6 ± 0.7 to 9.7 ± 0.5 mm Hg and VFP to 8.7 ± 0.3 mm Hg ($n=7$, $P<0.01$) six hours after occlusion. The pressure gradient between TP in the core and VFP increased gradually during the first three hours, then reached a plateau during the next three. The gradient was 5.3 mm Hg six hours after occlusion.

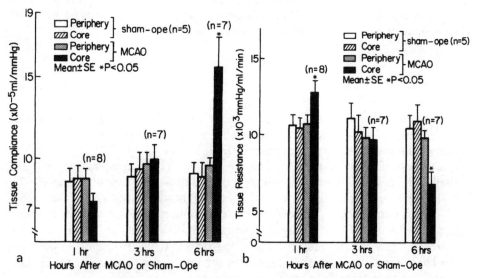

Fig. 1. Brain tissue compliance (**a**) and resistance (**b**) in the core and periphery 1, 3 and 6 hours after middle cerebral artery occlusion (MCAO) and sham operation. Tissue compliance increased markedly in the core 6 hours after MCAO. Tissue resistance increases 1 hour after occlusion and then decreases 6 hours

An increase in TP after MCA occlusion was directly related to the water content until the increase in water content reached 35 mg/g brain ($r=0.88$, $P<0.05$).

After MCA occlusion, TC in the core decreased slightly from $9.06 \pm 0.93 \times 10^{-5}$ to $7.41 \pm 0.53 \times 10^{-5}$ ml/mm Hg during the first hour. Then, TC rose gradually to control values three hours after occlusion and increased significantly to $15.75 \pm 1.84 \times 10^{-5}$ ml/mm Hg by six hours. There was no significant change in TC over six hours after occlusion in the periphery (Fig. 1a).

TR increased significantly from $10.49 \pm 1.03 \times 10^3$ to $12.84 \pm 0.82 \times 10^3$ mm Hg/ml/min in the core within the first hour after MCA occlusion. TR then gradually decreased over the next five hours and was reduced significantly to $6.68 \pm 0.93 \times 10^3$ mm Hg/ml/min six hours after occlusion. In contrast, TR did not change significantly in the periphery over six hours after occlusion (Fig. 1b).

An increase in water content caused a significant change in TC and TR. When water content increased slightly to 10.8 ± 0.7 mg/g brain one hour after occlusion, TC decreased slightly and TR increased significantly. In contrast, when the increase in water content was 40 mg/g brain 6 hours after occlusion, TC increased markedly and TR decreased. Comparisons of TR and TC showed a reciprocal relationship between the two.

Conclusions

We conclude that, at the initial stage of cerebral ischemia, low hydraulic conductivity and low compliance of ischemic cortical tissue limit the amount of edema fluid that can accumulate and prevents rapid movement of that same fluid. Later, as the ischemic injury progresses, edema fluid accumulates in highly compliant brain parenchyma, then migrates through highly conductive tissue into CSF spaces, driven by the pressure gradient that develops between the edematous tissue and the CSF.

References

Hatashita S, Hoff JT (1986a) Cortical tissue pressure gradients in early ischemic brain edema. J Cereb Blood Flow Metab 6:1–7

Hatashita S, Hoff JT (1986b) Role of a hydrostatic pressure gradient in formation of early ischemic brain edema. J Cereb Blood Flow Metab 6:546–552

Hatashita S, Hoff JT (1987) The effect of craniectomy on the biomechanics of normal brain. J Neurosurg 67:573–578

Hatashita S, Hoff JT, Salamat SM (1988) Ischemic brain edema and the osmotic gradient between blood and brain. J Cereb Blood Flow Metab (in press)

Marmarou A, Shapiro K, Poll W, Shulman K (1976) Studies of kinetics of fluid movements within brain tissue. In: Beks JWF, Bosch DH, Brock M (eds) Intracranial pressure III. Springer, Berlin Heidelberg New York, pp 1–4

After control measurements, the balloon was inflated in 0.5 ml increments (0.07 ml/s) at 15 min intervals during which all measurements were repeated. End-point of balloon expansion ($\simeq 5.5$ ml) was the onset of a flat EEG and arrest of lCBF over the compressed hemisphere, which was held constant for 15 min. Dogs that developed a distorted brain elastic response were excluded from this study, as this finding indicated major brain herniation (Walsh 1986). Thereafter the balloon was deflated (1 min) and the dogs were randomized into four equal groups: I was hyperventilated (room air and O_2) to a $PaCO_2 = 28 \pm 1$ mm Hg; II received furosemide (2.4 mg/kg) and nembutal (10 mg/kg) q8h; III received 20% Mannitol (1.4 gm/kg) i.v. bolus plus furosemide (0.5 mg/kg); IV received SOD (extra-pure) in i.v. dose of 15 mg (3500 units/mg) q15 min $\times$ 3 hours, beginning immediately after decompression. Evans blue (2%, 2 ml/kg) was given i.v. in the first 30 min of decompression. Measurements of lCBF and brain elastic parameters were repeated every 15 min for 240 min after decompression.

The animals were then ventilated overnight, sedated with fentanyl (2 mcg/kg/hr), and monitored. At 24 hrs the survivors were restudied and then euthanized (barbiturate). The brain was quickly removed, immersed in iced kerosene and examined for E.B. extravasation and intraparenchymal hemorrhages. Next, the brain was sectioned and samples (2 mm^3) were suspended in a kerosene-bromobenzene previously prepared column for specific gravity determination. Brain water content was calculated and expressed as percent water (Marmarou 1982).

Statistical significance among groups at each observation period was tested by the analysis of variance. A comparison of the means was performed with Tukey's Kramer test with level of significance at $p < 0.05$.

Results

The major physiological data are summarized in Figure 1. The changes in ICP were statistically not significant, even though ICP was the lowest (19.2 ± 6.2 mm Hg) in Group IV and the highest in Group I (40 ± 3.2 mm Hg) at 3 hours of decompression.

CPP tended to be higher in Group IV, but was statistically significant only at 60 min of reperfusion.

lCBF (decompressed hemisphere) was significantly higher ($p < 0.05$) in Group IV than in the other groups at 60 and 240 min of decompression. Beyond 240 min the data were skewed due to differences in survival rate (Table 1).

Recovery in G_0 paralleled lCBF recovery in all four groups (not shown). Recovery in $\bar{G}_0$ was significantly higher ($p < 0.05$) in Group IV at each observation period with 100% recovery at 3 hrs, and decreasing to 67% at 24 hrs. In Group I $\bar{G}_0$ fell to zero (loss in $\bar{G}_0$) after an initial 124% recovery (15 min). This suggested considerable edema (Schettini 1986). Group II followed an identical pattern, but with delay (240 min).

Table 1 summarizes the post-mortem findings and brain water content. In Group IV intraparenchymal perivascular hemorrhages and Evans blue extra-

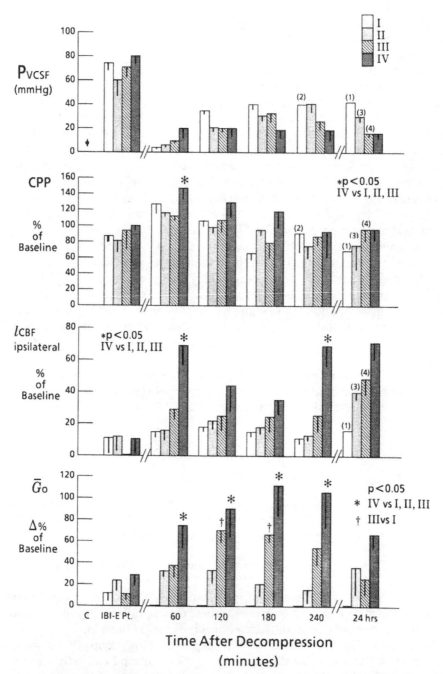

Fig. 1. Changes in ICP (*PVCSF*) in mm Hg (X±SD) and percentage (X±SE) of recovery in cerebral perfusion pressure (*CPP*), lCBF (decompressed hemisphere) and elastic curvature modulus (*G*) of the brain following decompression of an expanded extradural balloon in four groups of dogs (*n* = 5/group). *I* = hyperventilation; *II* = furosemide treatment; *III* = osmotic-loop diuresis; *IV* = superoxide dismutase (*SOD*) treatment. Statistical differences were assessed by analysis of variance, with the Tukey-Kramer procedure for comparison of the means. *C* = control; *IBI-EPt* = end-point of balloon expansion (5.5 ml) held for 15 min

Table 1. Influence of diuretics and superoxide dismutase (SOD) on 24 hour survival, intraparenchymal perivascular hemorrhages (PVH), dye extravasation and brain H_2O content following decompression of an expanded epidural balloon in the dog

Treatment group	24 h survival (%)	Evans blue extravasation (from lesion)			PVH[1]	Brain H_2O content (4% gm H_2O/gt)[2]				Con-tralat	Cere-bellum	Brain stem
		10 mm	15 mm	Con-tralat		Distance from lesion (mm)						
						0	5	10	15			
I Hyperventilation (n=5)	20	4+	3+	2+	3+	86.45 ±0.75	86.07 ±0.64	86.02 ±1.59	85.14 ±2.28	84.34 ±0.46	81.83 ±1.23	80.96 ±0.93
II Loop diuresis FSM (2.4 mg/kg) (n=5)	60	3+	3+	2+	2+	86.20 ±0.59	86.11 ±1.00	86.02 ±1.50	84.85 ±0.53	84.82 ±0.94	81.58 ±1.54	79.47 ±1.34
III Osmotic loop (Mann. 1.4 gm/kg) (FSM 0.5 mg/kg) (n=5)	80	3+	2+	+	2+	84.02 ±1.63	84.16 ±0.86	83.61 ±0.95	82.66 ±1.49	82.57 ±0.58	79.32 ±1.27ᶜ	78.80 ±1.57
IV SOD (60 mg/h × 3 h) (n=5)	100	2+	0	0	+	83.25 ±0.90ᵇ	82.84 ±0.81ᵃ	82.80 ±0.72ᵇ	82.45 ±0.56ᵇ	81.67 ±0.13ᵃ	79.81 ±0.70	79.97 ±1.67

1 = Intraparenchymal perivascular hemorrhages
2 = $X \pm SD$
Mann = 20% mannitol
FSM = Furosemide

Normal values (n=4): Cortical gray matter = 79.57±0.78
Cerebellum = 76.88±1.03
Brain stem = 75.77±0.54

Comparison by Tukey-Kramer procedure
$p < 0.05$
a = IV vs I, II, III
b = IV vs I, II
c = III vs I, II, IV

vasation was considerably less as compared to the other groups. Similarly, Group IV had significantly ($p < 0.05$) less edema in both the ipsi- and contralateral hemisphere (Table 1).

Discussion

Treatment with SOD resulted in higher recovery in cortical CBF and elastic curvature modulus, less cerebral edema and vascular damage, and 100% survival. Notwithstanding the limited number of dogs, this is strong evidence for an oxidative reaction initiated by the superoxide anion radical (O_2) during rapid decompression of an expanded extradural balloon.

The efficacy of SOD treatment implies that blood brain barrier (BBB) was disrupted with decompression and the O_2 radical was available extra-cellularly. Although oxidative reactions initiate as intracellular reactions O_2 radicals can escape, through anion channel, in the extracellular space (Kontos 1986); here, after dismutation (H_2O_2) it readily converts to the more reactive hydroxyl (OH·) radical, via the iron (reduced) catalyzed reaction. Free iron (low molecular weight complex) has been measured in the CSF (Halliwell 1984). The (OH·) radical is responsible for cerebral vascular injury associated with concussive brain lesion, and vasogenic edema following a freezing lesion (Kontos 1986, Chan 1985).

O_2 radicals may have originated from two sources: 1. Phospholipid degradation with accelerated metabolism of arachidonic acid (Aa) along the cyclooxygenase pathway with production of prostaglandins and O_2 in the presence of NADH (Kontos 1986); 2. the xanthine oxidase reaction occurring in cerebral microvessels, damaged by tethering during balloon expansion and decompression (Betz 1985, Busto 1984).

Three mechanisms during balloon expansion might have predisposed to oxidative reactions. First, vascular collapse of cortical vessels and as a result focal ischemia and reperfusion injury; secondly, direct trauma (tethering) to vascular endothelium of the microvessels around the expanding balloon; and thirdly, indirect trauma to vascular endothelium by hypertensive episodes (Kontos 1986).

Earlier studies have shown that the decompression following mild prolonged extradural brain compression alone causes cortical hypoperfusion, vasogenic edema, poor filling and extravasation of colloidal carbon from the cortical microvasculature of the decompressed area (Busto 1984, Yamaguchi 1976). The edema and the hypoperfusion were significantly reduced by glucocorticosteroids (Yamaguchi 1976), or α-tocopherol pretreatment (Busto 1984). Steroids might have acted as membrane stabilizers, and by stimulating the production of a lipoprotein, which is a phospholipase A_2 inhibitor, thereby preventing phospholipid degradation (Chan 1985). α-tocopherol is a natural anti-oxidant and a nonenzymatic scavenger of hydroxyl (OH·) radical. Focal ischemia (MCAO) is also associated with O_2 radical accumulation and cortical hypoperfusion during reperfusion, which could be markedly improved by SOD pretreatment (Davis 1987). These works and our data indicate that oxidative stress plays an important role in the cerebral vascular damage and edema in balloon decompression.

However, we do not imply that reperfusion injury is the sole mechanism for intracranial hypertension and cerebral edema following decompression of an expanded extradural balloon.

As the brain exhibits viscoelastic behavior, the expanding balloon causes brain tissue mass shift along the horizontal and/or vertical plane. When the vertical shift is predominant in our experimental model it can be recognized by the early onset of a distorted brain elastic response (Walsh 1986). For this reason we measured BER in order to avoid major brain herniation.

With major brain herniation the reperfusion injury is compounded by brain stem distortion and ischemia with or without hemorrhages (Thompson 1988); the resultant intracranial hypertension and cerebral edema may be unresponsive to dehydrating therapy and free SOD, even combined (unpublished data).

Acknowledgements. This research was supported by the VA Medical Research. We gratefully acknowledge Dr. H.A. Kontos' editorial assistance, and Mrs. Barbara Cook for typing the manuscript.

References

Betz AL (1985) Identification of hypoxanthine transport and xanthine oxidase activity in brain capillaries. J Neurochem 44:574–579

Busto R, Yoshida S, Ginsberg MD, Alonso O, Smith DW, Goldberg WJ (1984) Regional blood flow in compression-induced brain edema in rats: Effect of dietary Vitamin E. Ann Neurol 15:441–448

Chan PH, Longar S, Fishman A (1985) Oxygen free radicals. Potential edema mediators. In: Inaba Y, Klatzo I, Spatz M (eds) Brain edema. Springer, Berlin Heidelberg New York Tokyo, pp 317–323

Czernicki Z, Kozniewska E (1977) Disturbances in the blood brain barrier and cerebral blood flow after rapid brain decompression in the cat. Acta Neurochir (Wien) 36:171–187

Davis RJ, Bulkley GB, Traystman RJ (1987) Role of oxygen free radicals in focal brain ischemia. Fed Proc 46:2816

Halliwell B, Gutteridge JM (1984) Oxygen toxicity, oxygen radicals, transition metals and disease. Biochem J 219:1–14

Kontos HA, Wei EP (1986) Superoxide production in experimental brain injury. J Neurosurg 64:803–807

Marmarou A, Tanaka K, Shulman K (1982) An improved gravimetric measure of cerebral edema. J Neurosurg 56:246–253

Schettini A, Walsh EK, Beck J, Salton RA (1986) Brain elastic behavior and CSF dynamics in cold induced edema. In: Miller JD, Teasdale GM, Rowan JO, Gailbraith SL, Mendelow AD (eds) Intracranial pressure VI. Springer, Berlin Heidelberg New York Tokyo, pp 68–73

Thompson RK, Saleman M (1988) Dynamic axial brain stem distortion as a mechanism in the production of brain stem hemorrhages: role of the carotid arteries. Neurosurgery 22:629–632

Walsh EK, Schettini A (1984) Calculation of brain elastic parameters in vivo. Am J Physiol 247:R693–R700

Walsh EK, Schettini A, Beck J, Salton RA (1986) Brain elastic behavior and CSF dynamics during progressive epidural balloon expansion. In: Miller JD, Teasdale GM, Rowan JO, Gailbraith SL, Mendelow AD (eds) Intracranial pressure VI. Springer, Berlin Heidelberg New York Tokyo, pp 62–67

Yamaguchi M, Shirakata S, Yamasaki S, Matsumoto S (1976) Ischemic brain edema and compression brain edema. Water content, blood-brain barrier and circulation. Stroke 7:77–83

Fatal Brain Edema After Total Cerebral Ischemia in Man

H. Nihei[1], A. Tamura[2] and K. Sano[2]

[1] Department of Neurological Surgery, University of Virginia, Charlottesville, Virginia 22908 (USA)
[2] Department of Neurosurgery, University of Teikyo, 2-11-1 Kaga, Itabashi-ku, Tokyo (Japan)

Cardiac arrest produces global and complete ischemia in all organs of the body. Recently, great developments in the cardiopulmonary resuscitation technique have increased the number of patients who resume their cardiopulmonary function, but most of them remain unconscious; these cases are called post-resuscitation encephalopathy. The brain has been considered to be the most vulnerable organ, unable to tolerate even 10 minutes of ischemia. Although recent experimental results show the surprising reversibility of brain damage resulting from 1 hour of complete ischemia, it is rare to find cases showing clinically favorably recovery after a long period of cardiac arrest.

Therefore, we retrospectively reviewed our DOA (dead on arrival, patients who presented with cardiac arrest on admission) cases and analyzed what occurred in post-resuscitation encephalopathy.

Summary of Cases. Fifteen cases were chosen from 75 DOA cases occurring in the past 15 months, eliminating trauma, central nervous system disease, etc.

Five cases were resuscitated once, but died within 3 days due to respiratory or circulatory problems. Three cases were resuscitated successfully and recovered consciousness within 3 days. Another 3 cases died later from various complications.

The last 4 cases showed stable cardiopulmonary condition after resuscitation, but severe brain edema occurred later. Of these, 1 case which underwent bifrontal decompressive craniectomy remained in a persistent vegetative state and the remaining 3 cases died from cerebral herniation.

CT Scan. CT scans were performed on 9 cases and brain edema was observed in 4 of these cases (Fig. 1). Brain edema was not present on the day of admission, but it did appear during the following days. Cases with favorable outcome did not show any abnormalities on the CT scan.

ICP (Intracranial Pressure). ICP was monitored by ventricular catheter in 5 cases. Four cases showed increased ICP; 3 of these died, while one case received a decompressive craniectomy and survived in a persistent vegetative state. Another case with excellent recovery remained within the normal ICP range.

Other Findings. After resuscitation, spontaneous respiration and bilateral pupillary light reflex were observed in 13 of these cases. EEG and ABR (auditory

Eds.: J. T. Hoff and A. L. Betz
© Springer-Verlag Berlin Heidelberg 1989

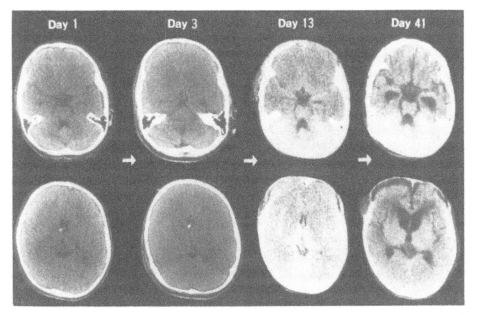

Fig. 1. Sequential CT scans of a 3-year-old girl whose heart arrested due to asphyxia. Decreased density of cerebral parenchyma and remarkable narrowing of lateral ventricles and cerebral cisterns were noted on day 3. This patient survived after bifrontal decompressive craniectomy but showed diffuse cerebral atrophy in the chronic stage

brainstem response) were examined in some cases, and it was confirmed that the brain was active electrophysiologically in the acute phase, even in the cases which later showed severe fatal brain edema.

Discussion. The reversibility of central nervous system damage following the ischemic insult still remains controversial. Contrary to the classical idea that the brain is so fragile that it is irreversibly damaged by less than 10 minutes of complete ischemia, recent experimental results show the surprising tolerance of neuronal function (Hossman and Kleihues 1973). Those experiments only reported the cerebral electrophysiological reversibility in the acute phase; there is no mention of what happens in the subacute or chronic stage of post-resuscitation encephalopathy.

We herein present fatal brain edema in the subacute stage after resuscitation. Brain edema occurred even though the findings of the CT scans were normal, activity in the EEG and ABR were noted, and spontaneous breathing and prompt pupillary light reflexes were observed. From these results, it is concluded that the functional reversibility after resuscitation does not always mean good outcome. We have no data to speculate on what such severe brain edema in the subacute phase depends, i.e., the neuron itself or the cerebral vessels. In other words, is it cytotoxic or vasogenic? In either case, there is a good possibility of saving these patients once the cerebral function is recovered after resuscitation. More extensive study should be done not only on cardiopulmonary resuscitation but also on cerebral resuscitation.

Conclusion

Fatal brain edema was observed in the subacute stage after cardiopulmonary resuscitation even after confirming normal brain CT scans, activity in EEG and ABR, prompt pupillary light reflex, and spontaneous breathing.

Reference

Hossmann KA, Kleihues P (1973) Reversibility of ischemic brain damage. Arch Neurol 29:375–384

Effect of Mannitol on Ischemic Brain Edema

A. Tamura, T. Kamiura, H. Kanemitsu, H. Nihei, N. Tomukai, and K. Sano

Department of Neurosurgery, Teikyo University School of Medicine, 2-11-1 Kaga, Itabashi-ku, Tokyo (Japan)

Introduction

Mannitol, an osmotic diuretic, is generally used in patients with brain edema for the purpose of reducing raised intracranial pressure (ICP) (Millson et al. 1981; McGraw et al. 1978; Muizelaar et al. 1984; Wise and Chater 1962). The remarkable and prompt effect of mannitol against raised ICP is widely recognized. However, its mode of action is still uncertain. Although experimental and clinical studies have shown that mannitol reduces blood viscosity and also increased cerebral blood flow (Kassel et al. 1981; Muizelaar et al. 1983), the effect of mannitol against brain edema itself, such as tissue water content, has been shown in several papers (Beks and ter Weeme 1967; Harbaugh et al. 1979; Nath and Galbraith 1986; Pappius and Dayes 1965, Takagi et al. 1984). In particular, there are few reports on its effect against edema caused by ischemia. The purpose of this study was to evaluate the effect of mannitol on ischemic brain edema following middle cerebral artery (MCA) occlusion in the rat.

Methods

Animal Preparation. Adult male Sprague-Dawley rats were anesthetized by halothane inhalation and a small polyethylene tube was introduced into the femoral vein. This catheter was connected to an infusion swivel device (Instech Co.). Using this system, rats could freely move and take food and water. Saline was continuously infused at a rate of 0.008 ml/min. The day after the catheterization, rats were anesthetized with halothane and the left MCA was permanently occluded via trans-retro-orbital approach (Tamura et al. 1981).

Measurement of Hemispheric Water Content. Six hours, 24 hours, and 72 hours after MCA occlusion, animals were decapitated and the brains were quickly removed. The wet weight of each hemisphere was measured on a chemical balance. After drying the brain in an oven at 110°C for five days, dry weight was measured and water content calculated. Mannitol was continuously infused through an intravenous catheter at a rate of 7.3 g/kg/hr for 2 hours. Thirty minutes after the end of mannitol infusion, rats were decapitated, then water content was measured. In the control group, saline injection was continued at a rate of 0.008 ml/min.

Intracranial Pressure VII 987
Eds.: J. T. Hoff and A. L. Betz
© Springer-Verlag Berlin Heidelberg 1989

Time sequential changes of water content following the mannitol treatment were evaluated 24 hours after MCA occlusion. The time intervals between the end of mannitol infusion and decapitation were changed. Animals were sacrificed at 30 minutes, 2 hours, 4 hours, and 6 hours after the two-hour mannitol infusion. The same dosage of mannitol was used.

Measurement of Regional Water Content. Regional water content was measured in the specimens obtained from six areas 24 hours after MCA occlusion. Thirty minutes after the same mannitol treatment, animals were decapitated and brains were cut into three coronal slices. Small specimens were taken from caudate nucleus, anterior part of cortex, and posterior part of cortex in each hemisphere. Water content of each sample was measured using a drying weighing method.

Results

In control animals, the values of water content of the MCA occlusion side 6 hours, 24 hours, and 72 hours after MCA occlusion were $80.84 \pm 0.28\%$ (mean $\pm$ sem), 82.49 ± 0.20, and 83.08 ± -0.40, respectively. In the treated group, they were 79.30 ± 0.28, 80.98 ± 0.20, and 81.47 ± 0.26 respectively. Therefore, the mannitol treatment significantly decreased the brain water content in each period ($p < 0.01$). Mannitol significantly decreased water content in the opposite side as well ($p < 0.01$). The values of water content of the contralateral hemisphere 6 hours, 24 hours, and 72 hours after MCA occlusion were 78.99 ± 1.04, 79.18 ± 0.08, and 79.40 ± 0.09, respectively in the control group. In the mannitol group, they were 77.97 ± 0.20, 77.96 ± 0.10, and 77.87 ± 0.17, respectively.

When the time interval between the end of infusion and the decapitation was changed, the mannitol treatment induced a significant reduction in water content

Table 1. Water contents 24 hours after left MCA occlusion in rats. Mannitol was continuously infused at a rate of 7.3 g/kg/hr for 2 hours. The time intervals between the end of mannitol infusion and the decapitation were changed. Each value in the mannitol treated group was compared with that of the saline control group. All values are indicated as mean $\pm$ SEM

Hemispheric water content (%) 24 hrs after MCA occlusion

Time interval after	Mannitol treated group	
	Ipsilateral (left)	Contralateral (right)
Mannitol infusion		
30 min ($n = 10$)	80.98 ± 0.19 ***	79.91 ± 0.11 ***
2 hrs ($n = 10$)	81.55 ± 0.20 **	77.96 ± 0.10 ***
4 hrs ($n = 8$)	81.43 ± 0.33 *	78.25 ± 0.18 ***
6 hrs ($n = 8$)	81.78 ± 0.30 +	78.43 ± 0.17 ***
Control group ($n = 13$)	82.49 ± 0.20	79.18 ± 0.08

+ $p < 0.1$, * $p < 0.05$, ** $p < 0.01$, *** $p < 0.001$. (Mean $\pm$ SEM).

988

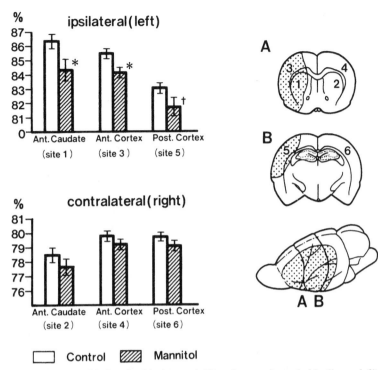

Fig. 1. Regional water content of ischemic side (*upper left*) and contralateral side (*lower left*) 24 hours after MCA occlusion. The regions are shown in coronal sections of rat brain (*right*). Areas of infarct are shown in *dotted areas*. All values are indicated as mean ± SEM. $^+p < 0.1$, $^*p < 0.05$

of the ischemic hemisphere until 4 hours after the treatment (Table 1). Six hours after infusion, a tendency of decreased water content was seen. In the opposite side, significant effects were observed in each period.

Figure 1 shows the effect of mannitol against regional water content in each area. Significant decreases in water content were observed in the ischemic core (ipsilateral caudate) and also in the peripheral zone (anterior part of cortex).

Discussion

It is a well known fact that mannitol possesses a remarkable effect of ICP reduction in clinical cases with brain edema. The most widely accepted mode of action has been considered to be reduction of brain edema by the creation of an osmotic gradient. There are many reports on its effects of increasing CBF, decreasing blood viscosity and improvement of microcirculation (Kassel et al. 1981; Muizelaar et al. 1984; Muizelaar et al. 1983). However, only a few studies have been done to evaluate the effect of hypertonic agents on brain edema itself. Pappius et al. (1965) reported using a cold injury model that hypertonic urea may reduce

ICP by extracting water by an osmotic gradient across the intact blood brain barrier in non-edematous brain. Similar results were obtained by other authors (Harbaugh et al. 1979; Wise and Chater 1962). Recently, Takagi et al. (1984), suggested in a cat infusion edema model, that mannitol may reduce by reducing cerebrospinal fluid volume. On the other hand, Beks and ter Weeme (1967), documented a significant reduction in the water content of white matter in the cold injured brain after administration of hypertonic agents. A recent clinical study in severe head injury has shown that mannitol increases the white matter specific gravity and probably does so by reducing brain water (Nath and Galbraith 1986). Thus, the mode of action of hypertonic agents on brain edema is still controversial. Information pertaining to the mechanisms of mannitol effect on ischemic edema is not available. In the present study, which used focal cerebral ischemia model in rats by occluding unilateral MCA, it has been clearly demonstrated that mannitol extracts water not only from the non-ischemic area but also from the core and periphery of the ischemic area.

The dosage of mannitol which we used in this study might be regarded as very high compared with other experimental studies or clinical use. However, dosage of drugs should be calculated in terms of surface area not body weight, particularly in the usage of blood volume expending agents. In fact, the clinical dosage in infancy and childhood is commonly calculated per surface area. This should be applied for experimental studies. The rate of 7.3 g/kg of mannitol, which we used in this study, is converted into 54.0 g/m^2 and this dosage corresponds to 1.4 g/kg in an average human adult, who is 170 cm in height and 66 kg in weight. Therefore, the dosage of mannitol in our study is not high and can be considered to be practical in clinical cases.

References

Beks JWF, ter Weeme CA (1967) The influence of urea and mannitol on increased intraventricular pressure in cold-induced cerebral edema. Acta Neurochir (Wien) 16:97–107

Harbaugh RD, James HE, Marshall LF, Shapiro HM, Laurin R (1979) Acute therapeutic modalities for experimental vasogenic edema. Neurosurgery 5:656–665

Kassel NF, Baumann KW, Hitchon PW, Gerk MK, Hill TR, Sokoll MD (1981) Influence of a continuous high dose infusion of mannitol on cerebral blood flow in normal dogs. Neurosurgery 9:283–286

McGraw CP, Alexander E Jr, Howard G (1978) Effect of dose and schedule on the response of intracranial pressure to mannitol. Surg Neurol 10:127–130

Millson Ch, James HE, Shapiro HM, Laurin R (1981) Intracranial hypertension and brain oedema in albino rabbits. Part two: Effects of acute therapy with diuretics. Acta Neurochir (Wien) 56:167–181

Muizelaar JP, Wei EP, Kontos HA, Becker DP (1983) Mannitol causes compensatory cerebral vasoconstriction and vasodilation in response to blood viscosity changes. J Neurosurg 59:822–828

Muizelaar JP, Lutz HA III, Becker DP (1984) Effect of mannitol on ICP and CBF and correlation with pressure autoregulation in severely head-injured patients. J Neurosurg 61:700–706

Nath F, Galbraith S (1986) The effect of mannitol on cerebral white matter water content. J Neurosurg 65:41–43

Pappius HM, Dayes LA (1965) Hypertonic urea. Arch Neurol 13:395–402

Takagi H, Saitoh T, Kitahara T, Ohwada T, Yada K (1984) The mechanism of ICP reducing effect of mannitol. Brain Nerve (Tokyo) 36:1095–1102

Tamura A, Graham DI, McCulloch J, Teasdale GM (1981) Focal cerebral ischemia in the rat. 1. Description of technique and early neuropathological consequences following middle cerebral artery occlusion. J Cereb Blood Flow Metab 1:53–60

Wise BL, Chater N (1962) The value of hypertonic mannitol solution in decreasing brain mass and lowering cerebrospinal-fluid pressure. J Neurosurg 19:1038–1043

Colloid Volume Expansion and Brain Edema

B. Tranmer [1], R. Iacobacci [2], and G. Kindt [2]

[1] Department of Clinical Neurosciences, University of Calgary, Calgary, Alberta T2N 2T9 (Canada)
[2] Division of Neurosurgery University of Colorado, Denver, Colorado (USA)

Introduction

Fluid management in the neurosurgery patient with brain edema can be quite difficult because of the risk of aggravating the edema and producing intracranial pressure (ICP) problems. In such situations, we have found colloid agents to be safer than crystalloid solutions. We report two experiments in which we studied fluid administration in animals with vasogenic brain edema. In Experiment 1, the effects of crystalloid and colloidal volume expansion on ICP and computerized EEG data are studied, and in Experiment 2, the effect of colloid volume expansion on local cerebral blood flow (CBF) and computerized EEG data are reported.

Materials and Methods

Experiment 1

Twenty adult mongrel dogs were anaesthetised with fentanyl, intubated and ventilated with 100% oxygen. Hemodynamic monitoring catheters were put in place and an 18 gauge spinal needle was passed stereotaxically through a burr hole into the left lateral ventricle. Twelve EEG electrodes were then embedded into the skull according to a standard 12 lead pediatric montage for collection of computerized EEG data. The EEG data was analysed as a power ratio index (PRI) which has been defined as the ratio of (delta + theta) power to the (alpha + beta) power (Tranmer et al. 1988). A liquid nitrogen cold lesion was then performed according to the technique described by Clasen (Clasen et al. 1953). Following the cold lesion, the animals were carefully monitored for six hours and then placed into one of four treatment groups; (1) control – maintenance fluid; (2) D5W – 30 cc/kg/hr; (3) 0.9% – NaCl 30 cc/kg/hr; (4) 6% hetastarch – 30 cc/kg/hr. These treatments were continued for two hours and then the animals were sacrificed and the brains were cut in coronal sections for examination.

Experiment 2

Adult mongrel dogs were anaesthetized with pentobarbital and a standard cold lesion was made on the parietal lobe as described in Experiment 1. The animals

Eds.: J. T. Hoff and A. L. Betz

were allowed to recover for 14 hours and then were reanaesthetized, intubated and ventilated on 100% oxygen. The cranium over the entire hemisphere on the side of the cold lesion was removed and local CBF electrodes and EEG electrodes were placed in the cortex surrounding the cold lesion. Local CBF measurements were performed by the hydrogen clearance technique, described previously by Willis (Willis et al. 1974). The animals were randomly placed into one of two treatment groups; (1) control group – maintenance fluid; or, (2) 6% hetastarch – 30 cc/kg for 2 hr.

Results (Table 1)

Experiment 1

In the control group, ICP and PRI values did not change significantly during the treatment. In the D5W gorup, ICP increased 141% ($p<0.001$) but the PRI value did not change. In the normal saline group, ICP increased 90% ($p<0.001$) and the PRI value increased 15% ($p<0.001$). In the 6% hetastarch group, ICP did not change and the PRI value showed improvement in the neuroelectric status as demonstrated by a significant decrease in the PRI value.

Experiment 2

In the control group, local CBF and the PRI value did not change significantly during the 2 hr treatment. In the 6% hetastarch group, local CBF increased 50%

Table 1

Experiment 1: Effect of hetastarch, 0.9% NaCl and D5W on ICP & power ratio index

	Control (25 cc/hr NaCl)	D5W (30 cc/kg/hr)	NaCl (30 cc/kg/hr)	Hetastarch (30 cc/kg/hr)
Intracranial pressure (mm Hg)				
Baseline	5±3	5±1	6±3	3±2
Post lesion	20±9*	17±5*	23±13*	17±4*
Post infusion	23±12	41±8*	44±19*	19±1
Power ratio index				
Pre-infusion	92±19	98±23	89±12	98±19
Post-infusion	86±32	104±41	102±20*	82±17*

Experiment 2: Effect of hetastarch on local CBF and power ratio index

	LCBF (cc/100 gm/min)	Power ratio index
Pre-infusion	30±15	109±30
Post-infusion	45±29*	87±28*

* $p<0.001$.

$(p<0.001)$ during the 2 hr hetastarch infusion. The PRI value decreased from 109 ± 30 to 87 ± 28 $(p<0.001)$ representing improvement in the neuroelectric status of the edematous hemisphere.

Discussion

These data suggest that colloid agents may be given safely to patients with cerebral edema and that crystalloid infusions should be held to a minimum in patients suspected of having intracranial pathology. These data also suggest that edematous brain tissue may have decreased perfusion levels and that augmentation of local CBF by colloidal volume expansion may be beneficial as demonstrated in these experiments by an improvement in the neuroelectric status of the brain.

References

Clasen RA, Brown DVL, Leavitt S et al. (1953) The production by liquid nitrogen of acute closed cerebral lesions. Surg Gynecol Obstet 96:603–616

Tranmer BI, Gross CE, Adey GR, Keller TS, Nagata K, Iacobacci RL (1988) Colloidal volume expansion during acute cerebral ischemia; Assessed by local CBF and computerized power ratio index. Neurol Res (in press)

Willis JA, Doyle TF, Ramirez A, Kobrine AI, Martins AN (1974) A practical circuit for hydrogen clearance in blood flow measurement. TN 74-2. Washington, DC. Armed Forces Radiation Research Institute

The Effect of IV Fluids on Cerebral Edema After Experimental Blunt Head Trauma

Y. Shapira, M. Muggia-Sullam, H.R. Freund, and S. Cotev

ICU, Department of Anesthesia, and Department of Surgery, Hebrew University-Hadassah Medical School, Jerusalem (Israel)

It is generally taught that parenteral fluid administration in patients with acute severe head injury (SHI) should be modest, or even restricted, so as to limit cerebral edema formation. This recommendation is based on the assumption that in regions of dysrupted blood-brain-barrier function, fluid efflux is determined primarily by the hydrostatic pressure gradient. Clinical or experimental evidence to support this recommendation is lacking.

At the same time, however, it had been shown that patients after SHI have prolonged intolerance to enteral feeding (Norton et al. 1988), while energy requirements are increased (Clifton et al. 1984). In fact, early management with total parenteral nutrition (TPN) seems to improve outcome after SHI (Young et al. 1987).

In this study we investigated the effect of large volumes of parenteral fluids, including TPN, on cerebral edema formation in our previously described model of experimental SHI in rats (Shapira et al. 1988).

Materials and Methods

Fifty five adult male Sabra rats (weighing 328 ± 73 g S.D.), which survived the acute effect of SHI induced by a weight-drop device (Shapira et al. 1988) over the exposed skull covering the left hemisphere, comprised the study population. The rats were randomly divided into 5 groups, as follows:

Group T ($n=8$) was traumatized but did not receive any further treatment.
Group C ($n=10$) was traumatized and a jugular venous cannula introduced (22 gauge silicone tubing). No parenteral fluids were administered.
Group G ($n=11$) was similarly treated, and a hydrolyzed gelatin/electrolyte (Haemaccel) solution given parenterally.
Group GNS ($n=12$) was treated as group G, but the IV fluid was 5% glucose/ 1/2 N saline.
Group TPN ($n=14$) was treated as group G, but the IV fluid was TPN, containing 25% glucose, 4.25% amino acids.

The latter 3 groups received the IV fluids by continuous infusion during 18 h post-SHI, at a rate of 10 ml/kg/h. All the rats were allowed to move freely in metabolic cages, and had free access to food and H_2O. A 4-point neurological severity score (NSS) was determined just prior to sacrifice of the rats at 18 h post-SHI. All rats were decapitated 18 h after trauma, their brains immediately (42 ± 5 sec) removed, and tissue samples (< 0.5 g) from the peritraumatized and corresponding contralateral regions obtained for specific gravity (SG) determination, using linear gradient columns (Marmarou et al. 1982).

Statistical methods included the two-way analysis of variance for each dependent variable, and Spearman's rank correlation for NSS and SG.

Results

The rats that received parenteral fluids did not consume H_2O or food until sacrificed, while the other rats consumed only minimal amounts (3–4 ml/18 h) of H_2O. Urinary output was 5.2 ± 2.7, 3.8 ± 1.8, 48.3 ± 13.5, 48.0 ± 19.0 and 36.7 ± 7.2 ml/18 h, respectively, for groups T, C, G, GNS and TPN.

Figure 1 demonstrates the SG of tissue samples from both hemispheres of all groups. There was a significant negative ($p = 0.697$) correlation between NSS and SG of the left hemisphere at 18 h post-SHI, indicating an association between the extent of left hemispheric edema and neurological dysfunction.

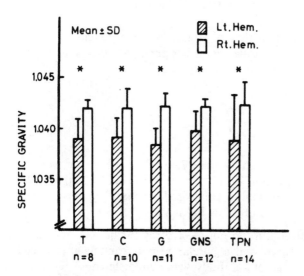

Fig. 1. Mean $\pm$ SD specific gravity (*SG;* specific gravity) of tissue samples from each hemisphere of all rats. In each group, SG of the left lobe was significantly ($p < 0.05$) less than that of the corresponding right hemisphere. There were no significant differences in SG of either lobe, between groups

Discussion

Our results suggest that brain edema and neurological dysfunction after experimental SHI are not aggravated by administration of even large volumes of parenteral fluids. Furthermore, hyperosmotic TPN may be given early to satisfy raised energy requirements after SHI. These findings are consistent with recent clinical data showing no effect on TPN on ICP after SHI (Young et al. 1987).

References

Clifton GL et al. (1984) The metabolic response to severe head injury. J Neurosurg 60:687–696

Marmarou A et al. (1982) An improved gravimetric measure of cerebral edema. J Neurosurg 56:246–253

Norton JA et al. (1988) Intolerance to enteral feeding in the brain-injured patient. J Neurosurg 68:62–66

Shapira Y et al. (1988) Experimental closed head injury in rats: mechanical, pathophysiologic, and neurologic properties. Crit Care Med 16:258–265

Young B et al. (1987) Effect of total parenteral nutrition upon intracranial pressure in severe head injury. J Neurosurg 67:76–80

The Effects of Nonsteroid Anti-Inflammatory Agent BW755C on Traumatic and Peritumoral Brain Edema

Y. Ikeda, K.L. Brelsford, and D.M. Long

Department of Neurological Surgery, The Johns Hopkins University, School of Medicine, 600 N. Wolfe St., Baltimore, Maryland 21 205 (USA)

Introduction

Recently the role of leukotrienes in the development of brain edema has come under increasing surveillance. BW755C (3-amino-1-[m(trifluoromethyl)phenyl]-2-pyrazoline) is a nonsteroid anti-inflammatory agent. BW755C inhibits the synthesis of both prostaglandins and leukotrienes by dual inhibition of cyclooxygenase and lipoxygenase pathways of arachidonic acid metabolism and is therefore considered to be a superior anti-inflammatory compound over the conventional cyclooxygenase inhibitors (Higgs et al. 1984). BW755C is also known to inhibit lipoxygenase predominantly over cyclooxygenase. In this study we evaluated the effect of BW755C on cold-induced edema and peritumoral edema, in an attempt to determine if leukotrienes could play a role in the development of vasogenic brain edema.

Materials and Methods

Cold-induced edema study: Vasogenic brain edema was produced in 18 cats by a standardized cortical freezing lesion. Animals were separated into 2 groups. Group-1: cold induced edema with sacrifice at 6 and 24 hr after the lesion. Group-2: this group was pretreated with BW755C (20 mg/kg) intraperitoneally 1 hr prior to the lesion and was sacrificed at 6 and 24 hr after the lesion.

Peritumoral edema study: Experimental brain tumor was produced by the injection of a 25 μl suspension of 3×10^5 viable VX2 carcinoma cells into the rabbit's brain. 17 rabbits were separated into 3 groups. Group-1: tumor free rabbits, Group-2: BW755C untreated tumor-bearing rabbits, Group-3: BW755C treated tumor-bearing rabbits; this group was treated with BW755C (10 mg/kg/day) intraperitoneally for 5 consecutive days from the 8th day following tumor transplantation and was sacrificed on the 13th day. Brain water contents were measured by the specific gravity (SG) method. BW755C was a gift of Wellcome Research Lab., Kent, England.

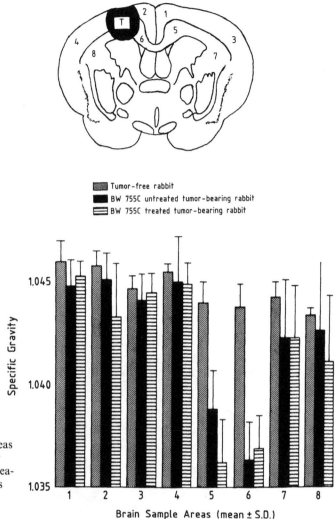

Fig. 1. Brain sample areas used for specific gravity (*SG;* specific gravity) measurement and SG values

Results

BW755C did not reduce the brain's water content of the injured side at 6 and 24 hr following cold injury. The peritumoral white matter of the affected hemisphere (area 6) and the adjacent white matter of the contralateral hemisphere (area 5) in BW755C untreated tumor-bearing rabbits showed no significant improvement of SG values in the peritumoral white matter of the affected hemisphere and the adjacent white matter of the contralateral hemisphere. BW755C had no effect on the other areas (Fig. 1).

Discussion

Leukotrienes, metabolites of arachidonic acid, are biologically active compounds and are known to increase vascular permeability, which may cause brain edema. Black et al. (1985) reported increased levels of leukotrienes in vasogenic brain edema. Dempsey et al. (1987) also proposed that leukotrienes mediate ischemic brain edema. This preliminary study indicates that BW755C had no beneficial effect on both types of brain edema, suggesting that leukotrienes do not contribute importantly to the development of brain edema in these two animal models. Leukotriene involvement can't be completely ruled out, because further studies are required for the hydrophilic properties of BW755C and species difference with respect to brain response and formation of leukotrienes (Ueno et al. 1981; Unterberg et al. 1987).

References

Black KL, Hoff JT (1985) Leukotrienes increase blood-brain barrier permeability following intraparenchymal injections in rats. Ann Neurol 18:349–351

Dempsey RJ et al. (1987) Moderate hypothermia reduces postischemic edema development and leukotriene production. Neurosurgery 21:177–181

Higgs GA et al. (1984) Inhibition of tissue damage by the arachidonate lipoxygenase inhibitor BW755C. Proc Natl Acad Sci USA 81:2890–2892

Ueno A et al. (1981) Species difference in increased vascular permeability by synthetic leukotriene C4 and D4. Prostaglandins 21:637–648

Unterberg A et al. (1987) Permeability and vasomotor response of cerebral vessels during exposure to arachidonic acid. Acta Neuropathol (Berl) 73:209–219

Effects of Recombinant Lipocortin on Brain Edema of Cytotoxic and Vasogenic Type

T. Mima [1], T. Shigeno [2], and K. Takakura [1]

[1] Department of Neurosurgery, University of Tokyo (Japan)
[2] Department of Neurosurgery, Saitama Medical Center, Tokyo (Japan)

Liberation of PUFA, in particular arachidonic acid, has been thought to be a major mediator of brain damage and edema formation. However, controversies still exist whether or not blockage of the liberation of arachidonic acid as well as inhibition of the subsequent cascade would ameliorate such harmful events in the CNS. As to the effect of glucocorticoids, evidence accumulates that they exert their action via *de novo* synthesis of protein designated as Lipocortin which, in turn, inhibits phospholipase A_2. An important aspect is that it requires several hours for the induction of this protein. Until we obtain Lipocortin, a steroid-induced anti-inflammatory protein, we have been studying the effect of high-dose dexamethasone, given 3 hours before ischemia, on edema formation, provided that Lipocortin could be induced in the CNS or incorporated into the brain from other organs. But the result is currently negative as far as early cytotoxic edema is concerned. Now, in this study, recombinant Lipocortin is in our hand so that we have done similar experiments by giving Lipocortin directly into the ischemic focus. We have further extended the use of Lipocortin in vasogenic brain edema after cold injury, because there are cellular reactions such as of leukocytes or macrophages where Lipocortin is supposed to be produced.

Material and Methods

Adult cats were anesthetized with halothane/N_2O/O_2 under controlled ventilation. Focal cerebral ischemia was produced by permanently occluding MCA. For direct intra-arterial perfusion within the ischemic area, we employed a technique of catheterization into the MCA distal to occlusion. Regional CBF was measured by the hydrogen clearance technique at six sites. After 4 hours of ischemia, the tissue specific gravity was determined and correlated with CBF values during ischemia. There were three groups of different treatments as follows: (1) control without any treatment ($n=9$), (2) control with initial BBB opening by perfusion of hypertonic mannitol ($n=4$), and (3) recombinant Lipocortin (10^{-7} M) given before and after ischemia into the ischemic focus ($n=4$) with prior opening of BBB by mannitol.

In rats, cold injury was given on the bilateral cortical surface via craniectomy for 1 min with cooled metal tip by liquid nitrogen. Twenty-four hours later, animals were sacrificed and the brain water content was measured in two ways in separate series of animals. One was by the microgravimetric technique where injury focus and the adjacent cortex were separately measured. In the other, brain water content was measured by drying-weighing in the whole cortical hemisphere. Animals were treated just before insult by intraventricular injection of either mock CSF alone or with Lipocortin.

Results

Mannitol perfusion had slight effect in increasing specific gravity, i.e., reducing ischemic edema formation. However, there was no beneficial effect of Lipocortin in either flow ranges of severe and moderate ischemia (Fig. 1).

Table 1.

	Core of cold injury	Periphery of cold injury
mock CSF	1.0251 ± 0.0014 ($n=8$)	1.0415 ± 0.0029 ($n=8$)
Lopocortin	1.0276 ± 0.0024 ($n=8$)	1.0434 ± 0.0014 ($n=8$)
	sig. $p < 0.05$	n.s.

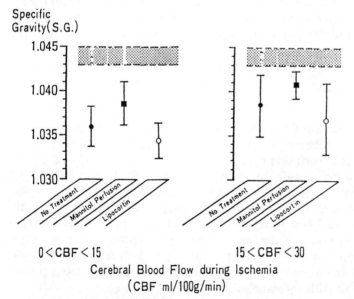

Fig. 1. Effects of Lipocortin perfused into the ischemic focus intra-arterially with transient BBB opening by mannitol. No effect can be seen in either severely ($0 < CBF < 15$ ml/100 g/min) or moderately ($15 < CBF < 30$) ischemic tissue

1002

Cold injury produced marked vasogenic edema as evidenced by Evans blue leakage. In the measurement of specific gravity, there was slight but significant amelioration of edema in the core lesion of injury after treatment of Lipocortin (Table 1). However, in the adjacent area, Lipocortin had no effect. By contrast when hemispheric water content was measured by drying-weighing, there was no effect of Lipocortin (data not shown).

Discussion

The innovative idea that glucocorticoids exert the action via *de novo* synthesis of protein designated as Lipocortin would have explained the previously reported ineffectiveness of glucocorticoids on ischemic brain edema. The reasons were: (1) not enough time is given for protein induction, (2) protein synthesis is disturbed in the ischemic tissue, (3) even though Lipocortin is produced outside the CNS such as macrophages, neutrophils, or renal cells, this protein cannot reach to the ischemic focus, because flow is interrupted and because BBB is still intact in the early ischemic stage. Our experiments so far conducted had purposes to solve these problems or questions. However, our previous studies under this idea did not lead us to success as far as glucocorticoid treatment was concerned. Further as shown in this study, it has to be concluded that even recombinant Lipocortin cannot affect ischemic edema formation.

The role of Lipocortin would be more suggested in vasogenic brain edema where cellular reactions such as with neutrophils and macrophages are involved. In the present study, however, the effect was limited within the lesion core which could only be detected by microgravimetric technique. Water content using whole brain did not detect such slight changes. Because edema progression in rats is limited mainly in the gray matter, use of large brains such as of cats should be done further. Tentatively, we may say that Lipocortin reduces vasogenic brain edema, but further investigations are required and currently on going in experimental brain tumor.

Anti-Edema Effect of Protease Inhibitors

M. Yamaguchi

School of Allied Medical Sciences, Kobe University, 7-10-2 Tomogaoka, Suma, Kobe 654-01 (Japan)

The activity of beta-glucuronidase (BGL), a lysosomal enzyme, increases in edematous brain (Bingham et al. 1971). Steroids are considered to be effective against the vasogenic type of brain edema. In this communication, I report that experimental brain edema is prevented by the administration of protease inhibitors (urinastatin or aprotinin) and that the increase in BGL activity of the edematous brain is also reduced by protease inhibitors.

Methods

Male Wistar rats of 250–350 g were used. Experimental brain edema was produced by the implantation of silver nitrate in the parietal region (Levine and Torrelio 1977). Normal saline, protease inhibitors, a free radical scavenger (AVS: N,N'-propylene bisnicotinamide), or steroid (betamethasone) were injected every 6 or 12 hr. Doses are shown in Table 1. The normal control group had neither insult nor injection. The water (Elliot and Jasper 1949), sodium (Na), and potassium (K) contents of the brain were estimated 24 hr after the implantation. Brain tissue was homogenized in ice-cold 0.25 M sucrose and used for the determination of free activity of BGL (Sigma Diagnostic Kit, # 325). Activity is expressed as μg of PP (phenolphthalein) liberated/mg of protein/hour. Protein measurements were performed according to the method of Lowry et al. (1951).

Results

The silver nitrate implantation produced an apparent blood-brain barrier damage, proved by Evans blue injection. The water content increased significantly in the right parietal region of the saline-injected group. This increase was reduced by the administration of drugs as shown in Table 1. Increased Na and decreased K were also observed in the edematous brain. Steroid administration appeared to prevent the Na increase. No definite effect was shown against K loss by any drugs. The free activity of BGL in the edematous brain increased significantly. This increase was prevented by the use of protease inhibitors, AVS, and steroid. However, urinastatin did not inhibit BGL in vitro (Table 2). When protease inhibitors

Intracranial Pressure VII
Eds.: J. T. Hoff and A. L. Betz
© Springer-Verlag Berlin Heidelberg 1989

Table 1. Water, electrolytes, beta-glucuronidase activity

Group	Side	Water content (% of wet wt.)	Na (mEq/wet wt.)	K (mEq/wet wt.)	beta-Glucuronidase (μg PP/mg/h)
Saline	R	82.52±1.26 (14)	41.4±7.3 (6)[b]	75.5±7.1 (6)[c]	0.428±0.096 (12)
(0.25 ml ×4)	L	80.00±0.80 (15)	30.2±4.2 (6)	104.9±5.0 (6)	0.146±0.071 (14)
Urinastatin	R	81.97±1.21 (9)*	30.8±5.1 (6)[+]	80.5±5.9 (6)[c]	0.145±0.046 (10)
(2,500 U ×4)	L	80.01±0.77 (9)	28.8±4.1 (6)	105.9±4.7 (6)	0.110±0.060 (10)
Urinastatin	R	80.96±0.69 (12)**	–	–	0.241±0.063 (6)
(10,000 U ×2)	L	79.36±0.50 (12)	–	–	0.185±0.095 (6)
AVS	R	80.59±0.67 (6)**	34.0±10.7 (6)[+]	83.8±9.6 (6)[c]	0.166±0.049 (12)
(100 mg/kg ×4)	L	78.41±0.46 (6)	23.5±5.9 (6)	113.0±4.7 (6)	0.167±0.059 (12)
Aprotinin	R	80.30±0.97 (6)**	40.2±3.7 (6)[c]	90.6±4.8 (6)[c]	0.216±0.075 (12)
(10,000 U/kg ×4)	L	78.47±0.41 (6)	26.2±3.5 (6)	113.4±2.1 (6)	0.157±0.036 (12)
Betamethasone	R	80.30±0.73 (4)**	25.6±5.4 (4)	87.4±4.8 (4)[+]	0.087±0.042 (8)
(5 mg/kg ×4)	L	79.23±0.39 (4)	25.9±4.8 (4)	107.4±4.2 (4)	0.055±0.020 (8)
Normal control		79.00±0.29 (8)	27.2±2.3 (4)	102.9±6.3 (4)	0.200±0.042 (10)

Statistical difference; [water] vs. R (edema) side of saline group: * not significant; ** $P < 0.01$; [Electrolyte] vs. Normal control: [+] not significant; [a] $p < 0.02$; [b] $p < 0.01$; [c] $p < 0.001$.

Table 2. Effect of Urinastatin (in vitro)

Addition	beta-Glucuronidase activity (µg PP/mg/h)
None	0.265±0.002 (3)
Urinastatin	
(0.1 Unit/ml)	0.270±0.013 (3)
(1 Unit/ml)	0.276±0.004 (3)
(10 Unit/ml)	0.275±0.011 (3)

Table 3. beta-Glucuronidase activity, without brain edema

Group	beta-Glucuronidase activity (µg PP/mg/h)	Significance vs. saline group
Saline (0.25 ml × 4)	0.080±0.016 (12)	–
Betamethasone (5 mg/kg × 4)	0.058±0.008 (8)	$P < 0.001$
Aprotinin (10,000 U/kg × 4)	0.092±0.024 (7)	n.s.
Urinastatin (10,000 U/kg × 4)	0.081±0.015 (8)	n.s.

n.s.: not significant

were given to the animals without brain edema, the activity of BGL was not changed while betamethasone significantly reduced the enzyme activity (Table 3).

Discussion

The anti-brain edema effect of aprotinin has been reported in several papers (Egami 1970; Czernicki 1979). Protease inhibitors may inhibit kinin-activating systems (Baethmann et al. 1980). Steroid significantly decreased BGL activity either in the normal or the edematous tissue, probably due to its membrane stabilizing action. Although protease inhibitors (urinastatin or aprotinin) prevented vasogenic brain edema formation, these substances did not directly inhibit BGL activity in vitro. With protease inhibitors there was no decrease of enzyme activity in normal tissue. Some proteolytic process, therefore, may exist before the lysosomal disruption stage of brain edema development. Studies with cathepsin and neutral protease will be important in the future.

Summary

When experimental brain edema was produced by silver nitrate implantation, the contents of water and sodium and the activity of beta-glucuronidase (BGL) were increased in brain tissue. Steroid, AVS (a free radical scavenger) or protease inhibitor (urinastatin or aprotinin) administration prevented the edema formation and the increase of BGL activity.

1006

References

Baethmann A, Oettinger W, Rothenfusser W, Kempski O, Unterberg A, Geiger R (1980) Brain edema factors: current state with particular reference to plasma constituents and glutamate. In: Cerevos-Navarro J and Ferszt R (eds) Advances in neurology, vol 28: Brain edema. Raven Press, New York, pp 171–195

Bingham WG, Paul SE, Sastry KSS (1971) Effect of steroid on enzyme response to cold injury in rat brain. Neurology 21:111–121

Czernicki Z (1979) Treatment of experimental brain edema following sudden decompression, surgical wound, and cold lesion with vasoprotective drugs and proteinase inhibitor "Trasylol". Acta Neurochir (Wien) 50:311–326

Egami T (1970) The effect of proteolytic enzyme inhibitor on experimental brain swelling. Bull Yamaguchi Med School 17:207–238

Elliot KAC, Jasper H (1949) Measurement of experimentally induced brain swelling and shrinkage. Am J Physiol 157:122–129

Levine S, Torrelio M (1977) Cerebral inflammation and edema: a model for testing antiinflammatory drugs. Exp Neurol 56:361–369

Lowry OH, Rosebrough NJ, Farr AL, Landall RJ (1951) Protein measurement with the Folin phenol reagent. J Biol Chem 193:265–275

Thromboxane Inhibition Does Not Prevent Brain Edema After Head Trauma

Y. Shapira, G. Yadid, S. Cotev, and E. Shohami

ICU (Department of Anesthesia) and Department of Pharmacology, Hebrew University-Hadassah Medical School, Jerusalem (Israel)

Introduction

Acute tissue damage caused by ischemia or trauma initiates a sequence of events which might lead to a focal increase in microcirculatory resistance. Prostaglandins (PG), in particular thromboxane (TXA_2), may play a role in this process. The concept that the balance of TXA_2 and PGI_2 (prostacyclin) levels has a role in the maintenance of normal blood flow is relevant in view of some reports on the beneficial effects of PGI_2 under these circumstances. The relative excess of PGI_2 over TXA_2 was shown to be protective in ischemic and hypoxic insults to various organs including the brain (Hallenbeck and Furlow 1979; Masuda et al. 1986). However, therapeutic attempts to induce such excess in stroke and head injury is still controversial.

We have previously shown that closed head injury (CHI) in rats induces local cerebral edema and increased production of PGs (Shohami et al. 1987). The synthesis of all measured PGs, was blocked by indomethacin but there was no effect on either neurological status or water content of the contused hemisphere after CHI.

In the present study we evaluated the effect in rats of a selective, specific thromboxane synthetase inhibitor, OKY-046, given during the early post-CHI period, on the outcome of injury.

Materials and Methods

CHI was induced in male Sabra rats by a weight-drop device falling over the left hemisphere as described in detail (Shapira et al. 1988). Rats were divided into 4 groups: Groups 1 and 2 were sham operated (skull exposure), and groups 3 and 4 were traumatized. Groups 2 and 4 received two i.p. doses of OKY-046, 100 mg/kg (kindly donated by ONO Pharmaceutical Co., Japan), immediately and 8 h after either trauma or sham. One hour after trauma, and just before sacrifice at 24 h, a neurological severity score (NSS) was determined to define the neurological status of the rats following CHI. The rats were decapitated, and samples of about 20 mg from each hemisphere were placed on top of linear gradient columns for determination of specific gravity (SG) (Marmarou et al.

1982). Cortical slices from the injured, temporo-parietal zone were extracted in Tris-NaCl buffer, containing EDTA, at pH 7.0, as previously described, and assayed by RIA (Shohami et al. 1987).

Results and Discussion

Figure 1 shows that PGs increased in the left, injured hemisphere (gr 3). OKY-046 inhibited the basal (gr 2) levels of TXB_2 only, as expected from a selective inhibitor of thromboxane synthetase. However, the augmented production due to CHI, of PGE_2 and 6-keto-$PGF_{1\alpha}$ was also abolished following OKY-046 (gr 4).

As vascular tone is affected, among other factors, by the local ratio of TXA_2 to PGI_2 concentrations, we have summarized this ratio for the different experimental groups (Fig. 1). In sham rats (gr 2), OKY-046 reduced this ratio due to selective inhibition of TXB_2 synthesis. CHI induced a selective increase of 6-keto-$PGF_{1\alpha}$ at 24 h after impact (gr 3); thus, the ratio in the injured zone was much lower than that in the corresponding hemisphere of sham rats. A further decrease in this ratio was reached after OKY-046 treatment (gr 4) due to a decrease in TXB_2 levels.

As a result of the injury, edema (decrease in SG) developed in the left hemisphere of traumatized rats (i.e., 3 and 4). In sham rats (gr 1), SG of both hemi-

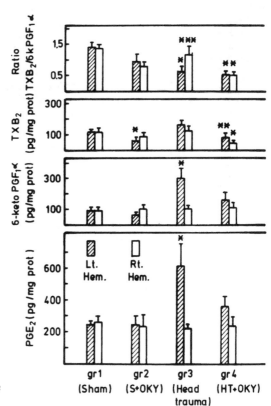

Fig. 1. Tissue levels of PGE_2, 6-keto-$PGF_{1\alpha}$ and TXB_2 and the TXB_2/6-keto-$PGF_{1\alpha}$ ratio in both hemispheres of the four experimental groups.
* $p < 0.02$ vs. gr 1 of the corresponding hemisphere;
** $p < 0.04$ vs. gr 3 of the corresponding hemisphere;
*** $p < 0.01$ vs. left hemisphere of the same group (*gr 3*) and vs. gr 4

1009

spheres were similar, and OKY-046 treatment did not affect it (gr 2). Thus, OKY-046 had no effect on SG of either sham or traumatized rats. Similarly, there was no significant difference in the NSS between groups 3 and 4, at either 1 or 24 h after CHI, implying that OKY-046 had no salutary effect on neurological function.

Vasoactive arachidonic acid metabolites are postulated to play a role in the maintenance of both normal CBF, and in the pathogenesis of cerebral ischemia (Pickard and Walker 1984). In line with preceding reports, we postulated that decreased TXB_2 and/or increased 6-keto-$PGF_{1\alpha}$ tissue levels might be followed by improved neurological status of rats after CHI. The results reported here demonstrate that although thromboxane synthesis and the TXB_2/6-keto-$PGF_{1\alpha}$ ratio decreased CHI rats treated with OKY-046, no changes in the NSS or SG could be observed. The role of the vasoactive eicosanoids in brain trauma remains to be elucidated.

References

Hallenbeck JM, Furlow TW Jr (1979) Prostaglandin I_2 and indomethacin prevent impairment of post-ischemic brain reperfusion in the dog. Stroke 10:629–637

Marmarou A et al. (1982) An improved gravimetric measure of cerebral edema. J Neurosurg 56:246–253

Masuda Y et al. (1986) Protective effect of prostaglandins D_2, E_1 and I_2 against cerebral hypoxia/anoxia in mice. Naunyn-Schmiedebergs Arch Pharmacol 334:282–289

Pickard JD, Walker V (1984) Current concepts of the role of prostaglandins and other eicosanoids in acute cerebrovascular disease. In: Mackenzie ET et al. (ed) L.E.R.S. vol. 2. Raven Press, New York, pp 191–218

Shapira Y et al. (1988) Experimental closed head injury in rats: mechanical, pathophysiological and neurological properties. Crit Care Med 16:258–265

Shohami E et al. (1987) Head injury induces increased prostaglandin synthesis in rat brain. J Cereb Blood Flow Metab 7:58–63

Is There No Way for the Treatment of Ischemic Brain Edema?

T. Shigeno, T. Mima, and K. Takakura

Department of Neurosurgery, Saitaman Medical Center, Department of Neurosurgery, University of Tokyo (Japan)

The first event which appears after cerebral ischemia is glial swelling, a feature of cytotoxic edema. At the time of later development of vasogenic edema, any treatment would be of no benefit in the presence of completely infarcted tissue. Thus, effort should be focused on how to manage early cytotoxic edema; otherwise, neurons would die. We therefore sought mechanisms, first at the brain capillaries which display BBB function, and second of the glial membranes which affect the milieu in and around neurons. The currently growing idea is that BBB, i.e., the capillary endothelium retains its morphology and function in cerebral ischemia. In particular, the entry of Na^+ in exchange with K^+ via Na^+, K^+-ATPase present at the antiluminal site of endothelium is of great importance in maintaining the extracellular environments for ions and contributing to cell volume regulation. On the other hand, at glial membranes ion antiport mechanisms operate once tissue acidosis has developed. Those ion channels are currently assumed to be Na^+/H^+ and Cl^-/HCO_3^- to remove H^+ from inside the cell, allowing influx of NaCl and H_2O. In the present investigations, we sought to elucidate if those mechanisms would be operating at the prenecrotic stage after ischemia, and if some pharmacological manipulations would be possible to relieve not only edema but also neuronal damage.

Material and Methods

To manipulate brain capillary function and inhibit presumed enhanced activity of the capillary Na^+, K^+-ATPase, we administered ouabain (10^{-5} M) directly into ischemic tissue via a catheter introduced just distal to MCA occlusion in cats. Perfusion was done intermittently every 2 min for 15 sec each so that naturally occurring circulatory conditions in the ischemic territory were not altered. We measured rCBF by the H_2 clearance technique, and subsequently compared flows with tissue specific gravity 4 hours later. Comparison was made between two groups receiving either ouabain or vehicle (Krebs-Ringer).

In another set of experiments, inhibitors of glial ion channels, such as for Na^+/H^+ and Cl^-/HCO_3^-, were superfused directly on the ischemic cortical surface. Indices for glial swelling and ionic environments were cortical impedance, pH and K^+. We used repeatable transient occlusion of MCA. After repeating control responses under exposure to mock CSF, a selective inhibitor to

Na^+/H^+, Amiloride, and inhibitors to Cl^-/HCO_3^-, ethacrynic acid and ONO-1016 were added in the superfusate.

Results

Ouabain perfusion within the ischemic focus significantly inhibited the decrease in specific gravity in both severely and moderately ischemic areas as shown in Table 1, indicating possible enhancement of capillary Na^+, K^+-ATPase in focal ischemia.

The brief ischemia caused by MCA occlusion was reproducible more than 6 times in each experiment. All three agents either alone or together had no effect on brain without ischemia. There was no change by one agent alone during ischemia as compared to changes under mock CSF superfusion. However, when inhibitors for both Na^+/H^+ and Cl^-/HCO_3^- channels were added together, the magnitude of impedance elevation was reduced, indicating resolution of glial swelling (Fig. 1). There was no change in the magnitude of K^+ elevation. The basic pattern of pH change was initial acidosis and subsequent brief alkaline shift at the time of recirculation, followed by normalization or slight acidic shift. However, with both antiporter inhibitors, the final acidic shift tended to be slightly enhanced.

Table 1

	Severe ischemia	Moderate ischemia
	$(0 < CBF < 15$ ml/100 g/min)	$(15 < CBF < 30$ ml/100 g/min)
Krebs-Ringer	1.0366 ± 0.0017 $(n = 14)$	1.0086 ± 0.0025 $(n = 15)$
Ouabain	1.0373 ± 0.0020 $(n = 9)$	1.0403 ± 0.0012 $(n = 11)$
	Sig. $p < 0.05$	Sig. $p < 0.01$

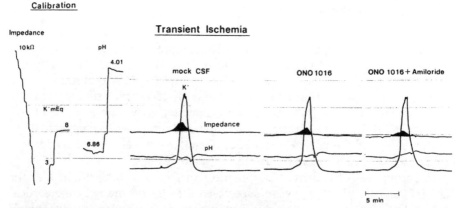

Fig. 1. Sequential changes in cortical impedance, K^+ and pH during and after ischemia. Note significant suppression of the increase of impedance during ischemia by superfusion with ONO-1016 and amiloride

Discussion

The primary ionic event after ischemia is a massive release of K^+ into the extracellular space from neurons. The enhanced activity of capillary Na^+, K^+-ATPase could, therefore, be to remove the increased extracellular K^+ into the blood stream. However, instead of removing K^+, there is an accumulation of Na^+ and H_2O in the brain. It is generally acknowledged that intracellular pH is controlled at the expense of cell volume via ionic channels located at cell membranes. The dominant ionic channel for extruding H^+ formed inside the cell during aerobic glycolysis or, more during anaerobic glycolysis, is Na^+/H^+ antiporter. Normally this does not cause cell swelling, but in acidic conditions, this causes cell swelling in simultaneous operation of Cl-HCO_3^- antiport, resulting in a net increase of NaCl inside the cell. We believe that this working hypothesis has been proven in early edema formation after ischemia, because glial swelling, can be reduced by the application of inhibitors for both channels. Thus, cytotoxic edema is a sort of protective mechanism intrinsic to glial cells for neurons suffering from lactoacidosis.

Taking both experimental results together, we conclude that glial swelling is an adaptive response against impending death of neurons. Therefore, therapy for ischemic brain edema should be focused, not on reducing water content, but on relieving ischemic cell damage itself. However, even treatment by Lipocortin to inhibit the release of arachidonic acid, did not show any effect on brain edema (Mima et al., this volume). This experimental hopelessness explains why there is currently no way to treat ischemic brain edema.

Acute Brain Swelling and Edema by Stimulation of the Medullary Reticular Formation in Cold Injured Brain

S. Nagao, M. Kawauchi, T. Ogawa, T. Ohmoto, and A. Nishimoto

Department of Neurological Surgery, Kagawa Medical School and Okayama University Medical School, 1750-1, Miki-Cho, Kita-Gun, Kagawa (Japan)

In severely head-injured patients with intracranial hypertension, irregular vital signs are frequently observed indicating medullary dysfunction. This study was carried out to investigate the effects of stimulating the medullary reticular formation on brain edema and ICP in a cerebral contusion model.

Method

The study was divided into two experiments.

Experiment 1 (28 Cats). The effect of stimulation of the medullary reticular formation on tissue water permeability was assessed using cold-induced edema. The cold injury was inflicted by applying a freezing probe of $-50°$ C directly on the dura for 1 min. Seventeen hours following cold-induced edema, animals were divided into 4 Groups. Group 1: cold lesion only, Group 2: intermittent electrical stimulation of the reticular formation of the medulla oblongata (P_{10}, $L_{\pm 2.5}$, $H_{-9.0}$) for 40 min, Group 3: medullary stimulation with C-2 cord transection to eliminate vasopressor response, Group 4: administration of Angiotensin II for 60 min. Water contents of the 4 groups were measured by a gravimetric technique from coronal slices across the lesion.

Experiment 2 (24 Cats). The ICP and local cerebral blood volume (CBV, photo-electric method) and BP were continuously recorded during stimulation of the medullary reticular formation in animals with cold-induced edema.

Results

Normal water content of the white matter was $67.7 \pm 0.9\%$. Seventeen hours following cold-induced edema, water content adjacent to the lesion increased to 74.2% and gradually decreased in tissue samples taken progressively further from the lesion area. There were no significant changes in water content in the contralateral hemisphere. Medullary stimulation produced a widespread significant increase in tissue water content in the injured hemisphere by 2.6 to 2.8%. In

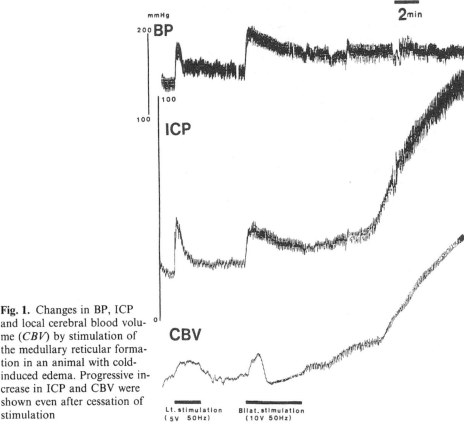

mmHg   2 min

200 BP

100

100

ICP

Fig. 1. Changes in BP, ICP and local cerebral blood volume (*CBV*) by stimulation of the medullary reticular formation in an animal with cold-induced edema. Progressive increase in ICP and CBV were shown even after cessation of stimulation

0   CBV

Lt. stimulation   Bilat. stimulation
(5V 50Hz)   (10V 50Hz)

animals with C-2 cord transection, stimulation resulted in a significant increment of water content by 1.6 to 1.9% without elevation of BP. In Group 2, water contents were significantly higher than those of Group 4 with induced hypertension by 2.1 to 3.0%.

The BP, ICP and CBV increased abruptly immediately after stimulation and response patterns were divided into 2 groups. In 15 of 24 animals (62%), temporary elevation of the ICP ranging from 10 to 25 mm Hg was observed after stimulation with a concomitant increase in CBV and BP. In 9 animals (38%), progressive increases in ICP and CBV were produced by stimulation and even after cessation of stimulation, ICP progressively increased up to 60 to 100 mm Hg (Fig. 1). Progressively increased ICPs were evoked with stimulation of the paramedian reticular formation of the medulla oblongata, that is, the region around the nucleus reticularis parvocellularis.

Discussion

Stimulation of the medullary reticular formation accelerated brain water permeability and increased CBV, consequently resulting in acute intracranial hypertension in an injured brain. We have reported that stimulation of the medullary reticular formation directly decreased the cerebral vasomotor tonus and increased CBV and ICP by intrinsic pathways of the central nervous system (Nagao et al. 1987). Decreased cerebral vasomotor tonus has been postulated to enhance water movement from the vascular space to the brain (Pappenheimer 1953; Starling 1896). Stimulation is thought to further decrease localized cerebral vasomotor tonus surrounding the lesion and elevate intraluminal pressure across the capillary. This is a proposed mechanism responsible for an increase in water content in the injured hemisphere. In preexisting intracranial hypertension and decreased compliance due to cold-induced edema, a rapid increase in CBV and water content with stimulation produced progressive intracranial hypertension (acute brain swelling) at a high rate. Thus preservation and stabilization of medullary function would become a therapeutic maneuver to control increases in intracranial hypertension.

References

Nagao S, Nishiura T, Kuyama H et al. (1987) Effect of stimulation of the medullary reticular formation on cerebral vasomotor tonus and intracranial pressure. J Neurosurg 66:548–554
Pappenheimer JR (1953) Passage of molecules through capillary walls. Physiol Rev 33:387–423
Starling EH (1896) On the absorption of fluids from the connective tissue spaces. J Physiol (Lond) 19:312–326

Time-Dependent Effects of Central Vasopressin Administration on Cold-Induced Vasogenic Edema in Cats

R.F. Reeder and E.E. Nattie

Dartmouth-Hitchcock Medical Center, Section of Neurosurgery, 2 Maynard Street, Hanover, New Hampshire 03 756 (USA)

Arginine vasopressin (AVP) containing neurons within the hypothalamus project to multiple extrahypophyseal sites (Buijs 1978). These neurons may participate in the regulation of cerebrospinal fluid (CSF) production/absorption (Liszczak et al. 1986; Noto et al. 1979), intracranial pressure (ICP) (Seckl and Lightman 1987), cerebral capillary permeability (Raichle and Grubb 1978), and brain water accumulation (Doczi et al. 1982). The authors have previously demonstrated that pharmacologic doses of intraventricular AVP increase the amount of cold-induced vasogenic edema measured 24 hr after lesion placement in cats (Reeder et al. 1986). Similar experiments examining edema spread 6 and 16 hr after lesioning were performed to clarify the time-course of this effect.

Methods

Animal Preparation. Adult cats ($n = 6$ for each treatment group, 24 animals total) were anesthetized with ketamine and xylazine infusion for the entire experiment. Animals underwent tracheostomy, were paralyzed with Gallamine, and were artificially ventilated to keep the end-tidal CO_2 between 26 and 30 Torr. Arterial blood gas determinations were made every 2 hr. The head was placed in a stereotactic frame and cannulae were placed for continual measurement of femoral arterial blood pressure, cisterna magna ICP, and infusions into the right cerebral ventricle. Infusion consisted of either AVP (40 pg/µl) or carrier solution (mock CSF) at a rate of 7.2 µl/min. Maintenance fluid of Lactated Ringer's solution was given and urine output was monitored via a cystostomy. A right frontal craniotomy was performed, and a transdural cold-lesion was made by placing a 4 mm cryosurgical probe against the dura for 3 min. The craniotomy was closed with Hygenic dental cement. One ml/kg of 2% Evans Blue dye was given intravenously. Animals were sacrificed at either 6 or 16 hr by rapid infusion of a saturated KCl solution.

Data Analysis. After brain removal, 3-mm thick coronal sections were made from the frontal pole to a distance 18 mm posteriorly (6 total slices). Each slice was photographed and the area of vasogenic edema marked by Evans Blue staining was obtained through computerized digital analysis (Laboratory Computer Systems, Inc., Micro-Plann II). Volume of edema spread was approximated by

Intracranial Pressure VII
Eds.: J.T. Hoff and A.L. Betz
© Springer-Verlag Berlin Heidelberg 1989

summing all stained areas and multiplying by 3-mm (slice thickness). White matter was dissected from gray matter in each slice and the water content was determined for the first three slices (adjacent to lesion) and the last three (distant from lesion) by wet and dry weight measurements. Samples of normal white and gray matter from the unlesioned hemisphere were similarly analyzed. Comparisons between treated and untreated groups at 6 and 16 hr were made using a Student's t-test. Values are reported as means $\pm$ the standard error of the mean.

Results

The central infusion of AVP had no demonstrable effect on arterial blood pressure, ICP, urine output, or serum sodium at 6 or 16 hr. Also, drug and fluid administration and arterial blood gases were not different between the groups. At 6 hr, mean CSF-AVP values for treated and control groups as determined by radioimmunoassay were 6300 ± 400 and 10.3 ± 1.3 pg/ml, respectively. Sixteen hour values were 3000 ± 300 and 18.9 ± 2.9 pg/ml.

At 6 hr, AVP administration led to a decrease in the water content of edematous tissue in adjacent (78.4 ± 0.3 versus $81.1\pm0.2\%$, $P<0.05$) and distant (69.5 ± 0.3 vs. $71.3\pm0.3\%$, $P=0.14$) samples, while normal white and gray matter water contents were not affected. Edema volume was also decreased by AVP infusion (0.995 ± 0.038 versus 1.310 ± 0.025 ml, $P<0.05$). At 16 hr, an opposite effect was seen. Animals infused with AVP had more water in edematous tissue adjacent (80.7 ± 0.2 versus $78.2\pm0.4\%$, $P<0.05$) and distant (72.3 ± 0.3 versus 69.5 ± 0.4, $P=0.06$); again, normal white and gray matter were not affected. Edema volume was increased by AVP administration at 16 hr (1.402 ± 0.050 vs. 1.048 ± 0.069 ml, $P=0.14$).

Conclusions

The authors demonstrate that pharmacologic doses of intraventricular AVP alter edema formation in a time-dependent manner. Specifically, AVP lessens vasogenic edema at 6 hr and increases it at 16 hr following the placement of a cryogenic lesion at the frontal pole of the cat brain. This effect appears to be mediated through central mechanisms (i.e. it is not secondary to changes in arterial blood pressure, fluid status, or acid/base balance). The factors that influence vasogenic edema formation and resolution are multiple and the site(s) of potential AVP interaction with this process can only be conjectural at this point. A time-dependent role of central AVP in the pathophysiologic development of vasogenic edema was previously suggested by the work of Doczi et al. (1984). In their study, whole brain water content of each cerebral hemisphere after experimental subarachnoid hemorrhage was compared between homozygous Brattleboro (AVP deficient) and Wistar rats at 6 and 24 hr after blood placement. Those investigators found that the AVP-deficient animals had less edema early, and more later;

1018

these findings are opposite of what might be expected from our observations in the cat. Unpublished data from our laboratory comparing amounts of early and late cold-induced vasogenic edema between Brattleboro and Long Evans rats have not indicated any differences. We feel the importance of the role of central AVP in both the physiology and pathophysiology of cerebral water balance remains unclear. Certainly, pharmacological effects of AVP on ICP, brain water content, and CSF production/absorption can be elicited (references noted above), but these effects may vary with time and/or site of action, and possibly with animal species as well. Potential clinical uses of centrally administered vasopressin agonists or antagonists await better understanding of this complex system.

Acknowledgements. This work was supported by a grant from the New Hampshire Chapter of the American Heart Association, and a grant from the Smith, Kline, and Beckman Co., Philadelphia, PA.

References

Buijs RM (1978) Intra- and extrahypothalamic vasopressin and ocytocin pathways in the rat. Pathways to the limbic system, medulla oblongata and spinal cord. Cell Tissue Res 192:423–435

Doczi T, Szerdahelyi P, Gulya K, Kiss J (1982) Brain water accumulation after the central administration of vasopressin. Neurosurgery 11:402–407

Doczi T, Laszlo FA, Szerdahelyi P, Joo F (1984) Involvement of vasopressin in brain edema formation: further evidence obtained from the Brattleboro diabetes insipidus rat with experimental subarachnoid hemorrhage. Neurosurgery 14:436–441

Liszczak TM, Black PMcL, Foley L (1986) Arginine vasopressin causes morphological changes suggestive of fluid transport in rat choroid plexus epithelium. Cell Tissue Res 246:379–385

Noto T, Nakajima T, Saji Y, Nagawa Y (1979) Effects of vasopressin and cyclic AMP on water transport at arachnoid villi of cats. Endocrinol Jpn 26:239–244

Raichle ME, Grubb RL Jr (1978) Regulation of brain water permeability by centrally-released vasopressin. Brain Res 143:191–194

Reeder RF, Nattie EE, North WG (1986) Effect of vasopressin on cold-induced brain edema in cats. J Neurosurg 64:941–950

Seckl JR, Lightman SL (1987) Intracerebroventricular arginine vasopressin causes intracranial pressure to rise in conscious goats. Brain Res 423:279–285

The Effect of Hyperglycemia on the Progression of Vasogenic Edema Following Cold Injury

L. Ott, D.J. Combs, D. Beard, R.J. Dempsey, D. Haack, and B. Young

Division of Neurosurgery, University of Kentucky Medical School, Lexington, Kentucky 40536 (USA)

Increased glucose availability can enhance cerebral ischemic damage (Pulsinelli et al. 1979; Rehncrona et al. 1981) and edema development (Myers 1979; Pulsinelli et al. 1979; Warner et al. 1987). Hyperglycemia is associated with poor prognosis following head injury (Merguerian et al. 1981) and the level of consciousness in head-injured patients has been correlated with fasting blood glucose levels (Pentelenyi et al. 1979). Traumatized brain may be susceptible to alterations in glucose availability as is ischemic brain. This study examined whether or not regional vasogenic edema development was altered over 24 hours in cold-injured rats of different glycemic states.

Methods

Sixty Wistar rats weighing 246–423 g were treated with 65 mg/kg i.p. of the diabetogenic drug streptozotocin or equivalent volume of vehicle prior to cold injury. Three to 13 days later, the fed diabetic or normal rats were anesthetized (87 mg/kg ketamine + 13 mg/kg xylazine, i.m.) and received either sham or cold-induced brain injury to the anterior left hemisphere. Body temperature was maintained at 37–38°C during anesthesia and blood glucose was measured at the time of sacrifice. Rats were reanesthetized with ketamine (140 mg/kg i.p.) and decapitated at 3, 6, or 24 hr post-insult. The brain was rapidly removed and dropped in kerosene. The olfactory bulbs and cerebellum were dissected away and three coronal slices made of the anterior portion of the brain. Slice 1 was made halfway between the frontal pole and the optic chiasm. Slice 2 was made at the optic chiasm and slice 3 through the midhypothalamus. Right and left cortical samples of brain (2 mm³) were taken from slices 1–3 and bilateral subcortical samples were taken from slices 2 and 3. Specific gravity was measured using the gravimetric technique. Specific gravity data for each region was expressed as the difference between the right hemisphere sample (uninjured) and the left hemisphere sample (cold or sham injury) and was designated as ΔSG. A positive ΔSG value for a particular sample (i.e., slice 1 cortex) indicates decreased specific gravity and increased tissue water in the left vs. right side of the brain. Analyses of specific gravity data and serum glucose levels were done by a three-way analysis of variance. Specific comparisons between groups were done using the Student's t-test with the error mean square from the corresponding analysis of variance.

Eds.: J.T. Hoff and A.L. Betz
© Springer-Verlag Berlin Heidelberg 1989

Results

Blood glucose levels were significantly greater in the SZ-treated rats at 6 and 24 hr post-insult (Table 1). No significant difference between blood glucose levels existed between SZ or V-treated rats at 3 hr. An additional eight rats (4 SZ-treated, 4 V-treated) rats were subjected to cold injury and immediately sacrificed to determine if blood glucose levels were, in fact, different at the time of insult. Blood glucose levels were greater in the SZ vs. V-treated rats at the time of insult but this difference was not quite significant (455 ± 66 vs. 300 ± 20, $P = 0.07$).

In all brain regions of both SZ and V-treated rats, sham-injured animals demonstrate ΔSG values of approximately zero. For cortical samples, ΔSG values were significantly increased by cold injury in both slice 1 and 2 ($P < 0.0001$, Fig. 1). Edema was maximal by 3 hr post-injury and remained constant over 24 hr. The values of ΔSG for slice 2 subcortex (Fig. 1) indicated a significant injury by time interaction ($P = 0.0003$) demonstrating a progressive spread of edema into this region over 24 hr in cold-injured rats. Edema development was not significantly altered in diabetic vs. nondiabetic rats in any of these regions. Little or no edema was detected in slice 3 and greater glucose availability did not increase brain edema.

Table 1. The terminal blood glucose levels (mg/dl) of diabetic and nondiabetic rats at different lengths of time following cold- or sham-injury. Since cold-injury did not significantly alter blood glucose levels, the blood glucose data has been pooled for SZ-treated ($n = 30$) and V-treated rats ($n = 30$)

Time post-injury	V-treated	SZ-Treated	Significance
3 hours	325 ± 10	342 ± 9	$P < 0.51$
6 hours	231 ± 16	365 ± 13	$P = 0.0006$
24 hours	132 ± 5	409 ± 20	$P < 0.0001$

Discussion

Despite the well-documented deleterious effects of hyperglycemia in cerebral ischemia, we found no enhancement of vasogenic edema over 24 hr in the SZ-treated vs. V-treated rats. Edema development in the cortical regions of slice 1 and 2 sample peaked before substantial differences in blood glucose existed possibly eliminating the chance of observing a deleterious effect. However, profound hyperglycemia produced by total parenteral nutrition (772 ± 57 mg/dl) does not alter edema development in fasted rats (160 ± 14 mg/dl), (unpublished observations, 1988). The lack of effect of hyperglycemia-inducing fluids over the first 4 hr following cold-injury suggests that profound hyperglycemia does not alter edema formation during this early period. Significant blood glucose differences over the final 18 hr of the experiment also failed to increase brain water in the edematous cortical regions of slice 1 and slice 2 cortex.

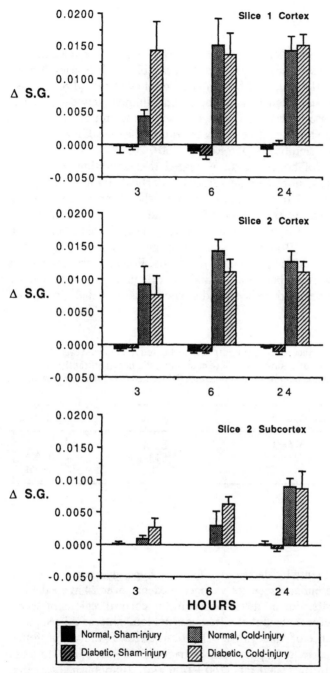

Fig. 1. ΔSG of the four treatment groups for the three most edematous regions at 3, 6, and 24 hr. Note the progressive nature of edema development in slice 2 subcortex compared to the relatively constant edema levels achieved in the two cortical samples; $n = 4$ or 5 for each bar plotted. See text for discussion of statistically significant effects

Unlike the cortical tissue samples, development of edema in the subcortical region of slice 2 was slower and progressive in nature. Blood glucose levels in diabetic vs. nondiabetic rats were significantly different over the final 18 hr of the experiment while edema was actively accumulating in slice 2 subcortex. Despite the differing blood glucose concentrations, edema development from cold injury was not altered in the diabetic rats compared to nondiabetics.

In conclusion, sustained increases in blood glucose levels over the 24 hr following cold-injury are not associated with enhanced edema development. This finding may not reflect so much the unimportance of blood glucose in fostering increased brain damage and edema as the distinctive characteristics of the cold-injury model as a model of traumatic brain injury.

Acknowledgements. This investigation was supported by Biomedical Research Support Grant # RR05374 from the Biomedical Research Support Branch, Division of Research Facilities and Resources, NIH.

References

Merguerian PA, Perel A, Wald U et al. (1981) Persistent nonketotic hyperglycemia as a grave prognostic sign in head-injured patients. Crit Care Med 9:838–840

Myers RE (1979) A unitary theory of causation of anoxic and hypoxic brain pathology. Adv Neurol 26:195–213

Pentelenyi T, Kammerer L, Stutzel M et al. (1979) Alterations of the basal serum insulin and blood glucose in brain-injured patients. Injury 10:201–208

Pulsinelli WA, Waldman S, Rawlinson D et al. (1982) Moderate hyperglycemia augments ischemic brain damage: a neuropathologic study in the rat. Neurology (NY) 32:1239–1246

Rehncrona S, Rosen I, Siesjö BK (1981) Brain lactic acidosis and ischemic cell damage: 1. biochemistry and neurophysiology. J Cereb Blood Flow Metab 1:297–311

Warner DS, Smith M, Siesjö BK (1987) Ischemia in normo- and hyperglycemic rats: effects on brain water and eletrolytes. Stroke 18:464–471

Effects of Arterial Hypertension and Jugular Vein Ligation on Edema Formation in Acute Brain Swelling Induced by Multiple Cold Lesions

T. Wang, H. Kuchiwaki, H. Ishiguri, and T. Kinomoto

Department of Neurosurgery, Nagoya University School of Medicine, Nagoya 65, Tsuruma-cho, Showa-Ku, Nagoya (Japan)

Introduction

Cold-induced edema has been used as a standard experimental model of cerebral vasogenic edema since Klatzo proposed it in 1967 (Klatzo 1967). However, few reports on experimental brain edema associated with both systemic arterial and intracranial venous hypertensions have appeared. This study was undertaken to evaluate the effect of arterial hypertension and bilateral jugular vein ligation on edema formation in acute brain swelling induced by multiple cold lesions in dogs.

Materials and Methods

The experiments were performed on 36 adult mongrel dogs weighing 9 to 14 kg. Under anesthesia with an intramuscular injection of Ketamine hydrochloride (15 mg/kg) the animals were intubated and breathed room air spontaneously. A femoral vein cannulation was maintained to infuse normal saline solution (20 ml/kg/hr) as well as Evans blue dye (60 mg/kg) 1 hr after inducing the cold lesions. The head of the animal was fixed in a stereotactic frame, and 5 burr holes were opened on the left cranium. The tip of a metal stick (8 mm in diameter) cooled by dry ice alcohol was placed on the exposed dura for 30 sec, twice. Then the burr holes were sealed with dental cement. Arterial hypertension was induced by repeated inflations of a balloon situated in the thoracic aorta and jugular vein ligations were performed both on the internal and external veins. The blood pressure was measured through the left brachial artery cannula and the ICP through an epidural pressure sensor fixed in the contralateral cranium. The monitoring period was 3 to 6 hr. Brain edema was estimated by brain tissue water content by wet/dry weights, the size of extravasation of Evans blue dye, and by microscope (hematoxylin-eosin and Kluver-Barrera stains). Evaluations were performed in following groups: group A (cold lesion with arterial hypertension) in 16 animals; group B (cold lesion with arterial hypertension and jugular vein ligations) in 12 animals; group C (cold lesion alone) in 6 animals; and a control group (group N) of 2 animals.

Intracranial Pressure VII
Eds.: J. T. Hoff and A. L. Betz
© Springer-Verlag Berlin Heidelberg 1989

Results

1. The mean values ($\pm$SE) of the maximal ranges of BP which continued for more than 30 min were as follows: $160\pm6.33/231.56\pm9.81$ mm Hg in group A ($n=16$); $172.1\pm5.13/269.58\pm3.28$ mm Hg in group B ($n=12$), and $83.33\pm4.94/176.67\pm6.67$ mm Hg in group C ($n=6$). The value of group B was significantly greater than those of others ($p<0.001-0.005$).
2. The mean values of the maximal ranges of ICP which continued for more than 30 min were as follows: $29.92\pm4.83/37.55\pm5.21$ mm Hg in group A ($n=16$); $40.07\pm3.922/53.38\pm5.64$ mm Hg in group B ($n=12$); $7.78\pm1.59/19.12\pm2.43$ mm Hg in group C ($n=6$). The mean values were also significantly different as $B>A>C$ ($P<0.001-0.005$).
3. The mean brain water contents ($\pm$SE) were as follows: in group A (the white matter, W: $72.6\pm1.07\%$; the grey matter, G: $83.34\pm0.5\%$) ($n=11$) in group B (W: $71.22\pm2.03\%$; G: $81.5\pm0.57\%$) ($n=7$), in group C (W: $70.80\pm0.48\%$, G: $81.11\pm0.38\%$) ($n=5$), and in group N (W: $66.37\pm0.34\%$, G: $79.89\pm0.28\%$) ($n=2$). There is a gradient of $A>B>C>N$. For both the white and the grey matters the values of groups A, B and C were significantly greater than those of group N. However, between groups A and B there is not significant difference ($p<0.2$).
4. The mean area of EB extravasation (SE) was measured with the largest (L) and the smallest (S) diameter of cold lesions in the brain surfaces, and largest depth into the white matter (D). The three measurements were as follows: in group

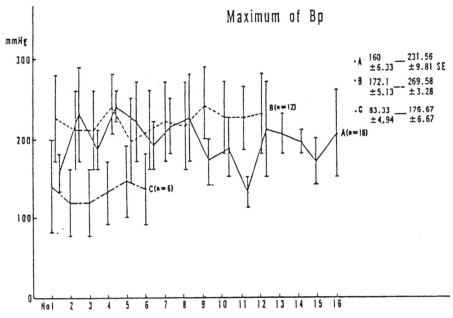

Fig. 1. Maximum values of (BP) of group A ($n=16$), B ($n=12$), and C ($n=6$) are indicated. The mean values ($\pm$ SE) are significantly different ($B > A > C$) ($p < 0.001-0.005$)

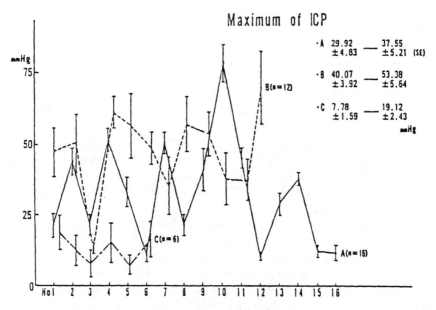

Fig. 2. Maximum values of ICP of group A ($n = 16$), B ($n = 12$), and C ($n = 6$) are presented. The mean values ($\pm$ SE) are also significantly different ($B > A > C$) ($p < 0.001 - 0.005$)

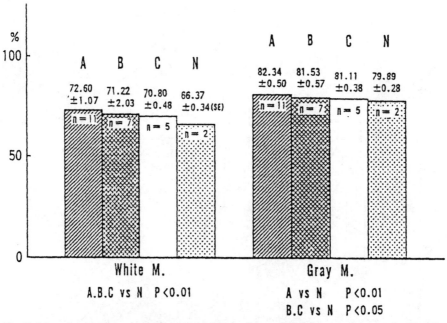

Fig. 3. Mean brain tissue water content ($\pm$ SE) is shown. There is a gradient as $A > B > C >$ both in the white and grey matters. Those values of group A, B and C are significantly greater than those in group N. However, there is no significant difference between group A and B ($p < 0.2$)

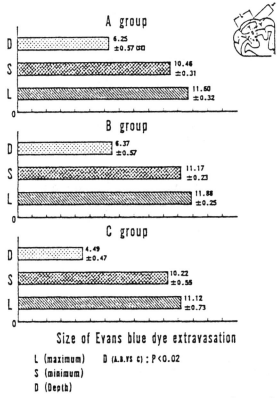

A group

D : 6.25 ±0.57 GM

S : 10.46 ±0.31

L : 11.60 ±0.32

B group

D : 6.37 ±0.57

S : 11.17 ±0.23

L : 11.88 ±0.25

C group

D : 4.49 ±0.47

S : 10.22 ±0.55

L : 11.12 ±0.73

Size of Evans blue dye extravasation

L (maximum)   D (A.B.vs c) : P<0.02
S (minimum)
D (Depth)

Fig. 4. Mean area of EB extravasation ($\pm$ SE) is presented. All three measurements of group B are greater than the others, the values of D are significantly different $(B>A>C)$ $(p<0.02)$

A (L: 11.60 ± 0.32, S: 10.46 ± 0.31, D: 6.25 ± 0.57 mm) $(n=11)$; in group B (L: 11.88 ± 0.25, S: 11.17 ± 0.23, D: 6.37 ± 0.57 mm) $(n=7)$; in group C (L: 11.12 ± 0.73, S: 10.22 ± 0.55, D: 4.49 ± 0.47 mm) $(n=5)$, respectively. Both in W and G, those values of groups A, B and C were significantly greater than those of group N $(p<0.01-0.05)$. However, between groups A and B there was no significant difference $(p<0.2)$.

5. The histological changes in the experiments showed that the most severe findings were seen in group B, such as marked degeneration, necrosis, and diffuse hemorrhages both in the surface of the cortex and the underlying white matters. Demyelination was observed using the KB stain. All changes mentioned above, except for the demyelination, were moderate in group A and mild in group C.

Discussion

In this experiment large areas of injuries were made in each hemisphere to obtain an acute model of diffuse brain swelling. In addition, a state of mechanical arterial hypertension was induced and jugular veins were ligated in our models (Hatashita et al. 1986). Using these procedures, our models were established with a high success rate in group B, in which ICP was raised above 50 mm Hg. Arterial hypertension increases intracranial blood volume by raising the intravascular pressure in the vascular bed injured by the cold lesions. An increased driving force in such a vascular bed aggravates accumulations of edema fluid.

Intracranial venous pressure may not be elevated by jugular vein ligation for as long a period of time as with intracranial sinus occlusion (Fujita et al. 1984) because there are abundant collateral venous drainages between extra- and intracranial venous systems. However, some effects of the disturbance of venous drainage appeared in group B in which maximum increases of BP and ICP were achieved. Thus, jugular vein ligation in the animals with cold lesions causes an increase in outflow resistance, a change in the regulation of cerebral blood flow, and the accumulation of metabolic products as well as other chemical substances. Explanation for the mechanisms involved in our models need further studies.

References

Fujita et al. (1984) Brain edema in intracranial venous hypertension. In: Brain edema. Springer, Berlin Heidelberg New York Tokyo, pp 228–234

Hatashita S, Hoff JT, Ishii S (1986) Focal brain edema associated with acute arterial hypertension. J Neurosurg 64:643–649

Klatzo I (1967) Presidential Address. Neuropathological aspects of brain edema. J Neuropathol Exp Neurol 26:1–14

Brain Edema and Calcium Content Following Closed Head Injury

E. Shohami, Y. Shapira, G. Yadid, and S. Cotev

Department of Pharmacology and ICU/Department of Anesthesia, Hebrew University-Hadassah Medical School, Jerusalem (Israel)

Introduction

Extension of cerebral dysfunction after severe head trauma is attributed, among other factors, to regional ischemia secondary to vascular disruption, vasospasm and intracranial hypertension (Graham et al. 1978). In cerebral ischemia, a cascade of pathophysiological processes is set in motion which had often been related to an initial intracellular accumulation of calcium ions (Raichle 1983). This calcium influx activates, among other enzymes, membrane phospholipases, with release of free fatty acids, including arachidonic acid. Vasoactive eicosanoids are synthesized, and oxygen free radicals released, with increased activity of Ca^{2+}-dependent proteases. Thus, secondary augmentation of damage after trauma may be associated with increased cerebral tissue Ca^{2+} content.

We previously described a rat model of severe closed head injury (CHI) (Shapira et al. 1988; Shohami et al. 1987). Edema was noted only in the contused hemisphere, as early as 15 min after trauma, which peaked at 18–24 hr. The edema gradually disappeared, and by 7–10 d water content of the tissue returned to normal. Activation of arachidonic acid metabolism was found after trauma in both pathways (i.e., cyclooxygenase and lipoxygenase) with a unique time course to each metabolic route. 5-HETE production was elevated (4-fold) at 15 min only in the contused hemisphere, and by 4 h post-injury it returned to normal and remained so throughout the course of the experiment (Shohami et al. 1988). On the other hand, PGE_2 synthesis peaked (4–6 fold) at 18–24 hr, and gradually returned to normal by 7–10 d. In the contralateral hemisphere, the increase in PGE_2 was significant, yet less pronounced, and it normalized faster than in the contused hemisphere. Since activation of the arachidonic acid cascade is Ca-dependent, we investigated in the present study tissue Ca content after CHI, and its temporal relationship to brain edema in the same rat model of CHI.

Material and Methods

CHI was induced after ether anesthesia on the exposed skull over the left hemisphere of rats, weighing 250–300 g, by a weight-drop device, as previously described (Shapira et al. 1988). One group (Sham-control), $n = 10$, was operated (i.e., skull exposure) but not traumatized. They were sacrificed at 24 hr post-sham. Thirty nine additional rats, who survived the initial effect of trauma, were randomly divided, and sacrificed by decapitation at 15', 1, 2, 4, 24 and 48 hr after CHI. The brains were removed immediately (<50 sec) after sacrifice, and tissue samples from the peritraumatized (left hemisphere), and corresponding contralateral zones were analyzed for specific gravity (SG), using linear gradient columns (Marmarou et al. 1982), H_2O content, by dry to wet weight ratio, and Ca content by atomic absorption spectroscopy (Rappaport et al. 1987).

Results and Discussion

Figure 1 shows the rise in tissue calcium content in both hemispheres (1 A) and the increase in water content (1 B) at the same time points. It is apparent that significant increase in Ca^{2+} content lags somewhat after the development of brain edema. Ca^{2+} content continues to rise at 48 hr post-trauma, while edema begins to subside. Furthermore, Ca^{2+} content rises at 24 and 48 hr also in the right, uninjured hemisphere, without an associated brain edema. However, over the whole time course of the experiment, a significant correlation was found between Ca^{2+} levels and water content (Pearson test, $p=0.36$, $p<0.001$, $n=48$) in both hemispheres.

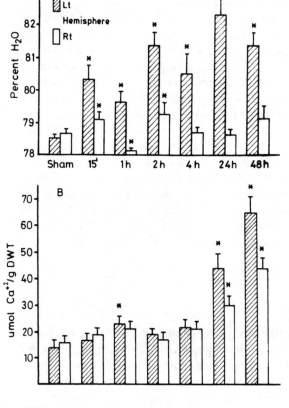

Fig. 1. **A** Mean ± SEM calcium content of the tissue samples from both hemispheres 24 hr after sham-operation, and 15' and 1, 2, 4, 24 and 48 hr after closed head injury over the left hemisphere. *$p<0.02$ as compared to the corresponding hemisphere in sham. **B** Mean ± SEM water content (Wet wt − Dry wt/Wet wt) of tissue samples from both hemispheres 24 hr after sham-operation, and 15' and 1, 2, 4, 24 and 48 hr after closed head injury over the left hemisphere. *$p<0.02$ as compared to the corresponding hemisphere in sham. The correlation between water and Ca was made by Pearson's test

The results indicate a massive increase in total tissue Ca^{2+} at 1–48 h after CHI. The source of this Ca is not known, but blood, CSF or brain tissue could each contribute to this progressive flux of Ca^{2+} ions into the injured area.

Measuring total tissue Ca^{2+}, as in the present study, does not identify the compartment which accumulates the Ca^{2+}, whether intra- or extracellular, and it does not distinguish between free and bound Ca^{2+}.

The possible role of Ca^{2+} in the pathophysiology of brain injury in the present model needs to be further studied.

References

Graham DI et al. (1978) Ischemic brain damage in fatal non-missile head injury. J Neurol Sci 39:213–234

Marmarou A et al. (1982) An improved gravimetric measure of cerebral edema. J Neurosurg 56:246–253

Raichle ME (1983) The pathophysiology of brain ischemia. Ann Neurol 13:2–10

Rappaport ZH et al. (1987) Regional brain calcium changes in the rat middle cerebral artery occlusion model of ischemia. Stroke 18:760–764

Shapira Y et al. (1988) Experimental closed head injury in rats: mechanical, pathophysiologic and neurologic properties. Crit Care Med 16:258–265

Shohami E et al. (1987) Head injury induces increased prostaglandin synthesis in rat brain. J Cereb Blood Flow Metab 7:58–63

Shohami E et al. (1988) Increased 5-HETE production in the brain following head injury. New York Academy of Sci. Proc. Symposium on AA metabolism in the nervous system (in press)

Elevated Brain Water During Urease-Induced Hyperammonemia in Dogs

L.H. Levin, R.C. Koehler, S.W. Brusilow, M.D. Jones Jr., and R.J. Traystman

Departments of Anesthesiology/Critical Care Medicine, and Pediatrics, The Johns Hopkins Medical Institutions, Baltimore, Maryland 21 205 (USA)

Liver dysfunction often results in elevated levels of plasma ammonium (hyper-ammonemia), which is thought to be one of several major factors contributing to hepatic encephalopathy. Either hyperammonemia alone or liver dysfunction cause pathological changes marked by astrocytic swelling (Gibson et al. 1974; Laursen 1982), and biochemical changes marked by glutamine accumulation in brain tissue (Bachmann and Colombo 1983; Mans et al. 1982). One major mechanism for ammonia detoxification in brain is glutamine formation from glutamate and ammonia by the enzyme glutamine synthetase (Cooper et al. 1979). Because this enzyme is localized in astrocytes, we speculated that brain swelling might be linked to glutamine accumulation as a biochemical marker of brain ammonia toxicity (Brusilow and Traystman 1986).

Increased brain water has been reported during fulminant hepatic failure, but plasma ammonium and brain tissue glutamine levels were not measured (Traber et al. 1986). Whether brain water increases with less severe liver dysfunction or with hyperammonemia alone is not clear (Pilbeam 1983). We determined if development of hyperammonemia over a 72 hr period in the absence of liver dysfunction increases brain water and if brain water correlates with glutamine accumulation.

Methods

Hyperammonemia was produced in eight mongrel dogs by intraperitoneal injection of urease (Sigma) twice per day. The daily dose varied from 0.75 to 3 units/day in order to achieve plasma ammonium levels between 400 and 1,000 µmols/liter. Plasma ammonium levels were measured twice per day using a cation exchange-colorimetric technique (Brusilow et al. 1982). After 72 hr of hyperammonemia, dogs were anesthetized with pentobarbital (25 mg/kg, i.v.), intubated and ventilated. Drill holes were made in the skull and the dura was retracted. Cortical biopsies were immediately freeze-clamped for analysis of glutamate and glutamine (Bergmeyer 1974; Hindfeldt et al. 1977) and glutamine synthetase activity (Rao and Meister 1971). Glutamine synthetase activity is reported in units of production of 1 µmol of gamma-glutamylhydroxamate from glutamine and hydroxylamine in 15 min per g of tissue. Biopsies of cortical grey matter were also obtained for assessing water content by the specific gravity technique

(Marmarou et al. 1978). The average of 6–8 specific gravity determinations was used in each animal. In addition to the eight urease-treated dogs, biopsies were obtained from six control dogs. All values are expressed as means ± SE.

Results

Baseline plasma ammonium levels were 18 ± 2 μmoles/liter. At 24, 48 and 72 hr of urease treatment, ammonium increased to 558 ± 137, 705 ± 214 and 761 ± 189 μmoles/liter, respectively. There was a small increase in plasma glutamine levels from 556 ± 72 to 660 ± 57 μmoles/liter and in plasma glutamate levels from 39 ± 3 to 49 ± 6 μmoles/liter. The animals became somewhat lethargic, but remained conscious, ate and drank.

Cortical specific gravity was lower in the urease-treated group (1.0412 ± 0.0010) than in the control group (1.0450 ± 0.0004), indicating increased brain water with urease treatment. The corresponding cortical glutamine levels were 11.13 ± 0.87 mmoles/kg in the urease group and 8.62 ± 0.29 mmoles/kg in the control group. Cortical glutamate was similar in the urease group (4.22 ± 0.25 mmoles/kg) and the control group (3.92 ± 0.11 mmoles/kg). Glutamine synthetase activity also was similar between the urease group (35.0 ± 1.1 units) and control group (34.9 ± 1.2 units).

Because there was considerable variation among animals in the levels of plasma ammonium and cortical glutamine that were achieved, linear regression analysis on pooled data from both groups was performed. Cortical glutamine correlated with plasma ammonium levels ($r = 0.51$). Cortical specific gravity also correlated with plasma ammonium levels ($r = 0.57$). However, the best correlation was cortical specific gravity with cortical glutamine levels ($r = 0.84$).

Discussion

This study demonstrates that hyperammonemia in the absence of gross liver dysfunction is capable of increasing water content in cortical grey matter. Moreover, the increase in brain water occurs at sub-comatose levels and durations of hyperammonemia. The animals usually became moderately lethargic between 24 and 72 hr, but remained generally alert and responsive. Whether the onset of lethargy coincides with the onset on increased brain water cannot be determined from this study. However, our results show that increased brain water precedes the onset of more severe behavioral manifestations of hyperammonemic encephalopathy.

Elevated levels of brain glutamine has been one of the most consistent biochemical changes observed in brain tissue during hyperammonemia. Glutamine synthesis from glutamate and ammonia in astrocytes is one of the primary pathways for ammonia detoxification in brain. Our data indicate that the increase in brain water is well-correlated with the increase in tissue glutamine concentration.

Thus, our results suggest that some process associated with glutamine metabolism may be linked to cerebral edema during hyperammonemia. In addition, the increase in glutamine in this model represents about 3 mosmoles/kg, which itself would increase brain water about 1%. Therefore, the increase in tissue glutamine without a depletion of glutamate may act as a source of intracellular osmoles and thereby directly contribute to the increase in brain water. Other metabolic alterations possibly linked to glutamine metabolism may also contribute to brain swelling.

Acknowledgements: Supported by grants from the National Institutes of Health (NS 25 275, NS 20 020 and HD 11 134) and the National Reye's Syndrome Foundation

References

Bachmann C, Colombo JP (1983) Increased tryptophan uptake into the brain in hyperammonemia. Life Sci 33:2417–2424

Bergmeyer HA (1974) L-glutamine, determination with glutamase and glutamate dehydrogenase. In: Methods of Enzymatic Analysis, 2nd Ed. Academic Press, New York, pp 1719–1722

Brusilow SW, Traystman RJ (1986) Letter to the Editor. N Engl J Med 314:786

Brusilow SW, Batshaw ML, Waber LJ (1982) Neonatal hyperammonemic coma. Adv Pediatr 29:69–103

Cooper AJL, McDonald JM, Gelbard AS, Gledhill RF, Duffy TE (1979) The metabolic fate of ^{13}N-labeled ammonia in rat brain. J Biol Chem 254:4982–4992

Gibson GE, Zimber A, Krook L, Richardson EP, Visek WJ (1974) Brain histology and behavior of mice injected with urease. J Neuropathol Exp Neurol 33:201–211

Hindfelt B, Plum F, Duffy TE (1977) Effects of acute ammonia intoxication on cerebral metabolism in rats with portacaval shunts. J Clin Invest 59:387–396

Laursen H (1982) Cerebral vessels and glial cells in liver disease: A morphometric and electron microscopic investigation. Acta Neurol Scand 65:381–412

Mans AM, Biebuyck JF, Shelly H, Hawkins RA (1982) Regional blood-brain barrier permeability to amino acids after portacaval anastomosis. J Neurochem 38:705–717

Marmarou A, Poll W, Shulman K, Bhagavan H (1978) A simple gravimetric technique for measurement of cerebral edema. J Neurosurg 49:530–537

Pilbeam CM, McD Anderson R, Bhathal PS (1983) The brain in experimental portal-systemic encephalopathy. II. Water and electrolyte changes. J Pathol 140:347–355

Rao SLN, Meister A (1972) In vivo formation of methionine sulfoximine phosphate, a protein bound metabolite of methionine sulfoximine. Biochemistry 11:1123–1127

Traber PG, Ganger DR, Blei AT (1986) Brain edema in rabbits with galactosamine-induced fulminant hepatitis. Gastroenterology 91:1347–1356

Study on FGP Cells in Cerebral Edema

M. Mato, S. Ookawara, and E. Aikawa

Department of Anatomy, Jichi Medical School, Tochigi-ken, 329-04 (Japan)

According to our studies on FGP cells (Mato and Ookawara 1981; Mato et al. 1986), they are localized in the perivascular space (Virchow-Robin space) of small cerebral blood vessels and originate from pial cells about one week after birth. The cells contain many round inclusion bodies with hydrolytic enzymes and are potent in their uptake capacity of endo- and exogenous materials. Recently, Sturrock (1987) and Jeynes (1985) discussed a possible biological role of FGP cells. In the present investigation, we focus our attention on the morphological changes of FGP cells in cerebral edema.

In the experiment, a group of 20 Wistar rats, 4 months old were subjected to a cold injury to the cerebrum. At intervals of 5, 16, 30, 48, 72 hr, 5 and 7 days after the injury, cerebral cortices (parietal region) were excised following a cardiac perfusion of a mixture of glutaraldehyde and paraformaldehyde buffered with phosphate or cacodylate solution (pH: 7.4). The specimens were then prepared for observation. Control specimens were prepared in the same manner. The regions adjacent to the damaged area were observed with a JEM 2000 EX.

At 5 hr after the injury, concomitant with the swelling of astrocytes, FGP cells appeared swollen and became pale, especially in the round inclusion bodies. Large vacuoles appeared in the cytoplasm and fused with each other (Fig. 1). Occasionally, the amorphous material, vesicles, mitochondria and a few intense inclusion bodies appeared unevenly localized in the cytoplasm. Only a small amount of HRP was detected in vesicles and inclusions, although HRP was widely dispersed in the cerebral cortices at a light microscopical level. At 16 hr, three kinds of FGP cells appeared. One was pale, with most of the cytoplasm occupied with pale inclusion bodies. A small amount of endoplasmic reticula and mitochondria were scattered in the cells. A second type of FGP cell looked dark. They possessed dark matrices and contained fairly intense inclusions, vacuoles and honeycomb like structures. They did not incorporate HRP. ACPase activity was detected throughout the cytoplasm. However, a third kind of FGP cell was slender and showed no marked change in cytoplasmic organelles. At 30 hr, the FGP cells were generally rich in vesicles and endoplasmic reticula, and included a discernible amount of pale vacuoles. Pseudopodia were frequently observed and some FGP cells appeared dark and degenerative. At 48 hr, the FGP cells appeared elongated and wrapped completely around the small blood vessels. The luminae of the blood vessels had become extremely narrowed. Pale vacuoles decreased in the cytoplasm, while dense inclusions and vesicles increased. HRP was detected in the vesicles and small inclusion bodies. Occasionally, the FGP

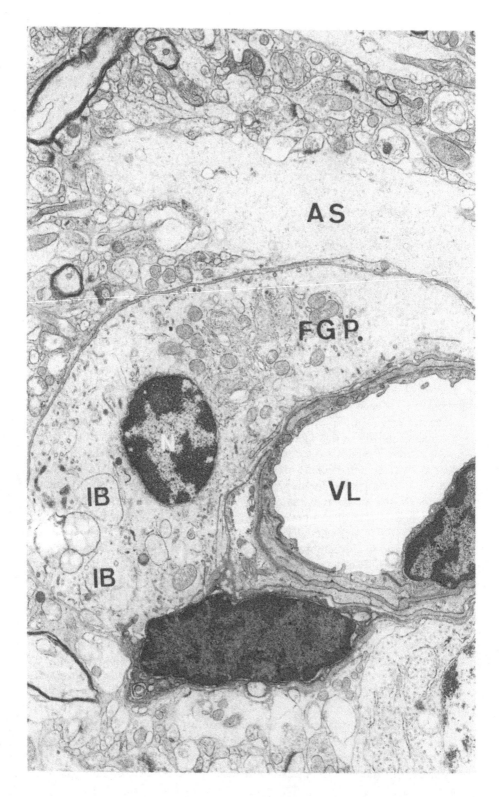

1036

cells were rich in endoplasmic reticula. At 72 hr, some of the FGP cells appeared markedly extended along the blood vessels. Migrating monocytic macrophages and leucocytes appeared close to the blood vessels. Sometimes, pale FGP cells were closely associated with the leucocytes.

At 5 days, the FGP cells decreased in number and contained inclusion bodies with various shapes. In some regions, pial cells appeared elongated in the perivascular space. At 7 days, the FGP cells were mingled with pial cell processes. The appearance of FGP cells at this stage was similar to that of the control. Astrocytes were still swollen.

From our observations, it is probable that the FGP cells take part in removing excessive tissue-fluid from the cerebral cortices. Swelling and wrapping of the FGP cells pinch the vascular wall which results in the narrowing of the vascular lumina. Next, the FGP cells appear to elongate along the blood vessel, with some cells showing degeneration. Finally, the processes of pial cells extend in the perivascular space and mingle with the FGP cells. These pial cells seem to be involved in the regeneration of FGP cells.

References

Jeynes B (1985) Reactions of granular pericytes in a rabbit cerebrovascular ischemia model. Stroke 16:121–125

Mato M, Ookawara S (1981) Influences of age and vasopressin on the uptake capacity of fluorescent granular perithelial cells (FGP) of small cerebral vessels of the rat. Am J Anat 162:45–53

Mato M, Aikawa E, Mato TK, Kurihara K (1986) Tridimensional observation of fluorescent granular perithelial (FGP) cells in rat cerebral blood vessels. Anat Rec 215:413–419

Sturrock RR (1987) Development of granular pial cells and granular perithelial cells in the spinal cords of mouse and rabbit. J Anat 153:113–122

◄ **Fig. 1.** The FGP cell becomes pale and contains pale inclusion bodies (*IB*). *AS;* astrocyte, *N;* nucleus, *VL;* vascular lumen

Intracranial Serum Proteins Under Several Blood-Brain Barrier (BBB) Conditions. Electrophoretographic Analysis

T. Uchizawa

Department of Neurosurgery, Hirosaki University, School of Medicine, 5 Zaifu-cho, Hirosaki 036 (Japan)

Intracerebral serum proteins in rats with altered blood-brain barrier (BBB) function were examined by a new method of electrophoretography. The rats were divided into 7 groups: controls ($n=5$), 6 hr of bilateral common carotid artery ligation ($n=10$), 6 hr of bilateral common carotid and right vertebral artery occlusion ($n=7$), 6 and 24 hr after cold injury ($n=6$ and $n=6$) and 6 and 24 hr after intracarotid injection of hypertonic solution (3 M urea) ($n=7$ and $n=6$).

A water soluble brain extract of each rat was concentrated and its protein composition was analyzed by cellulose acetate membrane electrophoresis. The serum of each rat was also analyzed on the paper as an indicator. Each electrophoretogram was calculated by densitometry.

Results

1) In all 5 control rats the β-globulin fraction was high and formed the most prominent band on the paper. 2) Among the 10 rats with 6 hr of bilateral common carotid artery ligation, the β-globulin fraction was high in 9 rats and the albumin fraction increased in one rat. 3) Among the 7 rats with 6 hr of common carotid and right vertebral artery occlusion the albumin fraction increased in 5 rats and the $\alpha 1$-globulin fraction increased in 2 rats. 4) Among the 6 rats tested 6 hr after cold injury the albumin fraction increased in 2 rats, the $\alpha 1$-globulin fraction increased in 2 rats, and the β-globulin fraction was high in 2 rats. 5) Among the 6 rats tested 24 hr after cold injury the albumin fraction increased in 5 rats and the $\alpha 1$-globulin fraction increased in 2 rats. 6) Among the 7 rats tested 6 hr after intracarotid urea injection the albumin fraction increased in 6 rats and the $\alpha 1$-globulin fraction increased in one rat. 7) In all 6 rats tested 24 hr after intracarotid urea injection the $\alpha 1$-globulin fraction was increased.

Discussion

Intracerebral serum albumin in the cold-injured brains appeared to be progressively increased for at least 24 hr. This suggests that BBB dysfunction in the cold injured brain is irreversible for at least 24 hr. However, the intracerebral serum

Eds.: J. T. Hoff and A. L. Betz
© Springer-Verlag Berlin Heidelberg 1989

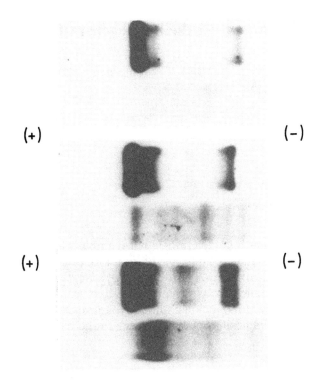

Fig. 1. Electrophoretograms of brain extracts and serum from a control rat (*upper*), a rat tested 6 hr after injection of hypertonic solution (*middle*), and rat tested 24 hr after that (*lower*). Each pair of electrophoretograms consists of serum (*upper*) and brain (*lower*). The most prominent protein band of the brain extracts is shifted from the albumin portion (6 hr after) to the γ-1 (24 hr after). This is probably because albumin inflow is restricted by a recovery of BBB function

protein pattern in the models injected with the hypertonic solution changed from an albumin-dominant pattern at 6 hr to an α1-globulin-dominant one at 24 hr. This indicates a recovery of BBB function, probably because of a restricted inflow of serum albumin. The increase in the albumin fraction in the group with 6 hr of bilateral carotid and right vertebral artery occlusion suggests BBB dysfunction in ischemic brains.

The difference in the intracerebral serum protein profiles may differentiate BBB disruption without edema from vasogenic brain edema. BBB destruction may play an important role in ischemic brain edema as well as in vasogenic edema.

Cerebral Endothelial Regeneration Following Brain Injury

T. Akimura, T. Orita, T. Kamiryo, Y. Furutani, T. Nishizaki, K. Harada, and H. Aoki

Department of Neurosurgery, Yamaguchi University School of Medicine, 1144 Kogushi Ubeshi, Yomaguchi-ken 755 (Japan)

Introduction

It has not been determined when and in which area regeneration of the cerebral endothelium occurs after brain injury (Orita et al. 1988). We therefore studied bromodeoxyuridine (BrdU) uptake by regenerating endothelial cells in two different groups of rats given cold lesions using immunohistochemistry employing anti-BrdU monoclonal antibody, anti-factor VIII-related antigen antibody and anti-glial fibrillary acidic protein antibody.

Material and Methods

Wistar rats (180–200 gm) were used. Under anesthesia, cold injury was produced on the right parietal cortex with a metal plate cooled to −70° C applied directly to the skull. According to metal plate area, they were divided into two groups; group I, 5.5 mm diameter and 70 sec duration and group II, 3.0 mm diameter and 20 sec duration. They were examined on day 1, 2, 3, 4, 5, 7 and 14, with the day after the operation counted as day 1.

Evans blue (2 ml/kg of a 2% solution) and BrdU (10 mg/kg; Sigma Chemical Co., St. Louis) were injected i.v. and allowed to circulate for 60 min. Rats were killed by perfusion and the brains removed. Sections were fixed in ethanol and stained by the biotinstreptoavidin method. Other serial sections were subjected to immunohistochemical staining with anti-factor VIII related polyclonal antibody and anti-GFAP using a PAP kit system.

Results

The extent of brain edema was estimated by the intensity and extent of the Evans blue stained area in the coronal brain slice. The lesion was maximal in extent on day 1 and its diameter was 4 mm in group I, and 2 mm in group II. It then showed a gradual decrease. The Evans blue-stained area disappeared on day 14 in group I, and on day 5 in group II.

Intracranial Pressure VII
Eds.: J. T. Hoff and A. L. Betz
© Springer-Verlag Berlin Heidelberg 1989

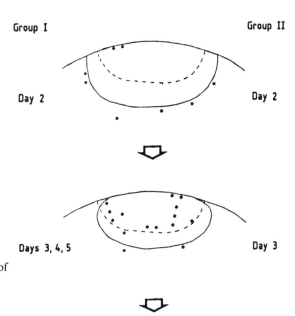

Group I   Group II

Day 2   Day 2

Days 3, 4, 5   Day 3

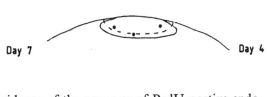

Fig. 1. Illustrations of distribution of
bromodeoxyuridine-positive endothelial cells in the lesions.
*; Bromodeoxyuridine-positive
endothelial cells
- - - - ; outer-most boundary of
macrophage layer
——; inner-most boundary of glial
fibrillary acidic protein-positive cell
layer

Day 7   Day 4

In both groups, the earliest evidence of the presence of BrdU-postive endothelial cells was observed on day 2, and the numbers of these cells increased most
markedly on day 3. They could no longer be detected on day 14 in group I and
day 5 in group II. There were significant differences between the number of
BrdU-positive endothelial cells in both groups from day 3 to 7.

In both groups, BrdU positive endothelial cells were always seen within Evans
blue stained areas. On day 2, most were observed at the periphery of the layer of
GFAP-positive cells and were not in contact with macrophages. After day 3,
BrdU-positive cells were seen in the macrophage layer – probably regenerated
from the edge toward the center of the lesion (Fig. 1).

Discussion

Anti-BrdU monoclonal antibody was used to localize BrdU, an analogue of
thymidine incorporated into the cellular nuclei at the time of mitotic DNA synthesis. It appeared that the earliest evidence of BrdU-positive endothelial cells was
observed on day 2 while injured endothelial cells regenerated from the periphery
toward the center of the lesion in both groups. Cancilla et al. (1979) reported that
the incorporation of ^{3}H-thymidine in the endothelial cells was first observed on

the 3rd day. But in their report, ^{3}H-thymidine was injected 24 hours prior to killing and we speculated their results would otherwise be the same as ours.

Up to now, macrophages were supposed to stimulate cerebral endothelial regeneration following cold injury (Cancilla et al. 1979). In our study, macrophages were observed from the 2nd day but BrdU-positive endothelial cells were not then in contact. From the 3rd day, BrdU-positive endothelial cells mingled with them and the number of macrophages greatly increased.

Since BrdU-positive endothelial cells were always found in the Evans blue stained area, we speculated that edema fluid may play an important role in endothelial regeneration. For example, an unknown substance may be present in the edema fluid or the edema fluid may be an important medium for transmission of stimulating substances from the macrophages.

References

Cancilla PA, Frommes BS, Kahn BS, DeBault LE (1979) Regeneration of cerebral microvessels. Lab Invest 40:74–82

Orita T, Nishizaki T, Kamiryo T, Harada K, Aoki H (1988) Cerebral microvascular architecture following experimental cold injury. J Neurosurg 68:608–612

Neurological Complications of Eclampsia

A.M. Richards, R. Bullock, and D.I. Graham

Departments of Obstetrics and Gynecology, Neurosurgery and Neuropathology,
Southern General Hospital, Glasgow G51 4TF (UK)

Introduction

Eclampsia and pre-eclampsia are the major cause of obstetric maternal mortality
in many countries, and neurological complications are the most important cause
of death in these patients (Gibbs and Locke 1976). The pathogenesis of these
complications – seizures, persisting coma, visual disturbance and hemiparesis
remains unknown.

Generalized vasculopathy, vasospasm and disseminated intravascular coagulation characterize the disease process outside the brain, and an imbalance between the vasodilator effects of prostacyclin and vasoconstrictor effects of thromboxane have been implicated as a cause of the vasculopathy (Moodley et al.
1984). Neurological complications of eclampsia are usually transient and cease
after the fetus is delivered.

Although older post mortem studies have shown intracranial hemorrhage in
60% of cases who die (Govan 1961), the pathophysiological processes responsible
for the neurological complications of eclampsia have not been studied in a large
series of patients.

Patients and Methods

Of 192 women with severe eclampsia and pre-eclampsia, presenting to the King
Edward VIII hospital in Durban, South Africa, 43 (22%) developed major neurological sequelae such as coma (lasting more than 6 hours after the last seizure),
hemiparesis and visual failure.

CT scans were performed as soon as possible after delivery, in these patients.

In six women in whom high ICP was suggested by CT scan features, ICP
monitoring was carried out and high ICP was managed by hyperventilation
($PaCO_2 \pm 28$ mm Hg) Mannitol 20% infusion, and sedation.

In two women CBF was measured using the Xenon enhanced CT method.
Neuropathological studies were performed in seven women who died.

Results

Edema: Thirty nine patients underwent CT scanning, and areas of low attenuation in white matter were present in 27 (69%). Three patterns of low attentuation (edema) were recognised:

Diffuse: Involving white matter throughout the brain; ($n = 5$).

Watershed: Involving parieto-occipital and fronto-parietal areas, corresponding to arterial territory watershed areas; ($n = 9$).

Occipital ($n = 13$).

The severity of edema correlated with the duration of seizures ($P < 0.001$ – Kruskal-Wallis Test) and patients who had no seizures (pre-eclampsia) had no edema. In 7 patients with seizures CT scans were normal, and intracerebral hematomas were present in 4 patients (10%).

ICP-Monitoring revealed transient high ICP in 5 of 6 patients monitored (Figure 1). ICP appeared to fall spontaneously after 24–36 hours.

Cerebral Blood Flow measurement (after sedation with benzodiazepines); revealed hyperperfusion in occipital, parietal, and watershed regions, 8 to 10 hours after the last seizure when compared with controls.

Neuropathological Examination: In 7 patients who died revealed widespread ischemic damage in 5 patients, and this was related to an episode of hypotension

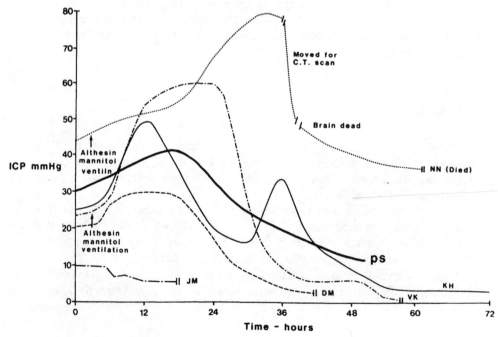

Fig. 1. ICP changes in 6 patients with CT demonstrated edema, after eclamptic seizures

1044

or high ICP in each case. Vasculopathy, as demonstrated by plasmatic vasculosis and fibrinoid necrosis, was present in 3 of the 7 patients, and fibrin thrombi occluding abnormal vessels, were seen in one case. Edema, perivascular microinfarcts and multiple small perivascular hemorrhages were also seen.

Discussion

We have demonstrated white matter edema, high ICP, and increased regional cerebral blood flow after eclampsia, and edema and high ICP were most marked in patients with the longest duration of seizures. In those who died, hematomas were uncommon, in contrast to older series (Govan 1961). Ischemic damage and vasculopathy were the most common histological findings.

Cerebral edema did not occur without multiple seizures in this series suggesting that it is not the cause of the "pre-eclamptic" prodrome of headache, vomiting and visual disturbance. Similarly, vasculopathy seems to be most marked when seizures have been frequent. The synergistic hypertensive effect of seizures, and the "eclamptic process" may result in loss of cerebral autoregulation, "breakthrough" vasodilation, vessel wall damage, and blood-brain barrier breakdown with consequent vasogenic edema.

Seizures, high ICP, and iatrogenic rapid reduction of cerebral perfusion pressure may have been responsible for the ischemic cerebral damage seen at post mortem (Richards et al. 1982). Our data have not shown an initial cause for seizures, but perivascular microhemorrhages maybe a factor.

References

Gibbs CE, Locke WE (1976) Maternal deaths in Texas 1968–1973. Am J Obstet Gynecol 126:687–691

Govan ADT (1961) The pathogenesis of eclamptic lesions. J Pathol Microbiol 24:561–575

Moodley J, Norman RJ, Reddi K (1984) Central venous concentrations of immunoreactive prostaglandins E, F and 6 Keto-prostaglandin F in eclampsia. BMJ 288:600–603

Richards A, Graham DI, Bullock R (1982) Clinicopathological study of neurological complications due to hypertensive disorders of pregnancy. J Neurol Neurosurg Psychiatry 51:416–421

Subject Index

L. M. Auer, Graz and Hannover; V. Van Velthoven, Gent

Intraoperative Ultrasound Imaging in Neurosurgery

Comparison with CT and MRI

1989. 466 figures. Approx. 180 pages. Hard cover
ISBN 3-540-50258-0

Intraoperative ultrasound is the first, and at present, only direct method available for depicting cerebral structures during neurosurgery. This atlas is a practical introduction to intraoperative ultrasound in neurosurgery and a guide to anatomy and pathomorphological diagnosis.
A short introduction to the technical basis of ultrasound is given first. It is followed by instructions for practical application of the method in the operating theater. The next, comprehensive chapter presents various intracranial pathomorphological changes in the ultrasound picture and compares them to the familiar computer tomography and MR images. A separate chapter deals with individual aspects of actual application during neurosurgical operations: ultrasound biopsy, puncture and endoscopy.

J. D. Miller, Edinburgh; G. M. Teasdale, J. O. Rowan,
S. L. Galbraith, A. D. Mendelow, Glasgow (Eds.)

Intracranial Pressure VI

1986. 361 figures, 127 tables. XIV. 798 pages. Hard cover
ISBN 3-540-16197-X

Contents: Traumatic Intracranial Hypertension; Causes, Consequences. – Pressure Volume Relationships. – Resistance to CSF Outflow. – Causes of Increased ICP: Autonomic, Vascular. – Methods of Measurement. - Pulse Wave Form Analysis. – Consequences of Raised ICP: Structural, Functional, Vascular. – Hydrocephalus/CSF Circulation. – Haemorrhage, Ischemia and Other Focal Lesions. – Therapy I: Osmotic and Other Agents. – Head Injury and Other Clinical Uses of ICP Monitoring. – Therapy II: Anesthesia, Pharmacology and Cerebral Metabolic Depressants. – Summaries. – Subject Index.

Springer-Verlag Berlin
Heidelberg New York
London Paris
Tokyo Hong Kong

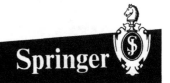

Springer

M. Samii, Hannover;
W. Draf, Fulda

Surgery of the Skull Base

An Interdisciplinary Approach

With a Chapter on Anatomy by J. Lang

1989. 289 figures in 840 separate illustrations. Approx. 560 pages. Hard cover ISBN 3-540-18448-1

Contents: Surgical Anatomy of the Skull Base. – Surgery of the Anterior Skull Base: Surgery of Malformations of the Anterior Skull Base. – Surgery of Traumatic Lesions of the Anterior Skull Base. – Surgery for Inflammatory Complications in the Region of the Anterior Skull Base. – Surgery of Space-Occupying Lesions of the Anterior Skull Base. – Surgery of Tumors of the Orbit and Adjacent Skull Base. – Special Operative Techniques. Surgery of the Middle Skull Base: Surgery of Traumatic Lesions of the Middle Skull Base. – Surgery of Inflammatory Disorders of the Middle Skull Base. – Surgery of Space-Occupying Lesions of the Middle Skull Base. – Surgery of the Posterior Skull Base: Surgery of the Internal Auditory Canal and Cerebellopontine Angle. – Surgery of Tumors of the Lateral Posterior Skull Base and Petrous Bone. – On the Problem of Paralytic Dysphagia Caused by Posterior Skull Base Tumors. – Surgery of the Clivus. – General Operative Techniques. – Surgery of the Craniocervical Junction. – Operative Technique. – Facial Nerve and Skull Base Surgery. – General Operative Techniques. – Special Operative Techniques.

This is the first text to consider the skull base as a whole and from an interdisciplinary point of view. It analyzes the wide spectrum of pathological entities which can affect this crossroad region, including anomalies, traumatology, tumors and infectious processes.
The book considers general as well as specific surgical aspects and offers a wealth of excellent drawings and pictures to complement the text.

Springer-Verlag Berlin
Heidelberg New York
London Paris
Tokyo Hong Kong

The reader will find himself equipped with a complete textbook on skull base surgery that emphasizes clinical applications and reflects valuable relevant experience from the fields of both ENT and neurosurgery.

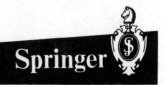

Springer

9 783642 739897